CRITICAL CARE

CLINICAL COMPANION

Contributors

Matthew L. Anderson, M.D., Ph.D.
Fellow, Department of Gynecologic Oncology
University of Texas
MD Anderson Cancer Center
Houston, Texas
Chapter 16

Juan Bartolomei, M.D.
Resident, Department of Neurosurgery
Yale University School of Medicine
Yale-New Haven Hospital
New Haven, Connecticut
Chapters 26 (Head Trauma), 35

Robert L. Bell, M.D.
Resident, Department of Surgery
Yale University School of Medicine
Yale-New Haven Hospital
New Haven, Connecticut
Chapters 3, 9 (Gastrointestinal Hemorrhage), 10, 11 (Cirrhosis and Ascites; Fever of Unknown Origins; Necrotizing Soft Tissue Infections; Pneumonia; Wound Infections), 13, 19, 30

Syed Ahmad Jamal Bokhari, M.D.
Department of Diagnostic Imaging
Yale University School of Medicine
Yale-New Haven Hospital
New Haven, Connecticut
Chapter 20

Michael Carrithers, M.D., Ph.D.
Fellow, Department of Neurology
Yale University School of Medicine
Yale-New Haven Hospital
New Haven, Connecticut
Chapters 12 (CNS Infections), 14

Pauline Chen, M.D.
Resident, Department of Surgery
Yale University School of Medicine
Yale-New Haven Hospital
New Haven, Connecticut
Chapters 11 (Fulminant Hepatic Failure, Portal Hypertension), 25 (Kidney Transplantation, Liver Transplantation, Pancreas Transplantation, Small Bowel Transplantation)

Michael A. Coady, M.D., M.P.H.
Resident, Department of
    Surgery
Yale University School of
    Medicine
Yale-New Haven Hospital
New Haven, Connecticut
*Chapters 4, 5 (Hemodynamic
    Monitoring and Alterations in
    Hemodynamics), 27 (Aortic
    Aneurysms)*

Christopher P. Coppola, M.D.
Resident, Department of
    Surgery
Yale University School of
    Medicine
Yale-New Haven Hospital
New Haven, Connecticut
*Chapters 7, 11 (Biliary Infections),
    12 (Catheter Maintenance),
    25 (Allograft Rejection, Cadaveric
    Donor Selection and Support,
    Immunosuppressive Therapy)*

Karynne O. Duncan, M.D.
Resident, Department of
    Dermatology
Yale University School of
    Medicine
Yale-New Haven Hospital
New Haven, Connecticut
Chapter 6

Steven J. Fleischman, M.D.
Resident, Department of
    Obstetrics and Gynecology
Yale University School of
    Medicine
Yale-New Haven Hospital
New Haven, Connecticut
Chapter 16

Thomas F. Higgins, M.D.
Resident, Department of
    Orthopaedics and
    Rehabilitation
Yale University School of
    Medicine
Yale-New Haven Hospital
New Haven, Connecticut
Chapter 18

Tanveer A. Janjua, MBBS
Resident, Department of
    Surgery
Division of Otolaryngology
Yale University School of
    Medicine
Yale-New Haven Hospital
New Haven, Connecticut
Chapter 2

Richard Kim, M.D.
Resident, Department of
    Surgery
Yale University School of
    Medicine
Yale-New Haven Hospital
New Haven, Connecticut
*Chapter 9 (Diarrhea in the
    Critically Ill Patient,
    Intraabdominal Abscess)*

Fotios A. Mitropoulos, M.D.
Resident, Department of
    Surgery
Yale University School of
    Medicine
Yale-New Haven Hospital
New Haven, Connecticut
*Chapter 12 (Fever of Unknown
    Origin, Fungal Infections,
    Urinary Tract Infections)*

Aldo J. Peixoto, M.D.
Fellow, Section of Nephrology
Yale University School of
    Medicine
Yale-New Haven Hospital
New Haven, Connecticut
Chapter 21

Frank G. Scholl, M.D.
Resident, Department of
    Surgery
Yale University School of
    Medicine
Yale-New Haven Hospital
New Haven, Connecticut
*Chapters 19 (Extracorporeal
    Membrane Oxygenation), 23,
    25 (Heart Transplantation), 27*

Seth A. Spector, M.D.
Resident, Department of
    Surgery
Yale University School of
    Medicine
Yale-New Haven Hospital
New Haven, Connecticut
*Chapters 1, 5 (Shock), 7, 8, 9, 11,
    15, 19 (Mechanical Ventilation),
    22, 24, 25 (Kidney
    Transplantation, Liver
    Transplantation, Pancreas
    Transplantation, Small Bowel
    Transplantation), 26, 29,
    31–34, 36–44, 46–49*

Edward R. Touhy M.D.
Fellow, Section of Cardiology
Yale University School of
    Medicine
Yale-New Haven Hospital
New Haven, Connecticut
Chapter 5

Anthony J. Vitale, BS, RPh
Clinical Pharmacist
Yale-New Haven Hospital
New Haven, Connecticut
Appendices D and E

CRITICAL CARE

CLINICAL COMPANION

EDITOR

SETH A. SPECTOR, M.D.

Department of Surgery
Yale University School of Medicine
Yale-New Haven Hospital
New Haven, Connecticut

ASSOCIATE EDITORS

CHRISTOPHER P. COPPOLA, M.D.

Department of Surgery
Yale University School of Medicine
Yale-New Haven Hospital
New Haven, Connecticut

ROBERT L. BELL, M.D.

Department of Surgery
Yale University School of Medicine
Yale-New Haven Hospital
New Haven, Connecticut

 LIPPINCOTT WILLIAMS & WILKINS

A **Wolters Kluwer** Company

Philadelphia • Baltimore • New York • London
Buenos Aires • Hong Kong • Sydney • Tokyo

Editor: Elizabeth Nieginski
Development Editors: Rosanne Hallowell, Lisa Bolger, and Martha Cushman
Managing Editor: Marette D. Magargle-Smith
Marketing Manager: Aimee Sirmon
Illustrator: Holly R. Fischer

351 West Camden Street
Baltimore, Maryland 21201-2436 USA

530 Walnut Street
Philadelphia, Pennsylvania 19106 USA

Printed in the United States of America

Library of Congress Cataloging-in-Publication Data

Critial care clinical companion / editor, Seth A. Spector; associate editors, Christopher P. Coppola, Robert Bell.
     p.; cm.
     Includes index.
     ISBN 0-683-30680-4
  1. Critical care medicine—Handbooks, manuals, etc. 2. Surgical intensive care—Handbooks, manuals, etc. 3. Intensive care units—Handbooks, manuals, etc. I. Spector, Seth A. II. Coppola, Christopher P. III. Bell, Robert, M.D.
    [DNLM: 1. Critical Care—Handbooks. WB 39 C9343 2000]
RC86.7.C716 2000
616'.028—dc21   99-057933

To purchase additional copies of this book, call our customer service department at **(800) 638-3030** or fax orders to **(301) 824-7390.** International customers should call **(301) 714-2324.**

00 01 02 03
1 2 3 4 5 6 7 8 9 10

Dedication

....

This book is dedicated to our wives,
Dena, Meredith, and Mona,
and to our children,
Sydney, Jared, Ben, Katie and Sydney.

Contents

PART III: PROCEDURES

APPENDICES

Foreword

....

An intensive care unit is merely a concentration of resources. The intensive care unit of today evolved from centralized recovery rooms during the 1940s. The Coconut Grove fire of 1942 proved the value of intensive care units, and showed that concentrating the critically ill into a single hospital space was an efficient use of limited resources. The polio epidemic of the 1950s expanded the role of the critical care unit to provide specialized care for the mechanically ventilated patient with respiratory failure. The first coronary care units appeared in the 1960s, improving outcome after myocardial infarction.

In the past two decades the widespread use of the critical care unit has come under closer scrutiny, with the recognition that health care is not an unlimited resource. Allocations of a large proportion of our health care resources are applied to extend the life of our most critically ill patients. The health care dollar is thus consumed by a small subset of patients, often in the last months of life.

ICU patients are typically the sickest population in the hospital. The medical and nursing staff is required to act rapidly and appropriately, as errors in management can have devastating consequences. A companion handbook such as this expedites the staff's ability to obtain essential reference material. Because the field of critical care changes very rapidly, up-to-date information is essential to those learning the nuances of ICU management. The authors of *Critical Care Clinical Companion* must be commended for their efforts to deliver crucial information to the bedside.

STEPHEN M. COHN, MD, FACS
Professor and Chief
Division of Trauma and Surgical Critical Care
Medical Director, Ryder Trauma Center
University of Miami School of Medicine

Preface

....

In an era of ever-changing and advancing technology, the ability to care for critically ill patients has become part of the mainstream. These patients compose a select group who require experienced management on a minute-to-minute basis. Critical care patients leave us essentially no time for delay or contemplation, and almost no room for error. They confront us with ultimate challenges in clinical diagnosis, judgment, and treatment. In the high-energy environment of the ICU, we are assaulted by data, rapid change, and uncertainty in spite of the abundance of information available.

In preparing the *Critical Care Clinical Companion,* we have made every effort to include the latest relevant information. The data provided in this handbook are not a summarization of any current textbook, but rather a synthesis of the latest medical literature. Although it is beyond the scope of this text to discuss all of the salient aspects of critical care in detail, we have attempted to provide the reader with a readily accessible information base. We have integrated our clinical practices with the medical literature and tried to point out and resolve any discordance.

The format of the text is user friendly. Charts, tables, algorithms, and illustrations are provided to allow the reader to rapidly assimilate the facts provided. While key basic science principles have been enumerated, special emphasis is placed on clinical diagnosis and management. There may be some variations in management among different institutions, but the goals and foundations of critical care are similar everywhere.

Ultimately, this book was written for the benefit of the critically ill patients who are encountered by medical students, physician assistants, residents, and medical staff. This book should be equally accessible and applicable to all medical personnel involved in the care of these patients.

Critical care is a constantly evolving field, which is why we view this undertaking as a work in progress. We welcome comments from our readers.

SETH A. SPECTOR, M.D.
CHRISTOPHER P. COPPOLA, M.D.
ROBERT L. BELL, M.D.
Department of Surgery
Yale University School of Medicine
Yale-New Haven Hospital
New Haven, Connecticut

Acknowledgments

....

We would like to express our appreciation to our mentors and teachers, who have imparted their wisdom and experiences to us and have taught us by example to care for patients with sincerity, sympathy, and compassion. They have shown us that caring for critically ill patients is a continuing commitment which necessitates an enlarging knowledge base and requires prompt attention to small fluctuations in patient condition. It was their encouragement and leadership that inspired us to produce this text.

PART I

Preoperative Evaluation

of the Surgical Patient

1

Preoperative Evaluation

of the Noncardiac

Surgery Patient

INITIAL SCREENING

I. **History.** A patient history is obtained to identify risk factors and comorbid disease.

II. **Physical examination.** A physical examination is performed to rule out unsuspected comorbidity.

III. **Screening Tests**

A. A **complete blood count** is obtained for:
1. Men over 40 years
2. Women of any age
3. Patients with known or suspected infection
4. Emergency admission patients

B. **Electrolyte, blood urea nitrogen (BUN), creatinine, and glucose levels** are obtained for:
1. Patients with diabetes
2. Patients with cardiac disease
3. Patients with renal disease
4. Patients taking medications that affect serum potassium levels
5. Emergency admission patients

C. **Prothrombin time and partial thromboplastin time** tests are indicated for:
1. Patients with a history of abnormal bleeding
2. Patients undergoing peripheral vascular surgery
3. All children

D. **Blood type and cross match** are required for any patient with anticipated blood loss of greater than 1 liter (or 20 cc/kg).

E. **Chest radiography** is indicated for:

  1. Patients older than 40 years
  2. Patients with known cardiac or pulmonary disease, including tuberculosis or history of positive purified protein derivative (PPD) test results
  3. Patients with high risk for postoperative pulmonary complications
  F. **Urinalysis** is indicated for patients with known or suspected diabetes, renal disease, or urinary tract infection.
  G. **Electrocardiography** is indicated for:
  1. Men older than 40 years
  2. Women older than 50 years
  3. Any patient with a history of cardiac disease
IV. **Methods for Calculating Risk of Perioperative Complications.** See **Tables 1-1, 1-2, and 1-3.**

CARDIOVASCULAR SYSTEM

  I. **Clinical Markers of Increased Risk for Perioperative Cardiac Events. Figures 1-1 through 1-3** are algorithms for preoperative cardiac assessment.
  A. **Major predictors**
  1. Unstable coronary syndromes (e.g., recent myocardial infarction [MI] with evidence of ischemic risk; unstable or severe angina)
  2. Decompensated congestive heart failure (CHF)
  3. Significant arrhythmia (e.g., high-grade atrioventricular [AV] block, supraventricular tachycardia)
  4. Severe valvular disease
  B. **Intermediate predictors**
  1. Mild angina
  2. Prior MI
  3. Compensated or prior CHF
  4. Diabetes mellitus
  C. **Minor predictors**
  1. Advanced age
  2. Abnormal ECG
  3. Rhythm other than sinus
  4. History of stroke
  5. Uncontrolled hypertension
  6. Low functional capacity
  II. **Functional Capacity.** The functional capacity of a patient is a reliable predictor of a cardiac event.
  A. Functional capacity is expressed in **metabolic equivalent (MET) levels.** Multiples of the functional capacity baseline can be used to express aerobic demands for specific activities.
  B. A **low capacity for exercise** is an **independent risk factor** for a cardiac event.
  C. The **Duke Activity Status Index (Table 1-4)** and other activity scales provide standard questions for determining exercise capacity.

Table 1-1. Goldman Criteria for Determining Independent Risk Factors for Noncardiac Surgery

Risk Factor	Points
History	
Age >70	5
MI in previous 6 months	10
Physical examination	
S_3 gallop or jugular venous distention (CHF)	11
Significant aortic valvular stenosis	3
ECG	
Nonsinus rhythm or premature atrial contractions	7
>5 premature ventricular contractions/min at any time preoperatively	7
Poor health ($Po_2 < 60$, $Pco_2 > 50$, K < 3, $HCO_3^- < 20$, BUN > 50, Cr > 3, abnormal SGOT, signs of liver disease, bedridden for noncardiac cause)	3
Operation	
Intraperitoneal, intrathoracic, or aortic surgery	3
Emergent	4
	53

Scoring:

Points	Class	Complication (%)	Mortality (%)
0–5	I	0.7	0.2
6–12	II	5.0	2.0
13–25	III	11.0	2.0
≥ 26	IV	22.0	56.0

These criteria were obtained by prospective multivariate analysis of 1001 patients over 40 years of age. (Adapted with permission from Goldman L, Caldera DL, et al: Multifactorial index of cardiac risk in non-cardiac surgical procedures. *NEJM* 297:845, 1977. Copyright 1977 Massachusetts Medical Society. All rights reserved.)
CHF = congestive heart failure; BUN = blood urea nitrogen; ECG = electrocardiogram; MI = myocardial infarction; SGOT = serum glutamate oxaloacetate transaminase.

III. Cardiac Stress Tests

    A. Previous stress tests. Determine whether a previous stress evaluation has been performed and, if so, when and why. Also, determine whether the previous stress test was an adequate test for ischemia.

    B. Exercise tolerance test. Administration of this test is limited to those patients with the ability (functional capacity) to exercise.

        1. This test yields **false-negative results** in patients who have **one-vessel cardiac disease.**

Table 1-2. Eagle Criteria for Predicting Postoperative Ischemic Events*

Clinical Factors	Odds Ratio	Points
Age > 70	—	Age × 0.077 −10
Angina	2.64	1.0
Q wave/previous MI by ECG	4.22	1.4
Ventricular ectopy requiring treatment	3.49	1.2
Diabetes	2.61	1.0
Ischemic ECG on dipyridamole thallium test	3.71	1.3
Thallium redistribution	9.78	2.3

Probability of an event $= e^{points}/(1 + e^{points})$

Scoring:

Clinical Factors	Thallium Stress Test	Event Risk (%)
0	Not performed	3.1
1–2	−	3.2
	+	29.6
≥ 3	Not performed	50.0
	−	33.0
	+	64.0

These criteria were obtained by retrospective analysis of 200 patients undergoing vascular surgery. (Adapted with permission from Eagle, et al: Combining clinical and thallium data optimizes preoperative assessment of cardiac risk before major vascular surgery. *Ann Intern Med* 110:859, 1989.)

ECG = electrocardiogram; MI = myocardial infarction; + = ischemic ECG or thallium redistribution during test; − = no ischemic ECG or thallium redistribution during test.

*Ischemic events include unstable angina, pulmonary edema, MI, or cardiac death.

  2. Results of this test are **less predictive in women** than in men.
  C. Dipyridamole (Persantine) thallium stress test
    1. Description. Dipyridamole **dilates the coronary vasculature** except in areas of significant stenoses which are already maximally vasodilated at rest.
    2. Sensitivity and specificity. This test is **60% to 90% sensitive** and **80% to 100% specific** for detection of coronary artery disease.
    3. Contraindications. This test is contraindicated in patients with **asthma** or **chronic obstructive pulmonary disease (COPD)**.

Table 1-3. American Society of Anesthesiologists Classification of Physical Status

Class	Physical Status
I	Normal, healthy patient with a localized abnormal process
II	Mild to moderate systemic disturbance caused by surgical condition or other process
III	Severe systemic disease that limits function but is not incapacitating
IV	Incapacitating systemic disease that is a constant threat to life
V	Moribund patient not expected to survive 24 hours without operation
VI	Organ donor

This classification system has been used to preoperatively stratify patients for risk, but has not been well validated. Emergency cases are designated by the addition of "E" to the classification number. (Adapted with permission from Owens WD, et al: ASA physical status classifications. *Anesthesiology* 49:239, 1978.)

    D. Dobutamine stress echocardiography
        1. Description. Dobutamine is administered, which induces tachycardia and increased myocardial oxygen demand. Echocardiography is then used **to assess induced myocardial wall motion abnormalities.**
        2. Risk. There is a risk of **myocardial infarction** with the induction of the ischemia.
IV. Surgery-Specific Risk for Perioperative Cardiac Events is related to the degree of hemodynamic stress associated with the procedure.
    A. High risk
        1. Major emergency surgery, particularly in the elderly
        2. Aortic and major vascular surgery
        3. Peripheral vascular surgery
        4. Surgery for which long intraoperative times and large fluid shifts are anticipated
    B. Intermediate risk
        1. Carotid endarterectomy
        2. Head and neck surgery
        3. Intraperitoneal and intrathoracic, orthopedic, and prostate surgery
    C. Low risk
        1. Endoscopic procedures
        2. Cataract surgery
        3. Breast surgery
V. Indications for Angiography
    A. Class I—helpful. Angiography is indicated in the following situations:

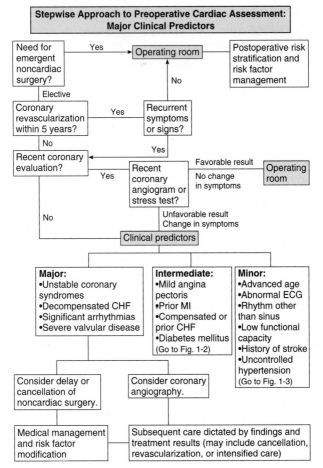

Figure 1-1. Universal algorithm for the stepwise approach to preoperative cardiac assessment: major clinical predictors. *CHF* = congestive heart failure; *ECG* = electrocardiogram; *MI* = myocardial infarction. (Adapted with permission from Eagle KA, et al: Guidelines for perioperative cardiovascular evaluation for noncardiac surgery. *Circulation* 93(6):1284, 1996, American Heart Association.)

1. When results of noninvasive testing indicate that there is a high risk of cardiovascular complications
2. When there is unstable angina pectoris
3. When there is angina pectoris that is unresponsive to medical therapy

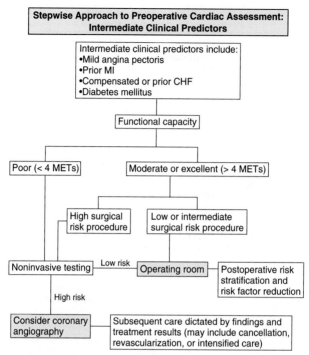

Figure 1-2. Universal algorithm for the stepwise approach to preoperative cardiac assessment: intermediate clinical predictors. *CHF* = congestive heart failure; *METs* = metabolic equivalents of the task; *MI* = myocardial infarction. (Adapted with permission from Eagle KA, et al: Guidelines for perioperative cardiovascular evaluation for noncardiac surgery. *Circulation* 93(6):1284, 1996, American Heart Association.)

      4. When there are nondiagnostic or equivocal noninvasive results in a high-risk patient undergoing a high-risk procedure

  B. Class II—may be helpful. Angiography may be indicated in the following situations:

      1. When results of noninvasive testing indicate that there is an intermediate risk of cardiovascular complications

      2. When there are nondiagnostic or equivocal noninvasive results in a low-risk patient undergoing a high-risk procedure

      3. In the case of urgent noncardiac surgery in a patient recovering from an acute MI

      4. In the case of a perioperative MI

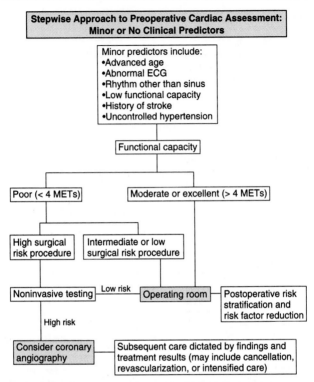

Figure 1-3. Universal algorithm for the stepwise approach to preoperative cardiac assessment: minor or no clinical predictors. *ECG* = electrocardiogram; *METs* = metabolic equivalents of the task. (Adapted with permission from Eagle KA, et al: Guidelines for perioperative cardiovascular evaluation for noncardiac surgery. *Circulation* 93(6):1284, 1996, American Heart Association.)

   C. **Class III—not necessary.** Angiography is not indicated in the following situations:
      1. In the case of low-risk noncardiac surgery in a low-risk patient
      2. For asymptomatic patients who have excellent exercise capacity after coronary revascularization
      3. For patients with mild, stable angina who have good left ventricular function and low-risk noninvasive test results
      4. For patients who are not candidates for revascularization owing to concomitant disease
      5. In patients who have had a prior adequate normal coronary angiogram (within the last 5 years)

Table 1-4. The Duke Activity Status Index*

Activity	Weight
1. Can you take care of yourself (e.g., eating, dressing, bathing, using the toilet)?	2.75
2. Can you walk indoors (e.g., around your house)?	1.75
3. Can you walk one or two blocks on level ground?	2.75
4. Can you climb a flight of stairs or walk up a hill?	5.50
5. Can you run a short distance?	8.00
6. Can you do light work around the house (e.g., dusting, washing dishes)?	2.70
7. Can you do moderate work around the house (e.g., vacuuming, sweeping floors, carrying the groceries)?	3.50
8. Can you do heavy work around the house (e.g., scrubbing floors, lifting or moving heavy furniture)?	8.00
9. Can you do yard work (e.g., raking leaves, weeding, pushing a power mower)?	4.50
10. Can you have sexual relations?	5.25
11. Can you participate in moderate recreational activities (e.g., golf, bowling, dancing, doubles tennis, throwing a football or baseball)?	6.00
12. Can you participate in strenuous sports (e.g., swimming, singles tennis, football, basketball, skiing)?	7.50

Reprinted from American Journal of Cardiology, Volume 64, Hiatky MA, et al: A brief self-administered questionnaire to determine functional capacity (The Duke activity status index), p. 652, Copyright 1989, with permission from Excerpta Media, Inc.)
*This is an indirect method of determining exercise capacity. It cannot replace exercise testing.

      6. For patients with severe left ventricular dysfunction who are not considered candidates for revascularization

      7. For patients unwilling to undergo revascularization

VI. Management of Specific Preoperative Cardiovascular Conditions

    A. Hypertension. Severe hypertension should be controlled before the procedure. The decision to delay surgery in order to obtain better control depends on the urgency of the procedure.

    B. Valvular heart disease

      1. Symptomatic stenotic lesions are associated with risk of perioperative severe CHF or shock. Patients with this condition often require **percutaneous valvulotomy or valve replacement** before noncardiac surgery to decrease cardiac risk.

      2. Symptomatic regurgitant valve disease is usually better tolerated perioperatively and may be stabilized preoperatively with **intensive medical therapy and monitoring.**

The valve may then be repaired definitively after the noncardiac surgery. **Exceptions** include severe valvular regurgitation with reduced left ventricular function, in which case valve replacement should precede noncardiac surgery.

C. **Myocardial disease.** Dilated and hypertrophic cardiomyopathies are associated with increased incidence of perioperative CHF. The goal is to maximize the patient's preoperative hemodynamic status and provide intensive postoperative medical therapy and surveillance. **Perioperative surveillance and prophylaxis** is as follows:

1. **Use of pulmonary artery catheters.** Their main value is for **assessing fluid status to avoid CHF.** This is particularly important in the following patients:
   a. Patients who have had a recent MI complicated by CHF
   b. Patients with significant coronary artery disease (CAD) who are undergoing procedures associated with significant hemodynamic stress
   c. Patients with systolic or diastolic left ventricular dysfunction, cardiomyopathy, and valvular disease undergoing high-risk operations

2. **Surveillance for perioperative MI.** Few studies have examined the optimal method for diagnosing a perioperative MI.
   a. In patients with known or suspected CAD undergoing high-risk procedures, **ECGs obtained at baseline,** immediately after surgery and over the first 2 days after surgery, appear to be cost effective.
   b. Use of **cardiac enzymes** (troponin I, CPK/MB) is best reserved for patients at high risk and those with clinical, ECG, or hemodynamic evidence of cardiovascular dysfunction.

VII. **Use of Beta Blockers.** In patients at risk for cardiovascular morbidity who have known coronary artery disease, one study indicated that the perioperative use of beta blockade resulted in a significant reduction in cardiac death through the first 2 years, with the principal effect at 6–8 months. In this study, atenolol was given prior to the induction of anesthesia, immediately after surgery, and daily through the patient's hospital stay (up to 7 days).

VIII. **Thermoregulation.** Maintenance of perioperative normothermia decreases the incidence of early postoperative cardiac morbidity.

RESPIRATORY SYSTEM

I. **Risk Factors for Postoperative Pulmonary Complications**
   A. Upper abdomen surgery poses a higher risk of pulmonary complications (40%–80%) than does lower abdomen surgery (20%).

    B. Vertical incisions are accompanied by a greater risk of atelectasis and hypoxemia than horizontal abdominal incisions.

    C. Prolonged surgical procedure

    D. Age over 65 years

    E. History of smoking, sputum production, wheezing

    F. Obesity

    G. ASA risk greater than Class I (refer to Table 1-3)

II. Preoperative Screening and Management

    A. Patients with underlying lung disease. Determine the type and severity.

    B. Smokers. Patients who smoke should discontinue smoking 2 months prior to surgery; this will improve mucociliary function.

    C. Patients who have asthma or COPD

        1. Bronchodilators should be taken the morning of surgery.

        2. Theophylline should NOT be taken the morning of surgery.

    D. Patients who have a productive cough. A preoperative course of antibiotics is indicated (ampicillin 250 mg PO qid × 10 days, or doxycycline 100 g PO qd × 10 days).

    E. Chest radiography should be ordered for all patients over 40 years and for those with pulmonary or cardiac disease.

    F. Pulmonary function tests (PFTs)

        1. The following patients should have preoperative PFTs:

            a. Patients with significant **COPD**

            b. Patients with **wheezes.** These patients should have preoperative PFTs (with and without bronchodilators) to determine whether therapy will improve the reactive airway disease.

        2. Maximum midexpiratory flow rate correlates with ability to cough and prevent postoperative pneumonia.

        3. Maximum voluntary ventilation (MVV) of less than 50% of predicted correlates with an increased incidence of postoperative pulmonary complications.

        4. Forced expiratory volume in the first second (FEV_1) of less than 1.5 liters, or less than 20% predicted correlates with high risk for postoperative complications.

        5. PFTs best predict outcome for **pulmonary resections (Tables 1-5 and 1-6).**

    G. Arterial blood gas (ABG)

        1. Consider obtaining ABG preoperatively in patients with any of the above six pulmonary risk factors (see I A–G) or those with poor PFTs.

        2. Carbon dioxide retention ($PaCO_2 > 45$ mmHg) correlates with the need for postoperative mechanical ventilation.

THE PATIENT WITH RENAL FAILURE

I. Goals of Preoperative Evaluation

    A. Determine whether renal failure is acute or chronic.

Table 1-5.   Pulmonary Function Tests (PFTs) and Pulmonary Resection

PFT	Prohibitive Risk	Normal Value
FEV_1	< 500 ml	40 ml/kg
FVC	< 1 L	30–50 ml/kg
FEV_1/FVC	$< 50\%$ predicted	$> 85\%$
FEF_{25-50}	<0.6 L/sec	3–4 L/sec
MVV	< 50 L/min	> 150 L/min

FEF = forced expiratory flow; FEV = forced expiratory volume; FVC = forced vital capacity; MVV = maximal voluntary ventilation

Table 1-6.   Acceptable Pulmonary Function Tests for Operability

	Pneumonectomy	Lobectomy	Wedge Resection
FEV_1	$> 1.7–2$ L	> 1.0 L	> 0.6 L
FVC	>2.1 L		
FEF_{25-50}	> 1.6 L/sec	> 0.6 L/sec	> 0.6 L/sec
MVV	$> 55\%$ predicted	$> 40\%$ predicted	$> 40\%$ predicted

FEF = forced expiratory flow; FEV = forced expiratory volume; FVC = forced vital capacity; MVV = maximal voluntary ventilation

      B. Determine the extent of renal failure (creatinine clearance).

      C. Prevent further renal damage.

      D. Minimize postoperative complications.

  II. Specific Management

      A. Closely monitor **intakes and outputs** and **daily weights.**

      B. Use a **Foley catheter** for patients who are not anuric.

      C. Institute **aggressive control of hypertension;** avoid angiotensin-converting enzyme (ACE) inhibitors.

      D. Check electrolytes frequently.

      E. Avoid nephrotoxic agents (e.g., aminoglycosides, radiocontrast agents).

      F. For patients on chronic hemodialysis:

         1. Dialysis should be performed the day before surgery.

         2. Check serum potassium prior to surgery.

THE DIABETIC PATIENT

  I. Preoperative Tests

      A. Electrocardiography

      B. Laboratory tests

1. Electrolytes
2. Serum glucose
3. Creatinine

II. Specific Management

A. **Patients with chronic hyperglycemia** may require intravenous hydration preoperatively.

B. Perioperatively, **patients with diabetes** should have their blood glucose checked by finger stick at least every 6 hours. Hyperglycemia should be treated with regular insulin and urine should be monitored for glucosuria.

C. **Patients with non-insulin-dependent diabetes**
1. Long-acting oral hypoglycemic agents (e.g., chlorpropamide, glyburide) should not be taken the day of surgery.
2. Metformin should not be taken the day of surgery.
3. Patients who require postoperative ICU monitoring or who will be NPO for more than 2 days should be converted to SQ insulin until PO intake is resumed.

D. **Patients with insulin-dependent diabetes**
1. Patients taking long-acting insulin preparations (e.g., ultralente) should be converted to an intermediate-acting preparation (NPH Insulin or lente insulin) 1 to 2 days prior to surgery.
2. On the morning of surgery, give patients one-half of their usual morning NPH or lente dose, and administer 5% glucose solution intraoperatively.

THE PATIENT WITH CEREBROVASCULAR SYMPTOMS

I. Postponement of Surgery

A. Surgery should be postponed for at least 6 weeks from the date of the stroke.

B. Surgery should be postponed in patients with ongoing transient ischemic attacks (TIAs). In addition:
1. Carotid duplex ultrasonography should be obtained.
2. If carotid stenosis of more than 70% is detected, endarterectomy should precede general or thoracic surgery.

II. Carotid Bruits.
A carotid bruit in an asymptomatic patient does not require further preoperative workup. Postoperatively, the patient should have carotid Doppler ultrasound.

THE PATIENT WITH MALNUTRITION. See also

Chapter 15, Nutrition.

I. History.
Determine the patient's usual body weight (i.e., body weight over the previous 3 to 6 months).

II. Physical Examination.
The following findings indicate malnutrition:

   A. Dry, scaly, atrophic skin
   B. Muscle wasting (especially temporal wasting)
   C. Presacral edema

III. Laboratory Tests
   A. Serum albumin (half-life = 20 days)
   B. Serum transferrin (half-life = 9 days)
   C. Serum prealbumin (half-life = 3 days)

IV. Specific Management
   A. Severe malnutrition
      1. Definition. Severe malnutrition is indicated by loss of more than 10% of usual body weight with serum albumin less than 2.5 g/dl and serum transferrin less than 150 mg/dl.
      2. Management. Patients with severe malnutrition should undergo 7 to 10 days of total parenteral nutrition (TPN). TPN should be continued postoperatively until the patient can tolerate oral feedings.

   B. Moderate malnutrition
      1. Definition. Moderate malnutrition is indicated by loss of 6% to 10% of usual body weight with serum albumin greater than 3.0 g/dl and serum transferrin greater than 200 mg/dl.
      2. Management
         a. Consider postoperative TPN if patient is to be NPO for many days postoperatively.
         b. Begin supplemental intestinal feeding for patients receiving preoperative chemotherapy or radiotherapy for head/neck, esophageal, or gastric neoplasms. (This may require operative feeding tube placement.)

PART II

Principles of

Management

2

Airway Management

I. **Definition.** Airway management involves securing the airway to relieve an obstruction or to maintain the airway for ventilation.

II. **History.** A patient history is used to obtain the following information.
   A. Is the problem lack of ventilation or airway obstruction?
   B. Is the obstruction mechanical or physiologic (e.g., laryngeal tumor versus syncope)?
   C. Is there history of trauma (e.g., trauma to larynx, facial skeleton, neck, or chest)?
   D. Is there history of a tumor (e.g., tumor in the larynx, oropharynx, esophagus, or thyroid)?
   E. Was a foreign body ingested? Was it witnessed or suspected?
   F. Is there history of a neurologic or cardiac event (e.g., syncope, seizure, cardiovascular accident, myocardial infarction)?
   G. Is there history of other medical problems?

III. **Physical Examination**
   A. In cases of suspected or obvious acute airway compromise, the first priority is assessment of the severity of the situation, which can be accomplished by determining **oxygen saturation.**
      1. Mild obstruction: 90%–95% oxygen saturation
      2. Moderate obstruction: 80%–89% oxygen saturation
      3. Severe obstruction: 70%–79% oxygen saturation
      4. Emergent obstruction: < 70% oxygen saturation
   B. After severity has been determined, check for the following:
      1. Sensorium
      2. Cyanosis
      3. Altered level of consciousness
      4. Hoarseness
      5. Stridor
         a. Inspiratory stridor indicates obstruction above the vocal cords.
         b. Expiratory stridor indicates obstruction below the vocal cords.

      c. Biphasic stridor indicates obstruction at the level of the vocal cords.

   6. Restlessness (sign of hypoxia)

   7. Drooling (caused by pain from an infection or tumor)

   8. Bleeding (caused by coagulopathy or trauma)

   9. Subcutaneous emphysema (indicates disruption of the aerodigestive tract)

   10. Palpable fracture (e.g., fracture of the facial skeleton or laryngeal cartilaginous framework)

IV. Diagnostic Tests

  A. Laryngoscopy is the most informative test if time allows and the expertise is available. The two methods are:

   1. Direct with a fiberoptic laryngoscope

   2. Indirect with a laryngeal mirror

  B. Relevant **radiographs** include:

   1. Lateral and anteroposterior views of the soft tissue of the neck to assess for epiglottitis, retropharyngeal abscess, and Pott's disease

   2. Chest radiograph to reveal pulmonary status, tracheal deviation, and pneumothorax

  C. A **CT scan** of the neck, with contrast, assesses for the presence of a tumor or abscess compressing the airway or a foreign body in the airway.

  D. ABG assesses tissue oxygenation in subacute airway obstruction only. These blood gases play no role in acute airway management.

V. Management depends on the diagnosis, severity of obstruction, and the expertise of the person managing the situation.

> **Intubation is the gold standard for securing and maintaining an airway. When in doubt, intubate!**

  A. Cricothyroidotomy (see Chapter 32) is preferred over tracheostomy in an emergency.

  B. Tracheostomy is used in an emergency if cricothyroidotomy is not a valid option (e.g., laryngeal fracture).

   1. Terminology

    a. Tracheotomy is the creation of a surgical opening into the trachea for the purpose of ventilation.

    b. Tracheostomy is the creation of a stoma (i.e., an epithelialized tract) from the neck skin to the trachea. The tracheostomy has the relative ability to stay open without an indwelling tracheostomy tube.

   2. Types of tracheostomy tubes

    a. Cuffed tracheostomy tubes

     (1) An inflatable cuff provides a 360° seal of the airway when inflated and is a prerequisite for adequate ventilation.

     (2) All of the tidal volume given by the ventilator is delivered without escaping around the tracheostomy tube.

   b. Noncuffed tracheostomy tubes
- **(1)** Noncuffed tracheostomy tubes are used for patients who are not on ventilators.
- **(2)** The tubes are made of plastic, metal, or Silastic material.

   c. Fenestrated tracheostomy tubes
- **(1)** Fenestrated tracheostomy tubes have a hole on the dorsal aspect of the superior portion near the flange so air can escape to the larynx.
- **(2)** In long-term use, fenestrated tubes promote growth of granulation tissue around the fenestration.
- **(3)** Fenestrated tubes should be used selectively.

3. Sizes of tracheostomy tubes
- **a.** Tracheostomy tubes are classified into three categories: neonatal, pediatric, and adult.
- **b.** The size can be measured in millimeters of outer diameter and inner diameter or the size scale used by the manufacturer.
  - **(1)** The outer diameter provides information about the size compatibility of the tracheostomy tube and the stoma.
  - **(2)** The inner diameter is the size of the actual hole through which the patient breathes.
  - **(3)** The brand-name tubes do not always have the same size units, as their numbers indicate.

4. Inner cannula of the tracheostomy tube
- **a.** The inner cannula provides a way to clean the tracheostomy tube without removing the entire tube.
- **b.** The inner cannula can be removed, cleaned, and reinserted or replaced.
- **c.** Both metal and plastic tubes can have inner cannulae.

5. Tracheostomy care
- **a. Tracheostomy care in the acute setting**
  - **(1)** A tracheostomy set should be placed at the bedside for the first 3 days for any emergencies.
  - **(2)** In the immediate postoperative period, the tracheostomy tube should be suctioned frequently because the irritation from a new foreign body produces more sputum.
  - **(3)** The cuff should be left inflated for the first 24 hours after insertion to avoid aspiration of blood or secretions.
  - **(4)** The inner cannula should be changed every day to every third day, depending on the amount of sputum production and mucus plugging.
  - **(5)** Povidone-iodine ointment should be applied to the tracheostomy stoma three times a day.
  - **(6)** The tracheostomy should be inspected every day for the first 7 days to look for infection, breakdown of neck skin from the tracheostomy

ties, signs of bleeding, and dislodgment of the tube.

(7) A tracheostomy mask with mist helps to avoid crusting and mucus plugging.

(8) If the medical and mental status of the patient allows, tracheostomy care should be taught from the first day.

(9) The first tracheostomy tube change should not be performed until 7 days after surgery.

b. Tracheostomy care in the chronic setting

(1) Clean the tracheostomy tube every day.

(a) Metal tubes can be cleaned with peroxide, water, and a steel brush.

(b) Plastic tubes should be cleaned with warm water and soap.

(c) Other tubes should be cleaned according to the manufacturer's instructions.

(2) Plastic tracheostomy tubes should be changed once every month.

(3) Silver nitrate cautery should be performed on any granulation tissue on the stoma.

(4) For any signs of infection, antibiotic ointment should be applied to the stoma three times a day.

(5) Patients should have a suction machine at home and should be instructed in its use before discharge. A room humidifier is also helpful.

(6) Patients cannot be discharged home unless they demonstrate the ability to care for the tracheostomy site and tube. They should also be instructed in the following steps in case of respiratory obstruction.

(a) If unable to breathe, cough strongly.

(b) If still unable to breathe, suction the tracheostomy tube using a suction machine and catheter.

(c) If still unable to breathe, take out and clean the inner cannula.

(d) If still unable to breathe, remove the entire tube and call for help.

(7) Patients who have had a laryngectomy can eventually be maintained without a tracheostomy tube.

6. Tracheostomy tube change

a. Tube change in a stable patient

(1) Make sure a head light is available and a tracheostomy set is at the bedside.

(2) Explain the procedure to the patient and make sure the patient does not have any active coagulopathy.

(3) Place the patient in the supine position.

(a) If the patient can tolerate it, place a shoulder roll under the shoulders.

      (b) Position the patient in the same fashion as required for performing a tracheostomy. This position lines up the tracheal hole with the hole in the skin by pulling up the trachea from the mediastinum.

  (4) Turn up the oxygen to 100% a few minutes before the tube change. Be sure to monitor the patient's oxygen saturation during the procedure.

  (5) Get the new tracheostomy tube ready along with lubricant jelly; peroxide to clean the stoma; gauze sponges; tracheostomy ties; a stiff, red rubber catheter; suction set up with endotracheal suction catheter and tonsil suction; scissors; a 10-ml syringe to deflate and inflate the cuff; and an assistant, if possible.

  (6) Suction the tracheostomy tube, standing on the right side of the bed if you are right-handed.

  (7) Deflate the cuff using the syringe and cut the tracheostomy ties and any stitches holding it to the skin.

  (8) Make sure the new tracheostomy tube is ready with its obturator (an introducer with a smooth, round end that prevents trauma) and that tracheostomy ties are in place.

  (9) Remove the tracheostomy tube anteriorly along its natural curve.

(10) Suction any secretions that are present on the stoma and clean the adjacent skin with peroxide-soaked gauze and sterile water.

(11) Inspect the stoma for erosion, bleeding, infection, or suture material and assess the newly formed track.

(12) Visualize the tracheal fenestration. Introduce the tube in a curved manner, and insert it with the obturator in place at a 90° angle to the neck.

(13) When inside the trachea, twist the tube 90° to its natural position inside the tracheal lumen. This maneuver prevents entrance into the pretracheal space.

(14) Remove the obturator and insert the inner cannula.

(15) Inflate the cuff if the patient is on a ventilator.

(16) Place the tracheostomy ties tight enough that you can slip two fingers under the ties without difficulty.

(17) Auscultate the chest to confirm good air entry and bilateral breath sounds.

(18) Remove the shoulder roll, elevate the head of the bed, and reduce the oxygen level.

b. Tube change in an unstable patient

(1) Follow the same steps for a tube change in a stable patient (see V B 6 a).

(2) A tracheostomy tube change can lead to fatal accidents in unstable patients; therefore, it is best for an experienced person to perform the tube change.

(3) Tube changes in unstable patients are often performed in the operating room in the presence of an anesthesiologist (especially for pediatric cases).

7. Complications

a. If **unable to introduce a tracheostomy tube,** do not panic.

(1) Look at the stoma and try it again while visualizing the stoma and the track. The tracheostomy tube will not find a track that you cannot, so do not push the tube.

(2) Try to pass a red rubber catheter in the stoma. If this works, thread the tracheostomy tube over it using the Seldinger technique.

(3) If you can see the stoma and track but the hole is deep, ask for an endotracheal tube.

(4) If still unsuccessful, call for help (i.e., anesthesiologist, otolaryngologist).

(5) While waiting for help, ask for intubation equipment.

(6) Continue to give the patient 100% oxygen. If the patient cannot breathe, start bagging the patient with a bag-valve-mask unit.

(7) Monitor oxygen saturation.

If you are ultimately unable to place or change a tracheostomy tube, just intubate.

---

b. Some **bleeding** is common after a traumatic attempt at introducing a tracheostomy tube.

(1) If the patient starts bleeding, auscultate the chest for bilateral breath sounds to confirm the position of the tracheostomy tube. Secure the tube if it is in the right place.

(2) If using a cuffed tube, inflate the cuff. If the bleeding persists, pack the stoma around the tracheostomy tube with absorbable hemostat (e.g., Surgicel).

C. Emergency airway management based on severity

1. Guarded condition

a. Immediately intubate the patient.

b. If the first attempt fails, perform emergent cricothyroidotomy (see Chapter 32).

2. Severe condition

a. Start mask bagging, call for help (e.g., anesthesiolo-

gist, otolaryngologist, surgeon), and ask for a tracheostomy set.
  - **b.** Attempt to intubate the patient.
  - **c.** If intubation fails, perform emergent cricothyroidotomy (see Chapter 32).
- **3. Moderate condition**
  - **a.** Discuss management options (e.g., intubation, observation, cricothyroidotomy) with the anesthesiologist.
  - **b.** Before attempting intubation, prepare for cricothyroidotomy (see Chapter 32).
    - **(1)** Place the patient in the supine position with both arms tucked, a shoulder roll across and under the shoulders, and the neck extended.
    - **(2)** Infiltrate the skin one to two finger breaths above the sternal notch with 5 ml of 1% lidocaine with epinephrine 1:100,000.
    - **(3)** Place the Bovie grounding pad on the patient.
  - **c.** If intubation is required, attempt fiberoptic intubation to avoid adding to the obstruction with blind intubation.
  - **d.** If intubation is unsuccessful, proceed with tracheostomy or cricothyroidotomy.
- **4. Mild condition**
  - **a.** Temporize with oxygen and perform a jaw-lift maneuver.
  - **b.** Consider mask bagging, mist, dexamethasone, cimetidine, careful observation in the ICU, racemic epinephrine, and nasal trumpet.
- **D. Airway management based on etiology**
  - **1. Trauma**
    - **a. Avoid bag masking** if there is a chance of skull-base fracture, because positive pressure ventilation can cause tension pneumoencephalus.
    - **b. Intubation** should be done only with **in-line stabilization** in the trauma patient.
    - **c.** If an orotracheal or nasotracheal tube cannot be placed safely or accurately, proceed to **cricothyroidotomy** (see Chapter 32).
  - **2. Tumor**
    - **a. Do not give any paralytics** unless you have confirmed that there is no trismus resulting from pterygoid muscle involvement.
    - **b.** Carefully **intubate** the patient. The first attempt is crucial because bleeding from a traumatic attempt makes it almost impossible to intubate.
    - **c.** In cases of subacute obstruction (e.g., tumors of the oral cavity, pharynx, or larynx), provide temporizing measures such as **oxygen, dexamethasone, mist,** and **mask ventilation** until further assistance is available.
    - **d.** In the presence of a previous tracheostomy scar, follow the scar and cut down.

3. For **infection** (e.g., epiglottitis, Ludwig's angina, neck abscess), **intubation** is the management of choice.

4. Foreign body
  a. If there is **partial obstruction, do not intervene.** It is important to encourage coughing.
  b. For **complete obstruction,** proceed as follows.
    (1) Perform a finger sweep.
    (2) Perform the Heimlich maneuver.
    (3) Perform cricothyroidotomy (see Chapter 32) for persistent, complete laryngeal obstruction.

5. Respiratory failure or insecure airway
  a. Always attempt **intubation** first.
  b. Surgical intervention is required after failed intubation attempts.
  c. Maintain oxygen saturation with mask ventilation while preparing for cricothyroidotomy (see Chapter 32) or tracheostomy.

6. Sleep apnea
  a. These patients should undergo **fiberoptic awake intubation.** During elective intubation, these patients can lose all muscle tone, go into laryngospasm on induction, and drop their oxygen saturation precipitously.
  b. Do not extubate these patients until they are fully awake.

7. Bilateral vocal cord paralysis is a rare occurrence that presents with stridor. It is amenable to **intubation.**

E. Tips for successful airway management
  1. When called for a **stat airway,** always remember **ATLS:**
    a. A—anesthesiologist, assistance
    b. T—tracheostomy set (ask nurses; do not leave patient)
    c. L—light, lidocaine (1% lidocaine with epinephrine 1:100,000)
    d. S—suction
  2. In an emergency, a cricothyroidotomy is preferred over tracheostomy.
  3. Never lose your calm.
  4. Never leave the patient.

3

Anesthesia in the ICU

NEUROMUSCULAR BLOCKADE

I. **General Indications for Neuromuscular Blockade**
   A. As an adjunct to general anesthesia
   B. For rapid sequence intubation
   C. As an adjunct to electroconvulsive therapy
   D. For symptomatic treatment of tetanus intoxication

II. **Indications for Neuromuscular Blockade in the ICU**
   A. For mechanical ventilation
      1. With inverse I:E ratio
      2. With controlled ventilation plus one of the following (despite maximal sedation): a combative patient, increased mean airway pressure, increased intracranial pressure
   B. To immobilize a patient for specific treatment (e.g., a patient undergoing a large skin graft, ventriculostomy placement)
   C. To decrease oxygen consumption

III. **Depolarizing Agents (Succinylcholine)**
   A. **Structure.** Structurally similar to acetylcholine (ACh), succinylcholine consists of two acetylcholine molecules attached by means of an acetate moiety.
   B. **Mechanism of action.** Succinylcholine binds to *N*-acetylcholine (*N*-ACh) receptors to produce an initial depolarization followed by desensitization of the membrane to subsequent stimulation. It will cause an increase in vagal stimulation.
   C. **Dosage and pharmacokinetics.** See **Table 3-1.**
   D. **Indications.** In the ICU, succinylcholine is used only for **rapid sequence intubation.**
   E. **Contraindications.** Succinylcholine is contraindicated for patients with the following:
      1. History of malignant hyperthermia
      2. Duchenne muscular dystrophy
      3. Hyperkalemia
      4. Burns, spinal cord injury, or crush injury (Succinyl-

Table 3-1. Neuromuscular Blocking Agents: Dosages and Pharmacokinetics

Drug	Dose (mg/kg)[1]	Metabolism	Onset	Action	BP	HR	ICP
Succinylcholine[2]	0.3–1.1	P	< 1 minute	1–2 minutes	↕	→	←
Pancuronium[3,4]	0.03–0.1 bolus, 0.02–0.1 maintenance	R	1–2 minutes	40–60 minutes	←	←	↕
Cisatracurium[3]	0.1–0.2 bolus; 0.12–0.24 maintenance	P	2–3 minutes	20–40 minutes	↕	↕	↕
Vecuronium[4,5]	0.08–0.1 bolus; 0.04–0.08 maintenance	H	2–3 minutes	30–40 minutes	↕	→	↕
Rocuronium	0.6–1.0	H	1–3 minutes	10–30 minutes	↕	←	↕
Mivacurium	0.2	P	1–2 minutes	15–20 minutes	→	←↕	↕

P = plasma, H = hepatic, R = renal
↑ = increased, ↓ = decreased ↔ = no change
[1]This dose may be used to initiate hourly infusion.
[2]Only depolarizing agent; used for rapid sequence induction.
[3]Active metabolites
[4]Prolonged effects in hepatic and renal insufficiency
[5]No vagolytic properties

choline may cause clinically significant hyperkalemia in these circumstances.)

Succinylcholine should not be used as a continuous infusion or given in repeated doses because of the high incidence of hyperkalemia, bradycardia, and asystole.

IV. **Nondepolarizing Agents (Pancuronium, Vecuronium, and Cisatracurium)**
   A. **Structure**
      1. Pancuronium and vecuronium are steroid derivatives.
      2. Cisatracurium is a curare derivative.
   B. **Mechanism of action.** The bulky molecules of these agents competitively inhibit ACh and prevent cell membrane depolarization.
   C. **Pharmacokinetics.** See Table 3-1.
   D. **Infusion guidelines.** See Table 3-1.

To dramatically reduce the incidence of adverse reactions, all patients with intravenous neuromuscular blockade should be monitored regularly with a twitch monitor. Infusion rates should be adjusted based on train of four (TOF) twitch response to maintain at least two twitches. Patients must be adequately sedated.

   E. **Drug selection**
      1. **Pancuronium** is the cheapest neuromuscular blocker. It should be used in patients who have normal renal and hepatic function and who can tolerate vagolytic side effects. It increases blood pressure, heart rate, and cardiac output. Its use results in mast cell degranulation.
      2. **Vecuronium** should be used in patients who have normal renal and hepatic function and who *cannot* tolerate vagolytic side effects. This drug does not induce mast cell degranulation.
      3. **Cisatracurium** should be used in patients who have renal or hepatic insufficiency or who are on concomitant steroid therapy. It has few or no cardiovascular side effects.
   F. **Precautions**
      1. Prior to initiating neuromuscular blockade, maximize opiates and benzodiazepines.
      2. NEVER use neuromuscular blockade without concomitant analgesia and sedation.
      3. ALWAYS monitor depth of blockade with a TOF monitor.
      4. Use the **lowest dose possible.**
      5. **Airway control and endotracheal suctioning are crucial** because the respiratory muscles are paralyzed and the cough reflex is abolished.
      6. Provide **ophthalmic lubricants** and passive **range of motion of joints and muscles.**

> **If no twitches are seen with a TOF monitor,
> then hold infusion until two twitches return,
> then resume infusion at a 20% decrease.**

V. **Reversal of Neuromuscular Blockade.** Reversal can be achieved through administration of an acetylcholinesterase inhibitor (**Table 3-2**).

Table 3-2. Neuromuscular Blockade Reversing Agents: Dosages and Pharmacokinetics

Drug	IV Dose	Time to Peak	Duration
Edrophonium	0.5–1.0 mg/kg	1 minute	45 minutes
Neostigmine	0.5 mg/kg (maximum 5 mg)	7 minutes	60 minutes
Pyridostigmine	0.25 mg/kg	12 minutes	100 minutes
Atropine	0.015 mg/kg	1.2 minutes	60–120 minutes
Glycopyrrolate	0.01–0.02 mg/kg	4 minutes	120–240 minutes

SEDATION AND ANALGESIA

I. **Indications.** Some form of sedation is used for virtually every patient in the ICU:
   A. To reduce patient awareness of the external environment (e.g., noise, physical restraints)
   B. To calm the patient (anxiolysis)
   C. To induce sleep
   D. As an adjunct for uncomfortable ICU procedures (e.g., endotracheal suctioning, cardioversion, endoscopy)
   E. As an adjunct to neuromuscular blockade
   F. As a treatment for alcohol withdrawal or status epilepticus (benzodiazepines only)

II. **Benzodiazepines**
   A. **Mechanism of action.** Benzodiazepines target benzodiazepine receptors on GABA-activated chloride channels in the CNS. They increase the frequency of channel opening, which decreases the excitability of neurons that receive GABA inputs. Benzodiazepines require the presence of GABA for efficacy.
   B. **Pharmacokinetics.** See Table 3-3.
   C. **Administration. Lorazepam** and **midazolam** may be given intravenously by bolus injection or continuous infusion. Always give a bolus dose prior to continuous infusion.
      1. **Guidelines for intravenous infusion**
         a. **Use lowest dose possible.** (See Table 3-3 for dosages.)
         b. **Continuously monitor patient** for desired level of sedation. The goal is to have an awake, communicative, comfortable patient.

Table 3–3.   Commonly Used Benzodiazepines: Dosages and Pharmacokinetics

	Lorazepam	Midazolam
IV dose	1–2 mg	1–5 mg
Intermittent IV dose	1–4 mg 4 hr	1–5 mg q 1–2 hr
Dose for continuous infusion	1–4 mg/hr	0.02–0.1 mg/kg/hr
Onset of action	20–30 minutes	1–5 minutes
Duration of action	6–10 hours	30 minutes–2 hours
Metabolism	Glucuronidation	Glucuronidation and oxidation
Active metabolites	No	Yes
Effects in renal insufficiency	Unchanged	Prolonged
Effects in hepatic insufficiency	Unchanged	Prolonged
Effects in elderly	Pronounced	Pronounced; use cautiously

      c. Although tachyphylaxis to benzodiazepines may occur, **attempt to decrease infusion rate daily.**

  2. Cessation of infusion

      a. Sedative effects may persist for 1 to 2 days after cessation of infusion.

      b. Withdrawal and addiction to benzodiazepines after ICU exposure **are rare.**

> **Patients who are on benzodiazepine infusions for more than 5 days should be tapered off the drug over a 3–5 day period.**

  D. Reversal. Reversal of benzodiazepine sedation can be achieved through the administration of **flumazenil.**

    1. Dosage is 0.1 mg q min to a total dose of 2 mg.

    2. For coma thought to be secondary to benzodiazepine overdose, give 5 mg IV.

    3. The half-life of flumazenil is 1 hour, so **repeated infusions may be necessary.**

    4. Use flumazenil with extreme caution. This agent may precipitate withdrawal.

III. Propofol

  A. Structure. Propofol is a derivative of phenol.

> **Like most phenols, the water solubility of propofol is poor. The commercial preparation of propofol uses a water-oil emulsion (10% lipid) that readily supports bacterial growth. Therefore, STRICT ASEPTIC HANDLING OF THE PROPOFOL PREPARATION AND A DEDICATED IV for infusion minimize septic complications.**

B. Mechanism of action. Propofol binds to the $GABA_A$-activated chloride ion channel; this increases the duration of channel opening (similar to barbiturates). Unlike benzodiazepines, propofol does not require GABA for channel opening.

C. Pharmacokinetics. Propofol has a unique pharmacokinetic profile.

1. **Metabolism** is hepatic and extrahepatic (possibly lung).
2. The pharmacokinetics are **not altered by renal or hepatic insufficiency.**
3. There is **no tachyphylaxis** to the sedative effect.
4. There is **no residual sedation** once infusion is discontinued.

D. Dosage

1. Administer 5 μg/kg/min initially.
2. Titrate infusion to desired level of sedation (**Ramsey Sedation Scale, Table 3-4**).
3. Decrease dose by 50% in the elderly.

E. Contraindications. Propofol is contraindicated in **hypovolemic patients.**

F. Effects independent of sedation

1. **Vasodilation.** This is mediated via inhibition of sympathetic vasoconstriction.

Propofol can cause profound hypotension in hypovolemic patients, and in elderly patients because of their limited cardiac reserve.

---

2. **Decreased tissue oxygen consumption and carbon dioxide production.** This may be beneficial in hyperdynamic patients.
3. **Long-term infusion.** Patients requiring long-term infusion of propofol should have periodic lipid profiles checked and the fat content of TPN should be adjusted accordingly.
4. **Elevated triglyceride levels.** Monitor if the patient is on the drug for more than 24 hours.

Table 3-4.   Ramsey Sedation Scale

1	Patient awake and anxious, agitated, or restless
2	Patient awake, calm, oriented, tranquil
3	Patient awake, responds to commands only
4	Patient asleep, brisk response to loud auditory stimulus or light glabellar tap
5	Patient asleep, sluggish response to loud auditory stimulus or light glabellar tap
6	Patient asleep, no response to loud auditory stimulus or light glabellar tap

IV. Opiates

    A. Mechanism of action. Opiates act at opioid receptors (mu, kappa, delta, sigma) in the thalamus, limbic system, and spinal cord to modulate nociceptive transmission and alter the subjective component of pain.

    B. Pharmacokinetics and dosage

        1. Opiates are metabolized by the liver and excreted though the urine.

> **The dose and frequency of administration should be decreased in elderly patients and patients with renal or hepatic insufficiency.**

        2. See **Table 3-5** for pharmacokinetics of the common opiates.

    C. Indications

        1. Opiates provide **analgesia** and **moderate sedation.**

        2. Opiates are **useful in combination with benzodiazepines or propofol** to achieve optimal sedation, especially in postoperative, mechanically ventilated, or paralyzed patients.

    D. Side effects and precautions

        1. Respiratory depression. Opiates decrease the medulla's response to carbon dioxide.

            a. The hypoxic drive (mediated by chemoreceptors of the carotid body and aortic arch) is unaffected. Therefore, **SUPPLEMENTAL OXYGEN MIGHT LEAD TO HYPOXIA.**

            b. The respiratory depressant and sedating effects of **fentanyl** may outlast the analgesic effects.

        2. Bronchoconstriction. This is related to endogenous release of histamine.

        3. Nausea and vomiting. Opiates stimulate the chemoreceptor trigger zone of the medulla.

        4. Miosis. This is caused by disinhibition of cranial nerve III.

        5. Urinary retention. Opiates stimulate release of ADH, increase ureteral tone, and decrease the urge to urinate.

        6. GI hypertonicity. This leads to constipation and sphincter of Oddi contraction.

        7. Dependence and withdrawal. Problems with dependence and withdrawal from narcotics administered in an ICU are rare.

    E. Reversal. Administer 0.1–0.4 mg IV of **naloxone** (an opiate antagonist) for suspected opiate overdose.

V. Butyrophenones (Haloperidol and Droperidol)

    A. Mechanism of action. The butyrophenones act by antagonizing D_2 dopamine receptors in the CNS, including mesolimbic and mesocortical projections (which has an antipsychotic effect) and in the medulla (chemoreceptor trigger zone, which has an antiemetic effect).

Table 3-5. Common Opiates: Dosages Pharmacokinetics

	Morphine	Fentanyl	Hydromorphone (Dilaudid)	Meperidine (Demerol)
IV dose	2–10 mg	50–100 μg	0.2–2.0 mg	25–75 mg
IV infusion	1–5 mg/hr	25–100 μg/hr[1]	—	—
Onset of action	10–20 minutes	2–5 minutes	—	10–20 minutes
Duration of action	4–6 hours	30–60 minutes[2]	4–5 hours	3–5 hours

[1]Initiate infusion with bolus of 1 μg/kg/hr.
[2]Prolonged administration increases duration of action to 9–16 hours.

B. Indications. The butyrophenones provides sedation to **agitated or delirious** patients.

The butyrophenones DO NOT provide sedation to patients with normal mental faculties, and in fact can cause extreme dysphoria in such patients.

C. Dosage and administration. The **IV dose** (for both haloperidol and droperidol) is 1–5 mg q 8 hr. Butyrophenones may be administered **every 30 minutes to acutely agitated patients** who fail to respond to the initial dose.
D. Side effects and precautions
   1. **Prolonged use** of butyrophenones can lead to **extrapyramidal side effects** (akathisia, dystonia, Parkinsonism, or Tardive dyskinesia) and **neuroleptic malignant syndrome.**
   2. The butyrophenones do not cause respiratory depression.
   3. Patients with low magnesium or concomitant drugs that prolong the Q-T interval are at risk for torsades de pointes. Obtain baseline ECG.

EPIDURAL AND INTRATHECAL ANESTHESIA AND ANALGESIA

I. Definitions
   A. Epidural anesthesia is regional anesthesia produced by injection of an opiate or a local anesthetic into the epidural space. The drug must penetrate the dura and enter into the cerebrospinal fluid (CSF) for efficacy.
   B. Intrathecal (spinal) anesthesia is regional anesthesia produced by injection of an opiate or a local anesthetic into the subarachnoid space. The drug is injected directly into the CSF.
II. Mechanism of Action of Epidural and Intrathecal Agents
   A. Opiates. After the drug enters the CSF, it enters the tissue of the dorsal horn of the spinal cord at a rate proportional to its lipid solubility. Highly lipid soluble opiates (e.g., fentanyl) have a more rapid onset but a shorter duration of action.
      1. Opiates **act at presynaptic receptors** to decrease neuronal transmission of the primary afferent (painful) stimulus.
      2. They also **act at postsynaptic receptors** to decrease the dorsal horn neuron response to stimulation.
   B. Local anesthetics
      1. They inhibit voltage-gated sodium channels.
      2. They block nerve fibers according to their size, i.e., the degree of myelination.
         a. Small delta A fibers (which modulate pain) are blocked before moderate-sized autonomic B fibers.

      b. The large A fibers that convey motor function are blocked last.

III. Clinical Use

  A. Intrathecal anesthesia and analgesia

    1. Advantage. Adequate analgesia can be achieved with a **small dose.**

    2. Disadvantages

      a. Post-procedure spinal **headache** may occur.

      b. An **indwelling intrathecal catheter is not feasible** because of potential complications from the catheter being in the subarachnoid space (infection and possible nerve damage).

    3. ICU role. Intrathecal anesthesia has a **limited role in the ICU setting.** Anesthesiologists sometimes administer intrathecal narcotics before abdominal operations.

  B. Epidural anesthesia and analgesia

    1. Advantages

      a. Can be administered via an indwelling catheter, which may be used for intermittent bolus injection, continuous infusion, or patient controlled epidural anesthesia (PCEA).

      b. Epidural anesthesia **provides significant relief of postoperative pain,** which allows for **improved pulmonary mechanics** and **earlier ambulation.** Studies show that epidural catheters are associated with a decreased incidence of pulmonary complications and a decreased incidence of deep venous thrombosis (DVT).

      c. Sympathetic block **increases blood flow to the viscera and extremities.**

        (1) With epidural anesthesia, there is a **lower incidence of ileus** after abdominal operations.

        (2) For **vascular bypass** operations, epidural analgesia improves extremity perfusion, although graft patency is NOT improved.

      d. Epidural analgesia is **associated with a shorter ICU and hospital stay.**

      e. Data are conflicting on the effect of epidural anesthesia on the **operative stress response** (e.g., production of catecholamines, cortisol, cytokines). Primary cardiac events are NOT reduced by use of epidural anesthesia.

    2. Disadvantages

      a. Epidural anesthesia requires a dedicated, 24-hour-a-day pain management team.

      b. Tubing and pump infusions may be cumbersome.

      c. The patient's respiratory rate must be monitored frequently.

    3. Complications

      a. Catheter related complications

        (1) Inadvertent dural puncture. The incidence is

about 1%. It results in spinal headache. Neurologic injury and meningitis are rare.

(2) **Epidural hematoma secondary to traumatic injury of the epidural vessels.** Symptomatic hematoma is rare (about 1 in 100,000). It can lead to permanent paraplegia. The incidence is not increased in patients receiving anticoagulants (e.g., IV heparin).

(3) **Catheter migration** may occur, leading to loss of analgesia.

b. **Opiate related complications.** See side effects and precautions on p. 33 for details.

(1) Respiratory depression

(2) Sedation

(3) Urinary retention

(4) Nausea and vomiting

c. **Local anesthetic related complications**

(1) Hypotension secondary to sympathetic blockade

(2) Weakness and pressure ulcers secondary to motor blockade

(3) Urinary retention secondary to motor or autonomic blockade

(4) Seizures or cardiac arrhythmias

4. **Drug selection and dosage**

a. **Bupivacaine** is the local anesthetic of choice because of its long half-life and minimal tachyphylaxis. It is administered as a 0.10–0.75% solution.

b. The **combination of a local anesthetic with an opioid** provides optimal analgesia while minimizing the side effects of the respective agents.

c. **Hydromorphone** is about 6 times more potent than morphine and has similar pharmacokinetics. **Respiratory depression is far less common** with hydromorphone than with morphine.

d. **Dosages and pharmacokinetics** of epidural narcotics are listed in **Table 3-6.**

Table 3-6. Epidural Narcotics: Pharmacokinetics and Dosages

	Morphine	Hydomorphone	Meperidine	Fentanyl
Lipid solubility	1.27	1.23	39	706
Duration of action	12–18 h	12 h	6 h	3–5 hours
Dose without bupivacaine	0.5 mg/hr	0.1–0.3 mg/hr	20 mg/hr	0.075 mg/hr
Infusion concentration with 0.1% bupivicaine	0.005%	0.0325%	0.1%	0.0005%

4

Cardiac Surgery

CARDIOPULMONARY BYPASS

I. **Definition.** Cardiopulmonary bypass (CPB) is the temporary diversion of blood flow from the heart through a heart–lung machine, which takes over the pumping and ventilatory functions of the heart and lungs during open heart surgery.

II. **Equipment: Heart–Lung Machine**
   A. **Basic components**
      1. One or more **venous cannulas** are used. They are inserted through the right atrial appendage or through the right atrium into the superior vena cava (SVC) and inferior vena cava (IVC).
      2. A **venous reservoir** is maintained.
      3. A **bubble or membrane oxygenator/heat exchanger** is used.
      4. **Roller or centrifugal pumps** are used to:
         a. Return oxygenated blood to the patient
         b. Operate cardiotomy suction or vent the left side of the heart
         c. Deliver cardioplegic solution
      5. An **arterial line filter** traps particulate matter and gaseous emboli.
      6. **Arterial cannulas** are usually placed in the ascending aorta just proximal to the innominate artery. **Femoral arterial cannulation** is often used for patients with dissecting aortic aneurysms, for patients who require reoperation, and in emergencies when rapid cannulation of the femoral artery and vein is necessary to establish circulation with partial CPB.
   B. **Subsystem components**
      1. The **cardiotomy suction system** aspirates blood from the open cardiac chambers and surgical field. It consists of two suckers, tubing, one roller pump, and a combined blood filter and reservoir unit. Blood is filtered, debubbled, and added to the perfusate.

2. The **cell saver system** is one in which diluted blood from the surgical field is retrieved. Red blood cells are concentrated and then returned to the perfusate.

3. The **cardioplegic delivery system** consists of a separate pump, reservoir, and heat exchanger. This system delivers cooled potassium-enriched blood or crystalloid solution to the coronary circulation.

4. The **left ventricular (LV) venting system** decompresses blood from the noncontracting heart and prevents LV distention. (Distention decreases myocardial contractility and produces lung damage from high pulmonary pressures.)

   a. Venting of the LV facilitates the exposure of the aortic root and valve.

   b. The LV may also be vented using a pulmonary artery catheter.

III. Cardiopulmonary Bypass Procedure

A. **Preparation of equipment.** The heart–lung machine is assembled 30 to 60 minutes before CPB. The machine is tested, primed with crystalloid, and recirculated for several minutes through filters that remove air bubbles. Two liters of priming solution (balanced starch solution) are required.

B. **Hemodilution.** Once the bypass begins, the hematocrit (HCT) is maintained at 20% to 25%. If the HCT drops below this level, homologous blood or packed red blood cells are added to the system.

1. **Advantages**

   a. Less blood products are required for the operation.

   b. Trauma to blood cells is reduced.

   c. Less plasma hemoglobin is produced secondary to reduced trauma.

   d. There is a lower incidence of renal acute tubular necrosis

   e. Flow characteristics improve.

2. **Disadvantages**

   a. Intravascular osmotic pressure is decreased.

   b. Interstitial edema is increased.

C. **Anticoagulation**

1. **Heparin administration.** Heparin is critical for CPB to prevent clotting. Heparin activates the natural plasma protein, antithrombin III, which is a protease inhibitor of factors IXa, Xa, and thrombin.

   a. The **initial dose** of heparin is **300 U/kg**.

   b. The **activated clotting time (ACT)** is used to monitor the degree of anticoagulation.

      (1) The ACT is checked 5 minutes after the administration of heparin, with a **goal of greater than 400 seconds ACT** before beginning CPB.

      (2) The ACT is checked at 20-minute intervals dur-

ing the bypass surgery. Additional heparin is administered to maintain an ACT of > 400 seconds.

2. **Protamine sulfate administration.** Protamine sulfate is given to neutralize heparin after the CPB has stopped.
   a. **Dosage is 1 mg for each 100 U of heparin**.
   b. **Complications** caused by protamine include **transient hypotension** (corrected with volume) and an **anaphylactic reaction** (rare).
3. **Heparin rebound.** Protamine sulfate may be cleared from the circulation faster than heparin can be removed; therefore, heparin rebound may occur. Treatment includes **additional protamine therapy**.

D. **Cardioplegia.** Cardioplegia, the temporary arrest of cardiac activity, is the **most popular method of myocardial protection** during heart surgery. Cardioplegia causes the heart to remain motionless, thus enabling the surgeons to perform the necessary procedure. The combination of arrest during diastole and cold cardioplegia **greatly decreases the oxygen demand of the heart**.
   1. The **cardioplegia delivery system** includes a reservoir that contains either blood or crystalloid plus K+ and other additives, maintained at 4°–12°C. The **active ingredient is K+**, which causes cardiac arrest during diastole.
   2. The **cold blood or crystalloid** is infused antegrade through the aortic root or retrograde through the coronary sinus. If the aortic root is opened, the cold blood or crystalloid may be delivered directly into the coronary arteries.
   3. **Perfusion pressure** is kept **below 40 mm Hg**.

IV. **Parameters of a Successful Bypass**

A. **Blood flow.** Pump flows are nonpulsatile and are usually between 1.5 L/min/m^2 (low flow) and 2.5 L/min/m^2 (high flow).
   1. High flow is maintained at normothermia and during cooling and rewarming.
   2. Low flow is used during hypothermia.

B. **Body temperature.** Body temperature is **lowered** during the CPB **to decrease metabolic activity and oxygen consumption**. Oxygen consumption decreases 50% for every 10°C decrease in body temperature.

C. **Blood pressure.** A mean arterial blood pressure should be maintained **between 50 and 80 mm Hg**. Sodium nitroprusside is used to control hypertension; phenylephrine (Neo-Synephrine) is used for hypotension.

D. **Arterial blood gases (ABGs)**
   1. The **pH** is maintained at **7.4**.
   2. The temperature-corrected **PCO_2** is maintained **between 35 and 40 mm Hg**.
   3. **ABGs are monitored every 15 to 20 minutes** after the initiation of CPB.
   4. **Venous blood saturation** is one of the best parameters for determining adequate tissue perfusion. It is measured

and maintained at **80% during hypothermia (65%–70% during normothermia)**.

E. Hematocrit
1. The hematocrit should be maintained **around 20**.
2. Any **drop in hematocrit should raise suspicion of blood loss** from a leg incision or into the pleural cavities.

F. Potassium should be kept within normal limits.

G. Urine output is a good reflection of systemic perfusion.
1. During CPB, urine output is **normally 3 ml/kg/hr**.
2. **If urine output falls** to < 1 ml/kg/hr, increase the flow rate or arterial pressure.
3. **Furosemide, mannitol, or dopamine** at a renal dose is reserved for **refractory low urine output**.

V. Discontinuation of Bypass. At the completion of the operative procedure:

A. Air is removed from the aorta and the cardiac chambers.

B. The heart is defibrillated, if necessary.

C. The temperature is checked to confirm rewarming, and ventilation of the lungs is begun.

D. CPB is gradually discontinued by progressive retardation of venous drainage.

E. Bypass flows are decreased as the heart fills and systemic pressure rises.

F. Cardiac function is measured by pulmonary capillary wedge pressure (PCWP) and cardiac output (CO). Depressed cardiac function may be improved by the administration of calcium; more severely depressed function is managed pharmacologically.

G. After CPB is discontinued, the atrial cannula or caval cannulas are removed.

H. Protamine sulfate is administered to reverse the effects of heparin. The ACT is measured to confirm that the effects of heparin are indeed reversed.

I. Blood from the oxygenator is infused through the arterial cannula, then this cannula is removed.

VI. Complications of Bypass

A. Intracompartmental fluid shifts and fluid retention

B. Multiple organ dysfunction

C. Embolic events

D. Bleeding

E. Activation of the coagulation system—both intrinsic and extrinsic pathways, complement, platelets, neutrophils, monocytes, and endothelial cells

F. Decrease in the total number of lymphocytes and inhibition of T cell function

G. Heparin-induced thrombocytopenia (2%–5%)

INTRA-AORTIC BALLOON PUMP

I. Definition. The intra-aortic balloon pump consists of an externally and **intermittently inflatable balloon attached to a pump**

console via a catheter. The balloon is placed into the **descending aorta (Figure 4-1).**

   A. The balloon is **inflated during diastole,** augmenting diastolic pressure and improving coronary blood flow and myocardial oxygen supply.

   B. The balloon is **deflated just before systole,** lowering systolic pressure in the aorta. This improves LV ejection and decreases LV workload and myocardial oxygen demand.

II. Equipment. Most intra-aortic balloon pumps used for adults consist of a catheter that is approximately 70 cm long with a 25-cm balloon at the tip. The catheter is attached to a console which coordinates inflation/deflation.

III. Physiology. Major determinants of myocardial oxygen consumption include pulse rate, transmural wall stress, and con-

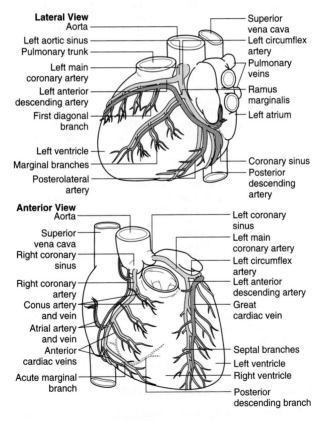

Figure 4-1. The coronary vessels.

tractile properties. The **physiologic effects of the intra-aortic balloon pump (IABP) [Figure 4-2]** are as follows:

A. The IABP modifies both LV ejection pressure and afterload. As a result:

    1. Transmural wall stress is decreased.

    2. Myocardial oxygen supply is increased by diastolic augmentation of coronary perfusion.

    3. Myocardial oxygen requirements are decreased through afterload reduction.

B. The correlate of coronary perfusion is equal to the **diastolic pressure time index (DPTI).**

    1. The DPTI is the time difference between the area under the diastolic aortic curve and the LV pressure curve.

    2. The IABP decreases the **tension time index (TTI),** or ventricular work, and increases the DPTI, or coronary perfusion (**Figure 4-3 and Table 4-1**).

C. The IABP requires a **minimum cardiac index of 1.2 to 1.4 L/min/m².**

IV. Indications for IABP

    A. Treatment of patients with intractable cardiac failure (35%–40% of bypass patients):

        1. Inability to discontinue cardiopulmonary bypass despite multiple interventions for more than 30 minutes

        2. Inadequate hemodynamics in the presence of inotropic support (**cardiac index** < 2 L/min/m², elevated left atrial pressure > 20 mm Hg, high peripheral vascular resistance)

        3. Preoperative cardiogenic shock secondary to a myocardial infarction (MI) or complications of an MI

        4. Persistent ventricular arrhythmias

    B. Treatment of patients with refractory angina despite maximal medical management (15%–25% of patients with angina). At least 80% of these patients obtain pain relief with IABP.

    C. Perioperative treatment of patients with complications of a myocardial infarction. Complications occur in 10% of patients and include acute ventricular septal defect (VSD), acute mitral regurgitation (MR), arrhythmias, and ventricular aneurysms.

    D. Treatment of patients with failed percutaneous coronary angioplasties

    E. As a bridge to a cardiac transplant

    F. Prophylactically for LV aneurysmectomy (combined with directed arrhythmia surgery)

V. Contraindications to IABP

    A. Severe aortic insufficiency. IABP enhances LV regurgitation and cardiac failure in patients with severe aortic insufficiency.

    B. Aortic dissection or severe aortoiliac disease

    C. Thoracic or abdominal aortic aneurysm. This is a relative contraindication.

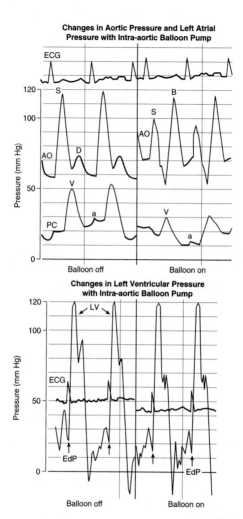

Figure 4-2. (*Top*) Changes in aortic pressure and left atrial pressure with the intra-aortic balloon pump. Both aortic and end-diastolic pressures decrease, suggesting a reduction in ventricular afterload. At the same time the diastolic aortic pressure (*D*) is enhanced (*B*). (*Bottom*) Changes in left ventricular pressure with the intra-aortic balloon pump. In a failing heart, the left ventricular end-diastolic pressure (*EdP*) greatly decreases with balloon pumping. *AO* = aortic pressure; *PC* = pulmonary capillary wedge pressure; *V* = ventricular wave; *a* = atrial wave; *LV* = left ventricular pressure. (Redrawn from Bolooki HK: *Clinical Applications of the Intra-aortic Balloon Pump.* Mt Kisco, NY, Futura Publishing, 1984.)

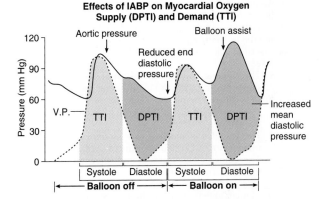

Figure 4-3. Effects of intra-aortic balloon pumping on myocardial oxygen supply and demand. During diastole, balloon assistance produced an elevated DPTI, suggesting an increase in myocardial oxygen supply. At the same time, ventricular work (TTI) decreased significantly. *DPTI* = diastolic perfusion time index; *TTI* = tension time index; *VP (dotted line)* = ventricular pressure; *solid line* = aortic pressure. (Redrawn from Bolooki HK: *Clinical Applications of the Intra-aortic Balloon Pump.* Mt Kisco, NY, Futura Publishing, 1984.)

Table 4-1. Functions of the Intra-Aortic Balloon Pump
Increases:
Aortic diastolic pressure
Coronary blood flow
Cardiac output
Renal perfusion
Decreases:
Aortic systolic pressure
LV systolic pressure
LV end-diastolic pressure
Cardiac afterload
LV wall tension
LV volume and stroke work
LV = left ventricular

    D. GI bleeding, thrombocytopenia, and bleeding diatheses are relative contraindications because of the need for anticoagulation.

VI. IABP Procedure

    A. Assessment. The arterial pulses, temperature, and color of the extremities are assessed and documented before and after IABP insertion and followed while the IABP is in place.

B. Anticoagulation. Anticoagulation therapy with IV heparin is initiated if the IABP is placed preoperatively. Some centers do not anticoagulate patients who have the IABP placed during the immediate postoperative period.

C. Insertion. The catheter is usually inserted **via the femoral artery**.

1. The **catheter length** is premeasured from the insertion site in the groin to just below the sternal notch.

2. The catheter is placed using the **Seldinger technique**. The tip of the balloon should be positioned just distal to the subclavian artery.

3. The catheter is attached to a monitoring console that provides an ECG reading or pressure tracing.

4. The guidewire is removed, and the central pressure is measured from the lumen.

5. The gas exchange lumen is purged.

6. The circulatory status of the limb should be monitored closely.

D. Timing. Inflation and deflation of the balloon must be carefully timed with an ECG or arterial pressure tracing (**Figure 4-4**).

1. **Inflation** takes place about 40 msec before the arterial dicrotic notch (more accurate) or with the ascending T wave on the ECG.

2. **Deflation** takes place during isovolumic contraction.
   a. On the ECG, deflation of the balloon takes place after the P wave and before the beginning of the QRS complex.
   b. Total deflation must occur before ejection of the R wave.

3. The **timing** of inflation and deflation **provides diastolic augmentation** (optimal afterload reduction and decreased aortic systolic and end-diastolic pressures).

4. **Fine tuning** of inflation is done by observing the arterial tracing. Deflation of the IABP rarely needs adjustment based on the arterial tracing.

E. Weaning should be gradual.

1. Pumping should be reduced from 1:1 (i.e., one IABP inflation for every heartbeat) to 1:2 to 1:4.

2. Inotropic agents are usually weaned before the balloon catheter is removed and before the balloon inflation ratio is lowered to 1:2.

3. The IABP is removed if cardiac function is satisfactory at 1:4. The pump should only be at 1:3 or 1:4 for a few hours. (There is increased risk of clot formation.)

F. Removal

1. **Heparin therapy is stopped** 6 hours in advance.

2. **Platelet and coagulation factors are corrected** as necessary.

3. **The balloon is fully deflated** to decrease the catheter size and minimize trauma when the catheter is removed.

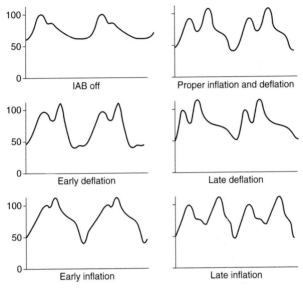

Figure 4-4. Slide switches on the IAB console permit proper timing of inflation and deflation during the cardiac cycle. (Redrawn from Cutler BS: The intraaortic balloon and counterpulsation. In *Irwin and Rippe's Intensive Care Medicine,* 4th ed. Edited by Irwin RS, Cerra FB, Rippe JM. Philadelphia, Lippincott Williams & Wilkins, 1999, p 118, Fig 9-6.)

  4. Pressure should be applied for 45 minutes after the catheter is removed.
  5. Distal pulses should be palpated or examined by ultrasound to prevent arterial thrombosis from occlusive pressure.

VII. Complications of IABP
 A. Limb ischemia from thrombosis, emboli, or vascular dissection
 B. Intra-abdominal or intrathoracic hemorrhage from vascular perforation or dissection
 C. Groin hematomas
 D. Lymph drainage
 E. Femoral artery pseudoaneurysm
 F. Wound infection
 G. Systemic sepsis
 H. Renal failure
 I. Device malfunction
 J. Paraplegia
 K. Thrombocytopenia

POSTOPERATIVE MANAGEMENT OF THE CARDIAC SURGERY PATIENT

I. **Arrival in the ICU**. A brief systematic examination of the patient is mandatory.
   A. **Airway and breathing**
      1. Check that the **endotracheal tube** is connected properly and securely to the ventilator.
      2. Assess the patient's **oxygen saturation level**.
      3. Observe **chest movement** and auscultate for **breath sounds**.
      4. Ensure that the **thoracostomy tubes** are connected to suction.
      5. Note the **ventilator settings**.
      6. Order an **ABG** along with the other lab tests.
      7. Order a portable supine **chest x-ray**. Assess for pneumothorax and mediastinal shift; position of endotracheal and nasogastric tubes; position of intravascular catheters; size and contour of mediastina silhouette; and pleural and extrapleural fluid collection.
      8. Assess **temperature** and correct to normothermia as soon as possible.
   B. **Connections.** Systematically review the various connections to ensure that nothing is overlooked.
   C. **Hemodynamic monitoring**
      1. Monitor the patient's blood pressure, pulse rate, CO/CI, PCWP, and systemic vascular resistance (SVR) at the bedside. Check that the patient's blood pressure remains adequate once the arterial line is transduced and calibrated.
      2. Auscultate for heart sounds; palpate the femoral and brachial arteries to confirm a satisfactory blood pressure.
      3. If a **pacemaker** is used, examine the connections and settings and confirm capture on an ECG.
      4. Initiate pacing if **bradycardia** or **heart block** is present. Keep in mind that **atrial fibrillation** can occur during atrioventricular (AV) pacing and may account for a fall in CO and blood pressure despite an acceptable ventricular pacing rate.
      5. Check that all **medications** (infusions) are properly labeled, dosed, and infusing at the correct rate.
      6. Re-examine the **thoracostomy tubes** for bleeding.
      7. Check a **12-lead ECG**.
      8. Assess **lab tests:** complete blood count (CBC), electrolytes, blood urea nitrogen (BUN), creatinine, calcium, magnesium, albumin, glucose, prothrombin time (PT), partial thromboplastin time (PTT), and platelet count. Redraw blood for lab tests every 3 hours. Measure ABGs, HCT, and K^+ as needed.

II. **ICU Monitoring**
   A. **ECG display.** Continuous bedside monitoring is critical for

immediate determination of rhythm changes. Any abnormality should be analyzed more thoroughly from a 12-lead ECG.

B. Arterial lines

1. Transduce radial or femoral catheters to the monitor.
2. Pay careful attention to perfusion of the hand; remove the arterial line immediately if ischemia develops.
3. Correlate the arterial line with cuff BP. Determine which is most accurate. Check BP in both arms.

C. Left atrial (LA) lines. LA lines are placed through the right superior pulmonary vein and passed into the left atrium during surgery. These lines may allow a **more accurate assessment of left-sided filling pressures**. LA lines are particularly useful in patients with severe pulmonary hypertension. Pulmonary vasodilators can be infused into the central venous circulation, whereas peripheral vasoconstrictors are infused into the LA line to maintain systemic resistance.

1. **Always aspirate before flushing** the line to ensure that no air or thrombus is present within the system.
2. These **lines should be removed when the chest tubes are still in place,** because bleeding may occur at the insertion site when they are removed.

D. Swan-Ganz catheter. This catheter is placed during surgery. It is useful for monitoring PCWP, CO, and SVR and for obtaining SvO_2. (See hemodynamic monitoring and abnormalities in Chapter 5.)

E. Pacing wires. Most surgeons place temporary atrial and ventricular epicardial pacing wires at the end of the cardiac surgical procedure. Make sure that all connections to the pacing box are correct and secure.

1. The atrial pacing wires may be connected to one ECG limb to obtain an atrial rhythm. This may aid in assessing atrial arrhythmias.
2. See PACEMAKERS AND IMPLANTABLE DEFIBRILLATORS in Chapter 5.

F. Endotracheal tube (ET). The ET is used for mechanical ventilation during the early postoperative period.

1. **Confirm bilateral breath sounds**
2. Order a **chest x-ray** to confirm proper placement of the tube.
3. **Suction every few hours** as necessary to keep the tube patent and free of secretions.
4. **Weaning** may be accomplished overnight, and **extubation** is generally done on the morning after surgery.

G. Chest tubes. Chest tubes are placed in the mediastinum and pleural spaces if they are entered during surgery.

1. An accurate **measurement of output** is essential.
2. The tubes should be connected to 20-cm water suction.

H. Nasogastric tubes. These tubes are useful for gastric decompression while the patient is intubated.

    I. Foley catheter. This catheter is useful for accurate measurement of urine output after surgery. It is removed on the first or second postoperative morning after diuresis.

    J. Hemodynamic monitoring. See HEMODYNAMIC MONITORING AND ABNORMALITIES in Chapter 5.

III. Guidelines for Removal of Lines and Tubes

    A. The **arterial line** should be removed after a stable post extubation ABG has been obtained. It should not remain in place for blood sampling.

    B. The **LA line** is removed in the ICU while the thoracostomy tubes are in place.

    C. The **Swan-Ganz catheter** is removed when inotropic support and vasodilators are no longer necessary and the patient is normovolemic.

    D. Chest tubes are removed when total drainage is less than 100 ml for an 8-hour period.

        1. Mediastinal tubes should be removed off suction to avoid damage to the grafts.

        2. A chest x-ray is not indicated after mediastinal chest tube removal but should be performed after pleural tubes are removed.

    E. The **Foley catheter** is left in place while the patient undergoes diuresis. It should be removed once the patient is out of bed and walking (usually on the second postoperative day).

    F. The **pacing wires** should be removed on the day before the patient is discharged from the hospital.

        1. The wires and skin are prepared with Betadine.

        2. The wires may be cut at the skin if significant tension is experienced while pulling them, to avoid possible bleeding and injury to the myocardium.

        3. The patient should be placed on a cardiac monitor for 4 to 6 hours after removal of pacing wires.

VALVULAR HEART DISEASE AND ENDOCARDITIS

I. Aortic Regurgitation

    A. Etiology

        1. Infectious endocarditis (most common etiology)

        2. Aortic dissection

        3. Chest trauma

        4. Bicuspid aortic valve and rheumatic abnormalities, predisposing the patient to infection and subsequent valve destruction

        5. Marfan's syndrome and hypertension as risk factors for an acute aortic dissection

        6. Rheumatic fever

        7. Annuloaortic ectasia

        8. Connective tissue diseases (systemic lupus erythematosus [SLE], aortitis, ankylosing spondylitis)

B. **Presentation**
   1. Acute congestive heart failure
   2. Diastolic murmur at the left sternal border
   3. Softening of S_1
   4. Apical diastolic murmur (Austin Flint murmur) leading to confusion with mitral stenosis
   5. Bounding, collapsing "water-hammer" pulses

C. **Diagnosis**
   1. A **chest x-ray** shows pulmonary congestion.
   2. An **echocardiogram** defines the presence and severity of aortic regurgitation and can rule out an acute aortic dissection.
   3. **Computed tomography, magnetic resonance imaging,** and **aortography** can define an acute dissection.

D. **Hemodynamics**
   1. The **severity** of aortic regurgitation is **graded from 0 to 4+** according to the rapidity and completeness of opacification of the LV after injection of dye into the aorta.
   2. PCWP is elevated and left ventricular end-diastolic pressure (LVEDP) is higher than 25 to 30 mm Hg.
   3. The aortic and LV diastolic pressures may equalize.

E. **Medical management**
   1. **Nitroprusside** may be used for afterload reduction.
   2. **β-Blockers** are used in the case of aortic dissection to decrease heart rate.
   3. **Oxygen** is given.
   4. **Diuretics** are used as necessary to maintain euvolemia.
   5. There is **no role for the IABP,** because it may worsen the LV volume overload.

F. **Surgical treatment.** Urgent operation is indicated for:
   1. Refractory heart failure
   2. Sepsis or embolization from endocarditis
   3. Aortic dissection

II. Mitral Regurgitation

A. **Etiology**
   1. Disorder of mitral valve (MV) leaflets (e.g., infective endocarditis, ankylosing spondylitis, or as a result of trauma)
   2. Disorder of MV annulus (e.g., connective tissue disorder, severe calcification)
   3. Disorder of chordae tendineae (e.g., infective endocarditis, rheumatic valvulitis, Marfan's syndrome, congenital aortic valve disease, SLE; may also be spontaneous or a result of trauma or pregnancy)
   4. Disorder of papillary muscle
      a. Dysfunction (e.g., ischemia, MI, left ventricular aneurysm or dilatation, amyloidosis, sarcoidosis, trauma, contusion)
      b. Rupture (e.g., trauma, acute MI, syphilis, myocardial abscess)
   5. Prosthetic valve malfunction

      a. Deterioration of leaflets or silastic disc
      b. Dislodgment of ball or disc
      c. Ring fracture
      d. Paravalvular leak
      e. Suture or pledget dislodgment
      f. Prosthetic valve endocarditis

B. Presentation
1. Dyspnea and hypotension
2. Sinus tachycardia
3. Cordal rupture (most dramatic presentation)
4. Loud holosystolic murmur audible at the apex, with radiation to the axilla

C. Diagnosis
1. An **ECG** may demonstrate an inferior or posterior infarct if papillary muscle rupture is the etiology.
2. An **echocardiogram** assesses the degree of mitral regurgitation.
3. **Coronary angiography** is useful for defining the lesions responsible for a possible ischemic event causing the acute MR.

D. Hemodynamics
1. Sudden dramatic afterload reduction due to approximately 50% ejection of LV volume into LA results in decreased ventricular wall tension.
2. Elevation in left-sided filling pressures occurs with the appearance of the ventricular (V) wave in the PCWP tracing.
3. Volume overload enlarges all chambers.

E. Medical management
1. **Vasodilator therapy** (e.g., sodium nitroprusside) reduces afterload and allows greater stroke volume to progress antegrade into the aorta.
2. **Nitroglycerin** is used for ischemic states.
3. **IABP** may be of great benefit.

F. Surgical treatment. Surgery is indicated for patients with **hemodynamically significant MR**. Treatment may include **valve repair or replacement**.

III. Tricuspid Regurgitation

A. Etiology
1. Rheumatic heart disease
2. Infectious endocarditis (IV drug abusers)
3. Myxomatous degeneration
4. Ebstein's anomaly
5. Carcinoid
6. Right ventricular infarction
7. Left-sided heart failure
8. Right-sided hypertension

B. Presentation
1. Dyspnea
2. Hepatic enlargement (from right-sided heart failure)
3. Peripheral edema

    4. Tachycardia

    5. Fever (with infectious endocarditis)

    6. Orthopnea

    7. Elevated pulsatile neck veins

    8. Holosystolic murmur at the lower left sternal border (increases with inspiration)

C. Diagnosis. An **echocardiogram** shows right ventricular enlargement and can provide accurate estimates of the severity of the tricuspid regurgitation. It may also reveal vegetations in endocarditis.

D. Hemodynamics

    1. Increased right atrial pressure

    2. Prominent V waves on the right atrial tracing

E. Medical management

    1. **Diuretics** correct volume excess.

    2. **Afterload-reducing agents** may be useful if tricuspid regurgitation has resulted from left-sided heart failure.

    3. **Nitroglycerin** is helpful if tricuspid regurgitation has resulted from an MI.

F. Surgical treatment. Surgery is indicated for:

    1. Refractory tricuspid regurgitation

    2. Valvular source of septic emboli

    3. Valve excision, repair, or replacement

IV. Aortic Stenosis

A. Etiology

    1. Bicuspid valve (in younger patients)

    2. Senile, degenerative, calcific stenosis (in older patients)

    3. Rheumatic heart disease

B. Presentation. There may be no symptoms until the late stage of disease.

    1. Angina

    2. Syncope

    3. Dyspnea

    4. Left ventricular failure

    5. Harsh, crescendo-decrescendo murmur heard best at the right upper sternal border, with radiation to the neck

    6. Aortic stenosis is often associated with a single second heart sound.

C. Diagnosis

    1. An **ECG** indicates left ventricular hypertrophy with strain.

    2. An **echocardiogram** defines the presence and severity of aortic stenosis.

D. Hemodynamics

    1. **LV pressures** are elevated.

    2. **CO** is depressed.

    3. The **valve area** is proportional to CO ÷ the square root of the valvular gradient.

        a. An **absolute valve area of less than 0.7 cm^2** is diagnostic of critical aortic stenosis, and **surgery is required** at this point.

      b. **Valve areas between 0.7 and 1 cm²** represent significant but subcritical aortic stenosis; **surgery may be necessary**.

E. Medical management

1. **Patients** with aortic stenosis **are preload or volume sensitive**. Low filling pressures are inadequate to distend the hypertrophied LV; however, high filling pressures may lead to pulmonary congestion.
2. **Pulmonary artery catheters are essential** to determine optimal fluid requirements.
3. In the case of a **mechanical obstruction to flow,** there is almost no role for drug therapy and **surgical treatment is required**.

F. Surgical treatment

1. **Critical aortic stenosis** (absolute valve area of < 0.7 cm²) requires surgical treatment.
2. Patients with **embolic phenomena** also require surgery.
3. **Percutaneous aortic valvuloplasty** may be useful for elderly patients who are not suitable surgical candidates.

V. Mitral Stenosis

A. Etiology. Rheumatic heart disease is the etiology.

B. Presentation

1. Progressive dyspnea on exertion
2. Hemoptysis (pulmonary apoplexy)
3. Loud S_1 with an opening snap

C. Diagnosis

1. A **chest x-ray** shows left atrial enlargement ("double density") and pulmonary congestion.
2. An **echocardiogram** defines the presence and severity of mitral stenosis.

D. Hemodynamics

1. An elevated PCWP reflects left atrial pressure (LAP).
2. The gradient between the PCWP and left ventricular end-diastolic pressure (LVEDP) reflects the stenosis.
3. Severe mitral stenosis is present if the valve area is less than 1 cm².

E. Medical management

1. The heart rate can be controlled with **digitalis, β-blockers, or calcium channel blockers.** This allows adequate time for filling of the ventricle during diastole.
2. **Diuretics** can be used judiciously for pulmonary edema.

F. Surgical treatment

1. **Percutaneous mitral valvulotomy** may be effective for mild mitral stenosis.
2. **Valve replacement** is necessary in cases of significant mixed regurgitation and stenosis or severe stenosis.

VI. Endocarditis. Endocarditis is an inflammation of the endocardium usually characterized by vegetations and often caused by microorganisms, especially bacteria or fungi. Heart valves are usually involved, but the infection may be on a septal defect or on the mural endocardium. Endocarditis is **usually fatal if left untreated**.

A. **Classification.** Endocarditis can be subdivided into three types: native valve endocarditis, endocarditis in drug abusers, and prosthetic valve endocarditis.

1. **Native valve endocarditis**
   a. **Microorganisms**
      (1) **Streptococcal infection** accounts for **60% to 80% of cases** in patients who are not IV drug abusers. *S. viridans,* a normal inhabitant of the oropharynx, is the most frequent infecting species. *S. pneumoniae* is another causative species.
      (2) *Staphylococcus aureus* accounts for 25% of cases.
      (3) Other causative bacteria include *Neisseria gonorrhoeae, Pseudomonas,* and *Salmonella.*
      (4) **Fungi rarely** cause native valve endocarditis.
   b. **Epidemiology**
      (1) The infection occurs **more frequently in men** than in women, and most patients are **older than 50 years** of age.
      (2) An identifiable **predisposing cardiac lesion** is present in **60% to 80%** of patients.
      (3) **Rheumatic heart disease** accounts for **30%** of cases.
      (4) The **mitral valve** is **most commonly involved,** followed by the aortic valve.
      (5) **Risk factors** include rheumatic heart disease, degenerative heart disease, calcific aortic stenosis, asymmetric septal hypertrophy, Marfan's syndrome, syphilitic aortic valve, and mitral valve prolapse.
      (6) **No underlying heart disease** can be recognized **in 20% to 40%** of patients.

2. **Endocarditis in drug abusers**
   a. **Infecting organisms**
      (1) *Staphylococcus aureus* is present in **more than 50%** of cases.
      (2) *Streptococcus* occurs in **more than 15%** of cases.
      (3) **Fungi** and **gram-negative bacteria** occur in **15%** of cases.
   b. **Epidemiology**
      (1) Mainly young male drug abusers are affected.
      (2) Only about 20% of addicts with their first episode of endocarditis have previously damaged heart valves.
      (3) The tricuspid valve is infected in more than 50% of cases; the aortic valve in 25% of cases; and the mitral valve in 20% of cases.

3. **Prosthetic valve endocarditis**
   a. **Infecting organisms**
      (1) *Staphylococcus epidermidis* and *Staphylococcus aureus* infections account for **more than 50%** of cases, with *S. epidermidis* occurring more frequently.

       (2) Gram-negative bacilli are present in **15%** of cases.

       (3) *Candida* infection occurs in **10%** of cases.

    b. Epidemiology. Any intravascular prosthesis predisposes to endocarditis. Prosthetic valve endocarditis accounts for 10% to 20% of all cases of endocarditis.

B. Pathogenesis

1. Disease arises secondary to the localization of microorganisms on sterile vegetations composed of platelets and fibrin. In 30% of cases there is a virulent organism but no prior sterile vegetation.

2. When **bacteremia** occurs, infection of a sterile vegetation is most likely.

3. Rapid destruction with consequent **valvular regurgitation** may occur.

4. **Vegetations may break off and embolize** to the heart, brain, and other organs.

C. Presentation

1. **Symptoms begin within 2 weeks** of the precipitating event.

2. The **onset is gradual** (with fever and malaise) **or acute** (with high fever).

3. A **cardiac murmur is almost always present,** except in patients with early endocarditis or in IV drug abusers with tricuspid valvular infection.

4. **Splenomegaly and petechiae** of the conjunctivae, palate, or buccal mucosa occur in 30% of cases.

5. **Embolic phenomena** may occur.

    a. Splinter hemorrhages (subungual) may occur.

    b. Roth spots (retinal hemorrhages) occur in less than 5% of cases.

    c. Osler nodes (tender nodules on finger or toe pads) occur in 10% to 25% of cases.

    d. Janeway lesions (hemorrhages on the palms and soles) may occur.

6. **Clubbing of the fingers** may be present.

7. **Mycotic aneurysms** occur in approximately 10% of patients.

D. Laboratory features

1. **WBC count** is often normal.

2. The **erythrocyte sedimentation rate** is elevated.

3. The **rheumatoid factor** is positive in 50% of cases in which disease is present for more than 6 weeks.

4. **Blood cultures** should be obtained; results are positive in more than 95% of cases.

E. Diagnosis

1. Disease is suspected when a murmur and unexplained fever occur, but a **definitive clinical diagnosis requires positive blood cultures.**

2. An **echocardiogram** will demonstrate the vegetation in up to 80% of patients with native valve endocarditis.

Table 4-2. Prophylaxis for Bacterial Endocarditis

Type of Procedure	Patient Status	Drug and Dosage
Oral, dental, respiratory, or esophageal	Standard (i.e., normal diet, no allergies)	Amoxicillin, 2 g PO given 1 hour before procedure
	NPO	Ampicillin, 2 g IM/IV given 30 minutes before procedure
	Penicillin allergy	Clindamycin, 600 mg PO; azithromycin, 500 mg PO; or clarithromycin, 500 mg PO given 1 hour before procedure
	NPO and penicillin allergy	Clindamycin, 600 mg IV given 30 minutes before procedure
GU or GI	Moderate-risk patient	Amoxicillin, 2 g PO; or ampicillin, 2 g IV given 30 minutes before procedure
	Moderate-risk patient and penicillin allergy	Vancomycin, 1 g IV over 1–2 hours; complete within 30 minutes of procedure
	High-risk patient	Ampicillin, 2 g IV and gentamicin, 1.5 mg/kg (max 120 mg) given within 30 minutes of procedure; 6 hours later give ampicillin, 1 g IV
	High-risk patient and penicillin allergy	Vancomycin, 1 g over 1–2 hours and gentamicin, 1.5 mg/kg (max of 120 mg) complete within 30 minutes of procedure

   3. Serial phonocardiography and cineradiography are use-
      ful when evaluating prosthetic valves.
F. Medical management. A cure for endocarditis requires the
   eradication of all bacteria from the vegetation. **Penicillins,
   cephalosporins,** and **vancomycin** are commonly used, depending on the culture and sensitivity results. Antibiotics are
   continued for several weeks (specific regimens exist for each
   antibiotic). Minimum inhibitory and bactericidal concentrations (MICs) should be determined.
G. Surgical treatment. Indications for valve replacement are:
   1. Appropriate microbicidal therapy not available (e.g., fun-
      gal endocarditis)
   2. Persistence or relapse of positive blood cultures despite
      therapy
   3. Heart failure secondary to severe valvular regurgitation
   4. Severe valve dysfunction
   5. Presence of a valve abscess
   6. Patient with aortic valve endocarditis who develops a first-
      or second-degree AV block
   7. Presence of a large vegetation (controversial)

Cardiovascular

Management

ADVANCED CARDIAC LIFE SUPPORT PROTOCOLS

See pages 122–129 (Figures 5-8 through 5-15).

ARRHYTHMIAS

I. **Clinical Assessment**
   A. **History**
      1. Is there a history of **organic heart disease,** either familial (e.g., hypertrophic cardiomyopathy) or congenital (e.g., Wolff-Parkinson-White syndrome)?
      2. Is there a history of **noncardiac diseases** that may have led to arrhythmia?
         a. Inflammatory diseases
         b. Infectious diseases (e.g., Lyme disease, Chagas' disease)
         c. Endocrinologic conditions (e.g., hyperthyroidism)
         d. Infiltrative diseases (e.g., sarcoid, primary or secondary amyloid)
      3. What is the **specific history?**
         a. **Symptoms.** Ask the patient whether he or she is experiencing palpitations, syncope, fatigue, anxiety, or feelings of impending doom.
         b. **Onset.** Ask the patient what brings on the symptoms.
         c. **Frequency.** Ask the patient how often the symptoms occur.
         d. **Duration.** Ask the patient how long the symptoms last.
         e. **Chronicity.** Ask the patient how long he or she has

had the problem (e.g., years, months, days, or no previous occurrences).

   f. Resolution. Ask the patient what makes the symptoms go away.

4. Is the patient taking any of the following **medications**?
   a. Digitalis
   b. β-adrenergic blockers
   c. Calcium channel blockers
   d. Antiarrhythmic agents

B. **Physical examination** should include the following:
   1. **Pulse.** Check the rate, intensity, and regularity.
   2. **Jugular venous pulsations.** Check for elevation, cannon a-waves of junctional ectopic beats, and atrioventricular (AV) dissociation.
   3. **Blood pressure (BP).** Check for orthostatic hypotension.
   4. **Heart**
      a. Find the location of the point of maximal impulse (PMI). Check for left ventricular (LV) hypertrophy.
      b. Determine whether an S_3 is present; this would be consistent with congestive heart failure (CHF).
      c. Determine whether an S_4 is present; this would be consistent with uncontrolled hypertension.
      d. Listen for systolic murmurs indicating aortic stenosis (AS) or mitral regurgitation (MR).
      e. Check for a parasternal or right ventricular (RV) heave that will indicate RV hypertrophy.
   5. **Lungs.** Listen for evidence of CHF or bronchospasm.

C. **Diagnostic tests**
   1. **Electrocardiograms.** Twelve-lead electrocardiograms (ECGs) taken during arrhythmia and as a baseline reading are essential for the diagnosis. A continuous rhythm strip recording is essential during any interventions.
   2. **Laboratory tests.** The following laboratory data are obtained:
      a. Serum electrolytes, including potassium, calcium, and magnesium
      b. Recent antiarrhythmic drug levels (if applicable)
      c. Thyroid function and thyroid-stimulating hormone (TSH) levels

D. **Management**
   1. **Cardioversion.** Synchronized direct current (DC) cardioversion is the **treatment of choice** for patients who are hemodynamically compromised from a re-entrant supraventricular tachycardia (SVT).
   2. **Pharmaceutical treatment. Adenosine** can be efective in both the diagnosis and treatment of SVTs.
      a. Mechanism of action. Adenosine produces profound conduction slowing in the sinus and AV nodal tissue; the effects resolve in seconds. Re-entrant circuit SVTs which involve nodal tissue will return to sinus rhythm in seconds after administration of adenosine.

    b. Dosage
- **(1)** Administer an initial dose of 6 mg by rapid IV push. If this is ineffective, use a dose of 12 mg.
- **(2)** If using central access or if the patient is on dipyridamole, the starting dose should be reduced to 3 mg.
- **(3)** In the presence of competitive inhibitors (e.g., caffeine, theophylline), increase the dose of adenosine.

    c. Relative contraindications include preexisting second or third AV block, sick sinus syndrome, and asthma.

II. Bradyarrhythmias

A. Sinus bradycardia
1. **Characteristics.** There is a P wave for every QRS.
2. **Etiology.** Causes of sinus bradyarrhythmias include:
   a. High vagal tone (in athletes)
   b. Infiltrative or inflammatory disease of the sinoatrial (SA) node
   c. SA nodal artery disease
   d. Hypothyroidism
   e. Drugs, such as β-blockers, narcotics, and phenothiazines

B. AV block
1. **First-degree AV block**
   a. **Characteristics.** There is a delay within the AV node that is prolonged so that the PR interval is > 200 ms.
   b. **Etiology.** This block may be caused by:
      (1) Antiarrhythmic drug effect
      (2) Myocardial ischemia
      (3) Increased vagal tone
      (4) Degenerative conduction system disease
      (5) Hyperkalemia
      (6) Cardiac tumor or infection (e.g., Lyme disease, Chagas disease)
2. **Second-degree AV block**
   a. **Mobitz type I (Wenckebach).** This block involves progressive prolongation of the PR interval. The disease is usually limited to the AV node. Group beating occurs (e.g., 2:1, 3:2, 4:3, 5:4).
   b. **Mobitz type II.** A dropped beat occurs without increased conduction time. The disease usually occurs below the AV node in the His-Purkinje system. This type of AV block is associated with a worse prognosis.
3. **Third-degree (complete) AV block.** In this type of AV block:
   a. No association exists between regular atrial and ventricular rates.
   b. The atrial rate is usually faster than the ventricular rate.
   c. The ventricular rate is faster than the atrial rate in benign competitive AV dissociation.

     d. Narrow complex beats reveal an escape focus in the His-Purkinje system.

     e. Wide complex beats suggest ventricular escape, which is unstable.

  C. Management

    1. If the patient is asymptomatic: There is no specific therapy, except in the case of a complete heart block.

    2. If the patient is symptomatic with syncope, lightheadedness, angina, or shortness of breath:

      a. Discontinue any antiarrhythmic agents or nodal-blocking agents.

      b. Give atropine, 0.5 mg IV; you may repeat this dose up to a total of 2 mg.

      c. If the patient does not respond to atropine, order a dopamine drip at a rate of 5–20 µg/kg/min.

      d. If the patient remains symptomatic, add an isoproterenol drip at a rate of 2–10 µg/kg/min.

      e. Pacemakers. An external transcutaneous pacemaker, a transvenous pacemaker, or a permanent pacemaker may be required (see pacemakers and implantable defibrillators).

III. Premature Complexes

  A. Premature atrial complex involves a shortened P-P interval with a compensatory pause.

  B. Premature junctional complex involves a premature narrow complex QRS interval.

  C. Premature ventricular complex involves wide complex beats that originate from the ventricle.

  D. Management

    1. Correct the underlying causes:

      a. Hypoxia

      b. Myocardial ischemia

      c. Electrolyte abnormalities

      d. Drug toxicity

      e. Catecholamine excess

      f. Excessive use of tobacco, caffeine, or alcohol

    2. No specific therapy is indicated except in the following instances:

      a. The patient is symptomatic. Premature ventricular complexes (PVCs) in couplets, triplets, and larger runs may be suppressed. Start **lidocaine** in a 1 mg/kg bolus, then start a lidocaine drip at a rate of 1–4 mg/min. Check the patient for signs of toxicity.

      b. The patient has coronary artery disease (CAD), in which case **β-blockers** should be given.

IV. Tachycardia

  A. Narrow complex tachycardia

    1. Sinus tachycardia. Therapy involves correcting the **underlying causes:**

      a. Increased sympathetic or decreased vagal tone

      b. Increased catecholamines

- c. Fever
- d. Myocardial ischemia or myocardial infarction (MI)
- e. Pulmonary embolism (PE)
- f. Hypovolemia
- g. Hypoxemia
- h. Pain
- I. Hyperthyroidism
- j. Drug withdrawal

2. **Atrial tachycardia**
   a. **Characteristics.** Atrial tachycardia is characterized by a heart rate of 130–200 beats/min with possible rate-related bundle branch block (BBB).
   b. **Subtypes**
      (1) **Paroxysmal atrial tachycardia (PAT).** There is a sudden increase in the patient's heart rate, with rates from 150–200 beats/min.
      (2) **Multifocal atrial tachycardia (MAT).** At least three different P wave morphologies must be present, along with irregular P–P intervals and an isoelectric baseline between phases. MATs are seen most commonly in patients with **chronic obstructive pulmonary disease (COPD).**
   c. **Etiology.** Underlying causes of atrial tachycardia include:
      (1) CAD with or without MI
      (2) Chronic lung disease
      (3) Alcohol intoxication
      (4) Digitalis intoxication
   d. **Management.** Therapy involves **correcting the underlying causes.** MAT is thought to occur as a result of depolarization, and may be further mediated by the patient's high adrenergic state.
      (1) Use **metoprolol** to control rate. (If there is a need to be able to quickly reverse these β-blocker effects, use esmolol.)
      (2) If metoprolol fails, use **calcium channel blockers** (e.g., verapamil, diltiazem) to slow atrial rate. Use **esmolol** to quickly terminate effects.
      (3) In MAT, if metoprolol fails, consider using **high dose magnesium.** The use of magnesium is limited in renal failure.
      (4) A disabling PAT that is poorly controlled by antiarrhythmic agents can be treated with **radiofrequency ablation.**

3. **AV nodal re-entrant tachycardia (AVNRT)**
   a. **Characteristics.** The heart rate is 150–250 beats/min.
   b. **Mechanism.** The AV node in these patients is functionally separated into two pathways: a slowly conducting path with a short refractory period and a rapidly conducting path with a long refractory period. A critically timed premature atrial contraction

(PAC) may block the fast path, travel down the slow path, and then proceed retrograde up the fast path, initiating a re-entrant SVT. In the atypical form, the impulse propagation is reversed.

  c. **Subtypes**

    (1) **Typical AVNRT** consists of a premature atrial beat followed by a prolonged PR interval, indicating conduction over the slow pathway. This is followed by initiation of a regular, usually narrow complex tachycardia. The retrograde P wave is obscured by the QRS complex.

    (2) **Atypical AVNRT** involves an inverted P wave within the T wave.

  d. **Etiology.** AVNRT is associated with physiologic stress, increased catecholamines, pain, fever, myocardial ischemia, and MI (involving the artery to the SA or AV node).

  e. **Symptoms** include palpitations, light-headedness, near-syncope or syncope, anxiety, and angina.

  f. **Management**

    (1) Attempt **vagal maneuvers.** Apply carotid massage or Valsalva maneuver.

    (2) If vagal maneuvers fail or if AVNRT recurs, give **adenosine,** 6–12 mg IV push (3–6 mg if via central line). This may convert the rhythm to sinus or enable better identification of the rhythm.

    (3) If the tachycardia continues, follow with **verapamil,** 5 mg IV every 5 minutes up to 3 doses.

    (4) If necessary, follow up with **diltiazem** in a bolus of 15–25 mg IV over 2 minutes up to 2 doses, or begin a continuous infusion.

    (5) **Electrophysiologic studies (EPS)** and **radiofrequency ablation** should be done if the medications do not have the desired effect in patients with a prolonged need for medication.

4. **AV junctional tachycardia**

  a. **Characteristics**

    (1) An atrial rate of 60–130 beats/min occurs with a normal or bundle branch-like QRS.

    (2) Competitive AV dissociation may occur with normal, nonconducted P waves at a rate lower than the ventricular rate.

  b. **Etiology.** AV junctional tachycardia occurs in MI, myocarditis, catechol excess, and digoxin toxicity.

  c. **Management. IV lidocaine or β-blockers** may be effective if the patient's condition is unstable.

5. **Orthodromic AV accessory pathway tachycardia**

  a. **Characteristics**

    (1) Rates of 150–250 beats/min are usually initiated by a premature atrial contraction (PAC) or a premature ventricular contraction (PVC).

      (2) Atrial contraction follows ventricular depolarization, and a retrograde P wave is seen at the end of the QRS complex.

      (3) Conduction is anterograde through the AV node and retrograde through the accessory pathway.

  b. Management. The patient is given **calcium, β-blockers,** or **antiarrhythmic agents. Radiofrequency ablation** is the treatment of choice and may obviate the need for chronic pharmacologic therapy.

6. Wolff-Parkinson-White (WPW) syndrome

  a. Characteristics

    (1) A pre-excited rhythm is present.

    (2) A short PR interval occurs with a δ wave (upsloping of the QRS).

    (3) Conduction may be through the AV node or via the accessory pathway.

  b. Management. Patients with WPW syndrome and atrial arrhythmias are managed as follows:

    (1) Patients with **regular narrow-complex tachycardia** associated with WPW syndrome may be acutely treated by lengthening AV node or accessory pathway retractions. Adenosine is the drug of choice, followed by verapamil and β-blockers.

    (2) Patients with **irregular wide-complex tachycardia (atrial fibrillation)** with conduction down the accessory pathway should not be treated by blocking the AV node because this may result in the atrial fibrillation degenerating into ventricular fibrillation. **Procainamide or quinidine** is given to slow conduction through the aberrant pathway.

    (3) Long-term **prophylactic treatment** should not be with AV blocking agents alone because they may precipitate rapid atrial conduction through the accessory pathway and, therefore, ventricular fibrillation. All adults with WPW and symptomatic SVT should have EPS studies and should be considered for ablation. There is no indication for prophylactic antiarrhythmic agents or for EPS studies in the asymptomatic patient.

7. Atrial fibrillation

  a. Characteristics. Atrial fibrillation involves **disorganized atrial activity:** an irregularly irregular rhythm without discernible P waves. Rates vary depending on the patient's current medications, but the rates are usually higher than 100 beats/min.

  b. Risk factors include hypertensive heart disease, coronary artery disease, valvular heart disease, cardiomyopathies, alcohol intoxication, theophylline toxicity, hyperthyroidism, pericarditis, acute MI, and pulmonary embolism.

  c. Symptoms include palpitations, irregular pulse, and

angina in patients with CAD, or CHF in patients with dilated and hypertrophic cardiomyopathies and aortic stenosis.

d. **Management.** Patients who are hemodynamically unstable should be cardioverted immediately with direct current.

(1) **Rate control** is the initial therapeutic goal.

(a) Correct the patient's electrolytes.

(b) **Calcium channel blockers** and **β-blockers** act quickly to control heart rate, but their use may be limited by hypotension. **Diltiazem** is often used as first-line therapy. Patients who have inadequate rate control with diltiazem and who have **preserved left function** respond to **verapamil**. β-blockers are useful in blocking catecholamines and slowing ventricular rate.

(c) **Digoxin** should be used in patients with moderate to severe LV dysfunction or borderline BP, or as an adjunct to other therapy.

(d) **Antiarrhythmic therapy** and **elective DC cardioversion** can restore the sinus rhythm. Electrical cardioversion may proceed immediately if transesophageal echocardiography excludes intracardiac thrombi, and if the patient has had anticoagulation therapy. Patients require anticoagulation for 3 weeks before and after cardioversion.

Antiarrhythmic therapy with quinidine and procainamide to convert a patient or to sustain sinus rhythm after cardioversion is associated with a 2½-fold increase in mortality.

---

(2) **Patients with new-onset atrial fibrillation** should be given 72 hours to correct to sinus rhythm, after which they should be started on aspirin or heparin therapy, and possibly cardioverted electrically.

(3) **Long-term anticoagulation** with warfarin (if not contraindicated) is recommended in **chronic and paroxysmal atrial fibrillation** to decrease the risk of embolic stroke in patients older than 60 years of age and in younger patients who have clinical evidence of primary cardiac disorder. The risk of stroke in non-anticoagulated patients is 4.5% per year and increases with age and other risk factors (e.g., hypertension, diabetes, LV dysfunction, enlarged left atria).

8. Atrial flutter

    a. Characteristics. Atrial flutter is a macro–re-entrant atrial circuit. Regular rhythm occurs with an atrial rate between 250 and 350 beats/min and a fixed AV block (2:1, 3:1), or a variable rate if conduction disease exists.

    b. Diagnosis

        (1) Jugular venous pulse shows **cannon A waves.**

        (2) ECG shows regular **sawtooth flutter waves.** Vagal maneuvers and adenosine can be used to increase the degree of AV block, which unmasks the flutter waves.

    c. Management is similar to that for atrial fibrillation, except that digoxin is less effective in controlling the ventricular rate. (See *7–Atrial fibrillation* above.)

        (1) DC cardioversion is the treatment of choice for **persistent atrial flutter.** Atrial thrombus must first be ruled out by transesophageal echocardiography (TEE). The patient must be on heparin prior to the procedure; heparin is continued for only 3 weeks if the patient remains in sinus rhythm.

        (2) Atrial flutter may be treated with **radiofrequency ablation** of the pathway or of the AV node itself, or with placement of a ventricular-inhibited (VVI) pacer.

B. Wide complex tachycardia

    1. Supraventricular tachycardia (SVT) with aberrant conduction

        a. If conduction disease exists, any of the above narrow complex rhythms may present as a wide complex.

        b. The **distinction between SVT and VT** depends on the patient's history. If the patient has had a prior MI or prior VT, or if AV dissociation or left-axis deviation is present, then VT is more likely to be present. If you are in doubt, treat the rhythm as a ventricular arrhythmia.

    2. Accelerated idioventricular rhythm

        a. Characteristics. When a bizarre QRS occurs with a rate of 60–100 beats/min, rare atrial capture is signified by a narrow complex beat after a normal P wave. This rhythm is self-limited

        b. Etiology. Accelerated idioventricular rhythm is usually caused by an **acute MI** or **drug toxicity.** If it occurs in the setting of thrombolysis, this rhythm heralds **reperfusion.**

        c. Management. No specific therapy is suggested unless the patient is symptomatic.

    3. Ventricular tachycardia (VT)

        a. Characteristics. The rate is higher than 100 beats/min with wide QRS.

      (1) Sustained VT. This type occurs for more than 30 seconds or drops the BP.

      (2) Monomorphic VT. All QRS complexes are the same.

      (3) Polymorphic VT. QRS complexes vary in appearance.

  b. Etiology. VT is usually associated with **CAD or MI** but may be seen in any structural heart disease, whether congenital or acquired. VT occurs rarely in patients with no structural heart disease.

  c. Management depends on hemodynamic stability.

      (1) If the patient is unstable, synchronized DC cardioversion is given.

      (2) If the patient is stable, pharmacologic therapy with lidocaine, procainamide, bretylium, or amiodarone by continuous infusion is indicated.

4. Ventricular fibrillation (VF)

  a. Characteristics. This rhythm is rapid and irregular with no P wave or QRS complex.

  b. Management

      (1) The **primary therapy** is immediate unsynchronized cardioversion.

      (2) Adjunctive therapy, first with epinephrine and then with lidocaine, should be initiated if cardioversion fails, in accordance with advanced cardiac life support (ACLS) protocol.

      (3) After the patient is stabilized, correct myocardial ischemia, hypoxemia, acidosis, electrolyte abnormalities, and drug toxicities.

      (4) Electrophysiologic studies. Because there is high risk for a recurrence of VF outside the setting of an acute MI, EPS should be done to determine the need for **antiarrhythmic drug therapy** or an **automated implantable cardiac defibrillator (AICD).**

5. Torsades de pointes

  a. Characteristics. This rhythm involves polymorphic VT with an undulating pattern of the QRS axis that shifts from positive to negative and back again.

  b. Etiology. Torsades de pointes may be associated with congenital long QT syndrome or it may be secondary to antiarrhythmic drug therapy (class Ia or class III agents).

  c. Management

      (1) The drug of choice is **magnesium sulfate** in a 1- to 2-g IV bolus.

      (2) Unstable patients should be **DC cardioverted** immediately.

V. Drug Therapy Tables. See **Tables 5-1 through 5-3.**

Table 5-1. Examples of Perioperative Arrhythmias with Likely Mechanism, Desired Antidysrhythmic Drug Action, and Useful Drugs

Arrhythmia	Probable Mechanism	Drug Action	Useful Drugs
Sinus tachycardia	Enhanced normal automaticity	Slow phase 4 depolarization	Esmolol, adenosine, edrophonium
Accelerated AV junctional rhythm (AVJR > 70 bpm)	Abnormal automaticity (with myocardial ischemia, hypoxia)	Treat ischemia, correct hypoxia; slow phase 4 depolarization	Nitroglycerine, esmolol, CCB*
Type I atrial flutter (Atrial rate < 300 bpm)	Macroreentry (atrium)	↑ atrial conduction and refractoriness	Procainamide, amiodarone
Atrial fibrillation	Microreentry (atrium)	↑ atrial and/or AV node conduction and refractoriness	Procainamide; amiodarone; esmolol; CCB†; digoxin†; AChE
Atrial tachycardia with digitalis toxicity	Triggered activity (DAD)	↓ Ca overload; oppose digitalis toxicity	CCB, phenytoin; digitalis antibodies
Torsades de pointes (polymorphic VT with long QT interval)	Triggered automaticity (EAD)	Abolish EAD; shorten potential duration	Mg; esmolol; CCB; positive chronotrope to ↑ heart rate‡
Monomorphic ventricular tachycardia	Macroreentry (ventricles)	Reduce or increase ventricular conduction time and refractoriness	Lidocaine, procainamide, bretylium, amiodarone

CCB = Ca^{+2} or calcium channel blocker (diltiazem, verapamil); AChE = anticholinesterase inhibitor (edrophonium); DAD/EAD = delayed/early after depolarizations; VT = ventricular tachycardia.
*By reversing comary spasm and/or opposing Ca current contributing to pacemaker potential.
†Not if patient is known to have ventricular preexcitation.
‡Temporary pacing is safer and more reliable.
(From Atlee JL: Perioperative cardiac dysrhythmias. *Anesthesiology* 86(6):1401, 1997.)

Table 5-2. Suggested Doses, Indications, and Precautions for Miscellaneous Drugs That Can Be Administered IV for Diagnosis or Management or Perioperative Arrhythmias

Drug	Dose (IV adult)	Indications	Precautions
Adenosine	6 mg (×2; then 12 mg (×2) if necessary	PSVT (including with WPW); diagnosis of wide or narrow QRS tachycardias	Give via large peripheral or central vein; transient flushing, bronchospasm, chest pain; dipyridamole potentiates, methylxanthines antagonize action
Atropine, glycopyrrolate	0.4–2.0 mg (0.2–1.0 mg)	Bradycardia or AV heart block (high vagal tone)	Excessive tachycardia; myocardial ischemia in patients with CAD
Digoxin	0.5–1.0 mg in divided doses over 12–24 hr	PSVT; ventricular rate reduction with atrial flutter-fibrillation	Halve dose in patients receiving quinidine; prodysrhythmia, especially with acute physiologic imbalance or toxicity
Edrophonium	5–10 mg (25–30 mg over 30 min); 0.25 mg/min infusion	PSVT (including with WPW); diagnosis of wide or narrow QRS tachycardias	Bronchoconstriction; increased airway secretions
Magnesium sulfate	1.0–2.0 g (5–60 min); 0.5–1.0 g/hr infusion	Torsades de pointes with CLQTS; adjunct therapy or dysrhythmias with hypomagnesemia	Hypotension; bradycardia, sinus arrest; potentiate muscle relaxants; additive or synergistic effects with volatile anesthetics, BB, CCB
Potassium chloride	10–40 mEq/hr infusion	Adjunct treatment for dysrhythmias with hypokalemia	Rapid central infusion; pain with peripheral infusion

PSVT = paroxysmal supraventricular tachycardia; WPW = Wolff-Parkinson-White syndrome; AV = atrioventricular; CAD = coronary artery disease; GI = gastrointestinal; SND = sinus node dysfunction; CLQTS = congenital long QT interval syndrome; BB, CCB = β or calcium channel blockers.
(From Atlee JL: Perioperative cardiac dysthythmias. *Anesthesiology* 86(6):1406, 1997.)

Table 5-3. Specific Antiarrhythmic Drugs Suitable for Parenteral Use in Acute Arrhythmia Management, along with Vaughan Williams Class Action, Dosing, Indications, and Precautions

Drug (Class)	Dose (IV adult)	Indications	Precautions
Procainamide (IA)	10–15 mg/kg loading; 2–6 mg/min infusion	Ventricular tachydysrhythmias; paroxysmal atrial tachycardias with WPW	Hypotension; worsen SND or AV heart block
Lidocaine (IB)	1–4 mg/kg loading (over 30 min); 1–4 mg/min infusion	Ventricular tachydysrhythmias; prevent recurrences of ventricular fibrillation	CNS toxicity (seizures); cardiotoxicity (AV heart block, bradycardia, hypotension)
Phenytoin (IB)	100 mg q 5 min until dysrhythmia controlled or 1.0 g given; infusion not recommended	Atrial or ventricular tachydysrhythmias (digitalis); ventricular tachydysrhythmias with adrenergic stress, CLQTS	Inject slowly into large peripheral or central vein (pain, sclerosis, thrombosis at injection site)
Esmolol (II)	0.5–1.0 mg/kg^{-1}/min^{-1} × 4 pm over 5 min; 50–200 µg/kg^{-1}/min^{-1} infusion	Slow ventricular rate with atrial flutter-fibrillation or automatic atrial tachycardia; inappropriate sinus tachycardia; stress-mediated tachycardias	Worsen heart failure; aggravate bradycardia or AV heart block with SND or impaired conduction; prolong SCh block
Metoprolol (II)	5–15 mg over 20 min (effect lasts 5–7 hr)	Same as esmolol	Same as esmolol; bronchospasm in patients with COPD or asthma
Propranolol (II)	1.0 mg/min × 3 if needed (effect lasts 3–4 hr)	Same as esmolol	Same as esmolol; bronchospasm in patients with COPD or asthma

continued

Table 5-3. Specific Antiarrhythmic Drugs Suitable for Parenteral Use in Acute Arrhythmia Management, along with Vaughan Williams Class Action, Dosing, Indications, and Precautions

Drug (Class)	Dose (IV adult)	Indications	Precautions
Amiodarone (III)	15 mg/kg × 10 min; 1 mg/min × 6 hr; 0.5 mg/min infusion (1,000 mg/24 hr)	Refractory ventricular tachydysrhythmias, paroxysmal SVT, atrial tachydysrhythmias	Potentiate hypotension or bradycardia with other drugs; AV heart block; worsen heart failure
Bretylium (III)	5–10 mg/kg q 10–30 min (maximum dose 30 mg/kg)	Ventricular tachydysrhythmias; prevent recurrences of ventricular fibrillation	Aggravate dysrhythmias (initial catecholamine release); hypotension
Diltiazem (IV)	20 mg initial dose; 25 mg repeat dose after 15 min	PSVT; ventricular rate reduction with atrial flutter-fibrillation	Caution with atrial flutter-fibrillation and accessory AV pathways
Verapamil (IV)	5–10 mg initial dose; 10 mg repeat dose after 30 min	PSVT; ventricular rate reduction with atrial flutter-fibrillation	Caution with atrial flutter-fibrillation and accessory AV pathways

PSVT = paroxysmal supraventricular tachycardia; WPW = Wolff-Parkinson-White syndrome; AV = atrioventricular; SND = sinus node dysfunction; CLQTS = congenital long QT interval syndrome; SCh = succinylcholine; COPD = chronic obstructive pulmonary disease. (From Atlee JL: Perioperative cardiac dysrhythmias. *Anesthesiology* 86(6):1402, 1997.)

CHEST PAIN MANAGEMENT (Figure 5-1). See also
MYOCARDIAL ISCHEMIA AND INFARCTION, pp 101–106.

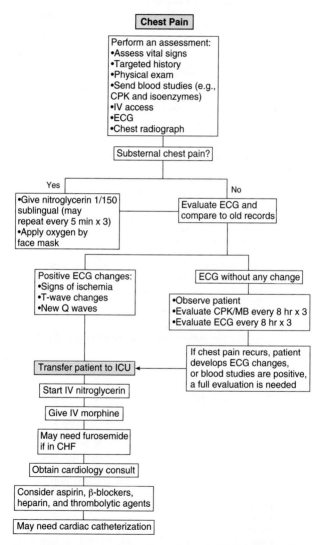

Figure 5-1. Algorithm for chest pain management. *CHF* = congestive heart failure; *CPK* = creatine phosphokinase; *ECG* = electrocardiogram.

I. Etiology

A. Pleuritic pain

1. **Cardiac causes**—pericarditis and Dressler's syndrome
2. **Pulmonary causes**—pneumothorax, PE, pneumonia, empyema, neoplasm, tuberculosis, bronchiectasis, and carcinomatous effusion
3. **GI causes**—liver abscess, pancreatitis, and Whipple's disease
4. **Subdiaphragmatic abscess**
5. **Body wall related disease**—costochondritis, chest wall trauma, rib fractures, myositis, soft tissue and bone tumors, herpes zoster, and muscle strain
6. **Collagen-vascular disease** with pleuritis
7. **Psychoneurosis**
8. **Familial Mediterranean fever (FMF)**

B. Nonpleuritic pain

1. **Cardiac causes**—myocardial ischemia, MI, myocarditis, mitral valve prolapse
2. **Esophageal causes**—spasm, rupture, esophagitis, ulceration, neoplasm, achalasia, diverticula, and the presence of a foreign body
3. **GI causes**—hiatal hernia, gastric neoplasm, peptic ulcer disease, cholecystitis, cholelithiasis, impacted gallstone, biliary neoplasm, and pancreatitis
4. **Dissecting or expanding aortic aneurysm**
5. **Dermatologic causes**—herpes zoster and mastitis
6. **Mediastinal tumors,** include lymphoma and thymomas
7. **Pulmonary causes**—infiltrates, PEs, and neoplasms
8. **Drugs** (e.g., cocaine)

II. Initial Evaluation

A. Take the patient's **vital signs.**

B. Evaluate with **continuous cardiac monitoring** and a **12-lead ECG.**

III. Specific History

A. Onset. When did the chest pain start? What was the patient doing at the time?

B. Provocative or palliative factors. What makes the pain get worse or better?

C. Quality. Is the pain sharp or dull? Is it a pressure or a pain? Is it a burning feeling, crushing feeling, or stabbing sensation?

D. Radiation. Does it radiate to the left or right arm, back, jaw, or abdomen?

E. Severity. How does the patient rate the level of pain on a scale of 1 to 10?

F. Timing. Is the pain constant or intermittent? How long does it last?

G. Associated symptoms. Is the patient experiencing diaphoresis, nausea, vomiting, headache, palpitations, dizziness, or lightheadedness?

H. Pleuritic or nonpleuritic. Is the pain pleuritic in nature?

IV. Past Medical History
  A. Cardiovascular disease
  1. Is there a previous ECG?
  2. Has the patient had a prior MI?
  3. Has there been a prior coronary artery bypass graft (CABG) or percutaneous transluminal coronary angioplasty (PTCA)?
  4. Has the patient had recent noninvasive testing such as a treadmill test or dipyridamole (Persantine) thallium scan?
  5. Are there cardiac risk factors such as age, sex, hypertension, diabetes mellitus, menopause, elevated cholesterol levels, smoking, family history, or obesity?
  B. Pulmonary disease. Does the patient have COPD, a history of deep vein thrombosis (DVT), or PE risk factors?
  C. Peripheral vascular disease. Is there a history of abdominal aortic aneurysm (AAA) or thoracic aortic aneurysm (TAA)?
  D. Cerebrovascular disease. Is there a history of carotid stenosis or a previous cerebrovascular accident (CVA)?
  E. Medications. Has the patient used aspirin, antihypertensive agents, or lipid-lowering agents?
V. Physical Examination
  A. Chest examination. Check for reproducible chest tenderness.
  B. Cardiac examination
  1. Check the **jugular venous pulse;** an elevation in jugular venous pulse indicates an approximately equivalent elevation in RA pressure.
  2. Check the **PMI;** lateral location indicates left ventricular hypertrophy (LVH).
  3. **Auscultate** for murmurs, rubs, or gallops.
  C. Lung examination. Listen for wheezes, crackles, consolidation, or a pleural rub.
  D. Extremity examination
  1. Look for evidence of peripheral vascular disease.
  2. Check for edema in the patient's lower extremities.
  E. Neurologic examination
VI. Diagnostic Work-up
  A. Obtain a **12-lead ECG.** Compare the results with a baseline reading for greatest accuracy.
  1. **ST segment elevation** is consistent with an acute MI or, if diffuse, with pericarditis.
  2. **ST segment depression** is consistent with subendocardial ischemia.
  3. **T wave inversion** is less specific but consistent with ischemia.
  B. Obtain a **chest radiograph.** Posteroanterior (PA) and lateral films are best. Portable x-ray machines can be used if necessary.
  1. **Infiltrate** is consistent with **pneumonia or a PE** if it is wedge shaped.
  2. **Effusions** are consistent with **CHF.**

      3. An enlarged heart is consistent with **LVH, pericardial effusion, or pericardial tamponade.**

   C. Check the patient's **arterial blood gases.**

   D. Order **routine blood work** including a complete blood count (CBC), platelets, electrolytes, BUN/creatinine, and serial CKs with MB fraction. If the results are nondiagnostic, Troponin I levels may be checked.

VII. Management

   A. Immediate therapy

      1. The patient should be given supplemental **oxygen.**

      2. An **aspirin** (325-mg tablet) should be chewed immediately unless it is strongly contraindicated.

      3. Sublingual nitroglycerin should be given; the patient's BP should be monitored closely.

      4. Topical nitrates can be given if the patient responds to sublingual therapy.

      5. If tolerated, IV or oral **β-blockers** are given (e.g., metoprolol 5 mg IV every 5 minutes up to 3 doses) to decrease myocardial oxygen demand.

   B. Further Management. The goal is to **ascertain the etiology** of the chest pain and rule out cardiac causes before proceeding with further workup.

      1. Noncardiac causes. If noncardiac causes are clearly identified and treated, a cardiac work-up may be deferred, unless incidental findings suggest a role for myocardial ischemia. If treatment of the noncardiac cause does not resolve the pain, a further work-up is necessary.

      2. Cardiac causes. A specific cardiac work-up should be pursued if anything suggests that CAD is the cause of the chest pain. Refer to MYOCARDIAL ISCHEMIA AND INFARCTION later in this chapter and to VALVULAR HEART DISEASE AND ENDOCARDITIS in Chapter 4.

CONGESTIVE HEART FAILURE

  I. Pathophysiology. CHF can be due to either systolic or diastolic dysfunction.

   A. Systolic dysfunction involves a decreased left ventricular ejection fraction (LVEF).

      1. Low cardiac output state occurs with a high wedge pressure and usually a low BP.

      2. The patient has a history of previous MIs or nonischemic cardiomyopathy.

   B. Diastolic dysfunction. LVEF is normal or elevated, usually with left ventricular hypertrophy and a noncompliant ventricle, as well as chronic and acute systemic hypertension.

  II. Initial Evaluation

   A. Assess the patient's **overall condition.** If no respiration or pulse is present, initiate ACLS.

   B. Assess the patient's **airway.** Check to see if adequate air exchange is present.

    C. Assess the patient's **breathing.** Assess the rate to see if it is rapid or slow, shallow or deep, easy or labored.

    D. Administer **supplemental oxygen** by either nasal cannula or face mask.

    E. Obtain the patient's **vital signs** and take a **pulse oximetry reading.**

    F. Initiate **cardiac monitoring** if possible.

    G. Obtain stat lab results, including those for **arterial blood gases, serum chemistries,** and a **CBC.**

    H. Obtain a **12-lead ECG** and a **portable chest x-ray** immediately.

III. History

    A. The **onset** can be rapid or insidious.

    B. Ask the patient about **prior episodes,** especially treatment of previous exacerbations.

    C. Assess the patient's **LV function** by prior echocardiography, multigated angiography (MUGA), or cardiac catheterization.

    D. Ask the patient about a history of **prior MI, cardiomyopathy, myocarditis, hypertension, valvular disease, endocarditis,** or **familial heart disease.**

    E. Inquire about **recent symptoms,** including chest pain, dyspnea on exertion, paroxysmal nocturnal dyspnea, orthopnea, palpitations, or viral illness.

    F. Ask the patient about **medications,** especially cardiac drugs, including diuretics.

    G. Inquire about a **history of noncardiac disease,** including thyroid disease, pulmonary hypertension, renal insufficiency or failure, Paget's disease, beriberi, or anemia.

    H. Ask the patient about **diet, medication patterns,** and **compliance** with doctor's instructions.

IV. Physical Examination

    A. **General.** Assess the patient's respiratory effort, level of consciousness, and pallor.

    B. **Neck.** Check the level of jugular venous pulsations and strength of carotid pulsations.

    C. **Lungs.** Assess air movement in and out of the chest and the presence of crackles or rales.

    D. **Heart.** Measure the heart rate, location of the PMI, intensity of the heart rate, murmurs, and gallops.

    E. **Abdomen.** Check for the presence of hepatojugular reflux.

    F. **Extremities.** Assess the degree of peripheral edema, distal warmth, and pulses.

V. Diagnostic Tests

    A. **Pulmonary artery (PA)/right-sided heart catheterization** yields valuable information about the etiology and allows guided and optimized diuretic therapy. It is less helpful in patients with mitral valve disease.

    B. **Echocardiography** allows a detailed structural view of the heart with information about valvular competency and LV and RV size and function.

C. **Radionuclide angiography** (equilibrium radionuclide angiography [ERNA] or MUGA) provides quantitative LV and RV ejection fractions (EFs) and information on diastolic compliance.

VI. Management

A. Initial stabilization is etiology independent.

1. **Nitrates** are used for immediate preload reduction. Employ **caution if aortic stenosis is present.**

   a. First give **sublingual nitroglycerin,** 0.3–0.6 mg SL every 5 minutes up to a total of 3 tablets.

   b. Then apply **nitropaste topically,** 1–2 inches to chest wall after the sublingual nitroglycerin has been given.

   c. If the topical therapy fails, give **IV nitroglycerin** at a rate of 5–300 μg/min. Titrate the IV nitroglycerin as tolerated by the patient's BP.

   d. If the patient is hypertensive and has a low EF, give **sodium nitroprusside.**

2. **Morphine** can be used to decrease the patient's anxiety and dyspnea.

3. **Diuretics** cause prompt venodilation with eventual decrease in preload.

   a. Treatment with **furosemide** IV should be started at 20 mg and increased, depending on prior exposure, dosing, and renal function.

   b. If there is no effect, the addition of **metolazone,** 2.5–10 mg 30 minutes before administration of furosemide, will augment diuresis.

   c. If the patient has **end-stage renal disease** (ESRD), consider prompt or emergent **hemodialysis.**

4. **Dobutamine.** In patients with systolic dysfunction, the addition of dobutamine increases cardiac output and augments diuresis.

Dobutamine should not be used during an acute MI.

---

5. **Vasodilators.** In refractory cases, phosphodiesterase inhibitors may be used.

B. Rule out myocardial ischemia with a 12-lead ECG and serial cardiac enzymes.

C. Long-term therapy. Long-term therapy of CHF is related to the pathophysiology and etiology.

1. **Systolic dysfunction** should be treated with diuretics, angiotensin-converting enzyme (ACE) inhibitors, and digoxin, and β-blockers should be cautiously added.

2. **Diastolic dysfunction** should be treated with calcium channel or β-blockers as well as diuretics to control both the heart rate and blood pressure, improve ventricular filling, and optimize performance.

3. **Underlying remediable etiologies,** such as ongoing myocardial ischemia and electrolyte disturbances, **must be corrected** to achieve success

HEMODYNAMIC MONITORING AND ALTERATIONS IN HEMODYNAMICS

I. **Goals of Hemodynamic Monitoring**
   A. To ensure **adequacy of perfusion** in stable patients
   B. To ensure **early detection and treatment of inadequate perfusion** in patients who become hemodynamically unstable
   C. To **titrate therapy to specific endpoints of resuscitation.** No one endpoint of resuscitation has been identified which can independently serve as a predictor of adequate tissue perfusion. Most physicians use a combination of the following endpoints to define adequate resuscitation:
      1. Heart rate
      2. Blood pressure
      3. Adequate urine output
      4. Central venous pressure
      5. Pulmonary capillary wedge pressure
      6. Oxygen delivery
      7. Oxygen consumption
      8. Lactate levels
      9. Mixed venous saturation

II. **Physiology of Cardiac Hemodynamics**
   A. **The Starling curve.** In 1914, E.H. Starling described the relationship between end-diastolic volume (EDV) and BP. Today's clinical correlate uses the relationship between stroke volume (SV) (rather than systolic pressure) and EDV. The slope of the ventricular function curve is determined by two factors: (1) contractile state of the myocardium and (2) afterload (**Figure 5-2**).
   B. **Frank-Starling mechanism.** The larger the diastolic volume of the heart, the more blood the ventricle will pump.
      1. An increase in end-diastolic pressure increases SV.
      2. Recall that

$$CO = HR \times SV = HR \times (EDV - ESV)$$

(CO = cardiac output, SV = stroke volume, EDV = end-diastolic volume, ESV = end-systolic volume)

   3. Beyond a certain point, further increases will not increase SV or cardiac output.

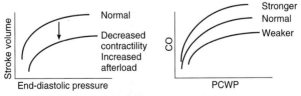

Figure 5-2. Frank Starling curves relating force of contraction to pressure (EDP or PCWP).

  4. A strong ventricle will have a higher cardiac output at lower filling pressures.
  5. A weak ventricle will have a lower cardiac output at higher filling pressures.

C. **Five factors affecting cardiac output.** Heart rate, preload, ventricular distensibility, contractility, and afterload all affect cardiac output. Most of these factors may be manipulated to optimize the Starling curve (increase the cardiac output). The **goal is to optimize the cardiac output.**

  1. **Heart rate.** To optimize the cardiac output, the heart rate must be adjusted to the range of 80 to 110 beats/min. Bradycardia and tachycardia may be treated with drug therapy.

  2. **Preload.** Cardiac output increases as preload is increased until the optimal preload on the Starling curve is exceeded.

  3. **Ventricular distensibility.** There is no way to manipulate this variable. A "stiff" ventricle may result from scarring or hypertrophy.

  4. **Contractility.** If the cardiac output is inadequate at normal filling pressures, the contractile strength of the heart may be inadequate. An inotropic agent may then be used to increase contractility. Recall that acidosis may severely depress the contractility of the heart.

  5. **Afterload**

   a. $SVR = \dfrac{80(MAP - CV)}{CO}$

   (SVR = systemic vascular resistance; MAP = mean arterial pressure; CVP = central venous pressure; and CO = cardiac output)

   b. A **decrease in afterload** may enable the ventricle to eject blood more easily, thus increasing the cardiac output.
    (1) While decreasing the afterload, keep the systolic arterial blood pressure between 100 and 140 mm Hg.
    (2) Afterload reduction is helpful in patients with aortic regurgitation, mitral regurgitation, and ventricular septal defect, and in those with low ejection fractions.

   c. **Augmentation of afterload** may decrease aortic pressure and coronary and other end-organ perfusion.

III. **Central Venous Catheter.** CVP monitoring elucidates the relationship between intravascular volume and RV function.

A. **Indications for CVP monitoring**
  1. Substantial fluid therapy
  2. Hemodynamic drug infusions

B. **Waveform analysis.** See **Figure 5-3.**
  1. An **a wave** is caused by atrial systole; this wave follows the p wave on the ECG.

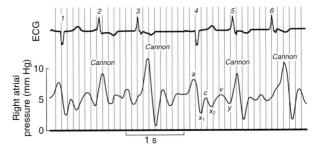

Figure 5-3. Right atrial pressure tracing showing a, c, and v waves, x descent, and y descent.

    2. A **c wave** occurs at the same time as tricuspid valve closes at the onset of systole and follows the QRS complex on the ECG tracing.

    3. The **x descent** is caused by relaxation of the atria and also by downward displacement of the AV junction (or the tricuspid valve) during the early part of systole.

    4. The **v wave** is caused by venous filling of the right atrium while the tricuspid valve is closed during late systole.

    5. The **y descent** is caused by rapid atrial emptying after the tricuspid valve opens.

  C. Pathologic conditions detected by CVP monitoring

    1. Atrial fibrillation. The a wave is absent.

    2. Tricuspid regurgitation. The v wave becomes prominent, the x descent is absent, and the y descent is steep.

    3. Tricuspid stenosis. There are large a waves caused by high pressure atrial contractions against the stenotic valve.

    4. Pericardial tamponade causes elevation and equalization of diastolic filling pressures. The y descent is dampened or absent owing to restricted ventricular filling.

    5. Constrictive pericarditis causes elevation and equalization of diastolic pressures with an early diastolic dip and a late diastolic plateau which is called the "square root sign." The a and v waves are followed by very steep x and y descents.

  D. Central venous catheter placement. See Chapter 49.

IV. Pulmonary Artery Catheter

  A. Indications

    1. General indications

      a. Shock

      b. To assess volume status

      c. To assess ventricular filling pressure

    2. Surgical indications

      a. Preoperative cardiovascular assessment and management

      b. Cardiac or major vascular surgery
      c. Perioperative cardiovascular complications
      d. Multisystem trauma
      e. Major burns
   3. Pulmonary indications
      a. To differentiate acute respiratory distress syndrome (ARDS) from cardiogenic pulmonary edema
      b. To monitor the patient's cardiovascular status while he or she is on intensive ventilatory support
   4. Cardiac indications
      a. Complicated MI
      b. Pulmonary hypertension
      c. Complicated CHF
      d. Evaluation of the effects of inotropic and vasoconstrictive drugs
      e. Evaluation of right and left heart function

B. Pulmonary artery catheter placement. See Chapter 44 for placement procedure. The placement of a PA catheter is guided by changes in wave forms as seen in **Figure 5-4.** There is progression from right atrium to right ventricle to pulmonary artery to a pulmonary capillary wedge pressure.

C. Factors affecting pressure readings
   1. The pulmonary capillary wedge pressure (PCWP) is an indirect reflection of left atrial pressure, which in diastole reflects LV end-diastolic pressure, which in turn reflects LV volume.
   2. Disease states that invalidate the presumption
      a. Mitral stenosis, which inappropriately increases left atrial pressure and volume (see **Figure 5-5**)
      b. Left atrial masses
      c. Pulmonary veno-occlusive disease, which causes in situ thrombosis in the pulmonary veins
      d. Cor triatriatum, where a membrane functionally divides the left atrium into two chambers
   3. Intrathoracic intravascular pressure measurements are

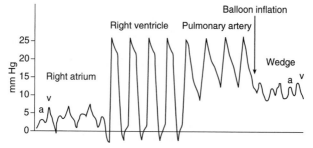

Figure 5-4. Standard sequence of tracings for placement of pulmonary artery catheter.

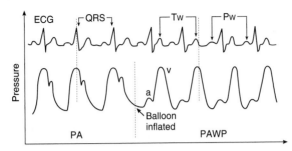

Figure 5-5. Mitral regurgitation. *a* = a wave, *ECG* = electrocardiogram, *QRS* = QRS complex, *PA* = pulmonary arterial pressure, *PAWP* = pulmonary arterial wedge pressure, *Pw* = P wave, *Tw* = T wave, *v* = v wave.

affected by respiration and change in dynamics of the thorax with respiration. Therefore, **all pressure measurements should be made at end-expiration.**

4. Note that in patients on high ventilator tidal volumes or on high positive end-expiratory pressure (PEEP), the filling pressures may be falsely elevated.

D. Mixed venous blood sampling

1. Blood is drawn from the distal port.
2. A **PvCO₂ < PaCO₂** suggests contamination by pulmonary papillary blood.
3. A mixed venous oxygen saturation should be higher than 65%; a lower value signifies increased unloading of oxygen in the periphery, usually owing to incomplete resuscitation, shock, or advanced disease process.

E. Central venous pressure readings. CVP measurements help in the diagnosis and management of right-heart failure, and are a crude estimate of circulating blood volume. CVP is measured through the proximal port of the PA catheter.

F. Pulmonary capillary wedge pressure readings. The PCWP measurement gives a good approximation of left ventricular end-diastolic volume (LVEDV).

1. **Factors affecting LVEDV approximation**
   a. The PCWP **overestimates** the LVEDV in patients with:
      (1) Increased airway pressure (PEEP)
      (2) Mitral valve disease
      (3) COPD
      (4) Pulmonary hypertension
      (5) Hypovolemia
   b. The PCWP **underestimates** the LVEDV when the ventricle is noncompliant.

2. **Procedure.** The PCWP is measured via the distal port of the PA catheter with the balloon inflated.
   a. The waveform is similar to that seen on the right atrial

tracing. Overwedging of the catheter tip is typically recognized by the loss of fluctuations in the pressure waveform (flat line).

b. Regional lung perfusion is determined by the relationship between pulmonary arterial, venous, and alveolar pressures. In vertical fusion, the alveolar pressure is constant whereas arterial and venous pressures change. Based on this, the lung was divided into three zones by West (**Figure 5-6**):

   (1) Zone 1: Alveolar pressure is greater than both arterial and venous pressures.

   (2) Zone 2: Arterial pressure is greater than alveolar pressure, which is in turn greater than venous pressure.

   (3) Zone 3: Arterial and venous pressures are greater than alveolar pressure.

   (4) The catheter tip should be placed in Zone 3 where the vesicular beds are persistent and do not collapse with balloon inflation. A lateral chest film may be used to check placement in supine patients, especially those on high PEEP pressures. The catheter tip should be at or below the level of the left atrium.

c. Mitral valve regurgitation (MR) may make floating a PA catheter difficult. With MR there are large v waves when the catheter is in the PCWP position. In the presence of severe MR, peak systolic v wave pressure can be equivalent to peak systolic pulmonary arterial pressure. This phenomenon may give the impression that the catheter is not wedging with the balloon inflated in the pulmonary artery. The way to determine

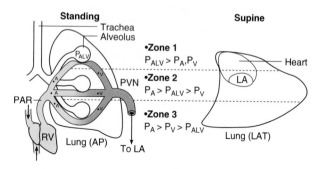

Figure 5-6. Zones of West. A = artery, AP = anteroposterior, LA = left atrium, LAT = lateral, P_A = arterial pressure, P_{ALV} = alveolar pressure, PAR = pulmonary artery, P_V = venous pressure, PVN = pulmonary vein, RV = right ventricle, V = vein. (Redrawn from Vallbhan R: Interpretation of Swan-Ganz catheter data. Baylor University Medical Center Proceedings 7[4]:16, 1994.)

the contribution of MR is to check an ECG, which will show that the peak systolic excursion of the pulmonary arterial pressure trading occurs after the QRS complex and the v wave occurs after the t wave (see Figure 5-5).

G. **Cardiac output.** Cardiac output is determined by thermodilution. A change in temperature is induced over a distance of the catheter and a thermodilution curve is generated. The computer integrates the area under the curve to determine the cardiac output.

1. **Preload** is defined by the LVEDV and is clinically evaluated by correlation of the PCWP. It is determined by the venovascular tone and the intravascular volume. As the preload is increased, the SV and cardiac output are augmented to a critical point after which a further increase in preload leads to a reduction in cardiac output and ventricular failure.

2. **Compliance**
   a. In myocardial oxygenation, ischemia results in decreased compliance.
   b. Fibrotic myocardial scarring (infarct) decreases compliance.
   c. Ventricular hypertrophy reduces compliance.

3. **Afterload** is defined by the tension in the ventricular wall during systole. It is determined by the vascular resistance and ventricular outflow. Afterload is the main determinant of cardiac output in a ventricle with reduced compliance.

4. **Contractility** is determined by the milieu of the myocyte, including the pH, oxygen tension, electrolytes, and temperature.
   a. **Reduced contractility** results from myocardial stunning after cardiac surgery and ischemia.
   b. **Increased contractility** occurs with ventricular hypertrophy (hypertension, idiopathic hypertrophic stenosis [IHSS], aortic stenosis).

H. **Pacing PA catheter.** This catheter is a temporary pacing device that is easy to place (see Chapter 44 for the procedure). The PA catheter should be used in all patients with known left bundle branch block and bifascicular block in case the placement of the catheter induces right bundle branch block and pushes the patient into complete heart block.

I. **Normal readings.** See Table 5-4.

J. **Right ventricular function assessment.** Right ventricular end diastolic volume index (RVEDVI) is the key measurement parameter which is an indicator of right ventricular preload. Several studies have shown that RVEDVI correlates better than CVP or PCWP with the cardiac index.

1. **Calculation:**
$$\frac{(CI/HR)}{EF}$$

Table 5-4. Normal Readings for Invasive Hemodynamic Monitoring (PA Catheter)	
Cardiovascular Parameter	**Normal Value Range**
Central venous pressure (CVP)	2–8 mm Hg
Right ventricle systolic/diastolic (RV)	25/2 mm Hg
Pulmonary artery systolic (PAS)	15–30 mm Hg
Pulmonary artery diastolic (PAD)	5–12 mm Hg
Mean pulmonary artery pressure	5–10 mm Hg
Pulmonary capillary wedge pressure (PCWP)	5–12 mm Hg
Cardiac output (CO)	4–7 L/min
Systemic vascular resistance (SVR)	800–1200 dynes/sec/cm^5

Note: These values must be used in conjunction with other information from the clinical setting.

(CI = cardiac index, HR = heart rate, and EF = ejection fraction)

2. Elevations in intrathoracic pressure (e.g., associated with mechanical ventilation, ARDS, and pulmonary hypertension) make assessment of PCWP difficult to interpret.

3. The RVEDVI is a better predictor of volume depletion and preload recruitable increases in cardiac index after fluid challenge. This index is not affected by increased levels of PEEP. A RVEDVI less than 140 ml/m^2 predicts that the patient would have a favorable increase in cardiac index after fluid challenge.

4. Critics argue that there is mathematical coupling between the RVEDVI and cardiac index. However, a volume challenge to a patient with a low RVEDVI will increase the cardiac index, whereas a volume challenge to a patient with a high RVEDVI will not affect the cardiac index.

K. Complications associated with insertion of the PA catheter occur in 5% of patients. They include:
   1. Arrhythmias
   2. Pulmonary artery rupture
   3. Pneumothorax, hemothorax
   4. Catheter knotting
   5. Incorrect placement

L. Complications associated with an indwelling PA catheter include:
   1. Heart block and arrhythmias
   2. Heparin-induced thrombocytopenia
   3. Infection (bacteremia, sepsis, endocarditis)
   4. Hemorrhage: pulmonary artery or right ventricle rupture
   5. Endocardial and valvular damage
   6. Venous thrombosis

V. Hemodynamic Instability

   A. Physiologic changes in shock states (Table 5-5)

      1. **Hypovolemic shock.** The primary problem is decreased ventricular filling (low PCWP), which leads to low cardiac output. Low cardiac output produces vasoconstriction and an increase in the SVR (**Figure 5-7**).

      2. **Cardiogenic shock.** There is a primary decrease in cardiac output, which leads to venous congestion (high PCWP) and peripheral vasoconstriction (high SVR). See Figure 5-7.

      3. **Septic shock.** Vascular tone is lost in the arteries (low SVR) and veins (low PCWP). Cardiac output is often elevated. See Figure 5-7.

   B. Etiology of shock

      1. Hypovolemia (bleeding, diuretics, third spacing, inadequate resuscitation)

      2. Elevated systemic vascular resistance

      3. Myocardial dysfunction (ischemia, acidosis, hypervolemia, hypothermia)

      4. Dysrhythmias

      5. Cardiac tamponade

      6. Increased intrathoracic pressure

   C. Clinical features of low cardiac output

      1. **Cool, clammy skin and slow capillary refill,** which occur as a result of sympathetic overactivity

      2. **Oliguria (low urine output),** one of the best indicators of inadequate tissue perfusion. If the urine volume is normal but contains large amounts of **glucose,** there may still be inadequate tissue perfusion.

      3. **Decreased mixed venous saturation**

      4. **Metabolic acidosis** (lactic acidosis)

VI. Hemodynamic Management

   A. General principles

      1. Identify the major hemodynamic problems.

      2. Look at the patterns in the Swan-Ganz readings (PCWP/CO/SVR).

      3. Institute fluid therapy and drug therapy to optimize the Starling curve.

   B. Heart rate and arrhythmias

      1. **Bradycardia**

         a. Etiology

            (1) Ischemia

            (2) Hypothermia

            (3) Use of β-blockers or calcium channel blockers

         b. Management

            (1) **Useful drugs** include:

               (a) Atropine

               (b) Isoproterenol

               (c) Calcium to reverse calcium channel blocker toxicity

               (d) Glucagon to reverse β-blocker toxicity

Table 5-5. Hemodynamic Measurements During Various Shock States

Diagnosis	BP	HR	CO	SV	PCWP	PAP	CVP
Normal	100–140/80	60–100	4–7	70	5–12	15–30/5–12	2–8
Septic shock							
Early	↓	↑	↑	←	→		↓
Late	↓	↕	↓	↕	←	↕	↑
Terminal	↓	↓↑	↓	↓	←	↑	
Cardiogenic shock							
LV infarct	↓/↓	↑	↓	↓↓	←	↑/↑	↑
Tamponade	↓/↓	↑	↓	↓↓	←	↑/↑	↑
Pulmonary hypertension	↓/↓	↑	↓	↓↓	↕	↑↑/↑↑	↑
RV infarct	↓/↓	↑	↓	↓↓	↕	↓/↑	↑
Hypovolemic shock							
Neurogenic	↓/↓ ↓	↕	↓	↓	→	↓↑/↓↓	↓
Anaphylactic	↓/↓	↑	↓	↓	→	↓↑/↓↓	↓
Adrenal insufficiency	↓/↓	↑	↓	↓		↓↑/↓↓	↓

BP = blood pressure; CO = cardiac output; CVP = central venous pressure; HR = heart rate; LV = left ventricle; PAP = pulmonary artery pressure; PCWP = pulmonary capillary wedge pressure; RV = right ventricle; SV = stroke volume.

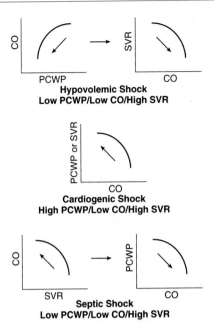

Figure 5-7. Frank Starling relationships in various shock states.

> (2) **Temporary pacemakers** may be used for heart block.

2. **Sinus tachycardia**

    a. **Etiology.** See p. 62.

    b. **Management**

    (1) Optimize the patient's volume status with crystalloid and colloid therapy.

    (2) Give the patient supplemental oxygen.

    (3) **Useful drugs** include:

    (a) Saline

    (b) Morphine or an anxiolytic agent

    (c) Esmolol (short-acting β-blocker)

Physiologic tachycardia should never be treated as a primary condition; a cause must always be pursued. β-blockers may precipitate heart failure in patients with marginal ventricular function.

C. **Preload. Optimize filling pressures** to yield an appropriate cardiac output without pulmonary edema.

1. **Decreased preload**

    a. Etiology
      (1) Hypovolemia
      (2) Vasodilation
      (3) Increased intrathoracic pressure
      (4) Cardiac tamponade
    b. Management
      (1) Put the patient in the Trendelenburg position to augment preload.
      (2) Use crystalloid and colloid therapy to replace volume.
      (3) Whenever possible, use fluid therapy rather than vasoactive drugs to raise the PCWP.
      (4) Control bleeding.
      (5) Monitor the patient's electrolytes and urine output.

2. Increased preload
    a. Etiology
      (1) Volume overload
      (2) Ventricular dysfunction
    b. Management
      (1) Minimal exogenous fluid therapy
      (2) Diuretics (furosemide, or bumetanide and chlorothiazide)
      (3) Low-dose dopamine

D. Afterload
  1. Normal afterload with insufficient cardiac output
    a. Etiology
      (1) Hypovolemia
      (2) Hypothermia
      (3) Low cardiac output (low heart rate and/or stroke volume)
    b. Treatment
      (1) Warm and hydrate the patient.
      (2) Start inotropic therapy (dobutamine, epinephrine).

  2. Increased afterload
    a. Etiology. Increased afterload is caused by hypertension, which may be related to pain, preeclampsia, pheochromocytoma, clonidine withdrawal, monoamine oxidase (MAO) inhibitors, or cocaine use.
    b. Management
      (1) Optimize the patient's **fluid status.**
      (2) Start vasodilator therapy. Vasodilators reduce preload or afterload, resulting in decreased myocardial oxygen consumption and improved EF. **Preload must be optimized** before starting a vasodilator.
        (a) Sodium nitroprusside (Nipride) is the drug of choice for afterload reduction.
        (b) Nitroglycerin therapy is adequate in large

doses. It also dilates the coronary artery and collateral vessels as well as the pulmonary vascular bed.

(c) **Esmolol** is a negative chronotrope, but it also results in afterload reduction.

3. Decreased afterload

a. Etiology

(1) Septic shock

(2) Neurogenic shock

(3) Uncompensated hypovolemia

b. Management

(1) Ensure adequate and rapid volume replacement based on the PCWP.

(2) Discontinue medications that may induce vasodilation (spinal anesthesia or analgesia, antihypertensive agents, sedatives).

(3) Start vasoconstrictive drug therapy.

(a) Dopamine (first-line agent for α-adrenergic stimulation)

(b) Epinephrine

(c) Norepinephrine

(d) Phenylephrine

E. Reduced contractility.
This is the final parameter to manipulate in hemodynamic management. It is best to first optimize heart rate, rhythm, preload, and afterload to maximize the cardiac output.

1. Etiology

a. Myocardial ischemia

b. Acidosis

c. Hypothermia

d. Hypercarbia

2. Management: inotropic therapy.
(See Appendix E for the effects of each drug.) Start with a first-line inotrope. If this is ineffective, add another first-line inotrope or change to a second-line agent.

Inotropes will increase myocardial oxygen demand and may have arrhythmogenic potential.

---

a. **Dopamine.** This first-line agent causes splanchnic and renal vasodilation and has a pressor effect at high doses.

b. **Dobutamine.** This first-line agent causes:

(1) Lower incidence of tachycardia

(2) Reflex vasodilation

(3) Pulmonary vasodilation and reduction in PCWP

(4) No impairment of coronary artery autoregulation

c. **Epinephrine.** This second-line agent may cause tachycardia.

d. **Amrinone.** This drug is indicated in refractory cases

or in right-sided heart failure or pulmonary hypertension.

e. Isoproterenol. This drug is indicated in pulmonary hypertension or right-sided heart failure.

VII. **Pressors and Inotropic Agents**

A. **Dopamine**

1. **Actions.** Dopamine affects both α- and β-adrenergic receptors, depending on the dose used. It stimulates adrenergic receptors both directly and indirectly through the release of norepinephrine.

   a. Dopamine produces **vasodilation** in renal, splanchnic, and cerebral circulations via discrete dopaminergic receptors.

   b. High doses produce **vasoconstriction** via peripheral α-receptor stimulation.

   c. Dopamine **increases pulmonary capillary hydrostatic pressure** through venoconstriction.

   d. Dopamine **increases renal sodium excretion,** independent of the effects on renal blood flow.

2. **Indications**

   a. Cardiogenic shock

   b. Septic shock

   c. Augmentation of urine output

3. **Adverse effects. Tachyarrhythmias** and **profound vasoconstriction** occur at high doses.

4. **Contraindications.** Dopamine is contraindicated in patients with **existing arrhythmias** when an alternative agent is available.

B. **Dobutamine**

1. **Actions**

   a. Dobutamine, as a selective β1 agonist, causes an increase in contractility (increased cardiac output). It also causes mild β2 stimulation, which results in peripheral vasodilation.

   b. A dose-related increase in cardiac output occurs with an infusion rate of 2–20 μg/kg/min. SVR decreases through reflex mechanisms; preload increases from improved cardiac output. The patient's heart rate is usually unchanged; however, tachycardia can be prominent when the patient is hypovolemic.

   c. As compared with dopamine, dobutamine produces a greater increase in cardiac output and is less arrhythmogenic.

   d. Short periods of dobutamine infusion can be associated with long-term (4-week) improvement in cardiac performance.

2. **Indications**

   a. Acute management of heart failure (inotropic agent of choice)

   b. Treatment of low cardiac output states (may be used with amrinone)

3. **Adverse effects**
    a. **Tachycardia** occurs in hypovolemic patients.
    b. **Ventricular arrhythmias** sometimes occur.
4. **Contraindications**
    a. Hypertrophic cardiomyopathy
    b. Myocardial infarction with cardiogenic shock
C. **Epinephrine**
    1. **Actions**
        a. Epinephrine functions as a **combined α and β agonist.** The predominant effect depends on the dose and regional circulation.
        b. This drug can produce **profound peripheral vasoconstriction,** particularly in the splanchnic and renal beds.
        c. Epinephrine **inhibits mediator release** from mast cells and basophils in response to antigen–antibody complexes in anaphylactic reactions.
        d. **Metabolic effects** include lactic acidosis, ketoacid accumulation, and hyperglycemia.
    2. **Indications**
        a. Anaphylaxis
        b. Hypotension resistant to conventional measures (second-line agent)
        c. When venous access is not readily available (epinephrine may be administered via an endotracheal tube)
    3. **Adverse effects**
        a. Acute MI
        b. Arrhythmias
        c. Lactic acidosis
        d. Acute renal failure
D. **Norepinephrine**
    1. **Actions**
        a. Norepinephrine is **predominantly an α agonist** but **can stimulate cardiac β receptors** in low doses.
        b. It produces **vasoconstriction** in all vascular beds, including the renal circulation. The addition of low-dose dopamine helps to preserve the renal blood flow.
    2. **Indications.** Norepinephrine can be used for septic shock when the patient is refractory to volume and dopamine therapies.
    3. **Adverse effects** include renal failure and other manifestations of peripheral vasoconstriction.
    4. **Contraindications.** Norepinephrine is contraindicated in patients who have hypotension associated with peripheral vasoconstriction because of the potential for hypovolemic shock.
E. **Trimethaphan camsylate (Arfonad).** This agent has no particular advantages over other vasodilators.
    1. **Actions**

      a. Trimethaphan camsylate blocks both sympathetic and parasympathetic ganglia.

      b. It dilates both arteries and veins.

      c. This drug is short acting and has its onset of action in 1 minute. The effect dissipates within 10 minutes.

  2. Indications

      a. Hypertension

      b. Acute aortic dissection (drug of choice)

  3. Adverse effects

      a. Paralytic ileus

      b. Urinary retention

  4. Contraindications

      a. Hypovolemia

      b. Autonomic neuropathy

      c. Bowel distention

F. Nitroglycerin

  1. Actions

      a. Nitroglycerin **promotes direct relaxation of the arteries and veins.** Venodilation predominates at low doses, whereas arterial vasodilation is predominant at high doses.

      b. Nitroglycerin **increases coronary flow.**

  2. Indications

      a. Myocardial ischemia

      b. Pulmonary hypertension

      c. Heart failure associated with an MI

  3. Adverse effects

      a. **Tolerance** (tachyphylaxis) develops because sulfhydryl groups are depleted within the vessel walls. **Acetylcysteine** (Mucomyst) can partially reverse tolerance.

      b. **Methemoglobinemia** can occur.

      c. **Hypoxemia** occurs in patients with pulmonary edema.

      d. **Resistance to heparin** is a side effect.

  4. Contraindications

      a. Increased BP

      b. Closed-angle glaucoma

      c. Hypovolemia

G. Sodium nitroprusside

  1. Actions

      a. Dilates systemic arteries and veins through direct action on the vessel wall

      b. Produces pulmonary artery vasodilation

      c. Increases SV without a change in heart rate

  2. Indications

      a. Hypertensive emergencies (best drug available for acute control)

      b. Hypertensive control in aortic dissection (combined with a β-blocker)

      c. Acute MI with septal or papillary muscle rupture

      d. Acute LV failure without hypotension

> **Generally, sodium nitroprusside should be used for no longer than 48 to 72 hours because of the buildup of toxic metabolites.**

    3. Adverse effects
        a. Cyanide toxicity
        b. Thiocyanate toxicity (in renal insufficiency)
        c. Changes in mental status
    4. Contraindications
        a. Vitamin B_{12} deficiency
        b. Renal failure

HYPERTENSION

  I. Hypertensive Crisis
    A. Definitions. The term *hypertensive crisis* refers to a **severe elevation in blood pressure** that is either a *de novo* or an acute exacerbation of chronic disease. The diastolic pressure is usually > 120 mm Hg; however, rather than relying on a specific number for diagnosis, you should consider the presence or absence of **acute and progressive target organ damage** as the determining factor.
      1. Hypertensive emergency is associated with ongoing CNS, cardiac, hematologic, or renal target organ damage.
      2. Hypertensive urgency indicates that there is potential for target organ damage if the blood pressure is not controlled.
      3. Malignant hypertension is a crisis with the presence of **retinopathy and papilledema.**
      4. Autoregulation serves to maintain blood flows in patients who have decreased systemic pressure, and to limit pressure-induced damage when systemic pressure rises.
        a. When systemic pressures are not controlled by autoregulation, **target organ damage** occurs. The pathophysiologic abnormality that causes target organ damage in most patients is an **increase in systemic vascular resistance,** which elevates blood pressure, overrides local autoregulation, and leads to organ ischemia and necrosis.
        b. **Elderly or chronic hypertensive patients** are able to tolerate elevated pressures because of an upward shift in cerebral autoregulation. (These patients have less tolerance of *hypo*tension because of changes in the vessel walls.)
    B. History and physical examination

> **It may be necessary to initiate antihypertensive therapy in the ICU prior to a comprehensive examination (see D 1 below).**

1. Determine whether the patient has diabetes or substance abuse/dependence, or has previously had hypertension, CAD, MI, or CVA.
2. Determine what medications the patient is currently taking.
3. Find out the patient's **baseline blood pressure** and recent trends during hospitalization.
4. **Confirm elevated blood pressure** in both arms using a manual cuff. A direct arterial catheter may be helpful.
5. Focus the patient history and physical examination on **end-organ manifestations** of hypertension.
   a. **Neurologic signs and symptoms:** headache, change in mental status, seizures, coma, focal deficits
   b. **Retinal signs and symptoms:** papilledema, hemorrhages, exudates, visual disturbances
   c. **Cardiac signs and symptoms:** pulmonary edema, myocardial ischemia or infarction, chest pain
   d. **Renal signs and symptoms:** hematuria, azotemia
   e. **Evidence of changes in organ perfusion and function**
6. Determine the patient's overall **fluid balance.** It may be necessary to review the patient's hospital charts for a complete assessment.

C. **Diagnostic tests**
   1. Obtain **ECG readings** to rule out ischemia.
   2. Obtain the following **laboratory test results:** serum electrolytes, BUN, creatinine, CBC with differential, cardiac enzymes, and urinalysis with sediment.

D. **Management**
   1. **Initial therapy** is aimed at **terminating the ongoing target organ damage** rather than returning the blood pressure to normal. Given that the cerebral circulation is the most sensitive to ischemia, neural autoregulation will determine the first stop point in lowering the blood pressure. If autoregulation has not occurred, therapy should be directed at lowering the blood pressure 25% below the initial MAP and lowering the SVR. In patients who have acute left ventricular failure, aortic dissection, or myocardial ischemia, both the cardiac output and the SVR should be lowered.
   2. **Acute left ventricular failure in the failing heart.** Attempt to decrease MAP and SVR in order to decease myocardial oxygen demand, cardiac work, and left ventricular wall tension.
      a. **Nitroprusside** is the agent of choice because of its ability to decrease preload and afterload.
      b. **Nitroglycerin** is an alternate therapy that has greater effect on the preload side.
      c. **ACE inhibitors** (e.g., enalaprilat) may be given intravenously to decrease afterload. These agents may help in converting from IV to oral therapy.
   3. **Myocardial infarction or ischemia.** Therapy should maintain local coronary arterial flow.

      a. Nitroglycerin is the therapy of choice.

      b. Beta blockers given IV also act to maintain coronary perfusion in the face of decreased systemic pressures.

  4. Aortic dissection. Once the diagnosis of proximal or distal dissection is made, it is imperative to **obtain maximum blood pressure control immediately** to limit extension of the dissection. The blood pressure should be as low as possible without signs of end organ damage. The therapy of choice is **nitroprusside.** Avoid tachycardia by instituting therapy with **β blockers.**

  5. Hypertensive encephalopathy occurs in the setting of severe hypertension, with blood pressure often above 250/150 mm Hg. Cerebral edema, petechial hemorrhages, and microinfarcts may occur. These patients usually have chronic untreated hypertension and slowly develop the neurologic symptoms over 48 to 72 hours. Treatment with **nitroprusside** should lead to rapid resolution.

  6. Cerebrovascular accident. Treatment of hypertension in patients with an acute CVA should be undertaken with great caution. Once ischemia occurs, a central core of dense ischemia is formed with a surrounding area of lesser ischemia that can be salvaged with adequate reperfusion.

      a. SBP should be treated only if the systolic pressure exceeds 220 mm Hg.

      b. If **thrombolytic therapy** is started, an easily titrated agent such as labetalol, captopril, or nicardipine should be used. The **target reduction is 25% of MAP.**

          (1) SBP > 180 mm Hg or DBP > 105 mm Hg: Use oral labetalol.

          (2) SBP > 230 mm Hg or DBP > 120 mm Hg: Use intravenous labetalol or nitroprusside.

II. Hypertension Without Hypertensive Crisis

  A. Continued therapy of chronic hypertension in the ICU. Rebound hypertension may occur in patients who have suddenly discontinued chronic therapy. Control is accomplished with β blockers and central agonists such as clonidine and methyldopa.

  B. New onset of hypertension in the ICU

      a. Evaluate the heart and fundus of the eyes for evidence of previously undiagnosed, untreated hypertension.

      b. Look for secondary causes of hypertension, such as pain, anxiety, hypoxia or hypercarbia, fluid overload, hypothermia, and rigors.

  C. Preoperative hypertension. Moderate chronic hypertension is a marker for potential coronary artery disease. Patients with preoperative MAP greater than 110 mm Hg, poor functional capacity, or hypovolemia are at risk for intraoperative hypertension with or without myocardial ischemia.

1. Regular blood pressure regimens should be continued up to the morning of surgery.
2. Pretreatment with β blockers before elective surgery can control blood pressure during anesthesia, intubation, and extubation, decreasing the risk of ischemia.

D. Postoperative hypertension
1. In the **immediate postoperative period** there are significant blood pressure fluctuations due to pain, hypothermia with shivering, hypoxia, and anxiety. Minute-to-minute blood pressure management may be required.
   a. **Nitroprusside or labetalol** are effective in controlling blood pressure in most patients.
   b. **Nitroglycerin** may be added or used as a single agent if the patient has **fixed coronary lesions.**
2. **During the 48 hours after surgery,** expansion of the intravascular volume occurs because of fluid mobilization, perioperative fluid administration, antidiuretic effects of anesthesia, and transient renal insufficiency, all of which may lead to hypertension.

III. Pharmacologic Agents Used to Manage Hypertension
A. Direct vasodilators
1. **Sodium nitroprusside** is the **most predictable and effective agent** for the control of hypertension.
   a. **Mechanism of action.** Sodium nitroprusside **dilates both the arterial and venous systems,** reducing preload and afterload and decreasing myocardial oxygen demand.
   b. **Pharmacodynamics and pharmacokinetics.** Sodium nitroprusside is rapidly decomposed to cyanide and then converted to thiocyanate in the liver. Thiocyanate is excreted renally and thus may accumulate with renal insufficiency, in which case it is removed by dialysis.
   c. **Clinical considerations**
      (1) Nitroprusside has a **rapid onset of action** and its effects can be terminated in an instant.
      (2) Thiocyanate **levels should be monitored;** they should remain below 10 mg/dl.
2. **Nitroglycerin**
   a. **Mechanism of action.** This drug predominantly **dilates the venous system;** it reduces left ventricular filling pressures and MAP without much change in stroke volume or cardiac output.
   b. **Clinical considerations.** Because nitroglycerin increases coronary flow through the collaterals, it should not be given to patients who have increased intracranial pressure or aortic or subaortic stenosis.
3. **Diazoxide**
   a. **Mechanism of action.** Diazoxide is a **potent arterial vasodilator** that reduces cardiac afterload, but it will induce a reflex tachycardia that can increase myocardial oxygen demand.

   b. **Clinical considerations**
      (1) Diazoxide is **contraindicated** in patients who have
          CAD, recent MI, aortic dissection, coarctation of
          the aorta, intracerebral hypertension, subarach-
          noid hypertension, CVA, or pulmonary edema.
      (2) Diazoxide **may cause sodium and water reten-
          tion,** which may necessitate diuretics. It **may also
          decrease cerebral blood flow.**
   4. **Hydralazine**
      a. **Mechanism of action.** Hydralazine is a direct arterial
         vasodilator that increases cardiac output and heart
         rate.
      b. **Clinical considerations.** Hydralazine is a good choice
         in eclampsia and left ventricular failure.
B. **β blockers**
   1. **Labetalol** is the agent most often used for hypertension
      in the ICU.
      a. **Mechanism of action.** Labetalol is a nonselective β
         blocker with selective α-1 antagonist. The ratio of β to
         α blockade is 7 to 1.
      b. **Clinical considerations**
         (1) Labetalol may be used to treat **pheochromocy-
             toma crisis** because of its α-1 blocker properties,
             and **aortic dissection** because of its β blocker
             properties.
         (2) There is no reflex tachycardia or changes in car-
             diac output. Myocardial oxygen consumption is
             reduced and coronary hemodynamics are im-
             proved.
         (3) It may be administered as a bolus or IV infusion,
             and can be titrated for effect.
   2. **Other agents.** Several β blockers—propanolol (β-1 non-
      selective), metoprolol (β-1 selective) and the short-acting
      esmolol (β-1 selective)—can be given by the IV route.
C. **Calcium antagonists**
   1. **Nifedipine** is administered orally or sublingually. The
      physiologic effects include decreased myocardial oxygen
      consumption, increased cardiac output and stroke vol-
      ume, decreased peripheral vascular resistance, and in-
      creased collateral coronary blood flow.

**The reduction in blood pressure is very unpredictable
with nifedipine. This drug should *not* be used to
treat hypertension in the acute setting.**

---

   2. **Nicardipine** is a rapid-acting systemic and coronary artery
      vasodilator that has minimal effects on cardiac contrac-
      tility or conduction. **Side effects** include tachycardia, hy-
      potension, nausea, and vomiting.
   3. **Verapamil**
      a. **Mechanism of action.** Verapamil is a potent arterial

vasodilator that has a significant effect on the atrio-ventricular conduction system, which is why it can be effective in treating tachyarrhythmias.

  b. Clinical considerations. Verapamil has a rapid onset of action but a pronounced negative inotropic effect. Administration is in small boluses or by continuous IV route. It may induce varying degrees of heart block and worsen CHF.

  4. Diltiazem is a potent arterial vasodilator that has significant effects on the atrioventricular conduction system. These effects tend to cause fewer conduction delays than does verapamil.

D. ACE inhibitors

  1. Captopril

  a. Mechanism of action. Captopril is rapidly absorbed as active drug with peak blood levels at 30 minutes. There is no change in cardiac output or reflex tachycardia.

  b. Clinical considerations. Captopril is effective in patients with CHF or recent MI. There is a **risk of hypotension or worsening renal function** in patients who are volume depleted or who have high-grade bilateral renal artery stenoses or high-grade stenosis in a single functioning kidney. **Other side effects** include bronchospasm, hyperkalemia, cough, angioedema, and rash.

  2. Enalaprilat is the only ACE inhibitor that may be administered parenterally. It is useful to substitute in patients who usually take oral ACE inhibitors, who have underlying poor left ventricular function, or who have had a recent MI.

E. Central agonists

  1. Clonidine is an α-2 central agonist that decreases peripheral vascular resistance by decreasing venous return and causing bradycardia that contributes to reduced cardiac output. It is available orally or as a transdermal patch that can last for up to 1 week. **Side effects** include rebound hypertension when discontinued, sedation, dry mouth, and orthostatic hypotension.

  2. Methyldopate hydrochloride is a central agonist that depresses central sympathetic nervous system outflow and decreases peripheral vascular resistance with no effect on cardiac output. It has a slow onset of action with IV administration.

F. α-adrenergic inhibitors. Phentolamine is a nonselective α-adrenergic blocking agent used to treat hypertension associated with excess catecholamine states such as pheochromocytomas, rebound hypertension, and hypertension associated with drug ingestion or withdrawal. The hypotensive effect of a single dose lasts 15 minutes and is associated with significant reflex tachycardia.

G. **Ganglionic blockers. Trimethaphan camsylate** blocks both adrenergic and cholinergic ganglia. It has a direct vasodilation effect, which increases its hypotensive effects without causing reflex tachycardia or change in cardiac output. **Side effects** include orthostatic hypotension, paresis of the bowel and bladder, blurry vision, dry mouth, and bladder retention.

IV. **Complications of Hypertension Management in the ICU.** See Table 5-6.

V. **Surgically Correctable Sources of Hypertension.** Patients with hypertensive emergencies where no primary cause is found may have secondary hypertension, which is due to a correctable condition. See **Table 5-7.**

MYOCARDIAL ISCHEMIA AND INFARCTION

I. **Etiology.** Myocardial ischemia is a consequence of an imbalance between myocardial oxygen demand and supply. In stable

---

Table 5-6. Complications of Hypertension management in the ICU

Overshoot hypertension
Infusion rate too rapid
Prolonged duration of effect
Additive drug effects
New cardiac disease (e.g., MI, tamponade)
Volume depletion or redistribution

Worsening neurologic function
Cerebral ischemia due to hypotension
Worsened intracranial hypotension or hepatic encephalopathy
Thiocyanate toxicity
New metabolic abnormality

Worsening of hypertension
Volume overload
Pseudotolerance
Cathecholamine excess and secondary hypertension
Poor medical regimen or compliance

Metabolic acidosis
Cyanide toxicity
Tissue hypoperfusion

Worsening renal function
Hypoperfusion
Volume depletion
ATN

Table 5-7. Surgically Correctable Sources of Hypertension
Aortic coarctation
Fibromuscular dysplasia or other renovascular disease causing stenosis
Pheochromocytoma
Primary aldosteronism
Cushing's disease

---

angina, the ischemia is a result of increased demand relative to the capability of supply. In acute ischemia, there is usually an abrupt decrease in coronary flow. Myocardia ischemia may be caused by any of the following:

  A. Abrupt decrease in coronary flow due to:
    1. Coronary thrombosis
    2. Coronary bypass graft occlusion
    3. Hemorrhage beneath an atherosclerotic plaque or unstable coronary lesion
    4. Coronary vasoconstriction or spasm
    5. Shock
  B. Increased myocardial demand due to:
    1. Tachycardia, especially ventricular tachycardia
    2. Uncontrolled atrial fibrillation

II. Presentation
  A. Substernal chest pain and tightness, with or without radiation to the neck or arm
  B. Nausea and vomiting
  C. Diaphoresis
  D. Tachycardia and hypotension
  E. Dyspnea
  F. Ventricular arrhythmia or PVCs

The key feature of unstable angina is new or more severe symptoms departing from the usual angina pattern, such as:
- **New onset of crescendo angina with chest pain at rest or at a lower threshold of exercise**
- **Prolonged chest pain poorly relieved by nitroglycerin**
- **Recurrence of angina after myocardial infarction**

III. Diagnosis of Myocardial Ischemia and Infarction
  A. 12-lead ECG
    1. An **ST segment elevation** greater than 2 mm in the precordial leads or 1 mm in the limb leads indicates a transmural infarction.
    2. An **ST segment depression** indicates subendocardial ischemia or reciprocal transmural ischemia.
    3. **T wave inversions** are nonspecific signs of ischemia.
    4. **Q waves** indicate irreversible myocardial necrosis.

   5. **New left BBB** renders the ECG uninterpretable but suggests an acute MI.
   6. The **location of the ischemia can be determined by the ECG leads affected.**
      a. Abnormal V1 and V2 readings indicate **septal location** and, if reciprocal, may indicate **posterior involvement.**
      b. Abnormal V3 and V4 readings indicate **anterior location.**
      c. Abnormal readings from leads V5, V6, I, and avL indicate **lateral location.**
      d. Abnormal readings from leads II, III, and avF indicate **inferior location.**
B. **Biochemical markers**
   1. **Creatine kinase (CK)** and **MB isoenzymes.** These biochemical markers rise within 8 hours of MI, usually peak within 24 hours, and then resolve. They are very sensitive to infarction but not to ischemia. Levels may also be elevated in renal failure, rhabdomyolysis, or trauma.
   2. **Lactate dehydrogenase.** This enzyme rises within 16 to 24 hours of MI and peaks in 3 to 6 days.
   3. **Cardiac troponins I and T.** The dynamics of these protein markers are similar to those of CK with a higher specificity and sensitivity. High levels may indicate a small amount of cell necrosis or a more severe myocardial ischemia.
C. **Echocardiography.** An echocardiogram taken during suspected ischemia may show wall motion abnormalities consistent with ischemia. Baseline function must be available for comparison.
D. **Nuclear scintigraphy.** A ^{99m}Tc sestamibi scan can be performed during a chest pain episode. Subsequent demonstration of a defect is highly specific for cardiac ischemia.
IV. **Management of the Patient with Myocardial Ischemia or Infarction**
   A. Administer **oxygen** via a face mask or nasal cannula.
   B. Maintain adequate **vascular access.**
   C. Provide **IV fluids** to maintain the patient's BP. Observe the patient for signs of pulmonary edema.
   D. Institute **antithrombotic therapy:**
      1. **Aspirin.** Administer 325 mg to be chewed unless absolutely contraindicated. The patient may be then maintained on 80–325 mg qd. **Ticlopidine,** 250 mg PO bid, may be used in patients with poor tolerance to aspirin. There is some delay in onset of effects of ticlopidine.
      2. **Heparin.** Heparin therapy reduces the risk of death, further infarction, refractory ischemia, and silent ST segment depression in the acute phase of an MI.
         a. Attempt to achieve an activated partial thromboplastin time of 2–2½ times control.
         b. Duration of therapy must be individualized.

      c. **Low molecular weight heparins** (dalteparin and enoxaparin) have been shown to be as effective as standard heparin therapy in reducing death rate, myocardial infarction, and recurrent ischemia. The advantage of these low molecular weight heparins is that therapy can be continued for 30 to 45 days on an outpatient basis.

E. Administer **nitroglycerin.**

    1. Give a **sublingual tablet** (0.15–0.6 mg) every 5 minutes, up to 3 doses.

    2. If this fails, order **IV nitroglycerin** starting at 50 μg/min and increase by 5 μg/min as tolerated.

    3. In low-risk patients, **topical nitrates** may be used to relieve pain and resolve ECG changes.

F. Administer **β-blockers** unless contraindicated. β-blockers reduce the risk of developing an MI and decrease myocardial work by reducing heart rate, blood pressure, and cardiac contractility. The goal is a basal heart rate of 60 beats/min.

    1. Agents and doses

      a. Atenolol can be given as 5 mg IV over 5 minutes up to 2 doses, then 25–50 mg PO q 12 hr up to a final dose of 100 mg PO qd.

      b. Metoprolol is given as 5 mg IV over 5 minutes up to 3 doses, then 25–50 mg PO q 6 hr up to a final dose of 100 mg PO q 12 hr.

    2. Contraindications

      a. The use of β-blockers may be limited because of their **blood pressure lowering effect.**

      b. β-blockers are relatively contraindicated in patients who have **moderate to severe LV dysfunction.**

G. Calcium channel blockers are the treatment of choice (with nitrates) for **Prinzmetal's variant angina. Diltiazem** induces a variable degree of reduced heart rate; **verapamil** has a negative inotropic effect. These agents do not prevent MI, but they can control recurrent angina.

H. ACE inhibitors have been shown to be helpful when started early in patients who have extensive MI, heart failure, or left ventricular dysfunction. Therapy should be initiated **within 24 hours** and continued for 4 to 6 weeks or longer.

I. Administer **IV morphine** to reduce pain and sympathetic stimulation.

J. Monitor electrolytes. Maintain the serum potassium level between 4.0 and 5.0, and the magnesium level > 2.0.

K. If the pain does not resolve or if it recurs, and if changes are consistent with an acute MI, consider **thrombolytic therapy or emergent cardiac catheterization.**

    1. Thrombolytic therapy. Aspirin should be administered with all thrombolytic agents. **IV heparin** should be administered with all thrombolytic agents and continued for 48 hours.

Thrombolytic agents should be administered under the direction of a cardiovascular or emergency medical specialist who is familiar with their indications and contraindications (Table 5-8).

    a. Streptokinase (SK) may be given to an individual only once in his or her lifetime.
      (1) Give the patient 1.5 million units over 1 hour.
      (2) Start heparin treatment 4 hours after SK therapy.
    b. Tissue plasminogen activator (t-PA) can be given up to a total dose of 100 mg.
      (1) Give the patient a 10-mg bolus.
      (2) Next give the patient 50 mg over 1 hour for the first hour.
      (3) Then give 20 mg/hr over the next 2 hours.
      (4) Start heparin therapy immediately.
      (5) **Complications of t-PA.** There is an increased risk of intracranial hemorrhage in patients older

---

Table 5-8. Thrombolytic Therapy: Indications and Contraindications

INDICATIONS FOR THROMBOLYTIC THERAPY

  I. Chest pain that lasts at least 30 minutes up to 12 hours, and ECG changes that are consistent with an acute MI, with an ST elevation of 2 mm or more in two contiguous precordial leads or 1 mm in limb leads of a contiguous territory (or new left BBB)

  II. Chest pain and ECG changes that do not resolve with standard therapy

ABSOLUTE CONTRAINDICATIONS TO THROMBOLYTIC THERAPY

  I. Acute Disease
    A. Active internal bleeding
    B. Heme-positive stool on a rectal examination (relative)
    C. Uncontrollable BP above 200/120 mm Hg
    D. Suspected aortic dissection

  II. Subacute or Chronic Disease
    A. Known cerebral arteriovenous malformation
    B. Tumor involving the spinal cord or cranial structures
    C. Hemorrhagic retinopathy
    D. Pregnancy
    E. History of hemorrhagic stroke
    F. Allergic reaction to streptokinase (SK) alone

  III. Recent Events
    A. Surgery, trauma, or suspicion of intracranial bleeding within the past 2 weeks (patient at risk for rebleeding)
    B. Spinal or intracranial procedure within the past 2 weeks
    C. Prolonged CPR (greater than 10 minutes)

than 65 years, those who weight over 70 kg, and those with hypertension.

    2. Emergent cardiac catheterization will help to identify any offending coronary lesions and may be able to stent or angioplasty these lesions to obviate the need for surgery.

L. If the pain persists without ECG changes, consider alternate causes.

M. Avoid antiarrhythmic therapy in patients who develop asymptomatic ventricular ectopy.

PACEMAKERS AND IMPLANTABLE DEFIBRILLATORS

I. Indications for a Permanent Pacemaker
    A. Sick sinus syndrome
    B. Third-degree heart block (not secondary to drug effects)
    C. Mobitz type II second-degree heart block with symptomatic bradycardia
    D. Bifascicular or trifascicular block with recurrent syncope
    E. Atrial fibrillation or flutter or SVT with a high-grade AV block
    F. Neurocardiogenic syncope with carotid hypersensitivity
    G. Advanced second- or third-degree block after an acute MI if there is a block within the His-Purkinje system

II. Indications for a Temporary Pacemaker
    A. Symptomatic second- or third-degree heart block due to drug toxicity or electrolyte imbalance
    B. Mobitz II, complete heart block, or bifascicular block during an acute MI
    C. Any of the permanent indications while the patient is awaiting pacer placement

III. Electrodes
    A. Transcutaneous electrodes. Because of the extreme discomfort associated with the high current output, electrodes are only used temporarily until a transvenous pacer can be placed.
        1. Placement. Electrodes (large external adhesive gel-coated pads) are placed on the skin of the anterior left chest and on the left side of the back (below and medial to the scapula).
        2. Pacing modes. See p. 107.
        3. Settings
            a. An **output** of 40–100 mA must establish capture and then decrease to the minimum reliable current.
            b. Rate. Any rate, usually between 60 and 100 beats/min can be used.
    B. Epicardial wires
        1. Placement. These wires are placed during cardiac surgery.
            a. Atrial electrodes are placed high on the atrium. They should be separated by 1 cm to allow atrial monitoring and bipolar pacing.

b. Ventricular electrodes are placed on the anterior surface of the right ventricle 1 cm apart; alternatively, one electrode can be placed with the other attached to the skin as a ground.

c. Wires are then tunneled out to exit the skin of the anterior chest wall and secured with a suture.

d. Atrial electrocardiograph. The ECG arm leads are attached to the two atrial wires. Leg leads are placed as usual.

  (1) Lead I provides a **bipolar atrial** tracing.

  (2) Lead II provides a **unipolar atrial** tracing.

2. Care

  a. Skin sites should be kept meticulously clean and covered with a dressing.

  b. Electrodes need to be coiled and protected from inadvertent electrical contact or removal.

IV. Placement of Transvenous Pacers

  A. Central venous access is achieved by a **standard subclavian or jugular approach** with an introducer sheath.

  B. The **flow-directed transvenous pacer** is introduced and **directed via fluoroscopy** into the distal right ventricle. The tip is lodged in the trabeculae of the myocardium. Alternatively, a pacing **PA catheter** may be placed such that the electrodes lie in the right ventricle.

> *Only under extreme circumstances* should transvenous pacers be placed without fluoroscopic guidance.

  C. Special care should be taken to **avoid ventricular rupture,** especially in the setting of an inferior wall MI.

V. Placement of Permanent Pacemakers

  A. The pacemaker is placed **under fluoroscopic guidance,** because wires typically are advanced into the right atrium and ventricle and screwed into place.

  B. A **skin pocket** is created near the insertion site, and wires are tunneled to the pacemaker pocket.

VI. Types of Permanent Pacemakers and Settings. See **Table 5-9.**

VII. Common Modes

  A. Asynchronous (atrial or AOO) mode. This mode is used with **epicardial wires.**

  1. There is **no sensing of atrial activity;** the set rate is paced.

  2. This mode is **dangerous** because the pacing spike can cause R on T phenomenon, leading to ventricular fibrillation.

  3. Leads are connected to positive and negative atrial electrodes.

  4. Settings

  a. Output. The output is slowly decreased from maximal output in order to find the threshold and is then set at double the threshold.

  b. Sensitivity. There is no sensitivity in the asynchronous mode.

Table 5-9. Permanent Pacemakers: Types and Settings

Chamber paced

V = ventricle
A = atrium
D = dual
S = single

Chamber sensed

V = ventricle
A = atrium
D = dual
0 = none

Modes of response

I = inhibited
D = dual
R = reverse
T = triggered
0 = none

Programmable functions

R = responsive
M = multiprogrammable
P = rate, output, or both
0 = none

Antitachyarrhythmic functions

P = programmable
S = shock
D = dual (P + S)
0 = none

---

      c. Rate. The rate is typically 60–100 beats/min.
  B. Demand (ventricular or VVI) mode. This is the only mode suitable for a patient with **atrial fibrillation.**
    1. The pacer **senses and is inhibited by ventricular electrical activity** (normal R wave); if no activity is present, the pacer paces the ventricle.
    2. This mode cannot increase the heart rate with physiologic stress.
    3. Pacemaker syndrome can occur in this mode. Ventricular pacing in response to sinus bradycardia leads to the loss of AV synchrony or retrograde atrial conduction.
  C. Dual mode (DDD). This is the most common and physiologic mode.
    1. The pacer **senses atrial and ventricular activity and is in-**

hibited by both, such that if atrial depolarization is not followed by ventricular depolarization, the ventricle will be paced. If neither one occurs, the atrium and ventricle will be sequentially paced.

2. The dual mode is usually combined with rate responsiveness (R) or a multiprogrammable (M) feature for the most physiologic pacing.

D. **Overdrive atrial pacing** may be used to capture the atrium in atrial flutter or fibrillation and restore sinus rhythm.

E. **Overdrive ventricular pacing** may be used to capture the ventricle in ventricular tachycardia and may then be slowed down to a normal sinus rhythm.

VIII. **Automatic Implantable Cardiac Defibrillators (AICDs).** These devices provide back-up pacing for both physiologic bradycardia as well as bradycardia following AICD discharge. Newer devices can provide pacemaker and AICD function in one unit.

A. **Indications.** AICDs are used:
   1. In patients following resuscitated "sudden death"
   2. In patients with ventricular tachycardia or fibrillation
   3. In patients with intractable SVT

B. **Antiarrhythmic drug therapy.** The AICD is usually used in combination with antiarrhythmic drug therapy to suppress ventricular arrhythmia and decrease the number of discharges.

C. **Placement.** The AICD is placed subcutaneously with transvenous electrodes inserted in the right side of the heart. These electrodes monitor electrical activity and also defibrillate the patient.

D. **Common modes.** The AICD can be programmed to allow several modes of therapy, including antitachycardic pacing (similar to overdrive pacing) to escape VT and as a last-resort defibrillation at increasing energies (to a maximum of 34 J).

IX. **Troubleshooting**

A. **Common causes of pacemaker malfunction**
   1. Electrocautery
   2. Transthoracic defibrillation
   3. Magnetic resonance imaging
   4. Extracorporeal shock-wave lithotripsy
   5. Transcutaneous electrical nerve stimulation
   6. Therapeutic radiation
   7. Electroconvulsive therapy
   8. Radiofrequency ablation
   9. Low battery
   10. Lead fracture, disconnection, or dislodgement
   11. Inappropriate settings

B. **ECG signs of pacemaker malfunction**
   1. Lack of pacemaker spikes or artifact
   2. Failure to capture, despite evident spikes
   3. Inappropriate pacemaker artifact (undersensing)
   4. Inappropriate pacemaker rate

C. **Management.** If a pacemaker is malfunctioning, a magnet may be applied to set the pacemaker to a rate of 60 without inhibition.

SHOCK

I. **Etiologic Categories.** Shock can be classified into four basic types: hypovolemic, cardiogenic, vasogenic, and neurogenic. The basis of all of these types of shock is **inadequate tissue perfusion.** Shock is caused by an oxygen debt, which leads to anaerobic metabolism and acidosis. Resuscitation involves correcting the balance between oxygen delivery and oxygen requirements.

II. **Classes of Shock.** See **Table 5-10.**

III. **Goals of Therapy**
   A. Restore adequate tissue perfusion and oxygen delivery.
   B. Improve oxygen delivery.
      1. Keep the arterial oxyhemoglobin saturation above 90%.
      2. In patients who do not respond quickly to fluid therapy, transfuse packed red blood cells (RBCs) to a hemoglobin of 11–13 g/dl.
      3. Optimize cardiac output. Keep the cardiac index above 2.5 L/min/m².
   C. Review HEMODYNAMIC MONITORING AND ALTERATIONS IN HEMODYNAMICS earlier in this chapter, p. 79.

IV. **Hypovolemic Shock.** Loss of body fluids occurs in an amount sufficient to cause intravascular volume depletion to the extent that compensatory mechanisms fail to restore normal perfusion.

Table 5-10.   Classes of Shock

Characteristics	Class 1	Class 2	Class 3	Class 4
Blood loss (ml)	<750	750–1500	1500–2000	>2000
Blood loss (%)	<15	15–30	30–40	>40
Pulse rate (beats/min)	<100	>100	>120	>140
Blood pressure	Normal	Normal	↓	↓
Pulse pressure	Normal/↑	↓	↓	↓
Capillary refill	Normal	+	+	+
Respiratory rate (breaths/min)	14–20	20–30	30–40	>35
Urine (ml/hr)	>30	20–30	5–15	Negligible
Mental status	Slightly anxious	Anxious	Confused	Lethargic
Fluid replacement	Crystalloid	Crystalloid	Crystalloid/ blood	Crystalloid/ blood

(Adapted with permission from ACS Committee on Trauma: *Advanced Trauma Life Support® Student Manual,* p 86. Chicago, American College of Surgeons, 1993.)

A. Physical examination and initial management
  1. **Airway.** Ensure that the patient's airway is open.
  2. **Breathing.** In severe shock, intubate.
  3. **Circulation.** Control hemorrhage.
  4. **Disability.** Perform a complete neurologic evaluation.
  5. **Exposure.** Perform a complete examination of all skin surfaces.
  6. **Gastric decompression.** Decompress the stomach using an orogastric tube.
  7. **Urinary catheter insertion.** After checking for possible pelvic fractures, insert a Foley catheter (this is not a priority).
B. Vascular access. Insert two large-bore peripheral IV catheters (a minimum of 14–16 gauge) because they have the highest flow rates. You may then proceed with central access.
C. Initial fluid therapy. All fluid and blood should be warmed or run through a high-flow/high-volume fluid warmer.
  1. **Begin** with the following:
     a. **Adult:** 2 L isotonic fluid
     b. **Child:** 20 ml/kg isotonic fluid
  2. **If the patient is still hypotensive** after the initial bolus, give blood.
  3. **Evaluate** the patient's response to fluid therapy.
     a. A **rapid response** usually indicates that only a small amount of blood was lost. If the patient remains hemodynamically stable after the initial bolus, change the fluid to a maintenance rate.
     b. If there is a **transient response,** fluids must be continued and blood must be replaced. The patient may need surgical intervention.
     c. **If the patient does not respond** to treatment with fluid or blood, **pump failure** must be considered. Immediate operative intervention may be needed to control exsanguinating hemorrhage.
D. If the patient does not respond to the initial fluid therapy (2 liters), begin packed RBC administration. If the need for blood is emergent, start with O-negative blood until type-specific and cross-matched blood is available. The goal is to maintain the patient's temperature and volume while avoiding coagulopathy.
  1. Heat the room and warm all fluids. You must **keep the patient warm.**
  2. After 6 units of packed RBCs have been transfused, check the patient's **prothrombin time** and transfuse fresh frozen plasma when necessary.
  3. After 8 units of packed RBCs have been given, check the **platelet count** and transfuse platelets if necessary.
  4. Follow the patient's **laboratory results** closely.
  5. **Calcium** may need to be administered in the case of a high-volume blood infusion.

    E. Determine whether the patient needs operative therapy or if the patient should go directly to ICU.

V. Cardiac Shock

  A. Compressive shock. Normovolemic patients will have **distended neck veins.** (Distended veins may not be seen in hypovolemic patients until they have been resuscitated with fluid.) Look for the following **causes** of compressive shock:

    1. Tension pneumothorax. The trachea shifts to the opposite side with decreased breath sounds. **Management** consists of inserting a 14-gauge angiocatheter in the second intercostal space, followed by **chest tube** placement.

    2. Cardiac tamponade

      a. Signs

        (1) Hypotension

        (2) Muffled heart sounds

        (3) Distended neck veins

        (4) Pulsus paradoxus: > 10 mm Hg drop in systolic blood pressure (SBP) with inspiration

      b. Management. Treat with **pericardiocentesis** (see Chapter 42 for technique) or a pericardial window.

    3. Positive-pressure ventilation. This is seen with tidal volumes > 12 ml/kg or a PEEP > 10 cm H_2O. Treat with **volume expansion.**

  B. Cardiogenic shock. This is usually caused by cardiac disease or by trauma when the heart is unable to generate an adequate cardiac output to maintain tissue perfusion.

    1. Etiology

      a. Arrhythmias

      b. MI

      c. Cardiomyopathy

      d. Valvular dysfunction

      e. Pulmonary vascular obstruction (embolus)

      f. Pericarditis

      g. Severe ventricular hypertrophy

    2. Management

      a. Optimize filling pressures.

      b. Provide inotropic support with dopamine, dobutamine, or epinephrine therapy.

      c. Use an intra-aortic balloon pump for refractory cases.

      d. Treat arrhythmias.

      e. Reduce vascular resistance with nitroglycerin or nitroprusside therapy.

      f. For an acute MI, use thrombolytic therapy and invasive treatment.

VI. Neurogenic Shock. This type of shock usually results from a **spinal cord injury, regional anesthesia,** or **autonomic blockade.** Isolated head injuries do not cause shock; you must look for other causes.

  A. Mechanism. There is a loss of vasomotor control and expansion of venous capacitance with inadequate ventricular filling and low cardiac output. The sympathetic nervous system fails to maintain normal vascular tone.

B. **Signs.** The patient may have warm, well perfused skin, low BP, normal to low urine output, low SVR, and a normal cardiac output. The patient with **spinal shock** may have the following:
1. Depressed spontaneous respirations
2. Diaphragmatic weakness
3. Decreased chest wall and lung compliance (Ineffective cough due to paralysis of the intercostal/abdominal musculature may result in lobar collapse.)

C. **Physical examination**
1. Give the patient a thorough neurologic examination at standard intervals.
2. Follow the ABCs of trauma assessment.

D. **Initial management**
1. Correct filling pressures with fluids.
2. Maintain Trendelenburg positioning.
3. Use vasoconstrictors (e.g., phenylephrine, norepinephrine) to restore venous tone.
4. Maintain the patient's body temperature.
5. If a **spinal cord injury** is present or suspected, proceed with the Solu-Medrol protocol:
   a. Give a bolus of 30 mg/kg of Solu-Medrol over 15 minutes.
   b. If the bolus is given **within 3 hours of injury,** follow up with a maintenance dose of 5.4 mg/kg/hr for 23 hours as a continuous infusion.
   c. If **more than 3 hours has elapsed** since the injury occurred, continue the infusion for 47 hours.

E. **Management in the ICU**
1. **Cardiovascular management** includes:
   a. Hemodynamic monitoring
   b. Arrhythmia precautions
   c. Inotropes
2. **Pulmonary management** includes:
   a. Frequent suctioning and incentive spirometry
   b. Ventilatory support with PEEP or large tidal volumes
   c. Bronchoscopy
3. **Gastrointestinal management** includes:
   a. Nasogastric suction for gastric atony, dilatation, and ileus
   b. Feeding tube

VII. **Vasogenic Shock.** Vasogenic shock includes systemic inflammatory response syndrome (SIRS), septic shock, traumatic shock, hypoadrenal shock, and anaphylactic shock. Endogenous or exogenous vasoactive mediators are believed to play a major role in the pathophysiology. Arteriolar and venous vasomotor tone are decreased.

A. **Clinical manifestations**
1. Hyperthermia or hypothermia
2. Leukocytosis or leukopenia
3. Tachycardia and tachypnea
4. Hypotension

     5. Metabolic abnormalities (e.g., lactic acidosis)
     6. Altered mental status
     7. Hypoxemia
     8. Oliguria
     9. Multiple organ dysfunction (see Chapter 13)

B. Predisposing conditions
     1. ARDS
     2. Major trauma or burns
     3. Diabetes mellitus
     4. Extremes of age
     5. Renal and hepatic failure
     6. Immunosuppression (organ transplantation, AIDS)
     7. Malignancy
     8. Malnutrition
     9. Indwelling catheters

C. Septic shock
     1. **Gram-positive bacteria—Clostridium, Staphylococcus, Enterococcus, and Streptococcus species**
          a. **Mechanism.** Massive fluid losses occur secondary to dissemination of cell wall components that initiate inflammation identical to that caused by gram-negative endotoxin or gram-positive exotoxin (often without bacteremia).
          b. **Clinical manifestations.** The patient may be hypotensive but have a normal urine output.
          c. **Management** involves IV antibiotics, fluids to correct volume deficit, and, most importantly, removal of the source.

     2. **Gram-negative bacteria—Escherichia coli, Pseudomonas, Klebsiella, Enterobacteriaceae, Serratia, and Bacteroides**
          a. **Mechanism.** Shock is initiated by endotoxin in the cell walls of these bacteria, which results in a diffuse increase in microvascular permeability. The source may be (in decreasing frequency) urinary tract, pulmonary, alimentary tract, burn, or soft tissue infection.
          b. **Clinical manifestations**
             (1) Increased fluid requirement
             (2) Hypermetabolism
             (3) Fever
             (4) Decreased blood pressure and perfusion of vital organs,
             (5) Increased cardiac output (low SVR)
             (6) Vasodilation
          c. **Risks.** The patient is at high risk for multisystem organ failure and acute respiratory distress syndrome (ARDS).
          d. **Management** involves identification of the source, placement of a PA catheter, and administration of IV fluids and vasopressors.

     3. **Fungi—Candida species.** Septic shock caused by fungi is

more common in neutropenic, immunosuppressed, multitrauma, and burn patients.

a. Risk factors include indwelling catheters, broad-spectrum antibiotics, and hyperalimentation.

b. Mechanism. *Candida* forms microabscesses in the microcirculation.

c. Clinical manifestations. The patient has high fevers and shaking chills, and may be hypothermic. Blood cultures are positive in 50% of patients.

d. Management involves fluconazole or amphotericin B as renal function permits.

4. **General management of the septic patient**

a. Hemodynamic management is done to optimize the patient's BP, volume status, and renal perfusion.

b. Consider **ventilatory support.**

c. Place a **PA catheter.**

d. Resuscitate the patient **with fluid.**

e. If volume resuscitation does not improve the patient's condition, start the patient on **vasoactive medications.**

(1) Start an infusion of **dopamine** at 3–5 μg/kg/min and increase the rate as needed to a maximum of 15–20 μg/kg/min.

(2) Determine the patient's **cardiac index** and **MAP.** If the cardiac index is below $2\ L/min/m^2$ and the MAP is appropriately elevated owing to the dopamine therapy, start an infusion of dobutamine at a rate of 1–2 μg/kg/min and then increase the rate as the patient's BP tolerates to a cardiac index > 2.

(3) **If the patient remains hypotensive** and has an adequate cardiac index, you will need to start a second agent.

(a) **If the patient's heart rate is > 120,** start therapy with **norepinephrine** at a rate of 2–4 μg/min and increase the rate as needed.

(b) **If the heart rate is < 100,** start therapy with **epinephrine** at a rate of 2–20 μg/min (0.025–0.3 μg/kg/min).

(c) Once these agents have begun, try to titrate the dopamine down.

f. Institute **stress ulcer prophylaxis.**

g. Prescribe the appropriate **antibiotics or antifungal agents.**

h. Begin **nutritional support** with early enteral feedings as soon as possible.

D. Anaphylactic and anaphylactoid shock

1. **Definitions**

a. Anaphylaxis is an allergic response, that is, the patient has been presensitized to an antigen (e.g., a drug, insect venom, a food item). Anaphylaxis is **mediated by immunoglobulin E (IgE)** antibody–induced mast cell degranulation.

b. **Anaphylactoid reactions** are **independent of IgE.** Types of anaphylactoid reactions include:

   (1) IgE-independent mast cell degranulation, which can occur with contrast media, opiates, and neuromuscular blockade agents

   (2) Complement mediated reactions (e.g., induced by blood products)

   (3) Reactions to NSAIDs, which biochemically favor leukotriene synthesis over prostaglandins

   (4) Idiopathic reactions

2. **Mechanism of action and clinical manifestations.** Release of mediators (e.g., kinins, histamine, prostaglandins) leads to various symptoms:

   a. Vasodilation

   b. Increase capillary permeability

   c. Bronchospasm

   d. Airway edema

   e. Circulatory collapse due to decreased MAP and cardiac output

3. **Management**

   a. Ensure an adequate **airway** and provide the patient with supplemental **oxygen.**

   b. Administer **epinephrine** to alleviate the hemodynamic effects of circulating mediators and to decrease mediator synthesis.

      (1) For **mild to moderate** reactions, treat the patient with 0.3–0.5 ml epinephrine in 1:1000 dilution subcutaneously. This dose may be repeated every 10 to 20 minutes.

      (2) For **severe reactions with hypotension:**

         (a) Provide the patient with fluid resuscitation.

         (b) Give the patient epinephrine at a rate of 0.5–5 µg/min continuous IV or a bolus IV of 0.1–0.2 ml of 1:1000 in 10 ml saline.

   c. Treat **bronchospasm** with an albuterol nebulizer.

   d. Administer **corticosteroids, aminophylline, and antihistamines** as secondary therapy.

   e. **If hypotension persists,** treat the patient with fluids and norepinephrine.

E. **Hypoadrenal shock** (shock due to adrenocortical insufficiency) is uncommon but may be considered in patients with a history of glucocorticoid therapy or hypotension of unknown etiology. A **high index of suspicion** is needed. For the diagnosis and treatment, see ADRENAL INSUFFICIENCY in Chapter 7.

SHORTNESS OF BREATH

I. **Initial assessment**
   A. **Level of consciousness.** If the patient has an altered mental status, initiate ACLS.
   B. **Airway.** Ensure airway patency, and intubate the patient if necessary.
   C. **Breathing.** Assess the patient's rate and quality of ventilation.
   D. **Circulation.** Identify the patient's pulse and its quality; if no pulse is present, initiate ACLS.

II. **Secondary assessment**
   A. **Initial treatment**
      1. Provide the patient with supplemental **oxygen** and monitor the patient's oxygen saturation level.
      2. **Elevate the head of the patient's bed** to improve respiratory mechanics.
      3. Obtain arterial **blood gases** and an immediate portable **chest radiograph.**
   B. **History**
      1. Ask the patient when and how the shortness of breath began and also what the patient was doing at that time.
      2. Obtain a pertinent medical history, including any history of cardiac and pulmonary disease.
      3. Ask the patient what medications he or she is currently taking.
      4. Ask the patient whether he or she has a history of smoking.
      5. Assess the patient's level of pain, dyspnea, and anxiety.
      6. Assess the patient's volume status.
   C. **Physical examination**
      1. **Airway.** Ensure that the patient has an adequate airway, and check for any upper airway compromise.
      2. **Lungs.** Listen for breath sounds bilaterally, and compare and identify any diminished breath sounds, focal consolidation, crackles, wheezes, or stridor.
      3. **Heart.** Assess the patient's heart rate. Be alert for any murmurs, rubs, or gallops, or the presence of a pulsus paradoxus. Note the location of PMI and the degree of jugular venous distention.
      4. **Extremities.** Assess the patient's pulses. Note the degree of edema and any cyanosis.
   D. **Diagnostic work-up**
      1. Evaluate the patient's chest radiograph and arterial blood gases.
      2. Draw blood for CBC, electrolytes, BUN, creatinine, and relevant drug levels, and obtain a urine sample.
      3. Ensure that the patient has adequate peripheral IV access.

III. **Etiology and Management.** Treatment depends on the established etiology.

A. Hypervolemia/CHF/pulmonary edema
1. Initiate diuresis with furosemide therapy.
2. Give the patient morphine if he or she is alert and normotensive.
3. Prescribe nitroglycerin if the patient's BP tolerates it.

B. Stridor secondary to an upper airway obstruction
1. Prescribe racemic epinephrine nebulizer therapy.
2. Intubate the patient immediately with an anesthesiologist's assistance if possible.
3. Order epinephrine 0.3–0.5 ml (1:1000) SQ.
4. Order high-dose steroids, such as Decadron 4–10 mg IV q 6 hr.

C. Pneumothorax. Place a thoracostomy tube immediately.

D. Anaphylaxis. Administer fluids and SQ epinephrine.

E. Asthma/COPD exacerbation
1. Give the patient albuterol and ipratropium therapy via a nebulizer as needed.
2. If the nebulizer treatment does not help, order a 125-mg bolus IV of Solu-Medrol followed by 40–60 mg q 6–8 hr IV.

F. Pneumonia. Initiate the appropriate antimicrobial therapy.

G. Bronchial mucus plugging
1. Ensure that the patient has adequate chest physical therapy and postural drainage.
2. Consider acetylcysteine nebulizer therapy to decrease sputum viscosity.

H. Aspiration
1. Institute NPO orders.
2. Do a formal evaluation of the patient's ability to swallow.
3. Observe the patient for development of aspiration pneumonia.

I. Pulmonary embolus
1. Initiate empiric heparin therapy.
2. Order either ventilation/perfusion scanning or a pulmonary angiogram to make the diagnosis.

J. MI. Initiate the appropriate therapy.

K. Anxiety. Administer anxiolytic agents.

SYNCOPE

I. Definition. Syncope is a sudden, transient loss of consciousness caused by diminished cerebral blood flow and associated with a loss of postural tone. Recovery is usually spontaneous.

II. Etiology. See **Table 5-11.**

III. History
A. Ask witnesses for their observations about the syncopal episode:
1. Did the patient have any **prodromal symptoms**?
2. Did the patient have **tongue biting or incontinence**?
3. Did the **body movements** occur **before or after the loss**

Table 5-11. Causes of Syncope

CARDIOVASCULAR CAUSES

I. Neurally Mediated Syncope
  A. Neurocardiogenic causes
  B. Situational causes
    1. Postprandial
    2. Tussive
    3. Valsalva-related (e.g., weight lifting, defecation, micturition)
  C. Syncope related to carotid sinus hypersensitivity
  D. Syncope related to autonomic insufficiency (orthostatic hypotension)

II. Neurally Independent Syncope
  A. Mechanical causes
    1. Aortic stenosis
    2. Atrial myxoma
    3. Pulmonary embolus or hypertension
    4. Prosthetic valve dysfunction
    5. Hypertrophic cardiomyopathy
    6. Cardiac ischemia or MI
    7. Aortic dissection
  B. Hypovolemia
  C. Arrhythmias

NON-CARDIOVASCULAR CAUSES

I. Neurologic Causes
  A. Vertebrobasilar insufficiency
  B. Normal pressure hydrocephalus
  C. Epilepsy
  D. Subclavian steal syndrome
  E. Drug or alcohol related

II. Psychogenic Causes
  A. Panic disorders
  B. Depression

---

of consciousness? (In syncope, the loss of consciousness precedes any tonic–clonic movement.)
  B. Obtain the patient's **medication history.**
  C. Obtain the patient's **cardiac and pulmonary history.**
  D. Ask about **chronic or underlying illnesses.**
IV. Physical Examination
  A. Do a complete physical examination, paying special attention to the list of **underlying etiologies** in Table 5-11 (to narrow the field of investigation and to determine management).
  B. Look for **carotid bruits.**

    C. Check **pupillary response** and **visual fields.**

    D. Do a complete **neurologic examination.**

V. Diagnostic Tests

    A. Obtain an **electrocardiogram** for evaluation.

    B. Order the following **laboratory tests:** CBC, platelets, electrolytes, BUN, creatinine, glucose, Ca, Mg, PO_4, and cardiac enzymes.

    C. Depending on the results of the electrocardiogram and laboratory tests, additional studies may be indicated, as follows:

        1. Holter monitoring and 30-day event monitoring

        2. Electrophysiologic studies

        3. Echocardiography

        4. Magnetic resonance angiography (MRA) of the vertebrobasilar system

        5. CT scan of the brain

        6. Carotid ultrasound

        7. EEG

        8. Tilt table testing (for diagnosis of syncope due to neurocardiogenic causes)

VI. Mechanism / Signs and Symptoms / Management. Signs and symptoms can help pinpoint the cause of the syncope, which will determine patient management.

    A. Syncope due to cardiovascular causes

        1. Neurally mediated syncope

            a. Neurocardiogenic causes. The trigger may be **pain, fear, or emotional stress.** Syncope typically occurs when the patient is standing. The patient may have a prodrome of nausea, warmth, lightheadedness, weakness, or visual disturbances. The treatment of choice is **β-blocker therapy.** If this treatment is not therapeutic, other drugs, such as oral theophylline, disopyramide, fluoxetine, or midodrine, may be used.

            b. Carotid sinus hypersensitivity. Patients with this diagnosis may develop symptoms of syncope with abrupt head turning, shaving, or wearing a tight collar. Treatment is **carotid sinus massage** performed at the bedside with the aid of ECG and blood pressure monitoring. A **permanent pacemaker** may be required for patients with chronic carotid sinus hypersensitivity.

        2. Neurally independent syncope

            a. Mechanical causes. Syncope due to obstructive disorders of the heart usually presents during exercise because of increased demands on the heart with fixed cardiac output. Syncope may be a sign of the following obstructive disorders:

                (1) Aortic stenosis. Syncope is a classic presentation. Treatment consists of aortic valve replacement.

                (2) Left atrial myxoma or clot. This mass may occlude the mitral valve and prevent left ventricular filling. Treatment is surgical removal.

                (3) Hypertrophic cardiomyopathy in young athletes.

Reduced myocardial blood flow during contraction results in myocardial ischemia and ventricular arrhythmias, often causing sudden death.

(4) **Pulmonary hypertension and pulmonary arterial spasm.** These conditions may lead to reduced left ventricular preload, which can cause sudden death.

(5) **Myocardial ischemia.** MI can result in cardiogenic shock or ventricular arrhythmias.

b. **Hypovolemic syncope.** This usually occurs secondary to massive hemorrhage or acute fluid loss. See *Hypovolemic Shock,* p. 110.

c. **Arrhythmias.** See p. 59.

B. **Syncope due to noncardiovascular causes**

1. **Neurologic causes.** Less than 5% of syncope cases are due purely to neurologic disorders.

a. **Vertebrobasilar insufficiency** occurring with a TIA may be due to compression from an intracranial tumor or atherosclerosis. Symptoms are due to temporary bilateral cerebral dysfunction and brain stem dysfunction, and include vertigo, diplopia, ataxia, dysarthria, weakness, and numbness. The vertebral arteries may be externally compressed from cervical ribs, osteoarthritis or cervical spondylosis, which results in syncope when the person turns or hyperextends the head. Severe hypoxemia, hypoglycemia, and hypercapnia may occur. This system must be assessed by MRA or conventional angiography.

2. **Psychogenic causes.** Panic disorder and depression may present with apprehension, motor twitching, and hyperventilation.

ADVANCED CARDIAC LIFE SUPPORT PROTOCOLS. See Figures 5-8 through 5-15.

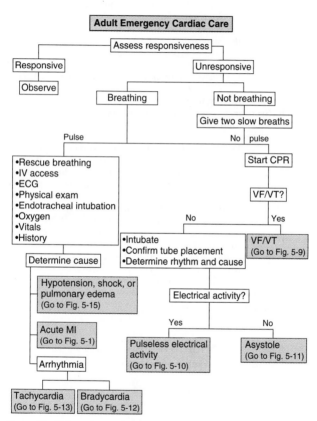

Figure 5-8. Universal algorithm for adult emergency cardiac care. *CPR* = cardiopulmonary resuscitation; *ECG* = electrocardiogram; *MI* = myocardial infarction; *VF/VT* = ventricular fibrillation/ventricular tachycardia. (Adapted with permission from Emergency Cardiac Care Committee, American Heart Association: Guidelines of cardiopulmonary resuscitation and emergency cardiac care. *JAMA* 268[16]:2216–2227, 1992.)

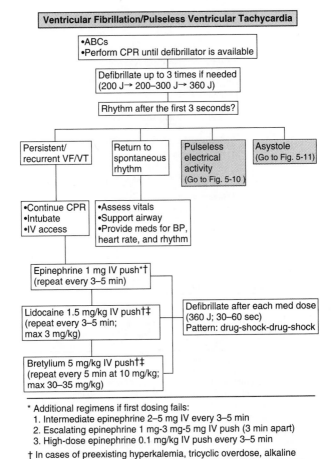

Ventricular Fibrillation/Pulseless Ventricular Tachycardia

• ABCs
• Perform CPR until defibrillator is available

Defibrillate up to 3 times if needed
(200 J → 200–300 J → 360 J)

Rhythm after the first 3 seconds?

Persistent/recurrent VF/VT

Return to spontaneous rhythm

Pulseless electrical activity
(Go to Fig. 5-10)

Asystole
(Go to Fig. 5-11)

• Continue CPR
• Intubate
• IV access

• Assess vitals
• Support airway
• Provide meds for BP, heart rate, and rhythm

Epinephrine 1 mg IV push*†
(repeat every 3–5 min)

Lidocaine 1.5 mg/kg IV push†‡
(repeat every 3–5 min; max 3 mg/kg)

Bretylium 5 mg/kg IV push†‡
(repeat every 5 min at 10 mg/kg; max 30–35 mg/kg)

Defibrillate after each med dose
(360 J; 30–60 sec)
Pattern: drug-shock-drug-shock

* Additional regimens if first dosing fails:
1. Intermediate epinephrine 2–5 mg IV every 3–5 min
2. Escalating epinephrine 1 mg-3 mg-5 mg IV push (3 min apart)
3. High-dose epinephrine 0.1 mg/kg IV push every 3–5 min

† In cases of preexisting hyperkalemia, tricyclic overdose, alkaline urine, and long arrest interval, use sodium bicarbonate 1 mEq/kg IV.

‡ In cases of torsades de pointes or severe refractory VF, use magnesium sulfate 1–2 g IV. In cases of refractory VF, use procainamide 30 mg/min (max 17 mg/kg).

Figure 5-9. Algorithm for the treatment of ventricular fibrillation and pulseless ventricular tachycardia (VF/VT). Note that hypothermic cardiac arrest is treated differently. *ABC* = airway, breathing, circulation; *CPR* = cardiopulmonary resuscitation. (Adapted with permission from Emergency Cardiac Care Committee, American Heart Association: Guidelines of cardiopulmonary resuscitation and emergency cardiac care. *JAMA* 268[16]:2216–2227, 1992.)

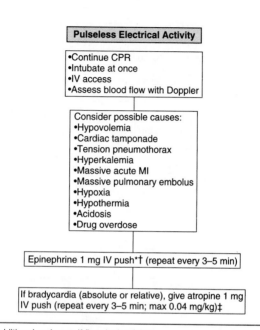

Pulseless Electrical Activity

•Continue CPR
•Intubate at once
•IV access
•Assess blood flow with Doppler

Consider possible causes:
•Hypovolemia
•Cardiac tamponade
•Tension pneumothorax
•Hyperkalemia
•Massive acute MI
•Massive pulmonary embolus
•Hypoxia
•Hypothermia
•Acidosis
•Drug overdose

Epinephrine 1 mg IV push*† (repeat every 3–5 min)

If bradycardia (absolute or relative), give atropine 1 mg IV push (repeat every 3–5 min; max 0.04 mg/kg)‡

---

* Additional regimens if first dosing fails:
 1. Intermediate epinephrine 2–5 mg IV every 3–5 min
 2. Escalating epinephrine 1 mg-3 mg-5 mg IV push (3 min apart)
 3. High-dose epinephrine 0.1 mg/kg IV push every 3–5 min

† In cases of preexisting hyperkalemia, tricyclic overdose, hypoxic lactic acidosis, alkaline urine, and long arrest interval, use sodium bicarbonate 1 mEq/kg IV.

‡ Shorter atropine dosing intervals may be helpful in cardiac arrest.

Figure 5-10. Algorithm for the treatment of pulseless electrical activity (electromechanical dissociation), which includes pseudoelectromechanical dissociation, idioventricular rhythms, ventricular escape rhythms, bradysystolic rhythms, and postdefibrillation rhythms. *CPR* = cardiopulmonary resuscitation; *MI* = myocardial infarction. (Adapted with permission from Emergency Cardiac Care Committee, American Heart Association: Guidelines of cardiopulmonary resuscitation and emergency cardiac care. *JAMA* 268[16]:2216–2227, 1992.)

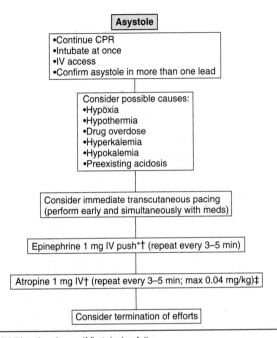

Asystole

- Continue CPR
- Intubate at once
- IV access
- Confirm asystole in more than one lead

Consider possible causes:
- Hypoxia
- Hypothermia
- Drug overdose
- Hyperkalemia
- Hypokalemia
- Preexisting acidosis

Consider immediate transcutaneous pacing
(perform early and simultaneously with meds)

Epinephrine 1 mg IV push*† (repeat every 3–5 min)

Atropine 1 mg IV† (repeat every 3–5 min; max 0.04 mg/kg)‡

Consider termination of efforts

---

* Additional regimens if first dosing fails:
  1. Intermediate epinephrine 2–5 mg IV every 3–5 min
  2. Escalating epinephrine 1 mg-3 mg-5 mg IV push (3 min apart)
  3. High-dose epinephrine 0.1 mg/kg IV push every 3–5 min

† In cases of preexisting hyperkalemia, tricyclic overdose,
hypoxic lactic acidosis, alkaline urine, and long arrest interval,
use sodium bicarbonate 1 mEq/kg IV.

‡ Shorter atropine dosing intervals may be helpful in cardiac arrest.

Figure 5-11. Algorithm for the treatment of asystole. *CPR* =
cardiopulmonary resuscitation. (Adapted with permission from Emergency
Cardiac Care Committee, American Heart Association: Guidelines of
cardiopulmonary resuscitation and emergency cardiac care. *JAMA*
268[16]:2216–2227, 1992.)

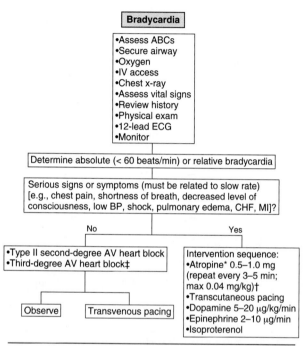

Bradycardia

•Assess ABCs
•Secure airway
•Oxygen
•IV access
•Chest x-ray
•Assess vital signs
•Review history
•Physical exam
•12-lead ECG
•Monitor

Determine absolute (< 60 beats/min) or relative bradycardia

Serious signs or symptoms (must be related to slow rate)
[e.g., chest pain, shortness of breath, decreased level of
consciousness, low BP, shock, pulmonary edema, CHF, MI]?

No — Yes

•Type II second-degree AV heart block
•Third-degree AV heart block‡

Observe — Transvenous pacing

Intervention sequence:
•Atropine* 0.5–1.0 mg
(repeat every 3–5 min;
max 0.04 mg/kg)†
•Transcutaneous pacing
•Dopamine 5–20 µg/kg/min
•Epinephrine 2–10 µg/min
•Isoproterenol

* Denervated, transplanted hearts do not respond to atropine.
Go straight to pacing and/or catecholamine infusion.

† Shorter dosing intervals may be used in severe clinical conditions.

‡ Never treat third-degree heart block plus ventricular escape
beats with lidocaine.

Figure 5-12. Algorithm for the treatment of bradycardia (the patient is not in
cardiac arrest). *ABC* = airway, breathing, circulation; *AV* = atrioventricular;
BP = blood pressure; *CHF* = congestive heart failure; *ECG* =
electrocardiogram; *MI* = myocardial infarction. (Adapted with permission from
Emergency Cardiac Care Committee, American Heart Association:
Guidelines of cardiopulmonary resuscitation and emergency cardiac care.
JAMA 268[16]:2216–2227, 1992.)

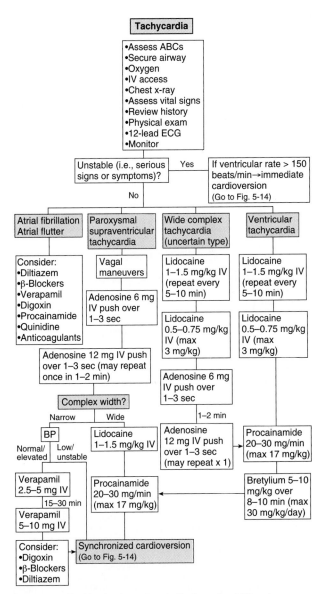

Figure 5-13. Algorithm for the treatment of tachycardia. *ABC* = airway, breathing, circulation; *BP* = blood pressure; *ECG* = electrocardiogram. (Adapted with permission from Emergency Cardiac Care Committee, American Heart Association: Guidelines of cardiopulmonary resuscitation and emergency cardiac care. *JAMA* 268[16]:2216–2227, 1992.)

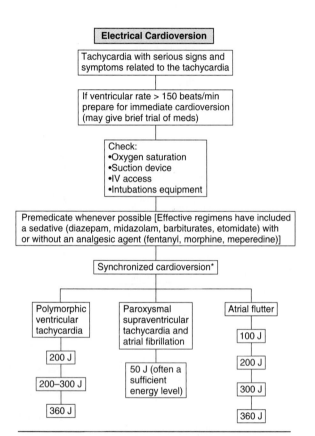

Figure 5-14. Algorithm for electrical cardioversion (the patient is not in cardiac arrest). (Adapted with permission from Emergency Cardiac Care Committee, American Heart Association: Guidelines of cardiopulmonary resuscitation and emergency cardiac care. *JAMA* 268[16]:2216–2227, 1992.)

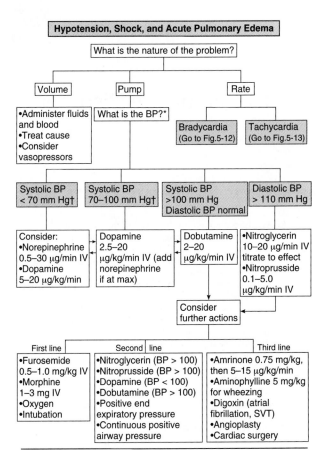

Figure 5-15. Algorithm for the treatment of hypotension, shock, and acute pulmonary edema. *BP* = blood pressure; *DBP* = diastolic blood pressure; *SBP* = systolic blood pressure; *SVT* = supraventricular tachycardia. (Adapted with permission from Emergency Cardiac Care Committee, American Heart Association: Guidelines of cardiopulmonary resuscitation and emergency cardiac care. *JAMA* 268[16]:2216–2227, 1992.)

6

Dermatologic Disorders

APPROACH TO THE DERMATOLOGIC PATIENT

I. History
   A. Ask the patient about the **onset** of the eruption.
   B. Inquire whether the **course** of the eruption has been intermittent, transient, or continuous.
   C. Ask about the **location** of the eruption at the onset and through its development.
   D. Ask about any **associated symptoms** (e.g., pruritus, pain, burning).
   E. Obtain a detailed pre- and post-admission **drug history.**
   F. Obtain the patient's **medical and dermatologic history.**
   G. Ask whether the patient has any **allergies.**
   H. Obtain the patient's **occupational, sexual, and travel history.**
   I. Ask whether the patient has a **family history** of dermatologic problems.

II. Dermatologic Examination
   A. Total body skin examination (TBSE). Do a general skin examination, including palms, soles, interdigital web spaces, mucous membranes, scalp and hair, nails, and external genitalia.
   B. Observation and palpation
      1. Note the **general condition** of the patient's skin.
      2. Note the **distribution of the eruption.**
      3. Describe the **primary lesion** (**Table 6-1**).
      4. Note the **shape of the primary lesion** (annular, targetlike, arciform, linear, round or oval, or umbilicated).
      5. Note the **arrangement of multiple primary lesions** (isolated, scattered, grouped or clustered, herpetiform, zosteriform, annular or arciform, linear, or reticulated).
      6. Note the **characteristics of the primary lesion.**
         a. Color
         b. Consistency or feel
         c. Presence of secondary change (scale, crust, excoriation, atrophy, or sclerosis)

III. Bedside Diagnostic Techniques. See **Table 6-2.**

Table 6-1. Common Skin Lesions

MACULE: Smaller than 1 cm
PATCH: Larger than 1 cm

Macule: a circumscribed, flat lesion without change in elevation or depression, which differs from the surrounding skin in color; its diameter is < 1 cm
Patch: a macule > 1 cm

PAPULE: Smaller than 1 cm
PLAQUE: Larger than 1 cm

Papule: a small, < 1 cm in diameter; solid, elevated lesion; the major portion of the lesion projects above the surface of the skin
Plaque: a mesa-like elevation that occupies a relatively large surface area compared with its height above skin level; often formed by a confluence of papules

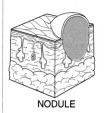

NODULE

Nodule: a palpable, solid lesion deeper than a papule; located in the dermis or subcutaneous tissue

VESICLE: Smaller than 1 cm
BULLA: larger than 1 cm

Vesicle: a circumscribed, thin-walled, elevated lesion that contains fluid; diameter < 1 cm
Bulla: a vesicle > 1 cm in diameter

continued

Table 6-1. Common Skin Lesions (*continued*)

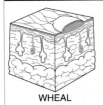

WHEAL

Wheal: a rounded or flat-topped elevated papule or plaque that disappears in hours

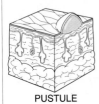

PUSTULE

Pustule: a circumscribed, raised lesion that contains purulent exudate

Abscess: a localized accumulation of purulent material deep in the dermis or SQ tissue; pus is not usually visible

Purpura: a nonblanching, purple discoloration in the skin due to extravasation of blood into the skin; may be palpable or nonpalpable

  Petechiae: purpura < 1 cm

  Ecchymosis: purpura > 1 cm

Erosion: a moist, circumscribed, usually depressed lesion; loss of all or a portion of the viable epidermis

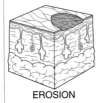

EROSION

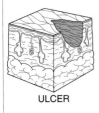

ULCER

Ulcer: a depressed lesion in which the epidermis and at least the upper dermis have been destroyed

Telangiectasia: a blanchable, small, superficial dilated capillary

Table 6-2. Dermatologic Bedside Diagnostic Techniques

Procedure	Indication	Technique	Findings
Diascopy	To distinguish erythema from purpura	Compress the skin lesion with a microscope slide.	Erythema blanches; true purpura has no blanching
Wood's lamp	To identify fluorescence	Examine the skin with low-intensity ultraviolet light in a dark room at a distance of 6 inches.	**Tinea capitis:** blue-green **Tinea corporis, versicolor** and **cruris:** faint green **Erythrasma:** coral-red **Pseudomonas:** yellow-green urine porphyrins **Porphyria cutanea tarda (PCT):** bright red
Potassium hydroxide (KOH)	To dissolve the keratin and allow clearer visualization of fungal elements	1. Scrape the border of the scaly lesion or the roof of the blister with scalpel. 2. Place the scrapings on the slide. 3. Add 2 drops of KOH for 2–5 min. 4. View under a microscope.	**Dermatophytes:** septae **Candida:** grape-like cluster of spores or a linear arrangement of spores forming pseudohyphae **Mycoplasma furfur:** a combination of short, septate hyphae and spores in clusters (i.e., "spaghetti and meatballs")
Gram's stain	To identify the bacteria	1. Wipe the target area. 2. Obtain pustular exudate with a scalpel. 3. Fix the material to slide by gently heating. 4. Apply crystal violet for	

continued

Table 6-2. Dermatologic Bedside Diagnostic Techniques (*continued*)

Procedure	Indication	Technique	Findings
		30–60 sec and rinse.	
		5. Apply iodine for 30–60 sec and rinse.	
		6. Rinse with alcohol for 5–10 sec.	
		7. Apply safranin for 30–60 sec and rinse.	
		8. Blot dry and view.	
Tzanck prep	Diagnosis of a bullous disease and cutaneous viral infections	1. Unroof the lesion and scrape the base with scalpel.	
		2. Allow to dry on a slide and fix with gentle heating.	
		3. Apply Wright stain for 60 sec.	
		4. Apply a Wright buffer and let mix for 60 sec.	
		5. Rinse, air dry, and view.	
Oil mount prep	Diagnosis of scabies	1. Scrape the skin and place the sample in immersion oil.	
		2. Place the sample oil on a slide and view.	
Skin biopsy		Obtain a small piece of tissue for histology.	

GENERAL DERMATOLOGIC ISSUES IN THE INTENSIVE CARE UNIT

I. **Soaps and Detergents.** Many soaps and detergents cause significant skin irritation. Use gentle cleansers, such as Dove soap or Cetaphil cleanser.

II. **Betadine Solution.** Any area of skin prepared with Betadine solution should be thoroughly washed following the procedure.

III. **Moisturizers.** Keeping the patient's skin well moisturized will help maintain the intact barrier function of the skin. Applying a moisturizer immediately after bathing will help seal in the moisture from the water.

IV. **Adhesives.** Adhesives may cause irritant contact and allergic contact dermatitis reactions.

V. **Pressure Sores and Decubitus Ulcers.** These may result from immobilization, sedation, neurologic deficit, muscle atrophy, older age, malnutrition, and debilitating medical disease.

> **Decubitus ulcers are a cause of significant morbidity and mortality, and are easier to prevent than treat.**

A. **Stages**
1. **Stage 1** involves nonblanchable erythema with intact skin.
2. **Stage 2** involves partial-thickness skin loss; an abrasion, blister, or shallow crater forms on the epidermis.
3. **Stage 3** involves full-thickness skin loss with damage or necrosis of the subcutaneous tissue that may extend to, but not through, the underlying fascia.
4. **Stage 4** involves full-thickness skin loss with extensive destruction, tissue necrosis, or damage to muscle, bone, or supporting structures.

B. **Prevention.** Preventing decubitus ulcers is of primary importance because they may lead to secondary infection, osteomyelitis, sepsis, amputation, and death.
1. To alleviate pressure points, **turn the patient frequently** in bed.
2. Use a **specialized bed** for prevention or alleviation of pressure points.
3. Place **lambskin or foam pieces** under pressure points.
4. **Examine the patient's skin daily,** paying particular attention to pressure points.
5. Maintain **adequate nutrition.**

C. **Management**
1. **Stage I lesions.** Pay attention to preventive measures and modification of risk factors.
2. **Stage 2 lesions.** Apply protective coverings (Duoderm).
3. **Stage 3 ulcers.** More extensive wound débridement and removal of adherent eschar is necessary.
    a. **Débridement** can be attained through whirlpool therapy; softening of the eschar with placement of Duoderm; or frequent soaks followed by the application of an antibiotic ointment.

  b. Healing. Once the lesion is débrided and the base of the ulcer is cleaned, the process of healing can begin. To encourage healing, the lesions should be cleaned with soaks twice a day, followed by the application of an antibiotic ointment and Vaseline gauze. Silvadene can be used in place of a topical antibiotic.

  4. Stage 4 ulcers should be treated the same as stage 3 ulcers, with a **surgical consultation** for extensive débridement, flaps, or skin grafting.

VI. Pruritus

 A. Etiology. A few common causes include dry skin, atopic dermatitis, scabies, systemic disease, and medications.

 B. Management. Guidelines for symptomatic management of pruritus are as follows:

  1. Investigate the underlying cause.

  2. Keep the skin well lubricated with a topical moisturizer.

  3. Use topical antipruritic agents frequently.

  4. Prescribe an antihistamine.

VII. Diaper and Incontinence Dermatitis. The eruption is characterized by redness, edema, scaling, papules, vesicles, and pustules distributed over the diaper area, sometimes extending up the abdomen and down the thighs.

 A. Evaluation includes an examination with a potassium hydroxide (KOH) preparation and a Gram's stain.

 B. Management

  1. The diaper should be changed frequently.

  2. The diaper area should be cleansed gently with water or a mild soap and patted dry.

  3. After each diaper change and cleansing, ketoconazole 2% cream should be applied to the area, followed by hydrocortisone 2.5% cream.

  4. If there is severe maceration or breakdown of the skin, a barrier ointment (e.g., Desitin, zinc oxide 20% ointment or 25% paste) can be applied over the ketoconazole and hydrocortisone creams.

  5. **Candidal infections** should be treated with ketoconazole and hydrocortisone therapy.

  6. Most **secondary bacterial infections** can be treated adequately with topical antibiotics.

NON–LIFE-THREATENING DERMATOLOGIC PROBLEMS

 I. Infections. See **Table 6-3** for types of dermatologic infections and their treatment.

 II. Dermatitis (inflammation of the skin). See **Table 6-4** for types of dermatitis and their treatment.

 III. Folliculitis is inflammation of the hair follicle caused by infection, chemical irritation, or physical injury. Folliculitis presents as a follicular pustule with surrounding erythema. See **Table 6-5** for types of folliculitis and their treatment.

Table 6-3. Non–Life-Threatening Dermatologic Infections

	Location and Predisposition	Clinical Signs	Treatment
Tinea corporis	Body; non–hair bearing skin	Erythematous ring-shaped (annular) scaly patches; vesicles or pustules	Topical antifungal bid for 3 wk*
Tinea pedis	Athlete's foot	Interdigital scaling/maceration; dry scaling with or without erythema; blistering eruptions; pruritus and pain	Topical antifungal bid for 2–4 wk*; may add corticosteroids for severely inflamed cases
Tinea manus	Hands or feet	Dry scaly rash with mild erythema	Topical antifungal bid for 2–4 wk*
Tinea cruris	Groin (jock itch); predisposed in opposed skin surfaces and wet areas	Single, red scaling patch in crural folds with an active advancing margin on the inner thigh, perineum, or perianal region	Topical antifungal bid for 2–4 wk*; may add mild topical steroids for severely inflamed cases
Tinea capitis	Scalp	Erythema, scaling, patchy alopecia; may have pustules or boggy plaques; highly contagious	Antifungal shampoo and griseofulvin for 6–8 wk
Tinea barbae	Beard; men who work with domestic animals; transmitted by an infected razor	Inflammation, swelling, pustules, crusts, and follicular nodules in the beard area	Topical antifungal bid for 2–4 wk*

(continued)

Table 6-3. Non–Life-Threatening Dermatologic Infections (continued)

	Location and Predisposition	Clinical Signs	Treatment
Tinea unguium (onychomycosis)	Fingernails and toe nails	Discoloration, thickening, and increased subungual debris	Oral antifungal agents
Tinea versicolor (pityriasis versicolor)	Chest and back in a christmas tree pattern; overgrowth occurs in the heat, humidity, pregnancy, hypercortisol states; also occurs in the immunocompromised	Small pink scaling macules that may coalesce to form large patches with pruritus	Topical ketoconazole cream bid for 2–4 wk. If widespread, apply selenium sulfide 2.5% and scrub vigorously in the shower for 3 wk; a one-time dose of oral ketoconazole
Cutaneous candidiasis	Skin (Candida albicans) Predisposing factors: obesity, diabetes, antibiotics, steroids, immunosuppression, and moist, warm environment	Presents in the skinfolds, axilla, groin, or fat; erythematous patches and plaques with surrounding satellite pustules	Topical antifungal bid for 2–4 wk*; may add mild topical steroids for severely inflamed cases
Thrush	Oral candidiasis; occurs in the mouth in patients on steroids, antibiotics; also occurs in infants and the immuno-compromised	Abnormal candidal overgrowth; white cheesy membrane on the mucosal surfaces (easily wiped off) with underlying inflammation and erythema	Nystatin swish and swallow qid for 2–3 wk or oral fluconazole

Vulvovaginal candidiasis	Perineum	Thick, white, cheesy plaques with underlying edema and erythema; curd-like vaginal discharge	Antifungal vaginal suppositories
Dermatophyte infections (ringworm)	Exposed areas of body	Itching; rings of erythema with a scaly border and central clearing; diagnose by KOH	Topical antifungals or oral griseofulvin (250–500 mg bid) for 4 weeks
Scabies (*Sarcoptes scabiei*)	Hands, feet, axilla, groin, and interdigital regions	Highly contagious inflammatory eruption with pruritus; papules, pustules, vesicles, nodules, and elongated or linear papules. Diagnose by a scraping of mites.	Apply lindane lotion over the entire body overnight; take antihistamines or topical steroids
Pediculosis (lice)	Head lice (*Pediculus humanus capitis*), body lice (*Pediculus humanus corporis*), and pubic lice (*Phthirus pubis*)	Appears as red puncta and excoriatings on the skin that may become papular and wheal-like; severe pruritus. Diagnose by scraping of lice.	Antihistamines; topical steroids; 1% lindane shampoos or permethrin 1% cream rinse; wash clothes in hot water.

*If recurrent or resistant to therapy, treat with oral antifungal agents for 2 to 4 weeks.

Table 6-4. Types of Dermatitis

	Etiology	Clinical Features	Treatment
Acute allergic contact dermatitis	Delayed-type hypersensitivity reaction; acquired from poison ivy, nickel, perfumes, cosmetics, or adhesive	Erythematous papules and plaques, to urticarial lesions, frank vesicles, or bullae; often arranged in linear, angulated; lesions may erode, drain the serous fluid and form crusts	Open the wet dressing (sheet in lukewarm water) for 10–15 min followed by topical steroid, qid for 3–4 days; antihistamines; systemic steroid for severe cases
Irritant contact dermatitis	Irritation of the skin from an outside process that destroys the barrier function; acquired from soaps, Betadine, moisture and urine in the diaper area, drooling, or fecal incontinence	Gradual onset: usually indistinct borders; diffuse erythema with dryness, cracking, and fissures	Avoid irritants; apply a topical steroid for 1–2 wk; daily lubrication of areas; open wet dressings for severe cases
Seborrheic dermatitis	Generally unknown; thought to be associated with genetic and environmental factors; can occur in immunocompromised patients	Chronic condition; redness and scaling in the scalp, eyebrows, base of eyelashes, nasolabial folds, external ear canal, sternum and posterior auricular folds	Frequent washing of the affected areas with selenium sulfide 2.5% shampoo—leave the lather in place for 5 min; apply topical ketoconazole on the face and chest

Asteatotic eczema	Aging, excessive dryness of the skin, cold weather, and an atopic diathesis	Eruption on the lower legs; dry and scaly skin with accentuation of skin lines; red plaques with thin long superficial fissures appear; in severe cases the fissures become deep and ooze; pain	**Mild:** lubrication bid **Severe:** open the wet dressing with moderate topical steroid
Statis dermatitis	Eczematous eruption in patients with venous insufficiency	Edema, varicose veins **Acute:** abrupt onset red, pruritic plaque that progresses to acute vesicular inflammation with weeping, crusts, and fissures **Subacute/chronic:** violaceous to erythematous plaque on the lower legs, fibrosis with skin thickening, brown discoloration of the skin with hyperpigmentation and a bumpy, cobblestone appearance	**Acute:** leg elevation, open wet dressings, high-potency topical steroid, antihistamines for pruritus and treat cellulitis **Subacute:** topical steroid every day bid until symptoms resolve **Chronic:** compression stockings

Table 6-5. Types of Folliculitis

	Distribution	Clinical Findings	Treatment
Acne vulgaris	Inflammatory disease of sebaceous follicles usually found on the face, chest, and back	Numerous lesions, follicular-based pustules, open and closed comedones, inflammatory papules, cystic lesions	Topical or oral antibiotic plus either benzoyl peroxide or tretinoin
Acne rosacea	A chronic, cutaneous eruption usually found in older individuals on the central face	Background flushing that progresses to persistent erythema and telangiectases. Superimposed on the central facial erythema are inflammatory papules, pustules and sometimes cysts	Topical metronidazole cream bid or PO antibiotics such as tetracycline for prolonged periods
Bacterial folliculitis	Infection of the hair follicle with *Staphylococcus aureus* or *Pseudomonas*	Follicular pustules with surrounding erythema. Diagnosis made after a culture of a pustule	Oral antibiotic

Demodex folliculitis	An inflammatory folliculitis usually seen on the face of older individuals with acne rosacea; caused by the hair mite, *Demodex folliculorum*	Cases of acne rosacea with pustules that have been resistant to the usual therapy Locate the organism using a KOH preparation	Crotamiton lotion, permethrin lotion, or lindane
Steroid acne	A form of papular acne found on the chest, back, upper extremities, and occasionally on the face as a complication of a high-dose of systemic corticosteroids	Characteristic monomorphous, perifollicular papular eruption in this distribution	Responds to withdrawal of steroids; if not, apply topical tretinoin cream
Eosinophilic folliculitis	A pruritic pustular folliculitis found usually in patients with HIV on the head, neck, and upper trunk	Pruritic pustular folliculitis; small skin-colored papules; pruritus Diagnosis made by a Tzanck preparation and skin biopsy	Ultraviolet B phototherapy

SERIOUS AND LIFE-THREATENING DERMATOLOGIC PROBLEMS

I. **Cutaneous Reactions to Medications.** These reactions constitute an estimated 19% of adverse events in hospitalized patients. Many of these eruptions are the typical morbilliform (maculopapular) eruption, urticarial reaction, or fixed drug eruption. **Table 6-6** lists clinical and laboratory findings indicating that a drug-induced cutaneous eruption may be serious. Serious and sometimes life threatening cutaneous reactions to medications are described below and summarized in **Table 6-7.**

A. **Stevens-Johnson syndrome (SJS) and toxic epidermal necrolysis (TEN)** are two interrelated mucocutaneous diseases. Patients may present with SJS, which then evolves into TEN; TEN has a poorer prognosis.

1. **Pathogenesis.** The pathogenesis of SJS and TEN is unknown, but most cases are thought to be induced by drugs (**Table 6-8**).

2. **Clinical presentation of SJS**

a. The patient often has **flu-like symptoms** for 1 to 3 days before the cutaneous eruption starts.

b. **Cutaneous symptoms** often include pain and a burning sensation on the skin. In 90% of cases, two **mucosal sites** are involved; in 10% to 30% of cases, the patient has a **fever** and mucosal involvement of the GI and respiratory tracts.

c. The **lesions** are **small blisters** on dusky, purpuric macules or purpuric targets. Small areas may progress to a confluence of lesions.

Table 6-6. Cutaneous Reactions to Medications: Clinical and Laboratory Findings Indicating Serious Problems

Cutaneous findings
Confluent erythema
Facial edema or central facial involvement
Skin pain
Palpable purpura
Skin necrosis
Blisters or epidermal detachment
Mucous membrane erosions
Urticaria
Swelling of the tongue
Laboratory findings
Eosinophil count > 1000/mm^3
Lymphocytosis with atypical lymphocytes
Abnormal liver function test

Table 6-7. Serious and Potentially Life-Threatening Cutaneous Reactions to Medications

	Skin Manifestations	Signs and Symptoms
Stevens-Johnson syndrome (SJS)	Erosions at > 2 mucosal sites; tiny vesicles; dusky, purpuric macules; atypical targets; < 10% body surface area detachment	Occasional fever (10–30%); even less frequent involvement of the respiratory and gastrointestinal tracts
Toxic epidermal necrolysis (TEN)	Individual lesions similar to those in SJS; confluent tender erythema; sloughing of necrotic epidermis in sheets with bright red denuded dermis exposed; > 30% of body surface area detachment	Almost all cases have fever, leukopenia, and greater likelihood of involvement of the respiratory and gastrointestinal tracts
Anticonvulsant and other hypersensitivity syndromes	Severe exanthematous eruption that often becomes purpuric; exfoliative dermatitis; other polymorphous skin eruptions	Many cases with fever, lymphadenopathy, facial swelling, hepatitis, nephritis, carditis, eosinophilia, atypical lymphocytes
Vasculitis	Palpable purpura, nodules, ulcerations, urticaria	Vasculitis of many internal organs such as the gastrointestinal tract; nephritis; fever; neuritis
Serum sickness and serum sickness-like reactions	Morbilliform eruptions, urticaria	Fever, arthralgias
Warfarin-induced necrosis	Distributed on fatty areas; painful erythema followed by purpura and then large areas of necrosis	
Angioedema	Urticaria and swelling; most often involves the central area of the face	Respiratory or cardiovascular distress

Adapted from Roujeau JC, Stern RS: *Severe adverse cutaneous reactions to drugs.* N Engl J Med 331(19):1272–1285, 1994.

Table 6-8. Drugs Associated with Stevens-Johnson Syndrome (SJS) and Toxic Epidermal Necrolysis (TEN)

Most Often Associated	
Sulfadoxine	Phenylbutazone
Sulfadiazine	Isoxicam
Sulfasalazine	Piroxicam
Co-trimoxazole	Chlormezanone
Hydantoins	Allopurinol
Carbamezapine	Amithiozone
Barbiturates	Aminopenicillins
Also Associated	
Cephalosporins	Tiaprofenic acid
Fluoroquinolones	Diclofenac
Vancomycin	Sulindac
Rifampin	Ibuprofen
Ethambutol	Naproxen
Fenbufen	Ketoprofen
Tenoxicam	Thiabendazole

From Roujeau JC, Stern RS: Severe adverse cutaneous reactions to drugs. *N Engl J Med* 331(19):1272–1285, 1994.

      d. Epidermal detachment occurs on less than 10% of the patient's total body surface area.
   3. Clinical presentation of TEN is often as described for SJS, with the following exceptions:
      a. TEN is distinguished from SJS by **epidermal detachment involving more than 30% of body surface area.** There is a sheetlike loss of epidermis, with many raised, flaccid bullae, which develop and spread progressively with mild cutaneous pressure. After detachment and loss of the tops of the flaccid bullae, an **exposed, red, oozing dermis** remains.
      b. Fever is common.
      c. There is a **greater likelihood of systemic involvement:**
         (1) Mucosal surface involvement with impaired urination, stomatitis, photophobia, and involvement of the synechiae and pseudomembranes in the eyes
         (2) Tracheal and bronchial involvement, resulting in epithelial sloughing and airway obstruction, epiglottal swelling, secondary pneumonia, and acute respiratory distress syndrome (ARDS)
         (3) GI tract involvement, resulting in esophagitis, bleeding, protein loss, and pseudomembrane development
         (4) Complications similar to those of burn patients,

including fluid losses, electrolyte imbalances, bacterial superinfections, and a hypercatabolic state.

(5) Sepsis

(6) Bone marrow involvement with anemia, leukopenia, and thrombocytopenia

4. **Mortality rates** are 30% for TEN and < 5% for SJS.

5. **Diagnosis** is based on a constellation of presenting symptoms, signs, and cutaneous features. A definitive diagnosis by skin biopsy will help to exclude other blistering diseases (e.g., *Staphylococcus* scalded skin syndrome or paraneoplastic pemphigus).

6. **Management**

   a. **Treatment of mild cases of SJS** includes withdrawal of the offending agent, evaluation for infection, meticulous mucous membrane hygiene, and supportive care. Systemic corticosteroid therapy is not indicated.

   b. **Treatment of severe cases of SJS and TEN** is similar to the care given to a burn patient.

      (1) Admit the patient to an **intensive care unit or burn unit.**

      (2) Give the patient **fluids and electrolytes.**

      (3) Adhere to **sterile precautions** and maintain **meticulous care of the skin and mucous membranes.** For the large denuded areas of skin, apply generous amounts of Vaseline or Aquaphor and Vaseline gauze.

      (4) Avoid adhesives.

      (5) Empirical antibiotics are not indicated, but **obtain bacterial cultures** when indicated. **Give antibiotics** promptly at the first sign of decompensation, sepsis, or positive blood cultures.

      (6) Consult an **ophthalmologist** and a **urologist.**

      (7) Institute early and aggressive **nutritional support.**

      (8) Provide adequate **pain control.**

      (9) Use of **systemic corticosteroid therapy** in severe cases of SJS and TEN **is controversial.**

B. **Anticonvulsant hypersensitivity syndrome (AHS)** can occur with phenytoin, carbamazepine, and phenobarbital.

   1. **Incidence.** The estimated incidence of AHS is 1 to 10 cases per 10,000 exposures. There is an increased incidence in African-Americans and in family members of affected persons.

   2. **Onset** is usually within 3 weeks to 3 months after anticonvulsant therapy is initiated.

   3. **Pathogenesis** is related to an inherited defect in the ability to detoxify the oxidative metabolites of aromatic anticonvulsant agents.

   4. **Clinical presentation**

      a. **Major clinical findings** include fever (100%), lymphadenopathy that is often tender, facial edema, hepatitis (51%), and pleomorphic skin eruption (87%).

  b. Minor clinical findings include diarrhea, interstitial nephritis (11%), pulmonary infiltrates (9%), anorexia, pharyngitis and myopathy.

5. **Laboratory results.** Laboratory tests may reveal eosinophilia (30%), atypical lymphocytes (6%), leukocytosis, Coombs' negative hemolytic anemia, thrombocytopenia, elevated liver function tests, elevated creatine phosphokinase (CPK), proteinuria, and hematuria.

6. **Management** involves prompt recognition of the syndrome and **discontinuation of the offending drug.** Systemic **corticosteroids** have never been shown to be beneficial in controlled trials; however, most physicians will institute empirical therapy. The patient should *never* be rechallenged with phenytoin, carbamazepine, or phenobarbital therapy; valproic acid and the benzodiazepines are safe alternatives.

7. **Clinical course.** The course of AHS varies; it can last for several weeks. A few patients develop lymphoma. Death is most often caused by hepatic necrosis or sepsis.

C. **Other hypersensitivity syndromes** involve specific, severe idiosyncratic reactions to such medications as sulfonamides, allopurinol, gold salts, and dapsone.

1. **Clinical presentation**

  a. The **onset** is 2 to 6 weeks after the initiation of the offending medication.

  b. A **severe morbilliform eruption** often occurs which may become purpuric and develop into an exfoliative dermatitis.

  c. In approximately 30% to 50% of cases, the patient also has fever, lymphadenopathy, hepatitis, nephritis, carditis, eosinophilia, and elevated atypical lymphocytes. Approximately 10% of such cases result in **death,** primarily caused by **hepatitis, nephritis,** and **carditis.**

2. **Diagnosis** is determined from the history, clinical features, and laboratory findings.

3. **Management** involves discontinuation of the offending medication and general supportive care. Systemic steroids are often administered, although there have been no controlled trials that prove their effectiveness. A rash and hepatitis may persist for weeks.

D. **Drug-induced vasculitis** is a subtype of hypersensitivity vasculitis that includes leukocytoclastic vasculitis and serum sickness. Drugs often associated with vasculitis include allopurinol, penicillin, sulfonamides, thiazides, pyrazolones, hydantoins, and propylthiouracil. Drug-induced vasculitis is often difficult to distinguish from other causes of vasculitis.

1. **Etiology** is unclear, but drug-induced vasculitis is thought to result from antibodies directed against drug-associated haptens.

2. **Clinical presentation**
   a. **Palpable purpura** is found most often on the lower extremities, although any cutaneous surface may be involved. There may be hemorrhagic blisters, urticaria, ulcers, nodules, and digital necrosis.
   b. The patient often has a **fever.**
   c. There may be **systemic involvement,** with vasculitis affecting the kidneys (glomerulonephritis) GI tract, liver, or central nervous system.
   d. **Death** occurs in less than 5% of cases; most deaths are **related to GI and renal involvement.**
3. **Diagnosis.** Rule out other possible etiologies. A **skin biopsy** may disclose leukocytoclastic vasculitis.
4. **Management.** Discontinue the offending medication, and administer systemic prednisone.

E. **True serum sickness.** In true serum sickness, a type III hypersensitivity reaction is mediated by the deposition of immune complexes in small blood vessels, by the activation of complement, and by the recruitment of granulocytes. Serum sickness-like reactions are not mediated by complement.
   1. **Offending agents** include serum preparations and vaccines. Serum sickness-like reactions have occurred with β-lactam antibiotics, β-blockers, and streptokinase.
   2. **Onset.** Serum sickness presents 1 to 2 weeks after the initial exposure to the foreign antigen.
   3. **Clinical presentation.** The patient first presents with **erythema** along the sides of the fingers, toes, and hands; this progresses to widespread morbilliform or urticarial eruption. In approximately 50% of cases, there is **systemic involvement** including rash, fever, constitutional symptoms, arthralgia, and arthritis.
   4. **Diagnosis.** In true serum sickness, complement levels (C3 and C4) are decreased.
   5. **Management.** Discontinue the offending agent and administer systemic corticosteroids.

F. **Warfarin-induced skin necrosis.** This rare and serious complication of warfarin therapy results from the formation of occlusive thrombi in the vessels of the skin and subcutaneous tissues.
   1. **Persons at greatest risk**
      a. Patients who have a hereditary deficiency in protein C or S are at greatest risk owing to a loss of the anticoagulant effect, which leaves them in a transient hypercoagulable state.
      b. Women
      c. Obese patients
      d. Patients who have been started on higher initial doses of warfarin
   2. **Onset.** This complication occurs usually 3 to 5 days after the initiation of warfarin therapy.
   3. **Clinical presentation. Sites of predilection** include the

breasts, thighs, hips, and buttocks. At an early stage, a **painful erythematous plaque** develops. This plaque later develops into a necrotic plaque with hemorrhagic blisters.

4. **Management**
   a. Discontinue warfarin therapy promptly.
   b. Initiate IV heparin therapy.
   c. Administer vitamin K.
   d. Consider treatment with monoclonal antibody-purified protein C concentrate.
   e. Initiate surgical débridement of necrotic tissue as needed.

G. **Angioedema.** Typically, an IgE-mediated, immediate hypersensitivity reaction causes the angioedema, but in many cases it results from non-IgE-mediated processes.

1. **Offending agents.** The most common offending agents are antibiotics (especially the penicillins), anesthetics, and radiocontrast media. Drugs that cause angioedema by non-IgE-mediated processes include angiotensin-converting enzyme (ACE) inhibitors, nonsteroidal anti-inflammatory drugs, radiocontrast agents, opiates, and curare.

2. **Onset** can occur from several minutes to several days after the initial exposure to the drug.

3. **Clinical presentation.** The patient has profound swelling of the deep dermal and subcutaneous tissues. Angioedema can be complicated by airway compromise and GI tract distress, and ultimately by anaphylaxis.

4. **Management.** Patients with **serious and complicated angioedema** may require treatment with SQ epinephrine. For **mild cases,** discontinue the medication and administer diphenhydramine every 6–8 hr until the patient is clinically improved.

II. **Infectious Diseases**

A. **Staphylococcal scalded skin syndrome (SSSS)**

1. **Susceptibility**
   a. This staphylococcal epidermolytic syndrome occurs most commonly among **children younger than 5 years of age,** who presumably lack immunity to the toxin and have a renal function that is too immature to dispose of the toxins. Seventy-five percent of persons older than 10 years of age are immune to the toxins.
   b. **Adult generalized SSSS** is associated with immunosuppression, abnormal immunity, and renal insufficiency.

2. **Clinical presentation**
   a. SSSS **starts as a** *Staphylococcus aureus* **infection** of the conjunctiva, nares, throat, or umbilicus.
   b. The disease **progresses to a diffuse, tender erythema** that is often attenuated in flexural and periorificial areas. The patient may have **sandpaper–like skin** and will often have a **fever.**
   c. Within 1 to 2 days of onset of the tender erythema, **the**

skin wrinkles, forms flaccid bullae, and peels off in large sheets, leaving behind a denuded surface. Minor pressure can induce more bullae.

  d. With healing, a **diffuse desquamation** appears.

3. **Clinical course.** Spontaneous remission occurs over 2 to 3 weeks. In children, death occurs rarely; in adults, the mortality rate may exceed 50%.

4. **Differential diagnosis.** The differential diagnosis is toxic epidermal necrolysis (TEN).

5. **Diagnosis**

  a. A definitive diagnosis is made after a **skin biopsy** has been taken. In SSSS, the epidermis is split in the upper layers of the stratum granulosum; in TEN, the split is in the subepidermal layer. To hasten a diagnosis, the plane of separation can be determined on a frozen section of the roof of a blister.

  b. A **culture** of material taken from the nares, eye, throat, umbilicus, or any other obvious site of infection may reveal an offending staphylococcal type-specific organism. A culture of skin scrapings or bullae contents will not grow any organisms.

  c. **Blood culture** results are often positive.

6. **Management**

  a. Give **IV antibiotics** (e.g., oxacillin).

  b. **Lubricate the patient's skin** with a bland moisturizer (Vaseline or Aquaphor) and cover the denuded areas with Vaseline gauze.

  c. Systemic corticosteroids are contraindicated.

B. **Ecthyma gangrenosum** is a rare but classic finding of *Pseudomonas* infection. It represents either cutaneous seeding from *Pseudomonas aeruginosa* bacteremia or a primary lesion without bacteremia. The disease is rare in septicemic patients, presenting in about 1.3% to 6% of patients with *Pseudomonas* sepsis. The mortality rate is high.

1. **Persons at risk**

  a. Immunocompromised patients

  b. Burn patients

  c. Malnourished patients

  d. Patients with diabetes

2. **Clinical presentation**

  a. **Location of lesions.** Lesions mainly occur in the gluteal and perineal areas, extremities, and, less often, on the trunk and face, although they can occur at any site on the skin.

  b. **Appearance of lesions.** Lesions consist of multiple noncontiguous ulcers or solitary ulcers that begin as isolated red, purpuric macules and become vesicular, indurated, and later, bullous or pustular. The central area of the pustular ulcer **becomes hemorrhagic and necrotic,** exhibiting a gun-metal gray discoloration. The lesion then **sloughs to form a gangrenous ulcer** with a gray-black eschar and a surrounding erythematous halo.

   c. Septicemic form. There are usually **fewer than 10 lesions.** Septicemic patients are quite ill; they exhibit **fever, hypotension,** and **tachycardia. Neutropenia** is a common finding. If the patient survives, the skin lesions heal slowly.

3. Diagnosis

   a. Blood cultures are taken.

   b. A **sterile skin biopsy** is taken for culture and sensitivity, and **another biopsy** is taken for routine hematoxylin and eosin (H & E) staining and other special stains to identify the organism.

   c. Needle aspiration of a lesion is done to make a rapid diagnosis through Gram's stain.

4. Management. IV antibiotic therapy includes a combination of an aminoglycoside and an antipseudomonal penicillin or cephalosporin.

C. Meningococcemia is caused by *Neisseria meningitidis.*

   1. Persons at risk. Most cases of this **potentially fatal disease** occur in **individuals younger than 20 years of age,** with approximately 50% of cases occurring in children younger than 5 years of age.

   2. Epidemiology. Meningococcemia occurs most frequently in the winter and spring; **epidemic outbreaks** occur when crowded conditions prevail.

   3. Transmission. Meningococcemia can be **spread via airborne droplets** from infected patients or from asymptomatic nasopharyngeal carriers.

   4. Onset is 3 to 4 days after exposure.

   5. Clinical presentation ranges from fever to shock.

     a. Lesions. Severe purpuric and ecchymotic lesions cover the skin and mucous membranes diffusely but **predominate on the trunk and lower extremities.** The lesions often begin sparsely over the sacral areas. In severe cases, bullae, ulcerations, necrosis, and sloughing of the skin occur.

     b. Systemic findings include stupor, shock, encephalitis, adrenal and pituitary involvement, and disseminated intravascular coagulation.

   6. Diagnosis is made on the basis of Gram's stain or culture of material from blood, cerebrospinal fluid, or nasopharyngeal scrapings. A quick diagnosis can sometimes be made after examination of a **skin biopsy** of the characteristic skin lesions.

   7. Differential diagnosis

     a. Rocky Mountain spotted fever (RMSF)

     b. Echovirus infection

     c. Coxsackievirus infection

     d. Toxic shock syndrome

     e. Gonococcemia and leukocytoclastic vasculitis, which

usually produce lesions that are elevated and palpable

8. **Management**
   a. Administer IV **ceftriaxone** (or chloramphenicol if RMSF is suspected) until culture results and sensitivities are available.
   b. Administer **penicillin G** to the patient as well as to persons who were in close contact with the patient. This is done to prevent nasopharyngeal carriage of the bacterial pathogen.

D. **Herpes simplex virus (HSV) infections** are caused by herpes simplex viruses type 1 (HSV-1) and type 2 (HSV-2).
   1. **Location of infection. HSV-1 infections** are localized primarily in the oral region, and **HSV-2 infections** are found in the genital region; however, either virus can cause infection in either location.
   2. **Phases.** HSV infections have two distinct phases: the primary infection and the secondary or recurrent infections.
      a. **Primary HSV infection** is acquired from another infected person or from an asymptomatic virus-shedding person.
         (1) **Transmission.** It is spread via respiratory droplets, by direct contact with an active lesion, or by contact with body fluid or secretions that contain the virus.
         (2) **Onset.** Symptoms occur from 3 to 7 days after the contact.
         (3) **Prodromal symptoms,** such as headache, fever, generalized aching, localized pain, and tender lymphadenopathy may occur. Prodromal symptoms at the site of inoculation that occur before the onset of lesions include tenderness, pain, mild paresthesias, and burning.
         (4) **Lesions.** The first lesions to surface are usually grouped, monomorphous vesicles on an erythematous base. These lesions then quickly erode, leaving umbilicated surfaces that crust over. The lesions may last for 2 to 6 weeks before they heal completely.
         (5) **Latency.** During the primary infection, the virus enters the nerve endings in the skin directly below the lesions and travels through peripheral nerves to the dorsal root ganglia, where it remains in its latent stage.
      b. **Secondary or recurrent HSV infection** occurs when the virus is reactivated under circumstances such as stress, immunocompromise, skin barrier breakdown, sun exposure, or illness. The reactivated virus travels down the peripheral nerves to the site of the initial infection and causes the characteristic focal, recurrent infection.

(1) **Prodromal symptoms**—localized pain, burning, and tingling—occur 2 to 24 hours before the onset of skin lesions.

(2) **Skin lesions** evolve rapidly from an erythematous base to erythematous papules to frank vesicles that soon umbilicate. Within 3 to 4 days, the vesicles rupture and form erosions that then become crusted.

(3) Systemic symptoms and lymphadenopathy are rare, unless a secondary infection occurs.

(4) The **frequency of recurrence** is variable, depending on the individual, the type of HSV infection, and the location.

3. **Clinical variants**

   a. **Immunocompromised host.** HSV infection in the immunocompromised host tends to be **more severe and long-lasting.** With orolabial infection, the disease may involve much of the oral mucosa with concomitant fever, malaise, lymphadenopathy, and dysphagia. Disseminated HSV infection can also be seen.

   b. **Dermatomal distribution.** HSV infection in a dermatomal distribution can also occur, making it **difficult to differentiate** HSV infection **from herpes zoster.** In dermatomal HSV infection, unlike herpes zoster, the vesicles are monomorphous in size and appearance.

   c. **HSV keratoconjunctivitis** can lead to **blindness** and therefore requires prompt ophthalmologic intervention.

   d. **Recurrent erythema multiforme** associated with recurrent HSV infection is a well-known phenomenon. At times the HSV infection may not be obvious, and only recurrent erythema multiforme lesions are present. In such cases treatment with **acyclovir** is indicated.

4. **Diagnosis.** A presumptive diagnosis can be made with **Tzanck preparation:** vigorous scrapings of the base of a vesicle are examined for characteristic multinucleated giant cells and acantholytic cells. A definitive diagnosis is made on **culture** of the vesicular fluid and vigorous scrapings from the base of a vesicle.

5. **Management.** HSV infections are **highly contagious** while the lesions are present; **contact isolation precautions** should be instituted. Treatment of the immunocompromised host must be prompt and aggressive to prevent dissemination of the disease.

   a. **First episode of genital herpes.** Treat with acyclovir, 400 mg PO tid for 7 to 10 days; famciclovir, 250 mg PO tid for 5 to 10 days; or valacyclovir, 1 g PO bid for 7 to 10 days.

   b. **Recurrence of genital herpes.** Treat with acyclovir,

400 mg PO tid for 5 days; famciclovir, 125 mg PO bid for 5 days; or valacyclovir, 500 mg PO bid for 5 days.

c. **Long-term suppression of genital herpes.** Treat with acyclovir, 400 mg PO bid; famciclovir, 250 mg PO bid; or valacyclovir, 500 mg PO bid.

d. **Mucocutaneous disease in immunocompromised patients.** Treat with acyclovir, 5 mg/kg IV every 8 hours for 7 to 10 days or until the lesions heal; or 400 mg PO 5 times per day for 7 to 10 days or until the lesions heal.

E. **Herpes zoster (shingles)** is a vesicular eruption resulting from the **reactivation of the varicella zoster virus (VZV)** that has been latent in the dorsal nerve root since the original infection with varicella (chickenpox). Most outbreaks occur in persons older than 40 years of age.

1. **Clinical presentation**

a. **Prodromal symptoms.** For 1 to 2 days there is a prodrome of pruritus, burning, paresthesias, tingling, and sometimes pain over the involved dermatome. Constitutional symptoms such as fever, malaise, and headache may be experienced during this period.

b. **Distribution of lesions.** The lesions are distributed **over a unilateral dermatome;** a few (up to 20) may be scattered outside the dermatome.

c. **Appearance and progression of lesions**

(1) The lesions usually begin as **erythematous papules** or **urticarial plaques.**

(2) The **classic lesions**—umbilicated vesicles on an erythematous base—develop 1 to 2 days later. The vesicles may be of various sizes and shapes, and can occur in small groups or large coalescent masses. Concomitant areas of erosions and crusting are often seen.

(3) **New vesicles** can develop for up to 1 week in normal hosts.

(4) Most vesicles become pustular within a few days before eroding and forming **crusts.**

d. **Complications** occur most often **in immunocompromised hosts** and include dissemination, chronic persistent infection, encephalitis, and pneumonia.

2. **Clinical variants**

a. **Ophthalmic zoster** involves the ophthalmic division of the trigeminal nerve. This variant is especially dangerous if the nasociliary branch of the ophthalmic division is involved, which is clinically evident by the presence of vesicles on the tip or side of the nose (Hutchinson's sign). **Ophthalmologic intervention is mandatory** to rule out the possibility of intraocular infection (e.g., uveitis or keratitis) and other sight-threatening complications.

b. **Ramsay Hunt syndrome** is a zoster infection that involves the geniculate ganglion. The clinical syndrome is a combination of herpes zoster oticus, facial nerve paralysis, and auditory symptoms. There is involvement of the sensory and motor divisions of the 7th cranial nerve (facial nerve), leading to possible facial paralysis, hearing deficits, and vertigo. Recovery from the motor paralysis is usually complete, but residual weakness can persist.

  c. **Disseminated zoster** occurs when many (arbitrarily > 20) lesions are present outside the primarily involved dermatome. Disseminated zoster is usually seen in **immunocompromised patients,** especially those with depressed cellular immunity (e.g., patients with Hodgkin's disease and HIV infection). Aggressive intervention with **antiviral agents** can be life-saving.

3. **Diagnosis** can often be made clinically.

  a. **Differential diagnosis.** Herpes zoster infection must be differentiated from dermatomal HSV infection, allergic contact dermatitis, and other blistering diseases.

  b. **Presumptive diagnosis** is made with a **Tzanck preparation.** Classically, one sees multinucleated giant cells and acantholytic cells that are identical to those found in HSV.

  c. **Definitive diagnosis** is made on **culture.** A diagnosis can be made even more quickly from the results of **immunofluorescent antibody stains.**

4. **Management**

  a. **Varicella (chickenpox).** Treat with acyclovir, 20 mg/kg (800 mg max) PO qid for 5 days.

  b. **Herpes zoster.** Treat with valacyclovir, 1 g PO tid for 7 days; famciclovir, 500 mg PO tid for 7 days; or acyclovir, 800 mg PO 5 times a day for 7 to 10 days.

  c. **Varicella or herpes zoster in immunocompromised persons.** Treat with acyclovir, 10 mg/kg IV every 8 hours for 7 days or until the lesions heal.

  d. **Acyclovir-resistant persons.** Treat with foscarnet, 40 mg/kg IV every 8 hours for 10 days.

  e. **Adjunct management**

   (1) **Open wet dressings,** followed by the application of an **antibiotic ointment** bid–tid, can help to remove serum and crusts, suppress bacterial growth, and soothe the cutaneous symptoms.

   (2) Treatment with PO **antihistamines** can relieve pruritus.

   (3) **Analgesics** may help to relieve pain.

   (4) Therapy with systemic **corticosteroids plus acyclovir** may help to accelerate the healing time.

III. Purpuric Lesions. Purpura is a condition characterized by visible hemorrhage into the skin. **Petechiae** are pinpoint hemorrhagic spots, usually less than 1 cm in diameter, whereas **ecchy-**

moses are more confluent and macular areas of hemorrhage usually greater than 1 cm in diameter. **Palpable purpura** is characterized by the presence of both hemorrhage and palpability.

A. **Nonpalpable purpura** signifies leakage of blood from the dermal vessels into the surrounding tissue. There is no palpable component because there is little or no inflammation. **Causes** include thrombocytopenia, functional platelet defects, coagulopathies, trauma, or weakened blood vessels.

B. **Palpable purpura** involves inflammatory destruction of the vessel walls of small vessels.

1. **Palpable purpura with early inflammation** may be due to any of the following conditions:

   a. **Hypersensitivity vasculitis (leukocytoclastic vasculitis)**, including the following types:

      (1) Schönlein-Henoch purpura

      (2) Drug-induced vasculitis

      (3) Infection-induced vasculitis

      (4) Vasculitis associated with malignancy

      (5) Vasculitis associated with connective tissue disease

      (6) Vasculitis associated with serum sickness

      (7) Urticarial vasculitis

      (8) Vasculitis associated with essential mixed cryoglobulinemia

   b. **Polyarteritis nodosa**

   c. **Granulomatous vasculitis,** including allergic granulomatous vasculitis (Churg-Strauss syndrome) and Wegener's granulomatosis

   d. **Erythema multiforme,** a small vessel injury that does not involve leukocytoclastic vasculitis

2. **Palpable purpura with bland occlusion and late inflammation** may be caused by the following conditions:

   a. **Embolic disorders**

      (1) Septic emboli

      (2) Acute bacterial endocarditis

      (3) Cholesterol emboli syndrome

      (4) Atheroembolic disease

   b. **Thrombosis and disorders of coagulation**

      (1) Disseminated intravascular coagulation

      (2) Protein C or S deficiency

      (3) Skin necrosis from warfarin therapy

      (4) Antiphospholipid antibody syndrome

      (5) Cutaneous calciphylaxis

      (6) Paroxysmal nocturnal hemoglobinuria

      (7) *Atrophie blanche* or livedoid vasculitis

   c. **Thrombosis caused by infectious organisms in vessels**

      (1) Vessel-invasive fungi

      (2) Ecthyma gangrenosum (*P. aeruginosa*)

   d. **Thrombosis caused by microvascular platelet plugging**

      (1) Heparin-associated thrombocytopenia syndrome

   (2) Polycythemia rubra vera

   (3) Other myeloproliferative disorders with thrombocytosis

   (4) Thrombotic thrombocytopenic purpura

  e. Thrombosis caused by cold agglutination or gelling

   (1) Cryofibrinogenemia

   (2) Monoclonal cryoglobulinemia

 3. Diagnosis

  a. Determine whether the lesions are purpuric and primary.

  b. If the lesions are caused by primary purpura, determine whether they are palpable.

  c. If the lesions are nonpalpable, etiologies for petechiae or ecchymoses should be pursued (see III A).

  d. If the lesions are early, palpable, and retiform with minimal surrounding erythema, see III B 1.

  e. If the lesions are early, palpable, and round, with prominent surrounding erythema, see III B 1.

  f. A dermatology consultation can be helpful.

IV. Other Serious Dermatologic Diseases

 A. Blistering diseases. Vesicles and bullae are the primary lesions in many diseases, several of which have previously been discussed.

  1. Dermatitis herpetiformis is a chronic, intensely pruritic vesicular cutaneous disease almost always **associated with a subclinical gluten-sensitive enteropathy.** This disease presents in young to middle-aged adults as a few pruritic vesicles or papules that are initially annoying and often attributed to insect bites or neurotic excoriations.

  2. Pemphigus is a rare, potentially lethal, autoimmune, intraepidermal blistering disease that involves the skin and mucous membranes. The exact etiology is unknown. The disease is characterized by circulating IgG autoantibodies directed against various epidermal intercellular (interkeratinocyte) components, resulting in disadhesion of epidermal keratinocytes and blister formation. Pemphigus vulgaris and pemphigus foliaceous are the two main subtypes.

   a. Pemphigus vulgaris (PV) is the **most common form.**

    (1) Clinical presentation. Oral erosions precede the onset of cutaneous bullae by weeks to months. Cutaneous lesions present as nonpruritic, flaccid bullae varying from 1 cm to several centimeters in diameter.

    (2) Diagnosis is made from the results of a skin biopsy, direct immunofluorescence of skin biopsies, and indirect immunofluorescence from serum.

    (3) Management. Give systemic corticosteroids and other immunosuppressive agents.

   b. Pemphigus foliaceous (PF)

- **(1) Clinical presentation.** PF often presents with localized or widespread areas of erythema, scaling, crusting, and only rarely bullae. Areas of predilection include the scalp, chest, back, and face.
- **(2) Diagnosis** is made from the results of a skin biopsy and immunofluorescence studies.
- **(3) Management** of PF is similar to that of PV. **PF can be fatal if left untreated.**

3. **Bullous pemphigoid (BP)** is a rare subepidermal blistering disease of unknown etiology. It is characterized by circulating and basement membrane-bound IgG autoantibodies. BP **occurs primarily among the elderly.**

   a. **Clinical presentation.** BP presents early with a localized area of erythema or with pruritic, urticarial plaques that progressively become more edematous and widespread. It is **often misdiagnosed as hives.** The eruption is usually generalized, although there is often a predilection for flexural surfaces. The palms and soles are also involved. Mucosal lesions, if present at all, are mild and transient. The **course** varies from localized, short-lived disease to generalized, persistent disease.

   b. **Diagnosis** is made from the results of a skin biopsy and immunofluorescence test.

   c. **Management.** First-line treatment involves systemic corticosteroid therapy.

B. **Generalized pustular psoriasis.** This rare form of psoriasis is serious and at times fatal.

   1. **Etiology.** Presumed precipitants include an abrupt withdrawal of systemic corticosteroids in a patient with psoriasis, underlying bacterial infection, hypocalcemia, and previous use of topical medications such as tar or anthralin.

   2. **Clinical presentation.** Generalized pustular psoriasis presents with the sudden onset of erythema on the flexural areas that progressively migrates over other body surfaces. Numerous tiny, sterile pustules form in these areas of erythema and then coalesce into "lakes of pus." The patient often appears toxic and febrile, and has a leukocytosis.

   3. **Management.** Systemic medications such as etretinate, methotrexate, or cyclosporine, are often used to achieve rapid control.

7

Endocrine Disorders

ADRENAL DISORDERS

I. **Normal Daily Cortisol Production.** Normal daily cortisol production is 12 mg/m^2/day, the equivalent of 25 to 30 mg of hydrocortisone PO.

II. **Hypercortisol State**

A. **Long-term glucocorticoid therapy** causes many of the **same complications as Cushing's syndrome,** such as obesity, edema, psychiatric disorders, and impaired wound healing. **Problems limited to synthetic corticosteroids** include benign intracranial hypertension, glaucoma, pancreatitis, aseptic bone necrosis, and panniculitis.

B. **Endogenous hypercortisolism** is associated with striae, purpura, hypertension, acne, hirsutism, impotence, and menstrual irregularities.

III. **Adrenal Insufficiency**

A. **Etiology**

1. **Primary adrenal insufficiency** can result from:
   a. Adrenal hemorrhage or thrombosis (Waterhouse-Friderichsen syndrome)
   b. Autoimmune adrenalitis (Addison's disease)
   c. AIDS-related infections such as cytomegalovirus (CMV) infection, tuberculosis, or fungal infection
   d. Metastatic carcinoma (lung, breast, or kidney)
   e. Isolated glucocorticoid deficiency
   f. Abdominal trauma
   g. Shock
   h. Tuberculosis
   i. Medication

2. **Secondary adrenal insufficiency (pituitary adrenocorticotropic hormone [ACTH] deficiency)** can result from:
   a. Long-term glucocorticoid therapy
   b. Postpartum pituitary necrosis (Sheehan's syndrome)
   c. Pituitary necrosis or bleeding into pituitary macroadenoma

  d. Head trauma affecting the pituitary stalk
  e. Pituitary or metastatic tumor
  f. Pituitary surgery or radiation
  g. Pituitary or adrenal surgery for Cushing's syndrome
  h. Hypothalamic tumor
  i. Sepsis (Cytokines may directly inhibit corticotropin release.)

B. Clinical presentation

1. Symptoms

  a. Fatigue, weakness, and mental depression
  b. Anorexia and weight loss
  c. Dizziness, orthostatic hypotension, and dehydration
  d. Nausea, vomiting, and diarrhea
  e. Headache and visual changes
  f. Symptoms of poor nutrition or immune deficiency (e.g., poor wound healing)
  g. Flank pain
  h. Vital sign instability

2. Signs

  a. Signs of **primary adrenal insufficiency** include:
    (1) Hyperpigmentation
    (2) Hyperkalemia
    (3) Vitiligo
  b. Signs of **secondary adrenal insufficiency** include:
    (1) Altered consciousness
    (2) Pale skin
    (3) Amenorrhea, decreased libido, and decreased potency
    (4) Scant axillary and pubic hair
    (5) Small testicles
    (6) Delayed puberty
    (7) Diabetes insipidus
    (8) Hyponatremia, hypoglycemia, neutropenia, and eosinophilia

C. Adrenal insufficiency in patients undergoing surgery

1. Effect of surgery on ACTH and cortisol release.
In stressful situations, circadian rhythm is temporarily lost, causing a change in cortisol feedback of ACTH release: either normal feedback is not in effect, or the central feedback has been reset at a higher level. Anesthesia and surgery, as well as trauma, fever, pain, and illness, normally increase release of cortisol and ACTH; this normal response maintains homeostasis. Absence of this response necessitates increased use of vasopressors, which leads to increased mortality rates.

  a. **After minor surgery,** approximate normal production of cortisol is 25–30 mg/24 hr.
  b. **After major surgery,** approximate normal production of cortisol is 75–150 mg/24 hr.

      c. **Levels return to baseline** 1 to 2 days after stress, but **circadian rhythm** is temporarily lost.

Etomidate, which is used for the induction of general anesthesia, has the side effect of 11α-hydroxylase inhibition. It is associated with lower intraoperative serum cortisol; it should be used with caution in ill patients.

---

    2. **To meet the stress response,** patients with adrenal insufficiency will require **exogenously administered steroids.**

      a. Administer hydrocortisone, 100 mg q 8 hr or as a continuous infusion, to provide 200–300 mg/24 hr.

      b. Taper steroids gradually following stress.

      c. Initiate prophylaxis against stress ulcers using sucralfate or histamine (H_2) blockers.

    3. **Patients on chronic steroid therapy** may require a change in steroid dosage.

      a. **In routine simple procedures,** there are lower perioperative cortisol levels but no measured increase in morbidity or mortality, so there is no need for stress dosing.

      b. **For minor procedures** (e.g., herniorrhaphy), administer 25 mg hydrocortisone/day for 1–3 days.

      c. **For moderate stresses** (e.g., open cholecystectomy, colectomy, total abdominal hysterectomy, lower extremity bypass), administer 50–75 mg hydrocortisone/day for 1–3 days.

      d. **For major stress** (e.g., Whipple's operation, abdominoperineal resection, esophagectomy), administer 100–300 mg hydrocortisone/day for 1–3 days.

      e. The **dosages** above may need to be tailored to the patient's routine dosage or the nature of the stress.

IV. Acute Adrenal Failure

    A. **Incidence.** Acute adrenal failure occurs in 2% to 3% of severely ill patients and in 0.01% to 0.7% of healthy patients after routine surgery.

    B. **Clinical presentation.** A high index of suspicion is required to diagnose acute adrenal failure, especially in the ICU where injury, shock, and alterations in routine steroid administration are common.

    1. **Hypotension** may occur secondary to hypovolemia and reduced arterial resistance. There is a decreased ability to modulate vascular tone in response to a decrease in cardiac output. **Refractory hypotension** is common, a result of the "permissive effect" of glucocorticoids on the vascular response to catecholamines.

    2. **Hemodynamic profile**

      a. **Low PCWP/low CI/low SVR** occurs in cardiovascular collapse which is a result of adrenal crisis.

      b. **Low PCWP/low CI/normal SVR** occurs with hypovolemia and the inability to vasoconstrict in response to a low cardiac output.

3. **Electrolyte abnormalities**
    a. **Hyponatremia** (decreased sodium resorption) is indicated by high urine sodium.
    b. **Hyperkalemia** (decreased potassium secretion) is indicated by low urine potassium.
4. **Hypoglycemia** may occur but is rare.
    5. **Fever, nausea, vomiting, and abdominal pain** may occur.
C. **Diagnosis.** The **cosyntropin stimulation test** (Cortrosyn Injection—synthetic ACTH 0.25 mg, mannitol 10 mg) is used to diagnose acute adrenal failure. This test can be done at any time of day or night, because diurnal variation in cortisol secretion is lost in the critically ill.
    1. **Procedure**
        a. Draw baseline serum cortisol.
        b. Inject Cortrosyn 250 μg IV.
        c. Draw serum cortisol 60 minutes later.
    2. **Results.** Cortrosyn stimulation should increase cortisol by an increment of 7 μg/dl, or to an absolute level of 18 μg/dl. Baseline cortisol below 10 μg/dl is abnormal during acute illness.
D. **Management**
    1. **Steroids** can be administered before checking for adrenal dysfunction when hypotension is severe or difficult to control. **Dexamethasone** is used because it does not interfere with the cosyntropin stimulation test; the recommended dose is 10 mg IV.
    2. **Aggressive fluid resuscitation** is also indicated when adrenal insufficiency is suspected, as long as there is no contraindication specific to the patient.
    3. **Cosyntropin stimulation test**
        a. **If results are positive,** start hydrocortisone 250 mg IV bolus, followed by 100 mg IV q 8 hr until the stress state is terminated.
        b. **If results are negative,** discontinue any steroid therapy. There is no need to taper if only 1 dose has been given.

GLUCOSE METABOLISM DISORDERS

I. **Diabetes Mellitus in the Critically Ill Patient**
    A. **Diagnostic criteria for diabetes**
        1. Fasting plasma glucose ≥ 126 mg/dl
        2. Random plasma glucose ≥ 200 mg/dl on 2 consecutive days
    B. **Complications associated with diabetes mellitus**
        1. Patients with type II diabetes are susceptible to **ketosis,** which is associated with **shock and dehydration.**
        2. Hyperglycemia, through its osmotic effect, causes the serum sodium to fall and may provoke an **osmotic diuresis** with development of symptomatic hyponatremia.

3. Hypocalcemia may predispose the patient to **arrhythmias.**

4. Uncontrolled hyperglycemia will impair **leukocyte function** as well as **wound healing.**

C. **Management.** The **goal of therapy** is to maintain **blood sugar between 150–250 mg/dl.** Treat blood sugar levels above 250 mg/dl. Blood glucose concentrations below 100 mg/dl may develop into **hypoglycemia.**

1. **Severity of diabetes.** Check whether the patient is hyperosmolar or ketoacidotic, and treat if necessary.

2. **Treatment of hyperglycemia**

   a. **Continuous infusion with regular insulin** is the best method for controlling hyperglycemia in the ICU. A blood glucose level of 75–150 mg/dl may not need to be treated initially; however, patients with type I diabetes require low levels of background insulin to prevent ketosis and catabolism.

   b. **Sliding-scale management is less beneficial** because it results in wide fluctuations in serum glucose, which can affect adequacy of treatment.

   c. **Increasing insulin requirements** are a sensitive indication of **progressive resistance** and may result from sepsis, occult infections, ischemia, vasopressors, hypoxia, and heart disease. **In stable patients,** increasing insulin requirements may be **secondary to increasing enteral or parenteral nutrition.** If large amounts of insulin are required hourly to maintain euglycemia (220 U/hr), it may be advisable to reduce the carbohydrate load. Target tissues may become desensitized to insulin when it is given at high levels, thus enhancing resistance.

II. **Diabetes Mellitus in the Perioperative Period.** Surgical patients with diabetes mellitus require close attention so that serious complications may be avoided. The stress of illness and surgery may cause an exacerbation of insulin deficiency or resistance, necessitating an increase in the dose of insulin or antihyperglycemic agents.

A. **Complications associated with diabetes mellitus**

1. Impaired wound healing

2. Impaired immune response leading to an increased risk of infection

3. Accelerated atherosclerosis with associated cardiovascular, cerebrovascular, and peripheral vascular disease

B. **Management of the diabetic patient undergoing minor outpatient surgery**

1. **Patients who will not miss any meals:**

   a. Instruct the patient to follow his or her normal dietary and insulin regimen.

   b. Closely monitor blood sugar during the procedure and in the immediate postoperative period.

2. **Patients who will miss a meal:**

    a. A patient who is not in the hospital should be scheduled for the first case of the day.

    b. A patient who is able to eat after the procedure should not take his or her regular insulin, but should take half of the usual dose of longer-acting insulin.

    c. A patient who is in the hospital preoperatively should be NPO and placed on a 5% dextrose solution. Blood sugar abnormalities should be treated appropriately.

C. Management of the diabetic patient undergoing major elective surgery

  1. Preoperative management. Optimize the patient's nutritional status and glucose control prior to surgery.

    a. If the patient is already in the hospital:

      (1) Discontinue oral hypoglycemic agents the day before surgery.

      (2) Monitor blood sugar and supply regular insulin as needed.

      (3) Ensure that the patient is NPO after midnight before surgery.

      (4) Start 5% dextrose IV fluid after the patient is NPO.

      (5) Give half the usual dose of NPH or lente insulin the morning of surgery, or give regular insulin and closely monitor the patient at scheduled intervals.

    b. If the patient is being admitted the day of surgery, adjust the diabetic regimen (diet and medication) as needed. It is better for the patient to be slightly hyperglycemic rather than hypoglycemic at the time of surgery.

  2. Intraoperative management. Monitor blood sugar frequently to avoid hypoglycemia and extreme hyperglycemia (> 250 mg/dl).

D. Management of the diabetic patient undergoing major emergency surgery

  1. Correct metabolic abnormalities as much as possible prior to surgery.

  2. Correct ketoacidosis preoperatively if possible; if this is not possible, provide vigorous fluid resuscitation and insulin replacement.

  3. Begin continuous insulin infusion.

  4. Monitor blood sugar frequently to avoid hypoglycemia and extreme hyperglycemia (> 250 mg/dl).

  5. Monitor electrolytes carefully; insulin administration may lead to severe hypokalemia.

  6. Optimize fluid status; this may be aided by a pulmonary artery (PA) catheter.

E. Postoperative management of the diabetic patient

  1. Intravenous fluid. Initiate volume resuscitation with normal saline or lactated Ringer's solution. Provide 5% dextrose for glucose source.

2. **Glucose monitoring.** Tightly control glucose (100–200 mg/dl) when possible. Monitor the urine frequently for glucose. A patient with mildly elevated blood glucose may be spilling sugar into the urine and thus may require more insulin to correct their glucosuria.

3. **Insulin administration.** The best route of administration for ICU patients is continuous IV; these patients must be observed closely to avoid hypoglycemia. The IV route is also preferable in patients with poor tissue perfusion and in those with peripheral edema. Once the patient is on a normal oral diet, the usual daily diabetic medication can be resumed, with insulin given by the subcutaneous route.

III. Diabetic Ketoacidosis (DKA)

A. Clinical presentation

1. Anorexia, nausea, vomiting, and polyuria
2. No fever unless infection is present
3. Kussmaul breathing, deteriorating mental status, hypotension, oliguria, and the progression of metabolic acidosis
4. Sweet, fruity odor on breath
5. Pleuritic chest pain
6. Abdominal pain that may be a result of the DKA or the precipitating factor in the DKA.

B. Diagnostic tests

1. Upon presentation, obtain blood glucose and ketones by finger stick, and urine ketones by urine dip analysis.
2. Order immediate biochemical evaluation as follows: CBC, electrolytes, Mg, Ca, phosphate, glucose, BUN/creatinine, blood and urine ketones, ABG, urine analysis, and blood cultures.
3. **DKA is indicated by the following test results:**
   a. Glycosuria and ketonuria
   b. Elevated plasma ketones (may continue to rise initially with treatment)
   c. Anion gap acidosis (pH < 7.3)
   d. Low serum bicarbonate (< 15 mEq/L)
   e. Hyperglycemia (serum glucose > 250 mg/dl)
   f. Moderate hyperosmolality
4. **Associated abnormalities** may include the following:
   a. **Serum sodium** is variable.
      (1) Large amounts of extracellular glucose have an **osmotic effect.** Sodium falls by 1.6 mEq/L for every increase of 100 mg/dl in serum glucose.
      (2) Factitious hyponatremia may occur secondary to hypertriglyceridemia.
   b. **Chloride abnormalities. Hyperchloremia** may represent a chronic ketoacidotic state or may occur during recovery. **Hypochloremia** may be due to vomiting.
   c. **Potassium abnormalities.** Even though serum potassium is elevated at presentation, all patients are at risk for severe hypokalemia.

    d. Ketone body measurements. These are useful for monitoring the resolution of DKA. In cases of severe acidosis, ketone body measurements initially rise rather than fall as the acidosis improves. Clearance is slow, so monitor q 12 hr.

C. Management. The patient should be admitted to an ICU. The goal of therapy is to restore normoglycemia. The serum glucose and osmolality must be lowered slowly to avoid shock, lactic acidosis, and cerebral edema.

  1. Fluid monitoring

    a. Monitor fluid status closely. Urine output is good indicator of fluid status; a PA catheter may be needed for accurate monitoring.

    b. Test urine for glucose. Glycosuria causes an osmotic diuresis and may disguise hypovolemia.

    c. Monitor electrolytes closely. Check glucose and potassium hourly, especially in patients with high insulin requirements.

  2. Insulin therapy

    a. The **loading dose** is 0.4 U/kg of regular insulin, half IV and half SQ.

    b. Begin constant infusion (30 U in 250 ml normal saline) at 50–100 ml/hr, or hourly injections of 5–10 U, IV.

    c. Plasma glucose may decline by 80–100 mg/dl/hr. Once it reaches 300 mg/dl, decrease the insulin infusion by half.

    d. Hyperglycemia will resolve faster than the ketosis and acidosis. Continue IV insulin until all ketones are cleared.

    e. When glucose reaches 200 mg/dl, change the route to SQ and administer q 2 hr until DKA is controlled, as evidenced by:

      (1) Serum glucose < 200 mg/dl

      (2) HCO_3 > 15 mEq/L

      (3) pH > 7.3

      (4) Negative serum ketones at 1:2 dilution

  3. Fluid resuscitation

    a. Use normal saline at 500–1000 ml/hr, with a bolus of 1 L in the first hour.

    b. As vital signs and urine output return toward normal, slow the IV fluid and change to 0.45% normal saline if serum Na > 140 mEq/L.

    c. As serum glucose approaches 300 mg/dl, add 5% dextrose to the IV fluid.

  4. Electrolyte correction

    a. Potassium. If K is < 3.5 mEq/L, add 40 mEq to the first liter of normal saline; then add 20 mEq/L if K is > 3.5 but < 5.5 mEq/L. Check serum potassium every 2 hours.

    b. Metabolic acidosis will usually be corrected with fluid resuscitation and insulin. If the pH falls below 7.0, give 1 ampule sodium bicarbonate; give 2 ampules if the pH < 6.9. Administer each ampule over 30 minutes with 15 mEq KCl. Check pH every 2 hours until it is > 7.2.

   c. **Phosphate** should be repleted in patients who are hypophosphatemic at initial presentation.

   d. **Bicarbonate.** Most physicians recommend that bicarbonate replacement should be undertaken in patients with an arterial pH < 7.1, in patients with depressed respiratory drive, and in patients with hypotensive shock who are unresponsive to rapid fluid replacement.

  5. Treatment of underlying cause. Determine and treat the underlying cause of the diabetic ketoacidosis (infection, myocardial infarction, pulmonary embolism).

  6. Complications

   a. **Hypotension and shock** are typically caused by volume depletion; normally, fluid replacement will reverse this condition. Persistent hypotension should prompt consideration of fluid shifts, bleeding, severe acidosis, hypokalemia, arrhythmia, myocardial infarction, sepsis, and adrenal insufficiency.

   b. **Thrombosis.** Activation of coagulation factors may result in thrombosis of cerebral vessels and stroke.

   c. **Cerebral edema** usually occurs after the initiation of hydration. Most often it is subclinical; if it becomes clinically apparent, it often results in permanent neurologic damage. Do not correct the serum glucose below 200 mg/dl in the first 12 hours to avoid precipitating cerebral edema.

   d. **Renal failure.** Hyperglycemic patients, after the initiation of hydration, should have brisk urine output. The most common cause of renal failure is postrenal obstruction.

   e. **Hypoglycemia**

IV. Hyperosmolar Nonketotic Coma. Hyperosmolar nonketotic coma usually occurs in elderly patients who have type II diabetes, and is essentially due to severe dehydration and volume contraction. Presentation is delayed owing to lack of ketosis and acidosis.

  A. Predisposing factors

   1. Infection

   2. Myocardial infarction

   3. High osmolar enteral feeds without adequate free water dialysis

   4. Stroke, hemorrhage, or trauma

   5. Burns

   6. Pancreatitis

   7. Dialysis

   8. Drugs such as thiazide diuretics, phenytoin, propranolol, cimetidine, and immunosuppressive agents

B. **Clinical presentation**
   1. Profound dehydration
   2. Azotemia
   3. Severe hyperglycemia, often > 1000 mg/dl
   4. Severe hyperosmolarity, often > 375 mOsm/L
   5. Tremors or fasciculations
   6. Obtundation, coma, seizures, or transient hemiplegia
   7. Hyperventilation
   8. Polyuria (urine losses equivalent to 0.45% normal saline solution with equal potassium and sodium)
   9. Increased levels of serum sodium, BUN, and creatinine because of intravascular dehydration

C. **Management**
   1. **Fluid resuscitation.** Fluid deficit is massive.
      a. Start with normal saline at 500–1000 ml/hr for 1–2 hours.
      b. As vital signs and urine output return toward normal, slow the IV fluid and change to 0.45% normal saline. Use the serum sodium as a guide; as long as it is still high, continue with normal saline to fill the intravascular space.
      c. As serum glucose approaches 300 mg/dl, add 5% dextrose to the IV fluid.
   2. **Insulin therapy.** Proceed as for DKA (see *2–Insulin therapy,* p. 167), but insulin requirements will be lower because the hyperglycemia will be corrected by rehydration. (It is important to rehydrate prior to aggressive insulin therapy.) The serum glucose will decrease with an increase in intravascular volume and increased renal function.
   3. **Electrolytes.** Correct electrolyte abnormalities.
   4. **Cerebral edema.** The onset of papilledema, headache, or persistent worsening obtundation during the administration of hypotonic fluids is suggestive of cerebral edema. Treat by terminating the hypotonic fluid and starting 10% dextrose normal saline.

V. **Hypoglycemia**
   A. **Etiology**
      1. Insulin overdose
      2. Prolonged effect of oral hypoglycemic agents
      3. Severe chronic pancreatic insufficiency from resection or zhronic pancreatitis
      4. Postprandial (associated with gastrectomy or gastrojejunostomy)
      5. Acute adrenal insufficiency (decreased insulin resistance)
      6. Acute hepatic failure (decreased gluconeogenesis or decreased clearance of oral hypoglycemics)
      7. Insulin-secreting tumor
      8. End-stage renal disease
   B. **Clinical presentation**

   1. Any change in mental status or responsiveness (confusion, somnolence, obtundation, coma, or seizures)
   2. Hypotension, diaphoresis, dysrhythmia, or cardiac arrest
   C. Diagnosis is by blood glucose level.
   D. Management
      1. Severe signs and symptoms. Give 50 ml of 50% glucose in water ($D_{50}W$) IV.
      2. Mild symptoms. Infuse 10% dextrose at 100–200 ml/hr.
      3. Underlying cause. Determine and treat the underlying cause of the hypoglycemia.

HYPERCALCEMIA

I. Overview
   A. Definition. Hypercalcemia is defined as serum calcium > 10.5 mg/dl.
   B. Physiology of calcium homeostasis. Calcium homeostasis depends upon a complex interaction of parathyroid hormone (PTH), vitamin D, calcitonin, and phosphate.
      1. Stimulation of PTH secretion. PTH secretion is stimulated by a fall in serum ionized calcium concentration.
      2. Effects of PTH. PTH increases renal tubular resorption of calcium, stimulates osteoclast and osteoblast activity, and increases renal conversion of 25-hydroxyvitamin D_3 to the active 1,25-dihydroxyvitamin D_3. PTH decreases serum phosphate and bicarbonate concentrations by increasing renal tubular secretion.
      3. Effects of vitamin D. 1,25-dihydroxyvitamin D_3 stimulates calcium absorption from the GI tract and phosphate resorption by the renal tubules; this enhances bone mineralization.
      4. Calcitonin and its effects. Calcitonin inhibits bone resorption and increases renal excretion of calcium. An elevated serum calcium level causes calcitonin to be released from the C cells of the thyroid.
   C. Incidence
      1. The incidence of hypercalcemia in **outpatients** is **0.1% to 0.5%.** Most of these cases are due to primary hyperparathyroidism.
      2. The incidence of hypercalcemia in **inpatients** is **5%,** with 67% of these cases due to malignancy.
      3. Prevalence is 0.1% to 0.5%.
   D. Etiology
      1. Laboratory error
      2. Hyperparathyroidism (see II below)
      3. Non-parathyroid endocrine causes
        a. Hyper- or hypothyroidism
        b. Adrenal insufficiency
        c. Pheochromocytoma
        d. VIPoma

4. Hereditary: familial hypocalciuria hypercalcemia (FHH)
5. Neoplastic
   a. Solid tumors or lytic bony metastases (breast, lung, kidney, esophagus, thyroid, multiple myeloma, lymphoma)
   b. Mediators of humoral hypercalcemia of malignancy (see **Table 7-1**)
      (1) PTHrP (secreted by squamous cell carcinoma of lung, cervix, and esophagus, and adenocarcinomas of the kidney, breast, and bladder)
      (2) PTH (secreted by lung, liver, and ovary)
      (3) Cytokines as part of humoral response to cancer (IL-1, IL-6)
      (4) Vitamin D (secreted by lymphoma)
6. Exogenous agents, including thiazide diuretics, lithium, estrogen, milk with absorbable antacids (causing milk-alkali syndrome), excess of vitamin A or D, aluminum, beryllium, and theophylline
7. Immobilization (bone resorption)
8. Granulomatous disease (tuberculosis, sarcoidosis, fungal infection)
9. Paget's disease
10. Idiopathic hypercalcemia of infancy (Williams syndrome)

E. **Clinical presentation**
   1. **Constitutional signs and symptoms** include weight loss, fatigue, weakness, myalgia, and anorexia.
   2. **Gastrointestinal manifestations** include nausea, vomiting, abdominal pain, constipation, pancreatitis, and peptic ulcer.
   3. **Renal manifestations** include polyuria, polydipsia, in-

Table 7-1. Comparison of Humoral Hypercalcemia of Malignancy and Primary Hyperparathyroidism

	Humoral Hypercalcemia of Malignancy	Primary Hyperparathyroidism
Bone resorption	Increased	Increased
Bone formation	Decreased	Increased
Gut absorption of calcium	Decreased	Increased
Serum 1,25-dihydroxyvitamin D_3	Decreased	Increased
Tubular absorption of HCO_3	Increased	Decreased
Serum chloride	Decreased	Increased
Plasma PTHrP	Increased	Normal
Plasma PTH	Decreased	Increased
Plasma phosphate	Decreased	Decreased

continence, uremia, renal colic, nephrolithiasis, and nephrocalcinosis.

4. **Neurologic manifestations** include personality disorders, psychoses, lethargy, headache, depression, hyporeflexia, memory loss, deafness, ataxia, confusion, coma, and seizures.

5. **Musculoskeletal manifestations** include myalgias and arthralgias, decreased deep tendon reflexes, bone pain, arthritis, and pathologic fractures.

6. **Dermatologic/ophthalmologic manifestations** include pruritus, conjunctivitis, and band keratopathy.

F. **Physical examination.** Findings may include hypertension, bony deformities, and neck mass (rare).

G. **Electrocardiogram.** Electrocardiographic changes may include bradycardia, shortened QT, widened T, and primary heart block.

II. Hypercalcemia Caused by Hyperparathyroidism

A. **Types of hyperparathyroidism**

1. **Primary hyperparathyroidism** involves abnormal secretion of parathyroid hormone with normal or elevated serum levels of calcium.

   a. **Pathology**
      (1) 80% to 85% solitary adenoma
      (2) 12% hyperplasia of all four glands
      (3) 1% parathyroid cancer
      (4) 3% have so-called multiple adenomas

   b. **Etiology**
      (1) Low-dose ionizing radiation to the neck
      (2) Genetic: multiple endocrine neoplasia (MEN) types 1 and 2 (hyperplasia due to defect in the neural crest stem cells)
      (3) Chronic stimulation of parathyroid glands which occurs in low-calcium or high-phosphate diets

2. **Secondary hyperparathyroidism** involves increased parathyroid hormone secretion in compensation for a chronically low serum calcium level. There is no intrinsic parathyroid abnormality.

   a. **Associated disorders**
      (1) Secondary hyperparathyroidism may occur in patients with **chronic renal failure;** it is secondary to phosphate retention, decreased conversion of 25-hydroxyvitamin D_3 to active 1,25-dihydroxyvitamin D_3, bone resistance to PTH, and decreased metabolic clearance of PTH.
      (2) Secondary hyperparathyroidism with a low or normal phosphate level may occur in patients with **malabsorption, rickets,** and **osteomalacia.**

   b. **Medical management.** Administer phosphate binders (calcium carbonate, calcium acetate) to lower serum phosphate and vitamin D levels.

   c. **Surgical management.** A few patients with hyperparathyroidism secondary to renal failure (5%–10%) will require subtotal parathyroidectomy because of:

(1) Noncompliance with medical therapy

(2) Failure of medical therapy to control serum calcium phosphate product

(3) Symptoms of pruritus, bone pain, fractures, or tissue calcification

3. **Tertiary hyperparathyroidism** occurs when:

a. Hypercalcemia develops in secondary hyperparathyroidism (autonomous function of parathyroid tissue)

b. Hyperparathyroidism and hypercalcemia persist after renal transplant with normal renal function

B. Clinical presentation of hyperparathyroidism

1. Hypercalcemia on screening blood work

2. Signs and symptoms of hypercalcemia (see *E–Clinical presentation,* p. 171).

3. Renal stones, decreased bone density (suggests cancer), musculoskeletal complaints, and pathologic fractures (fractures occurring after mild force or in unusual locations)

4. Rare: hypertension, pancreatitis, lump in neck, diabetes, bone disease

C. Evaluation of hyperparathyroidism

1. **History**

a. Has the patient experienced nephrolithiasis, previous fractures, or neuromuscular symptoms?

b. Does the patient complain of weakness, fatigue, constipation, depression, or memory loss?

c. Does the patient have associated conditions such as peptic ulcer disease, hypertension, gout, or pseudogout?

d. Does the patient have a history of childhood neck irradiation or a family history of hyperthyroidism?

e. Has the patient had previously diagnosed cancer or symptoms of malignancy?

2. **Physical examination.** Assess neck for masses and perform detailed neurologic and musculoskeletal examinations.

3. **Laboratory results**

a. **Parathyroid hormone.** Immunoradiometric or immunohistochemical assays for intact PTH are done. PTH is elevated in primary and ectopic forms of hyperparathyroidism. The increase in PTH in ectopic forms is usually lower than expected for calcium level because, in addition to PTH, these tumors secrete fragments of PTH-like hormones which are not detected on intact assay. In patients with **parathyroid adenomas** there is a correlation between the size of the adenoma and the PTH level.

b. **Calcium.** The calcium level in patients with hyperparathyroidism is > 10.5 mg/dl. Patients with a calcium level > 12 mg/dl require urgent treatment (see *B–Surgical treatment,* p 176). Remember the following:

(1) Correct the calcium level for albumin:

Corrected Ca = measured Ca + 0.8 × (4 − albumin)

(2) The serum calcium level of 20% of people with hyperparathyroidism is in the upper range of normal.

(3) Some patients have **normocalcemic hyperparathyroidism;** measure PTH and calcium simultaneously to identify this condition. PTH will be inappropriately high for calcium.

c. **Hypercalcemia with urine calcium** > 250 mg/day occurs in 75% of patients with primary hyperparathyroidism and hypercalcemia.

d. **Hypercalcemia with relative hypophosphatemia and hyperchlorhydria** usually indicates hyperparathyroidism.

e. Remember these **primary hyperparathyroidism laboratory pitfalls:**

(1) A low calcium and high phosphate diet may obscure mild hypercalcemia.

(2) Serum-intact PTH may be normal in 15% of patients with primary hyperparathyroidism.

(3) High calcium and PTH levels are seen in 20% of patients with FHH and in those with lithium hypercalcemia.

(4) High intact PTH is rarely seen in patients with malignancy, but hyperparathyroidism and malignancy can coexist (especially in breast cancer).

(5) High calcium and chloride levels may be seen in patients with thyrotoxicosis.

III. Hypercalcemia with Normal Parathyroid Hormone Levels

A. Diagnostic evaluation.

1. **Laboratory tests.** These tests will help narrow the differential diagnosis of the hypercalcemia:

a. CBC, platelet count, electrolytes, BUN/creatinine, and glucose

b. Calcium, magnesium, and phosphorous

c. PTH-related peptide (elevated in PTH-secreting tumors)

d. Protein electrophoresis in suspected multiple myeloma

e. Thyroid stimulating hormone (decreased in thyroid disease)

f. Arterial pH (may be acidotic secondary to bicarbonate excretion)

g. 24-hour urine collection for creatinine clearance to estimate glomerular filtration rate

2. **Diagnostic imaging**

a. Chest and abdominal radiographs may show abnormal calcifications or masses.

b. Bone densitometry will detect decreased bone density.

B. Management. See *V–Management of Hypercalcemia* below.

IV. **Hypercalcemic Crisis.** Life-threatening hypercalcemia (Ca > 14.5 mg/dl) may present acutely.

   A. **Symptoms**
      1. Weakness
      2. Nausea and vomiting
      3. Drowsiness, stupor, or coma
      4. Constipation
      5. Tachycardia

   B. **Immediate management**
      1. Hydrate aggressively.
      2. Administer furosemide for vigorous diuresis.
      3. Determine the cause of the hypercalcemia.
      4. Correct electrolyte imbalance.
      5. Avoid immobilization of the patient.
      6. Obtain a radiograph of the patient's hands.
         a. If subperiosteal resorption is present, the patient has hyperparathyroidism and needs urgent parathyroidectomy.
         b. If the radiograph is normal, malignancy is the most likely cause of the crisis.

   C. **Secondary management.** Proceed with medical or surgical treatment as outlined below.

V. **Management of Hypercalcemia**

   A. **Medical treatment**
      1. **Monitor electrolytes closely** during treatment.
      2. **Hydrate the patient** with 0.9% saline boluses followed by 0.9% saline with KCl, 20 mEq/L at 200–300 ml/hr as tolerated, to maintain a urine output of at least 100 ml/hr, optimally 3–5 L/day.
      3. **Administer furosemide** if the patient is fully hydrated; this promotes urinary calcium excretion and prevents volume overload.
      4. **Perform dialysis in patients with renal failure;** use low calcium dialysate.
      5. **Administer bisphosphates** (osteoclast inhibitors that take 24–48 hours for efficacy). Use in conjunction with other therapies.
         a. **Etidronate,** 7.5 mg/kg IV q 8 hr for 3–7
         b. **Pamidronate,** 30–90 mg IV over 24 hours, or 15–40 mg IV every day for up to 6 days by slow infusion
      6. **Administer calcitonin,** 1 U SQ test dose, then 4 U/kg SQ/IM/IV bid. The dose may be increased to a maximum of 8 U/kg every 6 hours. Calcitonin inhibits bone resorption and increases renal excretion of calcium. The effect is seen in a few hours but is short lasting.
      7. **Administer hydrocortisone,** 200–300 mg IV qd for 3–5 days, or prednisone 40–80 mg PO qd (adult dose), for the following disorders:
         a. Neoplastic etiology (breast, lymphoma, or multiple myeloma)

      b. Granulomatous disease

      c. Idiopathic hypercalcemia of infancy

  8. Administer gallium nitrate, which acts by inhibiting bone resorption. (Best results occur in patients with hypercalcemia of malignancy.)

      a. Administer 200 mg/m^2 for 5 days by continuous IV infusion.

      b. Side effects include **nephrotoxicity.**

Use gallium nitrate only after adequate hydration, and maintain urine output at 2 L/day during therapy. Avoid the use of aminoglycosides within 48 hours of treatment.

---

   9. Discontinue causative exogenous agents.

  10. Withhold dietary calcium.

  11. Mobilize the patient and administer a diuretic if hypercalcemia is secondary to immobilization.

B. Surgical treatment

  1. Indications for surgery are as follows:

      a. Markedly elevated serum calcium concentration (> 12 mg/dl)

      b. Previous episode of life-threatening hypercalcemia

      c. Reduced creatinine clearance (by 30%)

      d. Marked hypercalcuria (> 9.98 mMol/day or 400 mg/24 hr)

      e. Presence of kidney stones

      f. Markedly elevated 24-hour urinary calcium excretion (> 400 mg)

      g. Substantially reduced bone mass (> 2 standard deviations below mean for age, gender, and race)

      h. Patients in whom medical surveillance is neither desirable nor suitable

      i. Young patients (because of complications with long-term compliance with medical treatment)

      j. Age < 50 years

  2. Localization studies include the following:

      a. Neck ultrasonography for parathyroid adenoma

      b. Technetium sestamibi scanning of parathyroid glands

      c. Renal ultrasound for nephrocalcinosis

      d. Computed tomography for abdominal, thoracic, head, and neck tumors

      e. Bone scan for bony metastases

      f. Radiography for Paget's disease of bone or osteitis fibrosa cystica from hyperparathyroidism

      g. Biopsy of suspicious lesions

  3. Formal surgical neck exploration is the only treatment for patients with **newly diagnosed primary hyperparathyroidism.** Localization studies are not needed as long as there has been no prior neck surgery or radiation.

PHEOCHROMOCYTOMA

I. **Definition.** A pheochromocytoma is a tumor with unregulated growth and secretion that develops from the adrenal medulla.

II. **Review of Adrenal Anatomy and Physiology**

    A. **Anatomy of the adrenal glands.** The adrenal glands are flat, triangular glands, each weighing approximately 5 g, that lie at the top of each kidney. Each gland is made up of two parts: a medulla and a cortex (**Figure 7-1**).

        1. The **medulla** or **interior aspect** of the adrenal gland is of ectodermal origin (derived from the neural crest). It is composed of homogeneous sheets of cells organized into "nests" of secretory granules containing catecholamines.

        2. The **cortex** or **outer layers** of the adrenal gland is of mesodermal origin (derived from the adrenogenital ridge). It is composed of **three layers:**

            a. The **zona glomerulosa,** the outermost layer, produces aldosterone.

            b. The **zona fasciculata,** the middle layer, produces cortisol and adrenal sex hormones.

            c. The **zona reticularis,** the deep layer, stores cholesterol and produces cortisol and sex hormones.

    B. **Blood supply of the adrenal glands**

        1. The arterial supply is as follows:

            a. The superior adrenal arteries branch from the inferior phrenic arteries.

            b. The middle adrenal arteries branch from the aorta.

            c. The inferior adrenal arteries branch from the renal arteries.

        2. Blood passes from the cortex to the medulla.

        3. Blood leaves the adrenal glands by way of a cenral vein which empties into the vena cava on the right and the renal vein on the left.

    C. **Adrenomedullary physiology.** Stimulation of the adrenal glands may occur as a result of fear, stress, upright posture, pain, cold, hypotension, or hypoglycemia.

        1. Stimulation of preganglionic sympathetic fibers results in

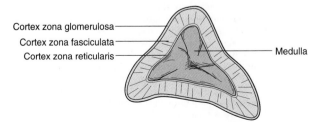

Cortex zona glomerulosa

Cortex zona fasciculata

Cortex zona reticularis

Medulla

Figure 7-1. Anatomy of the adrenal gland.

release of epinephrine (80% of secretion), norepinephrine, and dopamine.

2. Norepinephrine exerts negative feedback at preganglionic sympathetic neuron receptors.

3. Interruption of the sympathetic nervous system by injury or medication results in autonomic dystrophy with loss of adrenergic response.

III. Incidence and Risk Factors

A. The **incidence** of pheochromocytomas in the United States is 1 to 2 per 100,000 people.

B. In **hypertensive patients** there is an increased incidence, ranging from 0.01% to 1.0%.

C. The **peak incidence** is in people 30 to 50 years old.

D. The **male-to-female ratio** is 1:1.

E. Pheochromocytoma occurs predominantly in **Caucasians.**

F. Pheochromocytomas account for 1% to 9% of **incidentalomas.**

G. **Ten percent** of pheochromocytomas are:
1. Bilateral
2. Malignant
3. Extraadrenal
4. Familial
5. Found in children

IV. Associated Disorders

A. **Multiple endocrine neoplasia, type II (MEN-II)**

1. The **peak incidence** of pheochromocytoma associated with MEN-II occurs in a younger population (10–30 years of age).

2. **Eighty percent** of these pheochromocytomas are **bilateral.**

3. **Adrenal medullary hyperplasia** usually precedes pheochromocytoma.

4. **MEN-IIa (Sipple syndrome)** is characterized by medullary thyroid carcinoma, parathyroid hyperplasia, and pheochromocytoma.
   a. Pheochromocytoma occurs in 30% to 50% of patients.
   b. Pheochromocytoma predates thyroid cancer in 10% of patients.

5. **MEN-IIb (mucosal neuroma syndrome)** is characterized by medullary thyroid carcinoma, multiple mucosal neuromas, and pheochromocytoma.

B. **Neuroectodermal dysplasia syndromes**

1. **Von Recklinghausen's disease (neurofibromatosis).** Neurofibromatosis occurs in 5% to 10% of patients with pheochromocytoma, but pheochromocytoma occurs in < 1% of patients with neurofibromatosis.

2. **Von Hippel-Lindau disease.** Pheochromocytoma occurs in 53% of patients with this disease.

3. **Tuberous sclerosis**

4. **Sturge-Weber syndrome**

C. **Genetic abnormalities** (deletions from chromosomes 1p,

3p, 17p, or 22q) may be detected in patients with pheochromocytoma.

V. **Pathologic Features**

  A. **Size.** The median diameter of a pheochromocytoma is 7 cm and the median weight is 100 g, but it can be as large as 20 cm and 2 kg.

  B. **Location.** A pheochromocytoma may occur in any focus of neuroendocrine tissue including the adrenal medullae, ganglia of the heart, aorta, and bladder.

     1. **Adrenal sites.** Tumors of the right adrenal gland are more common than those of the left. Ten percent of adrenal pheochromocytomas are bilateral.

     2. **Extraadrenal sites.** The most common extraadrenal site is the organ of Zuckerkandl. Two percent of extraadrenal pheochromocytomas occur in the chest and one percent in the neck.

  C. **Malignancy**

     1. **Ten to twenty percent** of pheochromocytomas are malignant.

     2. Malignant pheochromocytomas are **three times more common in women.**

     3. **Extraadrenal tumors** are 2 to 3 times more likely to be malignant.

     4. **Diagnosis** of malignancy is by invasion of adjacent structures, nodal involvement, or metastasis.

     5. **Metastasis** may occur to bone, liver, lymph nodes, lungs, and brain.

VI. **Clinical Presentation.** Signs and symptoms are due to circulating catecholamines.

  A. **Hypertension** is the most consistent sign, occurring in 80% of patients.

  B. **Paroxysmal hypertension** occurs in 30% to 40% of patients.

  C. **Other signs and symptoms** include headache, palpitation, vomiting, abdominal discomfort, pallor, anxiety attacks, nausea, weakness, diaphoresis, angina, dyspnea, tremor, dizziness, visual disturbances, convulsions, flushing, itching, and paresthesias.

VII. **Diagnostic Tests**

  A. **Urine tests.** A 24-hour urine sample will show elevated catecholamines. Measurement of the urinary metanephrine level is the most accurate diagnostic tool (100% sensitivity, 80% specificity).

  B. **Blood tests.** Only 75% of pheochromocytomas will be detected by plasma epinephrine, norepinephrine, and dopamine levels. A glucagon 1–2 mg IV bolus precipitates a rise in plasma catecholamines to > 2000 pg/ml or > three times baseline in patients with pheochromocytoma.

  C. **Imaging studies.** CT, MRI, or ^{131}I-metaiodobenzylguanidine scintigraphy can be used to localize the pheochromocytoma.

VIII. **Management: Surgical Resection.** Pheochromocytoma is the indication for 22% to 43% of adrenalectomies. Perioperative mortality rates are 0% to 3%.

A. Perioperative hemodynamic management

1. **Initiate α-adrenergic blockade** for 1 to 3 weeks before surgery with one of the following drugs:
   a. Administer **phenoxybenzamine** 10–40 mg PO bid-tid, increasing the dosage by 10–20 mg/day until blood pressure is controlled.
   b. Administer **terazosin** 1–20 mg PO qd or **doxazosin** 1–16 mg PO qd.
   c. Administer **phentolamine** 5–15 mg IV bolus or 0.5–1 mg/min IV by continuous infusion every 4 hours (if patient cannot take PO).
   d. Administer **nifedipine** 10–20 mg PO tid or **nicardipine** 20–40 mg PO tid.
2. **Hydrate** the patient well.
3. **Administer β-blockers** for tachycardia. Avoid propranolol, which enhances the effect of norepinephrine.

> **Many patients will be on β-blockers for hypertension prior to the diagnosis of pheochromocytoma. For these patients, add the α blockade when diagnosis is made.**

B. Surgical approaches

1. The **anterior transperitoneal** approach allows a thorough exploration of both adrenal glands.
2. The **posterolateral** approach is not recommended for large, multiple, or extraadrenal tumors.
3. **Laparoscopic surgery** enables you to explore one adrenal gland at a time. It is contraindicated for large tumors.

C. Intraoperative management

1. Use a radial arterial line to monitor blood pressure.
2. Initiate aggressive volume replacement.
3. Be aware that anesthetic agents and morphine can stimulate catecholamine release.
4. Initiate sodium nitroprusside drip as needed.
5. Administer a short-acting β-blocker such as esmolol on demand.
6. Administer lidocaine for arrhythmias.
7. Use a PA catheter for patients with existing heart disease.

D. Postoperative monitoring in the ICU. Monitor for hypotension and hypertension.

THYROID DISEASE

I. Etiology and Precipitating Factors

A. Thyrotoxicosis (hyperthyroidism) may be due to:
1. Grave's disease
2. Toxic multinodular or uninodular goiter
3. Thyroiditis (subacute, silent, or postpartum)

    4. Drugs: amiodarone-induced or iodine-induced (Jod-Basedow phenomenon)

    5. Exogenous administration of thyroxine (T_4): thyrotoxicosis factitia

    6. Ectopic thyroid hormone production caused by struma ovarii or metastatic thyroid disease

    7. Pituitary adenoma

    8. Molar pregnancy

B. Thyrotoxic crisis (thyroid storm) is a life-threatening complication of hyperthyroidism. The mortality rate is 10% to 20%. **Precipitating factors** include:

    1. Infection

    2. Thyroid manipulation (surgery, palpation, change in thyroid medication, iodine, radiation)

    3. Metabolic disorders (diabetic ketoacidosis, hypoglycemia)

    4. Trauma

    5. Myocardial infarction or pulmonary embolus

    6. Labor and delivery

    7. Diagnostic procedures

    8. Drugs (T_4, haloperidol, digitalis, pseudoephedrine)

C. Congenital hypothyroidism may be due to:

    1. Thyroid dysgenesis

    2. Thyroid dyshormonogenesis

    3. Thyrotropin deficiency

    4. Iodine, drugs, or maternal antibodies (transient hypothyroidism)

D. Goiterous adult hypothyroidism may be due to:

    1. Drugs such as amiodarone, lithium, iodine, antithyroid medications, and cytokines

    2. Hashimoto's thyroiditis (chronic thyroiditis)

    3. Iodine deficiency

    4. Infiltrative diseases such as sarcoidosis, amyloidosis, and lymphoma

E. Nongoiterous adult hypothyroidism may be:

    1. Iatrogenic (due to thyroidectomy or radioiodine treatment)

    2. Transient (due to thyroiditis or nonthyroidal illness)

    3. Autoimmune idiopathic

F. Myxedema coma is an acute exacerbation of an underlying hypothyroidism. It is highly lethal, with mortality rates approaching 50%. **Precipitating factors** include:

    1. Cold exposure

    2. Cerebrovascular accident

    3. Congestive heart failure

    4. Drugs: narcotics, anesthetics, diuretics, phenothiazines, and sedatives

    5. Surgery or trauma

    6. Gastrointestinal hemorrhage or bowel obstruction

    7. Hypoglycemia, hyponatremia, hypoadrenalism

    8. CO_2 narcosis

    9. Febrile or infectious illness

     10. Seizures

     11. Drug overdose due to slow metabolism

II. Clinical Presentation

A. Thyrotoxicosis (hyperthyroidism)

    1. A palpable goiter is not necessarily present.

    2. **Systemic signs and symptoms** include unexplained fever, sweating, palpitations, nervousness, fatigue, and weight loss. Pain may be a symptom in subacute thyroiditis.

    3. **Cardiovascular signs and symptoms** include:

      a. Persistent sinus tachycardia

      b. Atrial fibrillation in the elderly

      c. High-output heart failure

      d. Hyperdynamic precordium

      e. Widened pulse pressure

      f. Systolic murmur

      g. Increased heart rate and cardiac output, and decreased systemic vascular resistance (SVR)

    4. **CNS signs** include persistent agitation, mental status changes, and other signs of CNS dysfunction.

      a. **Elderly patients with thyrotoxicosis often have no symptoms (apathetic thyrotoxicosis) and are diagnosed by a high index of suspicion.**

      b. **Many drugs mask the usual symptoms of thyrotoxicosis.**

B. Thyrotoxic crisis (thyroid storm)

    1. **Systemic signs:** temperature higher than 100°F (37.8°C) and profuse sweating

    2. **Cardiovascular signs and symptoms:** tachycardia, worsening angina, atrial fibrillation or flutter, high-output congestive heart failure, and hypotension

    3. **GI signs and symptoms:** nausea, vomiting, abdominal pain, and hepatic congestion

    4. **CNS signs and symptoms:** agitation, delirium, apathy, stupor, coma, and tremulousness

    5. **Progression:** As thyroid storm progresses, a stupor that leads to coma, hypotension, vascular collapse, and death may occur within 48 hours without treatment.

C. Hypothyroidism

    1. **Systemic signs and symptoms:** hypothermia, cold intolerance, hyponatremia, and weight gain

    2. **Dermatologic signs:** alopecia and coarse, dry skin

    3. **CNS and neurologic signs and symptoms:** apathy and lethargy, bradykinesia, depressed mental status, coma, and psychosis

    4. **Cardiovascular signs and symptoms:**

      a. Hypotension

      b. Unexplained cardiac dysfunction

      c. Bradycardia and angina

      d. Decreased CO secondary to decreased inotropy and chronotropy

      e. Increased peripheral vascular resistance with decreased intravascular volume

      f. Pericardial effusions

    5. Respiratory signs: hypoventilation due to decreased hypoxic and hypercapnic ventilatory drives

    6. Musculoskeletal symptoms: arthralgia and myalgia

    7. Other signs and symptoms: hoarseness, enlarged tongue, goiter, and periorbital edema

  D. Myxedema coma

    1. Systemic signs: hypothermia and non-pitting edema (doughy skin)

    2. CNS signs and symptoms: severe sensorial depression that may lead to coma

    3. Pulmonary signs and symptoms: airway obstruction, respiratory muscle weakness, decreased ventilatory drive

III. Diagnostic (Thyroid Function) Tests. See **Figure 7-2.**

  A. Serum triiodothyronine (T_3) and thyroxine (T_4) levels. T_4 is the major hormone secreted by the thyroid. T_3 is the active form produced by conversion from T_4. T_4 and T_3 are readily bound to carrier proteins.

  B. T_3 resin uptake. This test measures the abilities of carrier proteins to bind radiolabeled T_3 that is added to the sample.

    1. An **increase in T_3 resin uptake** indicates a decrease in protein binding due to occupation of carrier proteins by T_4 or a decrease in the number of carrier proteins.

    2. A **decrease in T_3 resin uptake** indicates less bound T_4 or an increased number of carrier proteins.

  C. Free thyroxine index (FTI). This is the product of the serum

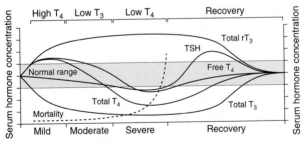

Figure 7-2. Alterations in thyroid hormone concentration with critical illness. Schematic representation of the continuum of changes in serum thyroid hormone levels in patients with nonthyroidal illness. These alterations become more pronounced with increasing severity of the illness and return to the normal range as the illness subsides and the patient recovers. A rapidly rising mortality accompanies the fall in total and free T_4 levels. (From Farwell AD: Sick euthyroid syndrome in the intensive care unit. In *Irwin and Rippe's Intensive Care Medicine,* 4th ed. Edited by Irwin RS, Cerra FB, Rippe JM. Philadelphia, Lippincott Williams & Wilkins, 1999, p 1310.)

T_4 and T_3 resin uptake. When T_4 and T_3 resin uptake change in the same direction, the diagnosis is thyroid disease. When the two change in the opposite direction, the diagnosis is a change in the level of carrier proteins.

D. Free T_3 and T_4. This test is a measure of unbound thyroid hormone.

E. Thyroid-stimulating hormone (TSH) levels. TSH is released by the anterior pituitary gland and is under negative feedback control. Serum levels of TSH are normally low (1–5 μU/ml). The levels rise to > 20 μU/ml in primary hypothyroidism; however, serum TSH can be low in secondary hypothyroidism.

F. Reverse T_3 levels. Reverse T_3, an inactive form of the active metabolite, is elevated in hyperthyroidism and in acute illness.

IV. Diagnosis. Thyroid disease is diagnosed by T_4 level (**Figure 7-3**).

V. Management of Thyrotoxicosis (Hyperthyroidism) and Thyroid Storm

A. Systemic support

1. Control fever with medications (other than salicylates) or

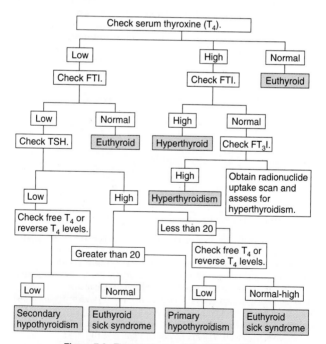

Figure 7-3. Thyroid disease diagnostic algorithm.

cooling blanket. Use chlorpromazine or meperidine, 25–50 mg q 4–6 hr to block shivering response.
2. Initiate fluid resuscitation.
3. For patients with infections, determine which organism is causing the infection. Avoid using empiric broad-spectrum antibiotics.
4. Identify and treat underlying illness.

B. **Medical therapy**
1. **For patients with severe concomitant medical illness who are at high risk for thyroid storm:**
   a. Treat with **antithyroid medication.**
   b. Use **β-blockers** or drugs that deplete catecholamine stores to control the peripheral effects of excess thyroid hormone. **Propranolol is the drug of choice.**
      (1) **Propanolol** (β_1–β_2 blocker), 1 mg/min IV for a total of 2–10 mg, then 40–80 mg PO q 4–6 hr.
      (2) **Metoprolol** (β_1 blocker), 5 mg IV q 6 h, then 100–400 mg PO q 12 h.
      (3) **Atenolol,** 50–100 mg PO qd.
      (4) **Esmolol,** bolus 500 mg/kg, then start continuous drip of 50–100 mg/kg/min.
      (5) **Reserpine,** test dose 0.25 mg IM, then initial dose 1–5 mg IM, then 1–2.5 mg IM q 4–6 hr.
      (6) **Guanethidine,** 1–2 mg/kg PO q 4–6 hr.
2. **To inhibit thyroid hormone synthesis and conversion of T_4 to T_3:** Administer **propylthiouracil (PTU).** Use an initial dose of 600–1200 mg PO followed by a dose of 200–300 mg PO every 6 hours, then taper to a routine dose of 100–200 mg PO tid.
3. **To inhibit thyroid hormone release,** administer one of the following agents:
   a. **Sodium iodide** (0.5 g every 12 hours), which blocks the release of preformed T_4 (can be given 1 to 2 hours after the loading dose of PTU)
   b. **Lugol's solution,** 3–5 drops PO tid
   c. **Supersaturated potassium iodide (SSKI),** 2 drops PO tid, **or potassium iodide,** 1 g over 30 min, PO every 8 hours.
4. **To inhibit peripheral conversion of T_4 to T_3,** use one of the following:
   a. **Corticosteroids** equivalent to 300–400 mg hydrocortisone daily (e.g., dexamethasone 2 mg IV q 6 hr)
   b. **Propranolol or metoprolol**
   c. **Propylthiouracil**
   d. **X-ray iodide containing contrast agents** (Telepaque or Oragrafin, 1 g IV qd)
5. **To remove thyroid hormone from circulation,** use one of the following methods:
   a. Plasmapheresis
   b. Peritoneal dialysis
   c. Cholestyramine, 4 g PO q 6 hr

> **SSKI inhibits the release of thyroid hormone, but should be given at least 1 hour after PTU because PTU can enhance hormone synthesis unless hormone release is blocked. Even if hormone release is blocked, the half-life of circulating T_4 is about 1 week, so symptoms may persist.**

6. **In severe cases of thyroid storm,** where glucocorticoid metabolism is accelerated and can cause a relative adrenal insufficiency, give **dexamethasone,** 2 mg PO q 6 hr.

7. **For severe tachyarrhythmias in patients with coronary artery disease:** Administer **propanolol,** 1 mg IV over 3–5 minutes. This can be repeated every 5–10 minutes until the desired effect is achieved. Alternatively, use 20–40 mg PO q 6 hr.

8. **For pregnant patients with thyrotoxicosis:** Use the **smallest possible dose** of antithyroid drug because these drugs can cross the placenta. **PTU is the drug of choice** because it is heavily protein-bound.
    a. **Patients with non–life threatening illness.** Give PTU until the FT_4 is at the upper limit of normal or mildly elevated.
    b. **Patients with life threatening illness.** Administer PTU, dexamethasone, and β-blockers acutely. Adjust doses as soon as the patient is more stable.

C. **Surgical therapy**
   1. **Indications**
      a. Large goiter
      b. Failed medical treatment owing to side effects of antithyroid medication or noncompliance
      c. Patient preference
      d. Toxic nodular goiter
      e. Grave's disease in pregnancy if antithyroid drugs are not tolerated (perform surgery in second trimester)
   2. **Surgical management**
      a. Render patient biochemically euthyroid with propylthiouracil before surgery.
      b. Give potassium iodide or Lugol's solution for 2 weeks before surgery to decrease thyroid vascularity and simplify resection.
      c. Perform subtotal thyroidectomy.
      d. Treat recurrent hyperthyroidism after surgery with radioiodine.

VI. **Management of Hypothyroidism**
   A. **Patients with mild hypothyroidism.** Treat with oral T_4 in a single daily dose of 50–200 μg.
   B. **Patients with severe hypothyroidism or myxedema coma.** It is wise to use IV therapy initially because of the impaired GI motility. T_3 is preferred because conversion of T_4 to T_3 is depressed in illness. Options include:

1. **T$_4$,** 300–500 µg IV initially and then 75–100 µg IV daily for days to weeks
2. **T$_3$,** 12.5–25 µg IV q 6 hr
3. **T$_3$ preparation** (may be the best choice for initial therapy in severe myxedema coma)
   a. Prepare 100 µg of T$_3$ in 2 ml of 0.1 N NaOH. Add this to 2 ml of 2% albumin solution. The final concentration is 25 µg/ml of T$_3$.
   b. Start with 0.0125 µg IV q 6 hr for 48 hours.
   c. If there is no response by HR, BP, or temperature after 15–21 hours, then increase the next 2 doses to 0.025 µg.
   d. If signs of myocardial ischemia develop, reduce the dose.
   e. If there is gradual improvement of metabolic parameters, taper T$_3$ and introduce T$_4$, starting with 0.05 µg IV q 24 hr.
4. **Combination treatment**
   a. T$_4$, 250 µg IV initial dose, 100 µg IV on day 2, and then 50 µg IV daily
   b. T$_3$, 12.5 µg PO every 6 hours
5. **Corticosteroids** (hydrocortisone, 100 mg IV q 8 hr). Some practitioners recommend corticosteroids as an additional treatment to exclude adrenal insufficiency.
6. **Provide systemic support.**
   a. Secure the patient's airway and mechanically ventilate if necessary.
   b. Passively warm the patient.
   c. Administer isotonic fluids to the patient with hypotension.
   d. Treat the underlying cause of the hypothyroidism.
   e. Institute water restriction for patients with hyponatremia, or use hypertonic saline if serum Na^{+2} < 110 mEq/L.

C. **Patients with hypothyroidism and coronary artery disease.** Start with T$_4$, 25–50 µg daily, and increase the dosage incrementally (12.5–25 µg) every month until the patient is euthyroid.

> **In patients with coronary artery disease, an increase in myocardial demand with thyroid replacement may precipitate ischemia. If angina develops, it must be considered unstable since the half-life of T$_4$ is several weeks.**

D. **Patients with hypothyroidism and concomitant adrenal insufficiency**

> **Rapid thyroid replacement can precipitate Addisonian crisis in patients with adrenal insufficiency.**

1. Critically ill hypothyroid patients should be tested for adrenal insufficiency and treated empirically with corticosteroids until adrenal insufficiency is excluded.
2. The examiner should be alert for signs suggesting hypogonadism (decreased libido, amenorrhea, diminished sex hormone dependent hair, or small testes), which would indicate that the hypothyroidism and adrenal insufficiency is secondary to pan-pituitary insufficiency.

8

Fluids and Electrolytes

ACID–BASE DISTURBANCES

I. **Analysis of Acid-Base Status.** Arterial **blood gas analysis** provides the values for the pH, partial pressure of carbon dioxide (PCO_2), and bicarbonate (HCO_3); this information is necessary for the evaluation of acid–base disorders. **Table 8-1** and **Figure 8–1** summarize the changes in pH, PCO_2, and HCO_3 in the various acid–base disturbances.

   A. **Acidosis vs. alkalosis.** The pH will generally define the disorder as acidosis or alkalosis.

      1. **Normal pH = 7.35 to 7.45.**

      2. **pH < 7.35 indicates acidosis.**

         a. **PCO_2 > 44 mm Hg** indicates a primary respiratory acidosis.

         b. **HCO_3 < 22 mm Hg** indicates a primary metabolic acidosis.

      3. **pH > 7.45 indicates alkalosis.**

         a. **PCO_2 < 36 mm Hg** indicates a primary respiratory alkalosis.

         b. **HCO_3 > 26 mm Hg** indicates a primary metabolic alkalosis.

   B. **Compensation.** Primary disturbances can be compensated, and thus correct the pH towards normal. Overcompensation cannot be achieved without exogenous mechanisms.

      1. The compensation for a primary metabolic disorder is respiratory change (change in PCO_2).

      2. The compensation for a primary respiratory disorder is metabolic change (change in HCO_3).

   C. **Metabolic disorders**

      1. **Characteristics**

         a. There is a change in HCO_3.

         b. The pH and PCO_2 change in the *same* direction.

         c. In **metabolic alkalosis,** the pH increases.

         d. In **metabolic acidosis,** the pH decreases. The anion

Table 8-1. Changes in Acid–Base Disorders

Disorder	Primary Change	Compensatory Change	Expected Compensatory Change
Metabolic acidosis	↓ HCO_3^-	↓ PCO_2	$PCO_2 = 1.5 \times HCO_3^- (8 \pm 2)$
Respiratory acidosis	↑ PCO_2	↑ HCO_3^-	
Acute			$\Delta pH = 0.008 (PCO_2 - 40)$
Chronic			$\Delta pH = 0.003 (PCO_2 - 40)$
Metabolic alkalosis	↑ HCO_3^-	↑ PCO_2	$PCO_2 = 7 \times HCO_3^- + (20 \pm 1.5)$
Respiratory alkalosis	↓ PCO_2	↓ HCO_3^-	
Acute			$\Delta pH = 0.008 (40 - PCO_2)$
Chronic			$\Delta pH = 0.017 (40 - PCO_2)$

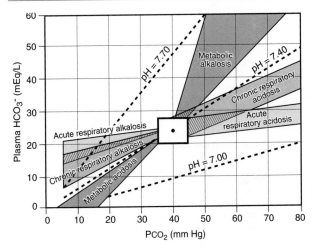

Figure 8-1. Graph used for determination of acid–base status. (Adapted with permission from Shapiro JI, Kaehny WD: Pathogenesis and management of metabolic acidosis and alkalosis. In *Renal and Electrolyte Disorders,* 5th ed. Edited by Schrier RW. Philadelphia, Lippincott-Raven, 1997, p 76.)

  gap may be normal or high depending upon the underlying disorder (see II A).

 2. Associated respiratory disorders

  a. For metabolic acidosis, the expected $P_{CO_2} = 1.5 \times HCO_3 + 8 \, (\pm 2)$.

  b. For metabolic alkalosis, the expected $P_{CO_2} = 0.7 \times HCO_3 + 20 \, (\pm 1.5)$.

  c. If the P_{CO_2} is greater than expected, a coexisting primary respiratory acidosis exists.

  d. If the P_{CO_2} is less than expected, a coexisting primary respiratory alkalosis exists.

D. Respiratory disorders

 1. Characteristics

  a. There is a change in P_{CO_2}.

  b. The pH and P_{CO_2} change in different directions.

  c. In **respiratory acidosis,** the pH > 7.45 and the P_{CO_2} > 40.

   (1) In **acute uncompensated respiratory acidosis,** the pH changes 0.008 U for every 1 mm Hg change in P_{CO_2}.

   (2) In **chronic compensated respiratory acidosis,** the pH changes 0.003 U for every 1 mm Hg change in P_{CO_2}.

  d. In **respiratory alkalosis,** the pH < 7.40 and the P_{CO_2} < 40.

        (1) In **acute uncompensated respiratory alkalosis,** the pH changes 0.008 U for every 1 mm Hg change in P_{CO_2}.

        (2) In **chronic compensated respiratory alkalosis,** the pH changes 0.017 U for every 1 mm Hg change in P_{CO_2}.

  2. Associated metabolic disorders

    a. A pH change lower than the calculated value is associated with a coexisting primary metabolic acidosis.

    b. A pH change greater than calculated value is associated with a coexisting primary metabolic alkalosis.

E. Mixed disorders. A normal pH with abnormal HCO_3 and/or P_{CO_2} indicates a mixed disorder.

II. Metabolic Acidosis

A. Etiology

1. Anion gap. To determine the etiology of metabolic acidosis, first determine the anion gap (AG), which is the difference between the sum of the measured cations and anions in the plasma or serum:

$$AG = serum\ Na - serum\ Cl - serum\ HCO_3$$

Note that a 50% reduction in serum albumin (**hypoalbuminemia**) will reduce the AG by 5–6 mEq/L.

2. Metabolic acidosis with normal AG is caused by the loss of bicarbonate-rich fluids from the GI tract or kidney. Use the mnemonic **HHARDUP** to remember the **possible underlying disorders:**

  a. **H**ypoaldosteronism

  b. **H**yperosmolar nonketotic coma

  c. **A**cetazolamide (carbonic anhydrase inhibitor)

  d. **R**enal tubular acidosis

  e. **D**iarrhea

  f. **U**reterosigmoidostomy, ileostomy

  g. **P**ancreatic fistula

3. Metabolic acidosis with high AG. The mnemonic **MUDPILES** will help you remember the **possible underlying disorders:**

  a. **M**ethanol use

  b. **U**remia (renal failure)

  c. **D**iabetic ketoacidosis (DKA)

  d. **P**oisons (**P**araldehyde, **P**henformin, **P**ropylene glycol)

  e. **I**ron, INH

  f. **L**actic acidosis

  g. **E**thanol or **E**thylene glycol use

  h. **S**alicylate use, **S**tarvation

B. Management

1. Correct the underlying disorder.

2. If the metabolic acidosis is mild to moderate, no immediate treatment is needed

3. If the pH < 7.20 or the HCO_3 < 15, correct half of the base deficit at a time with sodium bicarbonate (1 ampule = 50 mEq):

$$HCO_3 \ required = 0.4 \times wt \ (kg) \times (25 - measured \ HCO_3)$$

III. Metabolic Alkalosis

A. Etiology

1. Exogenous bicarbonate administration (lactate, citrate, acetate) may cause metabolic acidosis.
2. Chloride (saline)-responsive metabolic acidosis (urine chloride [U_{CL}] < 10–20 mEq/L) may be due to:
   a. Contraction alkalosis
   b. Diuretics
   c. Villous adenoma
   d. Gastric acid loss from large-volume vomiting or continuous gastric suction
3. Chloride (saline)-unresponsive metabolic alkalosis (U_{CL} > 10–20 mEq/L) may be due to severe potassium depletion or mineralocorticoid excess caused by any of the following (mnemonic **D. VAGA**):
   a. **D**iuretics
   b. **V**omiting
   c. **A**ldosteronism
   d. **G**astric drainage
   e. **A**lkali intake (antacids)

B. Management

1. Treat the underlying disorder.
2. Correct hypovolemia with normal saline.
3. Correct hypokalemia.
4. Administer acetazolamide (500 mg every 6 hours) to inhibit carbonic anhydrase, which restricts reclamation and synthesis of bicarbonate.
5. **If there is a chloride deficit,** replace chloride with 0.1N hydrochloric acid solution:

$$Chloride \ deficit = 0.4 \times wt \ (kg) \times (100 - measured \ Cl)$$

6. **In prolonged gastric suctioning,** use histamine-2 (H_2) antagonist to decrease gastric acid production.
7. **For patients who are volume overloaded and unresponsive to acetazolamide,** consider continuous hemofiltration (CAVH). This therapy must be combined with the infusion of chloride-containing fluid.
8. **For patients with chloride-unresponsive metabolic alkalosis,** use potassium replacement or mineralocorticoid antagonists (e.g., Aldactone).

IV. Respiratory Acidosis

A. Etiology.
Respiratory acidosis is caused by **acute or chronic hypercapnia due to inadequate ventilation,** which may be due to:

1. Upper or lower airway obstruction
2. Status asthmaticus, severe asthma, or COPD
3. Severe alveolar defects (pneumonia, pulmonary edema, ARDS)
4. CNS depression (sedatives, trauma, intracranial bleed)
5. Neuromuscular impairment
6. Ventilatory restriction (flail chest, rib fracture, pneumothorax)

B. **Management.** Improve alveolar ventilation by:
  1. Supplemental oxygen
  2. Aggressive pulmonary toilet
  3. Treatment of pneumonia
  4. Administration of bronchodilators
  5. Removal of obstruction (secretions, foreign body, misplaced endotracheal tube)
  6. Mechanical ventilation (Optimize minute ventilation with tidal volume and rate.)

V. **Respiratory Alkalosis**
  A. **Etiology.** Respiratory alkalosis is caused by **acute or chronic hyperventilation,** which can be due to:
    1. Metabolic encephalopathy
    2. Hepatic failure
    3. Anxiety
    4. Early sepsis
    5. Pulmonary embolism
    6. Hypoxia
    7. Congestive heart failure (CHF)
    8. Severe head injury
    9. Cerebrovascular accident (CVA)
    10. Mechanical overventilation
    11. Salicylate overdose
  B. **Management**
    1. Calm the patient.
    2. Have the patient do carbon dioxide rebreathing (paper bag treatment).
    3. Treat the underlying disorder.
    4. Administer a sedative as needed.
    5. Perform mechanical ventilation.

ELECTROLYTE CONCENTRATIONS IN BODY FLUIDS. Refer to **Table 8-2.**

ELECTROLYTE DISTURBANCES

> **When managing electrolyte disturbances, the rule of thumb is *replete and recheck***

I. **Potassium Imbalance**
  A. **Normal potassium levels** are in the range of 3.5–5.0 mEq/L.
  B. **Hypokalemia** is defined as **serum potassium (K) < 3.5 mEq/L.**
    1. **Etiology**
      a. **Shift of potassium into the cells** secondary to:
        (1) **Metabolic alkalosis** (potassium and hydrogen exchange across the cellular membrane)
        (2) **Increased activity of sodium–potassium adenosine triphosphatase (Na–K ATPase)** caused by

Table 8-2. Electrolyte Concentrations in Body Fluids

	Na$^+$ (mEq/L)	K$^+$ (mEq/L)	Cl$^-$ (mEq/L)	HCO$_3^-$ (mEq/L)	Vol/24 hr	IV Fluid Replacement
Saliva	20–60	10–20	15–30	30–50	1–2 L	D5¼NS + 20 KCl/L
Bile	130–145	4–6	95–105	20–40	0.1–1 L	D5NS + ½ amp HCO$_3$/L
Stomach	40–100	5–15	15–20	—	1.5–2.5 L	D5½NS + 20 KCl/L
Pancreas	130–140	4–6	40–75	80–115	1–2 L	D5½NS + 1 amp HCO$_3$/L
Small bowel	130–140	4–6	40–60	80–100	1–3 L	D5NS + 1 amp HCO$_3$/L
Colon	80–140	25–45	80–100	30–50	0.1–0.6 L	D5½NS + 20 KCl/L
Diarrhea	50–60	40–50	35–45	46–60	Variable	D5½NS + ½ amp HCO$_3$/L
Sweat	40–50	5–10	40–60	—	0.2–1.5 L	D5¼NS

β-receptor agonists (albuterol, epinephrine, dopamine) or insulin

b. Potassium depletion secondary to:

(1) Renal wasting

(a) Urine potassium (U_K) > 30 mEq/L and serum HCO_3 < 24 indicates renal tubular acidosis.

(b) U_K > 30 mEq/L and serum HCO_3 > 24

(i) With urine chloride (U_{Cl}) > 10 mEq/L. This may be caused by diuretics, steroids, low magnesium levels, or hyperaldosteronism.

(ii) With U_{Cl} < 10 mEq/L. This may be caused by nasogastric suction, vomiting, or hyperventilation.

(2) Extrarenal loss. U_K < 30 mEq/L). Causes include diarrhea, villous adenoma, or VIPoma.

c. Magnesium depletion. This impairs potassium reabsorption by the renal tubules.

2. Clinical presentation

a. Weakness (paralysis in extreme cases)

b. Cardiac arrhythmias such as premature ventricular contractions (PVCs), ventricular tachycardia (VT), or ventricular fibrillation (VF)

c. Increased likelihood of digoxin toxicity

3. Management

a. Oral supplementation. In a healthy patient, potassium can be regulated by diet and by oral supplements. Give potassium chloride, 10–40 mEq PO qd-bid (dose depends on deficit).

b. IV supplementation. In patients who are not eating or who are critically ill, potassium should be replaced intravenously.

(1) Administer potassium chloride, 10 mEq/100 ml IV peripherally, or 20 mEq/100 ml IV centrally.

(2) If more than 20 mEq is required at one time, split the doses between multiple peripheral veins to avoid a sudden influx of a large amount of potassium into the right heart (to prevent VT or VF).

c. Adjustment. Remember to adjust the potassium dosage according to renal function.

C. Hyperkalemia is defined as **K > 5.0 mEq/L. Pseudohyperkalemia** occurs when there is hemolysis during venipuncture or when there is potassium release during clot formation.

1. Etiology

a. Shift of potassium out of the cells. This may be secondary to any of the following (all except acidosis will have UK > 30 mEq/L in normal renal function):

(1) Myonecrosis. Destruction of cell membranes results in direct release of potassium.

   (2) Hypoinsulinemia. Insulin promotes potassium uptake in muscle and liver.
   (3) Acidosis. This results in a potassium–hydrogen shift across cellular membranes.
   (4) Digoxin toxicity. This damages the Na–K pump.
 b. Reduced renal excretion (U_K < 30 mEq/L) secondary to:
   (1) Severe renal insufficiency: glomerular filtration rate (GFR) < 10 ml/min, or urine output < 1 L/day
   (2) Adrenal insufficiency
   (3) Drugs such as angiotensin-converting enzyme (ACE) inhibitors, potassium-sparing diuretics, and nonsteroidal anti-inflammatory agents
 c. Exogenous causes such as
   (1) Diet rich in potassium
   (2) Use of potassium supplements
   (3) Blood transfusions
2. Clinical presentation
 a. Skeletal muscle weakness
 b. Cardiac conduction abnormalities
 c. ECG changes (occur in only 50% of patients):
   (1) Tall, narrow-base T wave in leads V2 to V4
   (2) Decreased P wave amplitude, and P-R interval that increases until the P wave disappears
   (3) QRS that becomes prolonged and results in ventricular asystole
3. Management. Treatment depends on the level of the hyperkalemia.
 a. Use one of the following agents **to promote potassium clearance:**
   (1) Polystyrene sulfonate resin (Kayexalate). This cation exchange resin is given orally, 30 g in 50 ml 20% sorbitol, or as a retention enema, 50 g in 200 ml 20% sorbitol.
   (2) Furosemide 20–40 mg PO. These agents are not effective in oliguric renal failure.
 b. To correct the transcellular shift, administer an **insulin–glucose infusion,** 10 U regular insulin IV in conjunction with 50 ml of 50% dextrose IV.
 c. For patients with ECG changes, arrhythmias, or K > 7.0 mEq/L, administer **calcium gluconate,** a direct membrane antagonist:
   (1) Give 10–20 ml of 10% solution IV over 3 minutes. This may be repeated in 5 minutes.
   (2) If the patient is on digoxin, add 10 ml of 10% solution to 100 ml NS and infuse over 20–30 minutes (to avoid digoxin toxicity by hypercalcemia).
   (3) Calcium increases the membrane threshold and

must be used in conjunction with another therapy that will reduce the hyperkalemia.

    d. Use dialysis for patients with chronic renal failure or in patients whose hyperkalemia is unresponsive to other measures.

    e. Remove all exogenous sources of potassium (e.g., from diet, IV fluids).

II. Calcium Imbalance

A. Normal calcium levels

    1. Normal total calcium = 8.5–10.2 mg/dl.

    2. Normal ionized calcium = 4.8–7.2 mg/dl or 1.1–1.3 mmol/L.

    3. Adjustment of total calcium for changes in serum albumin: For every 1 mg/dl decrease in albumin from 4.0, add 0.8 mg/dl to the total calcium.

B. Hypocalcemia is defined as **serum calcium (Ca)** < 8 mg/dl.

    1. Etiology. Hypocalcemia may be due to:

        a. Hypoparathyroidism

        b. Hypomagnesemia, which leads to decreased parathyroid hormone (PTH) release

        c. Alkalosis, which increases binding of calcium to albumin

        d. Renal failure secondary to phosphorous retention and defective conversion of vitamin D to its active metabolite

        e. Drugs such as aminoglycosides, heparin, theophylline, cimetidine, and furosemide

        f. Other causes such as pancreatitis, burns, fat embolism, massive blood transfusion, and cardiopulmonary bypass

    2. Clinical presentation

        a. Neuromuscular excitability, including hyperreflexia, tetany, and seizures

        b. Chvostek's sign. Have the patient open his mouth slightly and tap on the facial nerve. Jaw jerk is the positive finding. Chvostek's sign is present in 30% of patients who have hypocalcemia and in 25% of the general population.

        c. Trousseau's sign. Place the blood pressure cuff on the patient's upper arm; inflate the cuff and observe for muscle spasms.

        d. Cardiovascular signs, including peripheral vasodilation, hypotension, left ventricular failure, ventricular tachycardia, and prolonged QT interval

    3. Management. Treatment consists of intravenous calcium therapy.

        a. Calcium gluconate, 90 mg (4.5 mEq)/10 ml vial

            (1) For acute symptoms, give 100–200 mg Ca over 10 minutes until symptoms resolve. Monitor the patient closely; more medication may be required to relieve the symptoms.

   (2) Maintenance dose. Give 1–2 mg/kg/hr.
   b. Calcium chloride, 272 mg (13.6 mEq)/10 ml vial
C. Hypercalcemia is defined as **Ca > 11 mg/dl.** (See also HY-PERCALCEMIA, p. 170.)
   1. Etiology
      a. Hyperparathyroidism
      b. Malignancy (solid tumors, multiple myeloma, lymphoma)
      c. Thyroid disease
      d. Addison's disease
      e. VIPoma
      f. Pheochromocytoma
      g. Sarcoidosis
      h. Tuberculosis
      i. Drugs
      j. Exogenous causes
   2. Clinical presentation
      a. Altered mental status which can progress to coma
      b. Nausea, vomiting, ileus, pancreatitis, and constipation
      c. Hypotension and hypovolemia
      d. Polyuria and nephrocalcinosis
      e. Shortened QT interval on ECG
   3. Management
      a. Administer saline and loop diuretics.
         (1) Hypercalciuria causes an osmotic diuresis. Use an aggressive volume infusion of normal saline (200–300 ml/hr). Guard against dehydration.
         (2) Administer furosemide, 40–100 mg IV every 2 hours to promote calcium excretion.
         (3) Monitor urine output hourly and match the outputs with volume infusion.
      b. Administer calcitonin, which reduces serum calcium by inhibiting bone resorption. Use 4 U IM or SQ q 12 hr × 2 doses. If this is unsuccessful, the dose can be doubled after 2 days.
      c. Administer bisphosphates, which have an inhibitory effect on osteoclasts.
         (1) Give etidronate, 7.5 mg/kg IV over 4 hours qd x 3–7 days.
         (2) Give pamidronate, 90 mg IV over 24 hours, or 15–40 mg IV qd for up to 6 days by slow infusion.
      d. Dialysis is indicated only as a last resort prior to surgical intervention.
III. Phosphorous Imbalance
   A. Normal phosphorus levels range from 3 to 4.5 mg/dl. There is a diurnal variation.
   B. Hypophosphatemia
      1. Etiology
         a. Dextrose infusion, which may result in insulin-mediated transport of glucose and phosphorous into skeletal muscle and liver

  b. Overzealous carbohydrate feeding, especially in malnourished patients

  c. Respiratory alkalosis, especially in patients on mechanical ventilation

  d. β-agonist bronchodilators

  e. Diabetic ketoacidosis, in which glycosuria increases the urinary phosphate, and insulin therapy drives the remaining phosphorous into the cells

  f. Antacids, which contain aluminum hydroxide and bind phosphorous in the bowel lumen

 2. Clinical presentation. Hypophosphatemia is **usually asymptomatic,** but the following signs and symptoms may be evident:

  a. Reduced cardiac contractility

  b. Cardiomyopathy

  c. Hemolysis (uncommon)

  d. Decreased oxygen saturation through depletion of 2,3-diphosphoglycerate (shift of oxyhemoglobin dissociation curve to left)

  e. Muscle weakness caused by impaired ATP generation (ATP is needed for skeletal muscle to work)

 3. Management

  a. Administer **sodium phosphate,** 3 mmol PO_4/ml, and 4 mEq/ml Na; **or potassium phosphate,** 3 mmol PO_4/ml and 4 mEq/ml K. The dosage depends on the serum PO_4 level:

   (1) For the patient with serum PO_4 < 0.5 mg/dl, infuse 0.5 mmol/kg over 4 hours.

   (2) For the patient with serum PO_4 ranging from 0.5–1.9 mg/dl, infuse 0.16–0.25 mmol/kg over 4–8 hours.

  b. The patient may require **IV replacement therapy** for 5–7 days until intracellular stores are replenished.

  c. For otherwise healthy patients tolerating an oral diet, administer **Neutraphos,** 250–500 mg PO q 6 hr (8–16 mmol PO_4).

C. Hyperphosphatemia

 1. Etiology

  a. Renal failure or insufficiency

  b. Widespread cellular necrosis caused by rhabdomyolysis, tumor lysis syndromes, trauma, or acidosis

  c. Postoperative hypoparathyroidism

 2. Clinical presentation. Hyperphosphatemia is **usually asymptomatic,** but the following signs may be evident:

  a. Ectopic calcification if the calcium x phosphorus product (serum $Ca^{+2} \times PO_4^-$) is > 60

  b. Heart block

 3. Management

  a. Correct the underlying disorder.

  b. Restrict dietary phosphate.

      c. Increase urinary excretion with hydration and a diuretic (e.g., acetazolamide, 500 mg IV/PO q 6 hr).

      d. Administer phosphate binders (aluminum-containing antacids) such as Amphojel or Basaljel.

      e. Use dialysis in patients with extreme conditions such as ectopic calcification or cardiac disturbances.

IV. Magnesium Imbalance

A. **Normal magnesium levels** are in the range of 1.8–2.5 mg/dl.

B. **Hypomagnesemia (serum magnesium < 1.8 mg/dl)**

  1. Etiology

    a. **Decreased intestinal absorption** of magnesium due to malabsorption, malnutrition, diarrhea, or gastric aspiration

    b. **Increased renal excretion** of magnesium due to hypercalcemia, osmotic diuresis (such as in diabetes mellitus), or drugs such as loop diuretics, cyclosporine, and aminoglycosides.

  2. Clinical presentation

    a. Hypokalemia and hypocalcemia

    b. Hypophosphatemia

    c. Lethargy, confusion, nystagmus, tremors, tetany, and seizures

    d. Atrial and ventricular arrhythmias (VT, VF, torsades de pointes)

    e. Digitalis toxicity promoted by magnesium depletion

    f. The patient with **reactive CNS magnesium deficiency** may present with ataxia, slurred speech, metabolic acidosis, muscle spasms, seizures, progressive obtundation, excessive salivation, and reduced magnesium in the CSF.

  3. Diagnosis

    a. The patient with hypomagnesemia may have a normal serum level of magnesium.

    b. Check the **urine magnesium** for wasting.

    c. Perform a **renal magnesium retention test.** (This test is contraindicated in patients with cardiovascular instability, renal failure, or magnesium-wasting syndromes.)

      (1) Add 6 g $MgSO_4$ to 250 ml NS and infuse over 1 hour.

      (2) Collect urine for 24 hours. A total urine magnesium less than 12 mEq is evidence of total body magnesium deficiency.

  4. Management

    a. **Mild or chronic hypomagnesemia.** Administer magnesium oxide, 400 mg PO qd bid.

    b. **Moderate hypomagnesemia:** serum magnesium < 1 mEq/L or with associated electrolyte abnormalities

      (1) Add 6 g $MgSO_4$ to 250 ml NS and infuse over 3 hours.

(2) Then, add 5 g $MgSO_4$ to 250 ml NS and infuse over 6 hours.

(3) Continue with 5 g $MgSO_4$ every 12 hours (continuous infusion) for the next 5 days.

c. **Severe and life-threatening hypomagnesemia** associated with cardiac arrhythmias or seizures

(1) Infuse 2 g $MgSO_4$ IV over 2 minutes.

(2) Add 5 g $MgSO_4$ to 250 ml NS and infuse over 6 hours.

(3) Continue with 5 g $MgSO_4$ every 12 hours (continuous infusion) for the next 5 days.

C. **Hypermagnesemia (serum magnesium > 4 mEq/L or 7 mg/dl)**

1. **Etiology**

a. Renal insufficiency or renal failure, usually after treatment with magnesium containing antacids or laxatives

b. Exogenous magnesium

c. Hemolysis

2. **Clinical presentation**

a. **Neuromuscular signs and symptoms** include areflexia, lethargy, weakness, paralysis, and respiratory failure.

b. **Cardiac signs** include hypotension, bradycardia, prolonged PR, QRS, and QT intervals, complete heart block, and asystole.

3. **Management**

a. Remove the exogenous source of magnesium.

b. The patient who has **severe and symptomatic hypermagnesemia** should be treated with 10% calcium gluconate, 10–20 ml over 10 minutes, to temporarily antagonize the effects of the magnesium.

c. The patient in **renal failure** may need **urgent dialysis.**

INTRAVENOUS FLUIDS. Refer to Table 8-3.

SODIUM AND OSMOLALITY DISTURBANCES

I. **Hypernatremia (serum Na > 145 mEq/L)**

A. **Overview**

1. **Mechanism.** Hypernatremia may result from either of the following:

a. Loss of fluid with a low sodium concentration (< 135 mEq/L)

b. Gain of fluid with a high sodium concentration (> 145 mEq/L)

2. **Extracellular volume** in hypernatremia may be low, normal, or high.

a. **Low extracellular volume** occurs when there is a loss of hypotonic fluids (hypovolemic hypernatremia and hypoglycemic nonketotic syndrome). This may be caused by diuresis, vomiting, or diarrhea.

Table 8-3. Intravenous Fluid Composition

Fluid	Glucose (g)	Na$^+$ (mEq/L)	K$^+$ (mEq/L)	Cl$^-$ (mEq/L)	HCO$_3^-$ (mEq/L)	Osmolarity (mOsm/L)	Calories Kcal/L
D5W	50	0	0	0	0	252	170
D10W	100	0	0	0	0	505	340
D50W	500	0	0	0	0	2525	1700
0.45%NS	0	77	0	77	0	154	0
NS	0	154	0	154	0	308	0
D5/0.22%NS	50	38	0	38	0	329	170
D5/0.45%NS	50	77	0	77	0	406	170
D5/NS	50	154	0	154	0	560	170
LR	0	130	4	110	27	272	< 10
D5/LR	50	130	4	110	27	524	180
Albumin 5%	0	145	0	145	0	330	200
Albumin 25%	0	145	0	145	0	330	1000

Maintenance fluids: First 10 kg body weight = 100 ml/kg/24 hr = 4 ml/kg/hr
Second 10 kg body weight = 50 ml/kg/24 hr = 2 ml/kg/hr
Weight > 20 kg body weight = 20 ml/kg/24 hr = 1 ml/kg/hr
1.5 ampules of HCO$_3^-$ to 1 NS creates of pH of 7.4.
D = dextrose; LR = lactated Ringer's solution; NS = normal saline.

b. **Normal extracellular volume** occurs when there is a net loss of free water (diabetes insipidus).

c. **High extracellular volume** means a gain of hypertonic fluids.

B. Hypovolemic hypernatremia

1. **Etiology.** Hypovolemic hypernatremia can be caused by diuresis, vomiting, or diarrhea.

2. **Clinical concerns**

   a. Hypovolemia is **serious and life-threatening** because of the **risk of shock.**

   b. Hypertonicity leads to cellular dehydration, which leads to neurologic impairment. The degree of **mental status changes** is proportional to the magnitude of hyperosmolality and the time period of the change. **Seizures, focal neurologic deficits,** and **frank coma** may occur.

3. **Management** consists of fluid therapy.

   a. **Replace volume deficits rapidly** with normal saline to avoid hypovolemic shock

   b. **Replace free water deficits slowly** with normal saline over a period of 48 to 72 hours. Free water deficit is calculated as:

$$0.6 \times wt\ (kg) \times [(current\ Plasma\ Na/140) - 1]$$

C. Diabetes Insipidus (DI)

1. **Mechanism.** Impairment of renal water conservation results in the loss of large volumes of urine that is almost purely free water.

   a. **Central DI** is caused by inhibition of anti-diuretic hormone (ADH) release from the posterior pituitary. Polyuria occurs within 24 hours of the inciting event (see 2 a below). Urine osmolality is usually < 200 mOsm/L.

   b. **Nephrogenic DI** is caused by end-organ unresponsiveness to ADH. Urine osmolality is usually 200–500 mOsm/L.

2. **Etiology**

   a. **Central DI** may be idiopathic, or it may be caused by head trauma, neurosurgical procedures, brain tumors, intracranial aneurysms, meningitis, or encephalitis.

   b. **Nephrogenic DI** may be caused by sickle cell nephropathy, chronic pyelonephritis, multiple myeloma, hypercalcemia, hypokalemia, or drugs such as lithium, amphotericin B, methoxyflurane, and demeclocycline.

3. **Diagnosis**

   a. Obtain **urine osmolality** reading, then restrict fluids for 2 to 3 hours. Recheck urine osmolality; failure of the urine osmolality to increase more than 30 mOsm/L is diagnostic of DI.

b. Use the **vasopressin test** to determine whether the DI is central or nephrogenic. Check urine osmolality, then administer 5 U IV of aqueous vasopressin. Recheck the urine osmolality in 1 hour.

  (1) In **central DI,** urine osmolality increases abruptly by at least 50% of baseline.

  (2) In **nephrogenic DI** there is no response.

4. Management

  a. Replace free water deficits only (by oral intake or D5W).

  b. Monitor ongoing sodium and water losses and replace as needed.

  c. Strictly monitor urine outputs.

  d. For patients with **severe central DI,** administer vasopressin, 5–10 U SQ q 4–6 hr. Closely monitor serum sodium.

  e. For patient with **severe nephrogenic DI,** administer thiazide diuretics.

D. Hypervolemic hypernatremia is a rare condition caused by iatrogenic administration of hypertonic solutions.

1. Etiology

  a. Hypertonic saline resuscitation

  b. Sodium bicarbonate administration

  c. Excessive consumption of table salt

2. Management

  a. Patients with normal renal function. Intervention is not necessary because excess sodium will be excreted.

  b. Patients with impaired renal function who are taking furosemide for diuresis. The resulting urine contains approximately 75 mEq/L sodium, and excessive urine output will add to the hypernatremia. Therefore, the urine volume must be partially replaced with a more hypotonic solution.

E. Hyperglycemic nonketotic syndrome is a disorder of adults with mild or no diabetes who have adequate stores of insulin to prevent ketosis. Blood glucose is often > 900 mg/dl.

1. Mechanism. Persistent loss of glucose in urine precipitates an osmotic diuresis that can lead to severe volume loss.

2. Predisposing factors include infection, parenteral nutrition, β-blockers, diuretics, and steroids.

3. Clinical presentation. These patients usually have an altered mental status which may proceed to coma if the serum osmolality rises above 330 mOsm.

4. Glucose correction. Each increase in glucose of 100 mg/dl will cause a decrease in serum Na by 1.6 mEq/L in euvolemic patients, and 2.0 mEq/L in hypovolemic patients.

5. Management

  a. Correct intravascular volume deficits with normal saline.

  b. Replace free water deficits slowly. Make sure to adjust the measured serum sodium for the increased glucose.

c. Do not start insulin therapy until the hypovolemia is corrected. Use insulin cautiously, and monitor the blood sugar continually so that the insulin dose may be modified as needed. Insulin drip: 2–5 U regular insulin/hr.

II. Hyponatremia (serum sodium < 135 mEq/L)

A. **Hypotonic hyponatremia** is defined as an excess of free water relative to sodium in the extracellular space. **Volume status** is assessed to determine management.

1. **Hypovolemic hypotonic hyponatremia**

   a. **Mechanism.** There is a loss of fluid that is isotonic to plasma and replacement by hypotonic solution. This creates a net sodium loss, which creates a decrease in extracellular volume (ECV) and decreases extracellular sodium concentration.

   b. **Causes**

      (1) **Diuretics** (urine sodium > 20 mEq/L)

      (2) **Adrenal insufficiency** (urine sodium > 20 mEq/L)

      (3) **Secretory diarrhea** (urine sodium < 10 mEq/L)

2. **Isovolemic hypotonic hyponatremia.** There is a small gain in free water. **Causes** include:

   a. **Syndrome of inappropriate anti-diuretic hormone production (SIADH).** There is sustained release of vasopressin and inappropriately concentrated urine with hypotonic plasma:

      (1) Urine sodium > 40 mEq/L

      (2) Urine osmolality > 100–500 mOsm/kg water

   b. **Acute water intoxication (psychogenic polydipsia)**

      (1) Urine sodium < 10 mEq/L

      (2) Urine osmolality < 100 mOsm/kg water

3. **Hypervolemic hypotonic hyponatremia.** There is an excess of water over sodium. **Causes** include:

   a. **Heart failure** (urine sodium < 20 mEq/L)

   b. **Cirrhosis** (urine sodium < 20 mEq/L)

   c. **Renal failure** (urine sodium > 20 mEq/L)

B. **Severe hyponatremia** (serum sodium < 120 mEq/L)

1. **Mortality** can exceed 50%.

2. The major complication is a **metabolic encephalopathy** that may be irreversible and fatal, which can be accompanied by seizures and ARDS.

Rapid correction of severe hyponatremia can result in central pontine myelinolysis (a demyelinating brainstem lesion).

C. **Management**

1. Determine the volume status.

    a. The **hypovolemic patient** will have decreased BP, increased HR, decreased skin turgor, and weight loss.

    b. The **hypervolemic patient** will have edema, ascites, and weight gain.

2. Determine the sodium deficit:

$$0.6 \times bodyweight\ (kg) \times (130 - serum\ Na)$$
$$Use\ 0.5\ for\ women.$$

3. The **rate of correction** is dictated by the severity of the patient's symptoms.

    a. Symptomatic patients (patients with coma, generalized seizures, and respiratory arrest). Increase the serum sodium at a rate of 0.5 mEq/L/hr until a level of 125–130 mEq/L is reached. *Never* correct to normal levels with a rapid method.

    b. Alcoholics and malnourished patients. It is best to return these patients to 125 mEq/L.

4. For patients with **low ECV,** use 3% saline until the serum sodium is 125–130 mEq/L.

5. For patients with **normal ECV,** start with furosemide diuresis, then proceed with 3% saline for patients with severe symptoms, or isotonic saline in mild or no symptoms. Restrict fluid intake.

6. For patients with **high ECV,** use furosemide diuresis until the serum sodium rises to 125–130 mEq/L. Add hypertonic saline if the patient is symptomatic. Restrict fluid intake.

9

Gastrointestinal

Disorders

ACUTE ABDOMEN

I. **History**
   A. **Current medical history** should include information about:
      1. Patient setting (e.g., postoperative, trauma, organ failure)
      2. Mental status and ability to communicate symptoms
      3. Time of onset of pain
      4. Duration, acuity, and progression of pain
      5. Location at onset and movement of pain
      6. Radiation of pain (e.g., to the shoulder, groin, or back)
      7. Nature of pain (e.g., constant, intermittent, decreasing, increasing)
      8. Character of pain (e.g., sharp, dull, crampy)
      9. Effect of eating, vomiting, passing flatus, urination, respiration, movement, position, and eructation on pain
      10. Activities that make the pain worse or better
      11. Status of GI function and recent feeding history
      12. Last bowel movement
      13. Immunocompetence
      14. Coexisting disease possibly affecting presentation (e.g., renal failure, diabetes, atherosclerotic disease)
      15. Menstrual periods
      16. Alcohol, tobacco, and illicit drug use
      17. Medications [e.g., corticosteroids (use within the last year), cardiac medications, anticoagulants (length of and reason for use)]
   B. **Past medical history** should include information about:
      1. Similar episodes
      2. Previous surgery
      3. Cancer history (i.e., personal and family)

    4. Hernias

    5. Gallstones

    6. Cardiovascular disease [e.g., coronary artery disease (CAD), hypertension, myocardial infarction, congestive heart failure]

    7. Pulmonary disease (e.g., asthma, COPD)

    8. GI disease (e.g., ulcerative colitis, Crohn's disease)

    9. Kidney disease (e.g., renal insufficiency, dialysis, kidney stones)

    10. Neurologic disease (e.g., stroke, transient ischemic attack)

    11. Previous testing (e.g., endoscopy, radiographs)

II. Associated Symptoms

    A. Fever or hypothermia

    B. Chills

    C. Nausea and vomiting (e.g., bilious, feculent, food, blood, coffee-ground appearance)

    D. Chest pain

    E. Fluctuations in blood pressure

    F. Shortness of breath

    G. Change in bowel habits or caliber and color of stool (e.g., diarrhea)

    H. Obstipation (i.e., inability to pass flatus)

    I. Change in stoma output quantity or quality

    J. Drain output (volume and character)

    K. Penile or vaginal discharge

    L. Dysuria, hematuria

    M. Hematochezia (i.e., rectal bleeding), melena

    N. Anorexia, weight loss, early satiety

    O. Fatty food intolerance

III. Physical Examination

    A. Check the patient's vital signs and nutritional status.

    B. Examine the head, ears, eyes, nose, and throat for icteric sclera and signs of trauma and dehydration.

    C. Examine the neck for jugular venous distention and nodes. Also evaluate the thyroid and the position of the trachea.

    D. Examine the chest for equality of breath sounds and chest movements.

    E. Examine the heart, evaluating the rhythm and listening for murmurs and rubs.

    F. Perform a thorough examination of the abdomen.

        1. Inspect the abdomen for scars, signs of trauma, ecchymosis, wound discharge, and erythema. Also determine whether it is flat or distended.

        2. Auscultate the abdomen, listening for bowel sounds and bruits.

        3. Percuss the abdomen, evaluating for tympany and liver dullness.

        4. Palpate the abdomen to assess for rebound, rigidity, hepatosplenomegaly, masses, hernias, and fluid waves.

      a. Begin in the quadrant diagonally opposite to the area of pain and examine the painful area last.

      b. Palpate the flanks.

      c. Digitalize all stomas.

      d. Remove dressings and probe wounds.

    5. Evaluate the patient for signs associated with abdominal pain (Table 9-1).

  G. Examine the rectum for masses, tenderness, feces, and gross or occult blood.

  H. Perform a genital and pelvic examination to check for cervical discharge or tenderness, adnexal tenderness, uterine size, and masses.

  I. Examine the extremities for edema and cyanosis. Evaluate pulses and range of movement.

IV. Diagnostic Tests

  A. Laboratory tests

    1. Chemistry profile

    2. CBC

    3. Platelet count

    4. Liver function test

    5. Amylase and lipase

    6. Urinalysis

    7. β-Human chorionic gonadotropin (HCG)

    8. ABG

    9. Lactic acid

  B. Radiographs

    1. Posteroanterior and lateral chest radiographs

    2. Flat-plate and upright abdominal radiographs

  C. Imaging studies

    1. Ultrasound

    2. CT scan

    3. HIDA scan

    4. Endoscopic retrograde cholangiopancreatography (ERCP), if clinically indicated

V. Differential Diagnosis by Location (Figure 9-1)

VI. Common Surgical Diseases

  A. Abdominal aortic aneurysm (leak or rupture) [see p 629]

    1. History may include:

      a. Male with a family history of abdominal aortic aneurysm

      b. Abrupt onset of mild-to-severe lower abdominal, flank, or back pain

    2. Physical examination may reveal:

      a. Tachycardia

      b. Hypotension or hypertension

      c. Tender pulsatile abdominal mass

      d. Distention

      e. Guarding

      f. Rebound

    3. Diagnostic tests include:

      a. Abdominal ultrasound

Table 9-1. Signs Associated with Abdominal Pain

Sign	Finding	Associated Conditions
Murphy's sign	Inspiratory arrest with right upper quadrant pain	Cholecystitis
Charcot's triad	Right upper quadrant pain, jaundice, fever	Gallstones, cholelithiasis, choledocholithiasis, cholangitis
Reynold's pentad	Right upper quadrant pain, jaundice, fever, hypotension, mental status changes	Cholangitis
Courvoisier's sign	Palpable, nontender gallbladder with jaundice	Pancreatic malignancy
McBurney's sign	Tenderness at a point two-thirds the distance from the umbilicus to the anterior superior iliac spine	Appendicitis
Iliopsoas sign	Elevation of leg against examiner's hand causes pain	Retrocecal appendicitis
Obturator sign	Flexion and external rotation of the thigh causes pain	Pelvic appendicitis
Rovsing's sign	Manual pressure and release at left lower quadrant of the colon causes referred pain at McBurney's point	Appendicitis
Cullen's sign	Bluish periumbilical discoloration	Peritoneal hemorrhage
Grey Turner's sign	Flank ecchymoses	Retroperitoneal hemorrhage
Kehr's sign	Pain referred to left supraclavicular area	Splenic injury, subphrenic abscess

Right upper quadrant:
1. Cholecystitis
2. Cholangitis
3. Hepatitis
4. Duodenal ulcer
   (perforation, inflammation)
5. Gastritis
6. Pancreatitis (acute, chronic)
7. Abscess (subphrenic, hepatic)
8. CHF
9. Hepatomegaly
10. Fitz-Hugh–Curtis syndrome
    (gonococcal perihepatitis)
11. Pneumonia, effusion,
    empyema (right lower lobe)
12. Renal colic/stone
13. Urinary tract infection
14. Pyelonephritis
15. MI/ischemia
16. Pericarditis

Left upper quadrant:
1. Ulcer [duodenal (perforation,
   inflammation), gastric]
2. Gastritis
3. Pancreatitis (acute, chronic)
4. Spleen (enlargement, rupture,
   laceration, hematoma,
   infarct, aneurysm)
5. Subphrenic abscess
6. Pneumonia, effusion,
   empyema (left lower lobe)
7. Renal colic/stone
8. Urinary tract infection
9. Pyelonephritis
10. Ischemic colitis
11. MI/ischemia
12. Pericarditis
13. Aortic dissection
14. Intestinal obstruction

Diffuse:
1. Peritonitis
2. Pancreatitis (acute, chronic)
3. Intestinal obstruction
4. Early appendicitis
5. Mesenteric ischemia/infarction
6. Perforated duodenal ulcer
7. Perforated diverticulitis
8. Gastroenteritis
9. Inflammatory bowel disease
   (Crohn's, ulcerative colitis)
10. Colitis (pseudomembranous,
    ischemic, infectious)
11. Meckel's diverticulum
12. Aortic dissection
13. Abdominal aortic
    aneurysm (leak, rupture)
14. Acute urinary retention
15. Severe PID
16. Diabetic ketoacidosis
17. Uremia
18. Sickle cell crisis
19. Porphyria
20. Fecal retention

Right lower quadrant:
1. Appendicitis (acute,
   chronic, perforated)
2. PID
3. Ruptured ectopic pregnancy
4. Renal colic/stone
5. Urinary tract infection
6. Pyelonephritis
7. Perforation of cecal or
   ascending colon cancer
8. Crohn's disease
9. Intestinal obstruction
10. Cholecystitis
11. Pelvic/psoas abscess
12. Rectus sheath hematoma
13. Diverticulitis
14. Meckel's diverticulum
15. Ruptured graafian follicle
16. Ruptured corpus luteal cyst
17. Ovarian/fibroid torsion
18. Abortion (threatened, incomplete)
19. Endometriosis
20. Tubo-ovarian abscess
21. Fecal impaction

Left lower quadrant:
1. Diverticulitis
2. PID
3. Ruptured ectopic pregnancy
4. Renal colic/stone
5. Urinary tract infection
6. Pyelonephritis
7. Perforation of sigmoid/colon cancer
8. Crohn's disease
9. Intestinal obstruction
10. Abdominal aortic aneurysm
    (leak, rupture)
11. Pelvic/psoas abscess
12. Rectus sheath hematoma
13. Diverticulitis
14. Meckel's diverticulum
15. Ruptured graafian follicle
16. Ruptured corpus luteal cyst
17. Ovarian/fibroid torsion
18. Abortion (threatened, incomplete)
19. Endometriosis
20. Tubo-ovarian abscess
21. Fecal impaction
22. Appendicitis

Figure 9-1. The differential diagnosis of abdominal pain based on location.
CHF = congestive heart failure; *MI* = myocardial infarction; *PID* = pelvic
inflammatory disease.

      b. CT scan in hemodynamically stable patients

    4. Management. A patient with abdominal or back pain, a pulsatile abdominal mass, and hypotension must be taken directly to the operating room.

B. Aortic dissection

    1. History may include:

      a. Male > 40 years of age

      b. Hypertension

      c. Marfan's syndrome

      d. Previous surgical manipulation or coarctation

      e. Intense chest or upper abdominal pain with radiation to the neck, back, arms, and legs

    2. Physical examination may reveal:

      a. Diastolic murmur of aortic insufficiency

      b. Unequal carotid or distal pulses

    3. Diagnostic tests include:

      a. Chest radiograph (may show wide mediastinum, irregular aorta, left pleural effusion)

      b. Echocardiogram

      c. CT scan (may show a false or double lumen with IV contrast)

      d. Angiogram (will show a false or double lumen)

    4. Management. A patient with a wide mediastinum, a new aortic insufficiency murmur, and hypotension needs surgical intervention.

C. Appendicitis

    1. History may include:

      a. Abdominal pain in the midepigastrium and periumbilical region that subsequently localizes to the right lower quadrant (RLQ)

      b. Anorexia

      c. Nausea and vomiting

      d. Fever

    2. Physical examination may reveal:

      a. McBurney's point tenderness, Rovsing's sign, iliopsoas sign, and obturator sign (see Table 9-1)

      b. Rebound tenderness

      c. Abdominal rigidity

    3. Diagnostic test findings include:

      a. Increased WBCs

      b. Fecalith on abdominal radiograph

      c. Hyperemia, noncompressibility, and no peristalsis on abdominal ultrasound

      d. Localized fluid or an abscess on abdominal ultrasound if appendix is perforated

    4. Management involves surgical removal of the appendix.

D. Cholecystitis (acute) [see p 284]

    1. History may include:

      a. Overweight, multiparous female ≥ 40 years of age

      b. Excessive flatulence

      c. Fatty food intolerance

    d. Right upper quadrant (RUQ) or epigastric pain that radiates to the back or shoulder
    e. Fever
    f. Anorexia
    g. Nausea and vomiting
    h. Jaundice

> **In the ICU setting, acalculous and gangrenous cholecystitis occur with increased frequency.**

  2. Physical examination may reveal:
    a. RUQ or epigastric tenderness
    b. Guarding
    c. Palpable, tender gallbladder
    d. Murphy's sign (see Table 9-1)
  3. Diagnostic test findings include:
    a. Increased WBCs
    b. Increased liver function test
    c. Dilated, thick gallbladder; pericholecystic fluid; gallstones; and dilated common bile duct on ultrasound
    d. Nonvisualization on HIDA scan
  4. Management includes antibiotics and cholecystectomy. If the patient is unstable, place a cholecystostomy tube.
  5. Complications include cholangitis, gangrene or abscess, and empyema.
E. Mesenteric ischemia (see p 648)
  1. History may include:
    a. Male > 40 years of age
    b. CAD
    c. Decreasing weight
    d. Nausea and vomiting
    e. Diarrhea
  2. Physical examination may reveal pain out of proportion to physical findings. The pain may evolve into peritonitis with rebound tenderness and guarding.
  3. Diagnostic test findings include:
    a. Increased WBCs, hematocrit (HCT), and amylase
    b. Heme-positive stools
    c. Metabolic acidosis
    d. Bowel distention and gas in the portal circulation on abdominal radiograph
    e. Definitive diagnosis is provided by angiography.
F. Pancreatitis (acute) [see PANCREATITIS—ACUTE later in this chapter]
G. Peptic ulcer disease (see PEPTIC ULCER DISEASE later in this chapter)
H. Pelvic inflammatory disease
  1. History may include:
    a. Sexually active female
    b. Temperature to 104°F (40°C)
    c. Chills

      d. Bilateral lower abdominal pain (more common than unilateral)

      e. Dyspareunia

      f. Dysmenorrhea

      g. Purulent vaginal discharge

  2. Physical examination may reveal:

      a. Rebound

      b. Peritonitis

      c. Cervical motion and adnexal tenderness

  3. Diagnostic test findings include increased WBCs.

  4. Management

    a. Antibiotics

      (1) Mildly symptomatic patients may be treated as outpatients with PO ciprofloxacin and metronidazole or PO amoxicillin/clavulanate (Augmentin).

      (2) Patients with severe symptoms or those who are noncompliant or unable to take medication orally should be treated with IV cefotetan, cefoxitin, ampicillin/sulbactam (Unasyn), ticarcillin/clavulanate (Timentin), or piperacillin/tazobactam (Zosyn).

    b. Operative management

      (1) Indications

        (a) Ruptured or leaking tubo-ovarian abscess

        (b) Sepsis

        (c) Increasing fever, leukocytosis, or abdominal pain despite IV antibiotics

      (2) Procedure

        (a) Remove the source.

        (b) Adequately drain the abscess.

        (c) Copiously irrigate the abdominal compartment.

  5. Complications include abscess and infertility.

I. Pyelonephritis

  1. History may include:

      a. Fever

      b. Chills

      c. Dysuria

      d. Nausea and vomiting

  2. Physical examination may reveal flank and costal vertebral angle tenderness.

  3. Diagnostic test findings include:

      a. Increased WBCs

      b. Many WBCs, WBC casts, and bacteria on urinalysis

  4. Management involves administration of antibiotics.

J. Renal colic

  1. History may include severe intermittent flank, upper quadrant, or lower quadrant pain radiating to the back, testicles, or groin.

  2. Physical examination may reveal a benign abdomen.

  3. Diagnostic tests include:

    a. Urinalysis (shows variable RBCs)
    b. Abdominal radiograph with opaque density in the ureter or calyx
    c. IV pyelogram
    d. Spiral CT scan

  4. Management includes IV hydration and pain control. If the stone does not pass, lithotripsy or surgical extraction may be necessary.

K. Ruptured ectopic pregnancy

  1. History may include:
    a. Vaginal bleeding or abdominal pain 7–8 weeks after missed period
    b. Amenorrhea
    c. Nausea and vomiting

  2. Physical examination may reveal:
    a. Shock
    b. Sepsis
    c. Lower abdominal pain radiating to the shoulders
    d. Cervical motion tenderness
    e. Pelvic or adnexal mass
    f. Uterine bleeding

  3. Diagnostic test findings include:
    a. Decreased HCT
    b. Positive β-HCG
    c. Positive culdocentesis or ultrasound

  4. Management is surgical.

L. Sigmoid diverticulitis (see DIVERTICULAR DISEASE later in this chapter)

  1. History may include:
    a. Female or male > 35 years of age (female more common than male)
    b. Urinary symptoms
    c. Low-grade fever
    d. Variable left lower quadrant (LLQ) pain

  2. Physical examination may reveal:
    a. Guarding
    b. Rebound
    c. Radiation of pain to the back, flank, or groin

  3. Diagnostic test findings include:
    a. Increased WBCs
    b. Bowel thickening, fat stranding, and soft tissue mass or abscess on CT scan

  4. Management
    a. Mild symptoms and mild disease on CT scan requires:
      (1) Oral ciprofloxacin and metronidazole as an outpatient
      (2) Clear-liquid diet (advance as tolerated)
    b. Moderate-to-severe symptoms or significant disease or abscess on CT scan requires:
      (1) NPO
      (2) IV fluids

      (3) IV antibiotics (i.e., cefotetan, cefoxitin, cipro-floxacin and metronidazole, or ampicillin and gentamicin and metronidazole)

      (4) Parenteral analgesia

      (5) Percutaneous drainage of peridiverticular ab-scess

  c. Indications for surgical intervention include:

      (1) Failure to respond to medical management

      (2) Perforation

      (3) Colonic obstruction

      (4) Fistulation

  d. Many surgeons recommend elective resection after the acute episode has been treated. There is an increasing incidence of recurrence with each episode.

M. Splenic rupture (see Table 26-4)

  1. History may include:

    a. Trauma

    b. Rib fracture

    c. Spontaneous rupture with splenomegaly

  2. Physical examination may reveal:

    a. Left upper quadrant (LUQ) tenderness with some generalized abdominal tenderness

    b. LUQ mass

    c. Distention

    d. Guarding

    e. Rebound

  3. Diagnostic test findings include:

    a. Decreased HCT

    b. Increased WBCs

    c. Rib fracture on chest radiograph

    d. Gastric displacement and an immobile left hemidiaphragm on plain films of the abdomen

    e. Positive diagnostic peritoneal lavage

  4. Management is surgical (i.e., splenectomy or splenorrhaphy).

ACUTE VARICEAL HEMORRHAGE

I. Etiology

  A. Acute variceal hemorrhage is the principle life-threatening complication of **portal hypertension.**

  B. In patients with known varices, causes of UGI bleeds include:

    1. Varices (20%–50%)

    2. Gastritis (20%–60%)

    3. Peptic ulcer disease (6%–19%)

    4. Mallory-Weiss syndrome (5%–18%)

II. Diagnostic Tests. Esophagogastroduodenoscopy (EGD) is used to determine the site of the bleed and the presence of esophageal varices.

III. Management (Figure 9-2)

> **When managing an acute variceal hemorrhage, remember that in 8% of patients there are two sites of bleeding.**

A. Medical management

1. **Injection sclerotherapy**
   a. Injection sclerotherapy is the **preferred management of an acute variceal bleed,** and it is performed at the time of the first diagnostic endoscopy. When performed with endoscopy, the sclerosing agent is injected into the varix, causing thrombosis of the varix.
   b. **Effectiveness** of emergent sclerotherapy (maximum of two injections before further therapy) is as follows:
      (1) Overall success: 80%–90%
      (2) Single injection: 70%
      (3) Subsequent injection: 70% [required in rebleed cases (30%)]
   c. The **mortality** rate is 1%–2%.
   d. The **morbidity** rate is 20%–40% and is caused by:
      (1) Esophageal perforation
      (2) Exacerbation of hemorrhage
      (3) Esophageal ulceration
      (4) Fever
      (5) Pleural effusions

2. **Pharmacotherapy**
   a. **Vasopressin** (0.4 U/min) is a potent vasoconstrictor

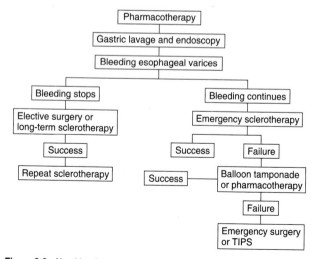

Figure 9-2. Algorithm for the management of suspected acute variceal hemorrhage.

that causes splanchnic vasoconstriction. It is useful in the acute setting. Side effects include myocardial and bowel ischemia.

  b. Nitroglycerin (SL/TD/IV) lowers portal pressure and counteracts the systemic side effects of vasopressin.

  c. Somatostatin (50-μg IV bolus followed by 50 μg/hr IV infusion) causes splanchnic vasoconstriction. It has fewer systemic side effects than vasopressin and is the preferred agent in many institutions.

3. Balloon tamponade (Sengstaken-Blakemore tube)

  a. The Sengstaken-Blakemore tube has three lumens:

    (1) Gastric aspiration port

    (2) Esophageal balloon inflation port

    (3) Gastric balloon inflation port

  b. Although the Sengstaken-Blakemore tube controls up to 80% of hemorrhages, 20%–50% rebleed after the balloon is deflated.

  c. Complications include:

    (1) Esophageal rupture

    (2) Esophageal ischemia

To minimize complications, do not use the Sengstaken-Blakemore tube longer than 48 hours.

---

4. Transjugular intrahepatic portosystemic shunt (TIPS)

  a. To place a TIPS, an 8- to 12-mm shunt is placed between a hepatic vein and a portal vein branch.

  b. Complications include:

    (1) Early rebleeding

    (2) Shunt stenosis

    (3) Shunt thrombosis

    (4) Postprocedure encephalopathy (10%–30%)

B. Operative management

  1. Indications

    a. Acute massive bleeding that fails to respond to non-surgical maneuvers

    b. Recurrent bleeding despite two endoscopic attempts to control bleeding

  2. Relative contraindications

    a. Pneumonia

    b. Moderate-to-severe encephalopathy

    c. Severe coagulopathy

    d. Severe liver failure

  3. Operative intervention

    a. Decompression of the portal venous system usually involves an end-to-side portacaval shunt or a mesocaval shunt. More than 95% stop bleeding; however, there is a high operative mortality rate. Complications include:

      (1) Hepatic failure from acute reduction of portal flow

          (2) Pneumonia
          (3) Delirium tremens
          (4) Renal failure
     b. Variceal ligation can be performed as direct ligation or esophageal transection.

DIARRHEA IN THE CRITICALLY ILL PATIENT

I. Definitions

    A. Diarrhea is defined arbitrarily as two to three loose stools for several consecutive days, or stools that consist of > 200 grams of fecal water.

    B. Nosocomial diarrhea is defined as the onset of acute diarrhea > 72 hours after hospitalization.

II. Pathophysiology. Diarrhea is primarily a disorder of water homeostasis. Several mechanisms may play a role in the pathogenesis of diarrhea.

    A. Osmotic diarrhea

       1. Under normal conditions, absorbable osmoles rapidly equalize across the small bowel.

       2. The presence of nonionic osmoles, such as undigested disaccharides in the small intestine, leads to the intraluminal flow of water and the development of diarrhea.

    B. Secretory diarrhea

       1. The majority of normal water absorption occurs along two pathways.

          a. In the small bowel, 8–9 liters are absorbed daily.

          b. The remaining 1–2 liters are absorbed by colonic mechanisms for a daily stool content of approximately 100 grams.

       2. In **acute bacterial infections** (e.g., *Vibrio cholerae,* enterotoxigenic *Escherichia coli*), toxin activates cyclic adenosine monophosphate (cAMP), which increases bicarbonate and chloride secretion into the bowel lumen.

       3. Increased GI hormones occur in several conditions and result in diarrhea.

          a. Vasoactive intestinal peptide (VIP) is increased in Verner-Morrison syndrome (VIPoma), resulting in watery diarrhea, hypokalemia, and achlorhydria.

          b. Gastrin is increased in Zollinger-Ellison syndrome and results in diarrhea secondary to:

             (1) Increased gastric acid secretion
             (2) Proximal intestinal villus damage
             (3) Inactivation of pancreatic enzymes at low intestinal pH (leads to steatorrhea)

          c. Increased amounts of substance P, serotonin, prostaglandins, and gastric inhibitory polypeptide may also result in diarrhea.

       4. Increased luminal bile acids stimulate colonic secretion.

       5. Laxatives (e.g., castor oil, docusate) stimulate cAMP.

      6. Secretory neoplasms (e.g., villous adenomas of the colorectum)

C. Altered motility

    1. Conditions that increase gut motility, such as hyperthyroidism, may decrease intestinal transit time and overwhelm colonic absorptive mechanisms.

    2. Similarly, conditions such as diabetes mellitus may decrease gut motility or increase transit time. This may also stimulate diarrhea by encouraging stasis of intestinal contents and overgrowth of bacteria.

III. Classification of Diarrhea

A. Ischemic diarrhea

    1. Etiology

      a. Ischemic diarrhea usually occurs in the setting of predisposing conditions, most commonly atrial fibrillation and prolonged hypotension.

      b. Reduced mesenteric blood flow may result in mucosal detachment and sloughing, resulting in bloody or blood-tinged diarrhea.

      c. Decreased supply of substrate may also interfere with energy-dependent absorption of water.

    2. Diagnostic tests

      a. Plain radiographs may show characteristic thumbprinting of the bowel wall or free air after perforation.

      b. CT scan may show thickened, edematous bowel walls.

      c. In cases of high suspicion, only mesenteric angiography can effectively rule out ischemic bowel.

      d. In unstable candidates, diagnostic peritoneal lavage is an extremely useful procedure. A tap positive for WBCs indicates full-thickness necrosis.

    3. Diagnosis

      a. Pain out of proportion to the physical examination is a classic finding.

      b. Diagnosis in an intubated, unresponsive patient is extremely difficult.

      c. Marked metabolic acidosis in the appropriate clinical setting should initiate work-up for ischemia.

B. Altered intestinal flora may be secondary to:

    1. Antibiotics

    2. Antacids (neutralization of gastric acid may allow bacterial overgrowth)

    3. Bowel preparations

    4. Enteral feedings

C. Malabsorption is perhaps the most common pathway leading to the onset of diarrhea. It can be caused by antibiotic therapy, lactase deficiency, sorbitol or fructose ingestion, enteral feeding, ileal and extended resections, vagotomy, and cholecystectomy.

    1. Malabsorption caused by antibiotic therapy

      a. Antibiotic use of any kind, any dose, and any method

of delivery may predispose to diarrhea caused by *Clostridium difficile.*

b. The inhibition of anaerobes by antibiotics has been shown to decrease the formation of short-chain fatty acids.

c. Management

  (1) Stopping or changing antibiotics may help alleviate symptomatic diarrhea.

  (2) In severe instances, the addition of lactobacillus may help recolonize intestinal flora.

2. Malabsorption caused by lactase deficiency and sorbitol or fructose ingestion

  a. In the setting of acute nosocomial diarrhea, lactose, sorbitol, and fructose should be removed from the diet.

  b. Halting ingestion of any diet may be both diagnostic and therapeutic for osmotic diarrhea.

3. Malabsorption caused by enteral feeding

  a. Starting and stopping tube feedings have both been implicated in nosocomial diarrhea. Certain formulations, such as Immun-Aid, have anecdotally led to a higher incidence of loose stools.

  b. Some evidence also suggests that elemental diets and formulations with > 30% of their total calories from fat are more likely to cause diarrhea.

  c. While fiber is essential for maintenance of healthy colonic enterocytes, altered intestinal flora from bowel preparations or antibiotic use may have a decreased ability to break down dietary fiber.

  d. Management

   (1) Gradually increasing feeding or starting at one-quarter or one-half strength dilutions has not conclusively been shown to decrease the incidence of diarrhea. However, in the setting of significant diarrhea, changing formulations, adding or removing fiber, or slowing or stopping enteral feeding should be considered.

   (2) Stopping feeding must be weighed against the proved immunologic and protective benefits of enteral feeding, both in terms of inhibiting bacterial translocation and protection of gastric mucosa.

4. Malabsorption caused by ileal and extended intestinal resections, vagotomy, and cholecystectomy

  a. In addition to short-gut syndromes and extended colon resections with high ileostomy output, ileal resections and cholecystectomy may alter the bile acid pool.

  b. Malabsorption of bile acids with increased delivery to the colon may increase colonic secretion of fluid and electrolytes. This may be particularly pertinent in the setting of altered intestinal flora, which may be less efficient at deconjugating bile acids. A decreased bile acid pool may also eventually lead to steatorrhea.

5. **Malabsorption caused by hypoalbuminemia.** Some studies show that very low serum albumin levels may lead to bowel wall edema, malabsorption, and diarrhea.

D. Acute infections

1. **Inflammatory diarrhea** with mucosal invasion by *Salmonella* species, *Shigella* species, and *Campylobacter* species results in mucosal sloughing, fecal leukocytes, blood-tinged diarrhea, and systemic signs of infection, including fever and leukocytosis.

2. **Noninflammatory diarrhea** usually presents with large volumes of watery diarrhea, is usually self-limited, and is caused by viral infection or occasionally *V. cholerae* or enterotoxic *E. coli*.

E. Drug-induced diarrhea occurs via a variety of mechanisms, including magnesium, laxatives, quinidine, digoxin, cimetidine, theophylline, cytotoxic chemotherapy, and radiotherapy.

F. *C. difficile* diarrhea

1. **Incidence.** Colonization occurs in approximately 10% of hospitalized adult patients on antibiotics or undergoing chemotherapy.

2. **Pathology.** On gross examination, there is a toxin-mediated inflammatory response characterized by pseudomembranes or plaques composed of leukocytes, fibrin, and epithelial cells with underlying inflamed mucosa.

3. **Pathophysiology.** *C. difficile* diarrhea is attributed to the combined effects of the elaborated toxins A and B, which damage the colonic mucosa.

4. **Risk factors** include:
   a. Age (Colonization is more frequent in the young; disease is more frequent in the elderly.)
   b. Severe illness
   c. Adjuvant therapy
   d. Previous history of *C. difficile* diarrhea
   e. Renal insufficiency
   f. Recent hospitalization
   g. GI surgery
   h. Antibiotics in the previous 2 months via any route or dose, especially broad-spectrum penicillins, cephalosporins, and clindamycin

5. **Signs and symptoms** include:
   a. Fever
   b. Severe, cramping abdominal pain
   c. Profuse, watery, green, foul-smelling, bloody diarrhea
   d. Leukocytosis
   e. Abdominal distention or pain with diarrhea

6. **Diagnosis** of *C. difficile* diarrheal syndromes
   a. The diagnosis of *C. difficile* colitis should be suspected

in anyone with diarrhea who has received antibiotics in the previous 2 months or whose diarrhea began ≥ 72 hours after hospitalization.

    b. When the diagnosis of *C. difficile* is suspected, a single stool specimen should be sent to the laboratory for testing for the presence of *C. difficile* or its toxins.

    c. If the results of laboratory tests are negative, but the diarrhea persists, one or two additional stools can be sent for testing with the same or different tests.

    d. Endoscopy is reserved for special situations, including:

        (1) Rapid diagnosis needed and test results are delayed

        (2) Test is not highly sensitive

        (3) Patient has ileus and a stool is not available

        (4) Other colonic diseases are in the differential diagnosis

7. Management of *C. difficile* diarrhea or colitis

    a. Antibiotics should be discontinued, if possible.

    b. Nonspecific supportive therapy should be given, and is often all that is needed in treatment. Specific antibiotics should not be given routinely.

    c. When the diagnosis of *C. difficile* diarrhea is confirmed or highly suspected before laboratory diagnosis and specific therapy is indicated, metronidazole (PO) is preferred.

    d. If the diagnosis of *C. difficile* diarrhea is highly likely and the patient is seriously ill, metronidazole (IV) may be given empirically before the diagnosis is definitely established.

    e. Vancomycin (PO) is reserved for therapy of *C. difficile* diarrhea when one or more of the following conditions are present:

        (1) The patient failed to respond to metronidazole.

        (2) The patient's organism is resistant to metronidazole.

        (3) The patient is unable to tolerate metronidazole, is allergic to metronidazole, or is being treated with ethanol-containing solutions.

        (4) The patient is either pregnant or is < 10 years of age.

        (5) The patient is critically ill because of *C. difficile* diarrhea or colitis.

        (6) There is evidence suggesting the diarrhea is caused by *Staphylococcus aureus*.

    f. Dosages

        (1) Antibiotics, except in the setting of *C. difficile,* are not indicated.

        (2) The usual dosing for *C. difficile* diarrhea is as follows:

            (a) Metronidazole, 500 mg PO/IV q 6 hr

         (b) Vancomycin, 250–500 mg PO q 6 hr
         (c) Cholestyramine, 4 g PO q 8 hr

IV. Diagnostic Tests

  A. In the setting of acute diarrhea with no suspicion of mesenteric ischemia, a single stool sample should be sent to test for *C. difficile.*

  B. In the routine patient, there is no indication for testing for ova and parasites.

V. Management of Diarrhea

  A. Supportive care

    1. Nosocomial diarrhea is predominately iatrogenic, usually drug-induced (e.g., antibiotics) or due to enteral feeding. Replace fluid losses parenterally and remove the offending source.

    2. Infectious diarrhea requires careful replacement of fluid and electrolytes. Replacement of potassium is the hallmark of care because most cases are self-limited.

  B. Antimotility agents are generally not indicated and are specifically contraindicated in the setting of *C. difficile* colitis.

  C. Tube feedings

    1. Change to a lower fat formulation (may be effective).

    2. When fluid and electrolyte issues become significant, decrease enteral feedings to a baseline of 20 cc/hr to maintain mucosal integrity.

    3. Reduce osmolality by using isotonic feeding solutions. It may also be necessary to reduce the volume of the feedings.

    4. Use intragastric feedings to slow gut transit time and reduce osmolality.

    5. Reduce the infusion rate and then increase it very slowly, allowing the bowel to regain its absorptive properties.

    6. Avoid complete bowel rest whenever possible.

    7. If the *C. difficile* toxin assay is negative, take the following steps and do not hesitate to repeat the assay.

      a. Start kaolin with pectin, 30 ml PO q 3 hr for 48 hours.

      b. If there is no response, consider opiates (e.g., paregoric, 1 ml/100 ml formula for 24 hours).

      c. If diarrhea continues, give fiber formula and kaolin with pectin, 30 ml PO q 3 hr for 72 hours.

      d. If the diarrhea still continues, start total parenteral nutrition.

DIVERTICULAR DISEASE

I. Definitions

  A. Diverticulum—an outpouching or sac arising from a hollow viscus

  B. Diverticulosis—presence of at least one diverticulum

  C. Painful diverticular disease—symptoms without inflammation

  D. Diverticulitis—symptoms with inflammation; severity related to extent of colonic involvement (Table 9-2)

Table 9-2.	Stages of Acute Diverticulitis
Stage	**Description**
1	Microabscesses of colonic wall, peridiverticular inflammation
2	Small, well-defined microabscesses within the mesentery or epiploic appendages
3	Larger pericolic abscesses and pelvic abscess secondary to perforation
4	Generalized peritonitis secondary to a perforated abscess or fecal leakage

II. Incidence
    A. Diverticular disease occurs equally in males and females.
    B. Diverticular disease is more prevalent in western cultures.
    C. Prevalence increases with age such that 65% of persons > 80 years of age have diverticula.
    D. Bleeding occurs in 5% of persons with diverticula. Although 70% of diverticular bleeding stops spontaneously, 25% of patients have recurrent bleeding.
    E. Incidence based on the location of disease is as follows:
        1. Disease limited to the sigmoid: 65%
        2. No disease in the sigmoid: 1%–4%
        3. Disease in the right colon: 5%–10% (usually 30–50 years of age)

III. Pathology
    A. Diverticula occur at points of weakness in the antimesenteric wall (e.g., entry points of perforating blood vessels, between longitudinal fibers of the taenia coli).
    B. Most colonic diverticula are false diverticula (e.g., mucosal herniations).
    C. Diffusely distributed lesions are shallow and wide; lesions limited to the sigmoid typically are deep with a narrow neck.

IV. Pathogenesis
    A. Muscular hypertrophy results in increased intraluminal pressure.
    B. Low stool bulk results in low radius and segmentation of the colon during contraction.
    C. Increased fecal bile acids result in increased colonic motor activity.
    D. Muscular hypertrophy, low stool bulk, and increased bile acids work in concert to exert pressure on the bowel wall according to Laplace's law, which states that pressure varies inversely with the radius and directly with wall thickness.
    E. Diverticulitis may be due to microperforation of a diverticulum secondary to increased intraluminal pressure or fecal impaction.

V. Risk Factors
    A. Marfan's syndrome and other collagen disorders may result in a younger onset of disease.

B. A low-residue diet increases the risk of disease; therefore, vegetarians have a lower incidence of diverticular disease.

C. Diverticular disease is associated with varicose veins, CAD, colon cancer, and granulomatous colitis.

VI. Signs and Symptoms

A. Although 80%–85% of patients with **diverticulosis** are asymptomatic, symptoms can include:

1. Diarrhea or constipation (62%)
2. Flatulence (50%)
3. Heartburn (33%)
4. Nausea and vomiting (20%)
5. Mass (20%)
6. Distention (14%)
7. Urinary symptoms (13%)
8. Epididymitis, scrotal inflammation

B. Symptoms of **painful diverticular disease** are present in 75% of patients and include:

1. Colicky lower abdominal pain (left side > right side)
2. Pain that worsens after meals and is relieved after passing flatus

C. Diverticulitis develops in 10%–25% of patients with diverticulosis. Patients with diverticulitis present with:

1. Acute, severe, and persistent LLQ abdominal pain
2. Anorexia
3. Fever
4. Chills
5. Absent bowel sounds

VII. Diagnosis

> **When evaluating a patient for diverticular disease, always rule out the possibility of cancer.**

A. Obtain a history and perform a physical examination. If there is no fever or leukocytosis, the diagnosis can be made clinically. After the episode has resolved, perform the following evaluations:

1. Barium enema (double contrast gives a higher yield but has an increased risk of perforation)
2. Colonoscopy

B. Perform anoscopy to evaluate for hemorrhoids.

C. Obtain a CBC, prothrombin time (PT), partial thromboplastin time (PTT), electrolytes, BUN/creatinine, and urinalysis.

D. Obtain an abdominal radiograph to rule out free air.

E. If there are signs of inflammation or if diverticulitis is likely and moderate to severe (see Table 9-2), perform the following evaluations:

1. CT scan with PO and IV contrast (Some institutions give rectal contrast, but not in the acute setting.)
2. Technetium-99m (^{99m}Tc)-labeled leukocyte scan to assess for abscess and phlegmon

F. If patient has rectal bleeding, follow the protocol for GI hemorrhage (see GASTROINTESTINAL HEMORRHAGE later in this chapter).

VIII. Management

 A. **Asymptomatic outpatients** should be directed to increase the amount of fiber in their diets.

 B. **Early, mild diverticulitis**

  1. Administer oral antibiotics (i.e., ciprofloxacin/metronidazole) for 7–14 days.

  2. Keep the patient on a clear-liquid diet until the pain resolves. Then begin a diet high in fiber.

  3. Evaluate the patient's progress daily.

  4. Hospitalize the patient if he or she is unreliable or if there is evidence of systemic illness.

 C. **Acute diverticulitis** (i.e., moderate-to-severe diverticulitis)

  1. Hospitalize the patient with complete bowel rest, IV fluids, and a nasogastric (NG) tube for drainage.

  2. Administer broad-spectrum antibiotics for 7–10 days:

   a. Cefoxitin, 1.0–1.5 g IV q 6 hr

   b. Ampicillin and gentamicin and metronidazole

   c. Cefotetan, 2 g IV q 12 hr

   d. Ampicillin/sulbactam (Unasyn)

   e. Ciprofloxacin and metronidazole

   f. Ticarcillin/clavulanate (Timentin)

   g. Imipenem/cilastatin

  3. Use analgesics with caution.

  4. Delay operative therapy until the disease is quiescent.

   a. Indications for operative therapy include:

    (1) Failure to progress

    (2) Complications (e.g., perforation, fistula)

    (3) Second episode

    (4) Diabetic patient

   b. Operative mortality rate is 17%–22% during an acute episode, and there is a 10% recurrence rate after surgery.

   c. Operative options (Table 9-3)

 D. **Isolated diverticular abscess** (stage 3 disease; see Table 9-2)

  1. CT- or ultrasound-guided percutaneous drainage is the treatment of choice for an isolated diverticular abscess.

  2. Percutaneous drainage is useful for elderly or unstable patients and may help avoid a multiple-stage procedure.

  3. There is a 71%–88% success rate for percutaneous drainage with a subsequent single-stage procedure (see Table 9-3).

 E. **Diverticular hemorrhage**

  1. Resuscitate and stabilize the patient with invasive monitoring in an ICU setting.

  2. Follow the protocol for a LGI hemorrhage (see GASTROINTESTINAL HEMMORHAGE later in this chapter).

 F. **Fistulae** require resection by a single- or two-stage procedure (see Table 9-3).

IX. Complications of Diverticulitis

Table 9–3.   Operative Options for the Treatment of Acute Diverticulitis

Type of Procedure	Steps in Procedure	Indications
Single-stage	Resection* and primary reanastomosis	Uncomplicated disease; no signs of inflammation, infection, or contamination
Two-stage	Resection*, end colostomy, and Hartmann's pouch	Free colonic perforation complete obstruction
	Surgery for reanastomosis (allow at least 6 weeks between operations)	
Three-stage	Diverting colostomy Resection*, end colostomy, and Hartmann's pouch	Complete obstruction, peritonitis, unstable on presentation, complicated cases
	Surgery for reanastomosis	

*Resection should include any colon with acute disease or large numbers of diverticula, and it should extend to the peritoneal reflection.

A. **Fistulae**
1. Fistulae can form to the bladder (50%), vagina, skin, small bowel, or ureter.
2. Fistulae occur in 12%–25% of patients, and they are more common in males because the uterus is a barrier to fistula formation.
3. A colovesical fistula can cause pneumaturia and fecaluria.
B. **Obstruction**
1. Obstruction occurs in 2% of cases of diverticulitis.
2. Obstruction can cause large or large and small bowel obstruction.
C. **Perforation**
1. Risk of perforation increases with the use of nonsteroidal anti-inflammatory drugs (NSAIDs) and corticosteroids.
2. The mortality rate from perforation is 6%–26%.
D. **Bleeding**
1. Bleeding is a late complication usually due to perforating vessels.
2. Bleeding is most commonly from the right colon.
3. Although 70% of patients stop bleeding spontaneously, 3%–5% of patients require transfusion.
4. There is a 22% chance of rebleed after the first bleed and a 50% chance of rebleed after the second bleed.
E. **Giant colonic diverticulum** (i.e., 3–35 cm) is a rare complication.

FULMINANT COLITIS

I. Definitions

A. Fulminant colitis is the combined development of acute colitis marked by severe, usually bloody diarrhea and systemic manifestations of sepsis. It may occur as an acute exacerbation of inflammatory bowel disease (IBD) or it may occur during the initial presentation of IBD.

B. Toxic megacolon is characterized by massive colonic distention and is thought to precede perforation. Approximately 5%–15% of patients with IBD develop toxic megacolon.

II. Etiology

A. Acute infectious diarrhea, such as diarrhea caused by *Salmonella* species or cytomegalovirus (common in HIV-positive patients), may precipitate onset of fulminant colitis in previously quiescent disease.

B. Recent discontinuation of medical therapy or previous antibiotic use may predispose to toxic colitis.

III. Diagnosis

A. Clinical criteria for diagnosis

1. Six or more bloody stools daily
2. Mean evening temperature of $> 99.5°F$ ($> 37.5°C$) or a temperature of $> 100.0°F$ ($> 37.7°C$) on at least 2 of 4 days
3. Tachycardia > 90 beats/min
4. Anemia (i.e., hemoglobin < 9 g/dl)
5. Erythrocyte sedimentation rate > 30 mm/hr

B. Diagnostic tests

1. Send stool specimens for culture, ova and parasites, and *C. difficile* toxin to rule out infectious colitis.
2. Obtain serial abdominal radiographs daily to check for free air and increasing distention of the transverse colon.

IV. Management

A. Medical management

1. Give patient IV fluid and replace electrolytes.
2. Give patient blood transfusions as necessary.
3. Keep the patient NPO, using a NG tube when necessary.
4. Give the patient total parenteral nutrition only in Crohn's disease or in previous nutritional depletion.
5. Administer the appropriate medications.
   a. Hydrocortisone (100 mg IV q 8 hr) should be given to patients who have been on corticosteroids in the recent past (i.e., within 6 months).
   b. IV antibiotics are also an option in the treatment of fulminant colitis.
   c. Some institutions report a response to high-dose IV cyclosporine in steroid-unresponsive patients.
   d. Currently, there is no role for sulfasalazine or mesalamine in the acute setting.
   e. Avoid the use of narcotics, antidiarrheals, and anticholinergics.

   6. Some physicians suggest placement of a long intestinal tube by interventional radiology to help decompress the transverse colon.

B. Operative management

   1. Absolute indications for emergent surgery include:
      a. Free perforation
      b. Massive hemorrhage (i.e., patient requires $> 6–8$ units of PRBCs and is still actively bleeding)

   2. Indications for colectomy include:
      a. Free air on abdominal radiograph
      b. Increasing distention of the transverse colon past 7–9 cm on abdominal radiograph
      c. Initial attack of toxic colitis (25%–50% of these patients require colectomy)

   3. If the patient's condition has not significantly improved after 24–48 hours of conservative management, aggressive surgical intervention is required and will decrease the chance of colonic perforation.

   4. Some physicians manage toxic megacolon conservatively for 7–10 days with careful observation and long intestinal tubes and only refer those with progressive or worsening symptoms for surgery.

   5. Postoperative mortality
      a. Overall: 10%–15%
      b. Emergent surgery: 9%
      c. Perforated colon: 27%–44%

GASTROINTESTINAL HEMORRHAGE

I. Upper Gastrointestinal (UGI) Hemorrhage

   A. Definition. UGI hemorrhage is bleeding from a source proximal to the ligament of Treitz.

   B. Etiology

   1. Peptic ulcer disease (duodenal ulcer, 24%; gastric ulcer, 21%) [see PEPTIC ULCER DISEASE later in this chapter]
      a. About 20% of patients present with bleeding, and 20% bleed during the course of the disease.
      b. Factors that increase mortality include age > 65 years, > 5 units of blood transfused, and multiorgan failure.

   2. Gastritis (14%) may be secondary to:
      a. Stress (e.g., sepsis, burns, head injury)
      b. Ethanol consumption
      c. NSAIDs
      d. *Helicobacter pylori*

   3. Variceal hemorrhage (11%)
      a. Portal hypertension can cause a variceal hemorrhage.
         (1) Increased resistance to blood flow to the liver causes the opening of portosystemic collaterals.
         (2) Esophageal varices develop from collaterals between the left gastric vein and the azygos vein.

       b. Varices can be found in 25%–70% of cirrhotics.

       c. Bleeding occurs in 33% of patients with varices. The mortality rate is 25%–50% after the first hemorrhage.

       d. In up to 50% of patients with known varices, bleeding will be from another source (e.g., gastritis, peptic ulcer disease).

  4. Mallory-Weiss syndrome (9%)

       a. These patients (most commonly binge drinkers) present with a history of forceful vomiting or retching, which results in a mucosal tear near the gastroesophageal junction (usually on the gastric side).

       b. Only 50% of cases have the classic history of vomiting and retching.

  5. Less common causes of UGI bleeding include:

       a. Esophagitis

       b. Neoplasia

       c. Angiodysplasia

       d. Aortoenteric fistula (usually follows aneurysm or vascular surgery)

       e. Hemobilia

       f. Osler-Weber-Rendu disease

       g. Dieulafoy's lesion

       h. Marginal ulcer

C. Signs and symptoms

  1. Hematemesis (bright-red blood or coffee-ground emesis)

  2. Melena (dark, tarry stools)

  3. Hematochezia (bright-red blood from the rectum; seen with massive UGI bleeds)

D. Diagnostic tests

  1. Laboratory tests include:

       a. Type and cross-match blood for 6 units

       b. CBC

       c. PT and PTT

       d. Electrolytes

       e. BUN/creatinine

       f. ABG

  2. An **ECG** and **chest radiograph** aid in management.

E. Management

  1. UGI hemorrhage from unknown cause

       a. Ensure adequate airway, breathing, and circulation.

       b. Start two large-bore (i.e., $\geq$ 16-gauge) IVs and infuse lactated Ringer's solution or normal saline as needed. The amount of fluid required to resuscitate the patient should be based on heart rate, blood pressure, and urine output.

       c. Restore blood volume and reverse shock, if present.

       d. Insert a NG tube and lavage with 400 ml of fluid.

         (1) Hematemesis or a bloody aspirate clearly implicates an UGI source. For grossly positive aspirates, an attempt should be made to clear the stomach of blood with warm saline lavage before endoscopy.

(2) An aspirate that returns heme-negative bile is considered negative for an UGI source. Bile must be seen.

e. Admit all patients with active bleeding to the ICU.

f. Empiric medical therapy involves the administration of a histamine (H_2) blocker (e.g., cimetidine, ranitidine, famotidine) by continuous IV infusion.

g. EGD identifies the source of UGI bleed in 90%–95% of cases if performed within 48 hours.

Do not attempt an EGD until the patient has been resuscitated and ECG rules out myocardial ischemia.

---

(1) EGD should be performed for positive or inconclusive NG-tube aspirates and in patients with risk factors for duodenal ulcer disease.

NG aspirates will be free of blood in 10% of bleeding duodenal ulcers.

---

(2) EGD may prove therapeutic (electrocautery or injection of bleeding vessel).

2. UGI hemorrhage from peptic ulcer disease

a. Within 48 hours, 75% of hemorrhages from peptic ulcer disease stop bleeding spontaneously.

b. The first line of therapy is via EGD.

c. Operative therapy

(1) Indications

(a) Massive bleed (i.e., > 5 units) that does not respond to endoscopic treatment

(b) Patient at significant risk for rebleed (i.e., age > 65 years, hemoglobin < 8 g/dl, visible vessel at ulcer base)

(2) Procedures

(a) For a duodenal ulcer, perform a suture ligation of the bleeding vessel with or without vagotomy. Vagotomy may not be necessary in the era of *H. pylori* treatment.

(b) For a gastric ulcer, perform a suture ligation of the bleeding vessel with or without vagotomy and biopsy the ulcer to rule out malignancy.

(c) For a distal gastric ulcer, perform an antrectomy with Billroth II reconstruction.

3. Esophageal variceal bleeding

a. EGD is used for diagnosis and treatment by injection or rubber-band ligation.

b. Pharmacologic treatment is used to lower portal venous pressure.

      (1) Vasopressin (0.1–0.4 U/min IV infusion) controls 60%–75% of variceal bleeding. Concomitant use of nitroglycerin (IV/SL) allows for the use of higher doses.

      (2) Octreotide (50-μg bolus followed by 50 μg/hr IV for 5 days) is more effective than vasopressin in randomized trials. It has become the drug of choice in many institutions.

   c. Balloon tamponade via a Sengstaken-Blakemore tube or a Minnesota tube should be used in cases with a high rate of rebleeding or bleeding uncontrolled by pharmacologic or endoscopic therapy. Balloon tamponade has a high rate of esophageal perforation, esophageal necrosis, and aspiration.

   d. Operative therapy

      (1) Indications

         (a) Uncontrolled hemorrhage

         (b) Persistent rebleed despite maximal medical therapy

      (2) Procedures

         (a) A TIPS is an effective yet temporary measure to lower portal venous pressure. This procedure should only be performed in transplant candidates.

         (b) A distal splenorenal (Warren) shunt should be used for stable patients who are not candidates for transplantation.

         (c) Central portacaval shunt, suture ligation of bleeding varices, and esophageal transection should be used for unstable patients who are not candidates for transplantation.

II. Lower Gastrointestinal (LGI) Hemorrhage

  A. Definition. LGI hemorrhage is bleeding from a source distal to the ligament of Treitz.

  B. Etiology

    1. Diverticular disease (see DIVERTICULAR DISEASE in this chapter)

    2. Angiodysplasia refers to abnormal arteriovenous communications that result from precapillary sphincter incompetence. Lesions are mostly of the right colon but can occur anywhere in the GI tract.

      a. Incidence is 2%–6% in the general population and 25%–50% in the elderly.

      b. Massive LGI bleed is a presentation in 10%–15% of patients.

      c. In 90% of patients, bleeding stops spontaneously.

      d. The rebleeding rate at 1 and 3 years is 25% and 45%, respectively.

    3. Colon carcinoma (or polyp) usually presents with occult bleeding. It is rarely a cause of massive LGI bleeding.

4. **Ischemic bowel disease** can occur secondary to mesenteric embolus, thrombus, or low-flow state.
   a. Patients are typically elderly with a history of abdominal aortic aneurysm repair, atrial fibrillation, or hypotension.
   b. Bleeding is usually intermittent; 75% stops spontaneously.
5. **IBD** presents with bright-red blood from the rectum in almost all patients with ulcerative colitis and in approximately 25% of patients with Crohn's colitis.
   a. Massive LGI bleed occurs in 1%–5% of patients with IBD.
   b. Bleeding usually resolves spontaneously.
6. Less common causes of LGI bleed include:
   a. Massive UGI bleed
   b. Meckel's diverticulum
   c. Aortoenteric fistula
   d. Infectious colitis
   e. Hemorrhoids

C. **Signs and symptoms**
1. Hematochezia (passage of bright-red blood or clots from the rectum)
2. Melena (seen with slow bleeding from proximal colon)

D. **Management**

Always keep in mind the question, "Is the patient still bleeding?" Melena and clots can be passed from the rectum days after bleeding has stopped.

---

1. Follow the **initial management of UGI hemorrhage** (see p 232).
2. Insert a **NG tube** to rule out an UGI source, followed by EGD if the aspirate is positive. Up to 10% of patients with suspected LGI bleed have an UGI source.
3. Perform bedside **anoscopy** (or rigid sigmoidoscopy) to rule out anal and rectal lesions (e.g., polyp, hemorrhoid).
4. Perform studies to **localize blood loss.**
   a. **Colonoscopy** is the diagnostic (and sometimes therapeutic) procedure of choice and will identify the bleeding site in > 70% of cases.
      (1) Endoscopic visualization is obscured by bleeding of > 1 ml/min.
      (2) Electrocoagulation controls active bleeding in 20% of cases.
      (3) It is necessary to have adequate bowel preparation.
   b. **Angiography** detects active **bleeding of > 1 ml/min** and may reveal only some of multiple bleeding sites. Findings are negative in 50% of patients that require emergent operation.

        (1) Therapeutic **arteriography** includes embolization (microcoils, autologous clotted blood, gel-foam) and the use of vasopressin (0.2–0.4 U/min).

        (2) Of LGI bleeds controlled by vasopressin, 40% rebleed and 30% require emergent operation.

        (3) The complication rate of arteriography is 10%; only 8% undergo segmental (not subtotal) colectomy based on arteriographic findings.

    c. Nuclear imaging with ^{99m}Tc-labeled RBCs can detect **bleeding as slow as 0.1 ml/min.** "Tagged" RBCs persist in the circulation for 24 hours, so serial examinations are possible.

        (1) A positive scan should be followed by angiography (or surgery).

        (2) A negative scan should be followed by colonoscopy.

  5. Determine the need for **operative intervention** (Figure 9-3).

Frail and elderly individuals tolerate an operation much better than blood loss.

E. Prognosis

  1. The overall mortality rate is 10%–15%.

  2. Predictors of poor outcome include age > 60 years, > 5 units of blood loss each day, shock, rebleed, coagulopathy, and comorbid disease.

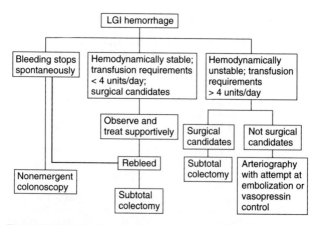

Figure 9-3. Algorithm for the treatment of lower gastrointestinal (LGI) hemorrhage.

INTESTINAL OBSTRUCTION

I. **Etiology**
A. **Mechanical obstruction**
1. **Luminal obstruction** can result from tumors, intussusception, meconium, gallstones, and impaction (e.g., feces, barium, bezoars, parasites, foreign objects).
2. **Intrinsic bowel lesions** include:
a. Congenital lesions (e.g., atresia and stenosis, imperforate anus, duplications, diverticulum, Hirschprung's disease)
b. Traumatic lesions (e.g., hematoma)
c. Inflammatory lesions (e.g., regional enteritis, diverticulitis, ulcerative colitis)
d. Neoplastic lesions (e.g., polyps and other tumors), circumferential lesions
e. Strictures (postoperative or a result of resolving perforation or inflammation)
3. **Extrinsic bowel lesions** can result from neoplasms, annular pancreas, anomalous vessels, abscesses, and hematomas.
a. Volvulus can be congenital (midgut), cecal, or sigmoid.
b. Adhesions are the most common cause of extrinsic bowel lesions, with an overall prevalence of 67% after laparotomy. They can occur within 1 week after surgery, and obstruction occurs in 3%–26% of cases.
c. Hernias (internal and external) can obstruct when incarcerated.
d. Ladd's bands are peritoneal bands that result from incomplete intestinal rotation. These bands may cause obstruction and usually occur in pediatric patients.
B. **Functional obstruction** (paralytic ileus)
1. Postoperative state
2. Trauma (e.g., spine fractures)
3. Retroperitoneal hematomas
4. Peritonitis
5. Electrolyte imbalance (especially hypokalemia)
6. Ischemia
7. Shock
8. Renal failure
9. Ascites
10. Abscess
11. UTI
C. **Idiopathic pseudo-obstruction** [i.e., chronic illness characterized by recurrent symptoms of intestinal obstruction with no evidence of mechanical obstruction (e.g., Ogilvie's syndrome)] may be due to COPD, electrolyte disturbances, or polypharmacy.
II. **Classification of Obstruction**
A. **Small bowel obstruction**

      1. **Pathogenesis**

         a. Fluid and gas accumulate proximal to the obstruction. The gas predominantly results from swallowed air.

         b. There is an abundance of nitrogen that cannot be absorbed by the intestine.

         c. As the bowel becomes distended, it loses its ability to absorb water and electrolytes; thus, it fills with fluid and becomes more distended. In addition, the bowel becomes prosecretory.

         d. There is a rapid proliferation of bacteria within the obstructed bowel.

      2. Proximal obstruction causes more vomiting and results in greater losses of water and electrolytes than distal obstruction.

    B. Obstruction by strangulation

      1. Blood flow to the obstructed bowel segment is impaired.

      2. Blood flow in the distended bowel remains normal until an intraluminal pressure of 20 cm H_2O, at which point blood flow becomes compromised.

      3. Closed loop syndrome occurs when the proximal and distal ends of an affected loop are obstructed and there is decreased blood flow.

    C. Colon obstruction

      1. The colon acts as a closed loop and is prone to perforation. If the ileocecal valve is competent, there may not be any small bowel distention.

      2. There is less fluid and electrolyte disturbance as compared to small bowel obstruction.

      3. The most common cause of colon obstruction is cancer. The obstruction usually perforates near the cancer.

      4. An incompetent ileocecal valve will allow small bowel distention.

III. Signs and Symptoms

    A. Obstruction

      1. Abdominal pain (usually crampy) and distention

      2. Nausea and vomiting [bilious (high obstruction) versus feculent (low obstruction)]

      3. Obstipation (severe constipation with failure to pass flatus)

      4. Diarrhea (usually persists until fluid and stool distal to the obstruction is passed or in cases of partial obstruction)

      5. Difficulty initiating or advancing feedings

      6. High gastric residuals

    B. Strangulation

      1. Tachycardia (with hypotension may indicate dehydration)

      2. Fever (may be caused by peritonitis or ischemia)

      3. Abdominal distention and tenderness

      4. Presence of a mass

      5. Leukocytosis

      6. Peritonitis

IV. Physical Examination
  A. Check vital signs. Alterations can indicate systemic complications of obstruction such as sepsis or shock.
  B. Perform an abdominal examination.
    1. A distended, tympanitic abdomen with localized tenderness, involuntary guarding, percussion tenderness, and rebound are signs of peritonitis caused by perforation and strangulation.
    2. Evaluate for hernias, masses, and old scars.
  C. Perform a pelvic examination on all women with abdominal pain.
  D. Perform a rectal examination, which may reveal masses and occult blood in the stool.
V. Diagnostic Tests
  A. Laboratory tests
    1. CBC and platelet count
    2. Electrolytes
    3. BUN/creatinine
    4. Calcium, magnesium, and phosphorus
    5. Alkaline phosphatase, liver transaminases, and bilirubin
    6. PT and PTT
    7. Lactic acid
    8. Amylase and lipase
  B. Radiographs (supine abdomen, upright abdomen, chest)
    1. Look for free air.
    2. Determine the gas pattern and the associated bowel.
      a. For small bowel obstruction, colonic air denotes partial process.
      b. Large bowel obstruction with small bowel dilation is associated with an incompetent ileocecal valve.
      c. Look for the air cutoff sign in the large bowel to determine possible location of the obstructing source.
    3. Check for distended bowel.
      a. Small bowel have valvulae conniventes (i.e., lines across the entire diameter of the bowel).
      b. Large bowel have haustra (i.e., small indentations on the lumen).
    4. Check the location of the bowel.
      a. The small bowel is usually central.
      b. The large bowel is usually peripheral.
    5. Check air–fluid levels.
  C. Hypaque enema
    1. Hypaque is used to identify a large bowel obstruction instead of barium because of the risk of present or impending perforation and subsequent barium peritonitis. There is also a risk of barium getting caught proximal to an incomplete obstruction and getting impacted.
    2. A hypaque enema allows visualization of intraluminal masses, strictures, and volvulus. It can often reverse a volvulus.
  D. UGI contrast examination with small bowel follow through

delineates the pathology of the UGI tract and is often able to localize the area of obstruction.

E. CT scan helps identify abdominal pathology such as free air, free fluid, masses, and inflammation.

VI. Management

A. Identify the area of obstruction.

B. Identify **partial versus complete obstruction.**

C. Resuscitate the patient, which involves:

    1. Liberal rehydration using lactated Ringer's solution

    2. Placement of a NG tube to relieve the propagation of obstruction through swallowed air and to relieve vomiting

    3. Placement of a Foley catheter to monitor urine output

    4. Repletion of electrolytes

D. Determine the need for operative therapy.

    1. Nonoperative treatment is appropriate under the following conditions; however, if these conditions do not resolve, surgery is required:

      a. Postoperative obstruction

      b. Pediatric intussusception (hydrostatic reduction)

      c. Sigmoid volvulus (colonoscopy or sigmoidoscopy)

      d. Partial obstruction (hydration, electrolyte repletion, and bowel decompression; close observation is imperative to notice progression of partial-to-complete obstruction)

      e. Recurrent small bowel obstruction (may ultimately require definitive surgical therapy)

    2. If **operative therapy** is required, attempt to normalize electrolytes, hydration, vital signs, and urinary output. Then determine the timing of the procedure.

      a. The procedure should be performed as soon as possible for a complete obstruction.

      b. Patients with a short course of illness may undergo surgery immediately, whereas patients with metabolic derangements may do better with 12–18 hours of resuscitation.

    3. There are surgical options for small and large bowel obstructions.

      a. Small bowel obstructions are primarily treated with resection and primary anastomosis.

      b. Complete large bowel obstructions caused by colorectal cancer, diverticulitis, or volvulus require urgent celiotomy and treatment of the offending lesion.

        (1) The most conservative approach is resection of the obstruction and end colostomy with Hartmann's pouch.

        (2) If the patient is critically ill and requires immediate operative therapy, a loop colostomy is an option.

        (3) If the patient has a right-sided lesion, primary anastomosis after obstruction is an option. Although it is more accepted on the right side, this procedure is controversial. It is determined by the quality of the tissues, the amount of dilation of the bowel, and the overall metabolic status of the patient.

(4) For left-sided lesions, resection and Hartmann's pouch is appropriate. If the bowel integrity appears good, some physicians may try to do a primary repair.

(5) Another option for left-sided lesions, especially cancerous lesions, is complete resection of the colon back to the ileum and an ileocolonic anastomosis. These patients may have significant diarrhea, which may improve and is partially dependent on the length of remaining colon distal to the resected lesion. The benefit of an ileocolonic anastomosis is one operation and, if cancerous, less extensive surveillance.

INTRAABDOMINAL ABSCESS

I. **Definitions of Intraabdominal Compartments.** Several anatomic recesses in the abdomen lead to localization of fluid with specific implications for therapy. Though the pelvic and bilateral subphrenic spaces are the most dependent portions of the supine abdomen, the RLQ and LLQ are the most common areas of abscesses.

A. The **right suprahepatic or subphrenic space** is defined by the diaphragm superiorly, the dome of the liver inferiorly, and the posterior attachment of the coronary and triangular ligaments posteriorly and medially. The lateral aspect freely communicates with the infrahepatic space.

B. The **right infrahepatic space** is defined by the liver superiorly, the transverse mesocolon inferiorly, and the duodenum and the hepaticoduodenal ligament medially. The deepest portion of this space is Morison's pouch.

C. The **left subphrenic space** is defined by the diaphragm superiorly, the transverse mesocolon inferiorly, the falciform ligament medially, and the phrenicocolic ligament laterally.

D. The **left anterior infrahepatic space,** defined by the posterior surface of the left lobe anteriorly and the surface of the stomach posteriorly, communicates with the left subphrenic space.

E. The **left posterior infrahepatic space** contains the anatomical lesser sac, which is in direct communication with the right subhepatic space via the foramen of Winslow.

II. **Pathophysiology**

A. **Flow of peritoneal fluid**

1. Lymphatic lacunae along the inferior surface of the diaphragm reabsorb peritoneal fluid and drain directly into the thoracic duct. This is particularly pertinent in the

supine position because respiratory variation creates hydrostatic flow in the cranial direction.

2. The peritoneal fluid ascends equally along both lateral colic gutters.
   a. Forward flow along the left side is impeded by the phrenicocolic ligament.
   b. Flow along the right side continues unimpeded in direct continuity with both the supra- and infrahepatic spaces.
3. Consequently, abscess formation occurs preferentially on the right side rather than the left side of the abdomen.

B. **The role of infection**
1. Clearance of intestinal infection depends on mechanical clearance by peritoneal fluid dynamics and basic cellular mechanisms of inflammation.
2. Resident macrophages begin the process with phagocytosis, elaboration of chemotactic cytokines, and activation of the complement cascade.
3. When bacterial contamination overwhelms lymphatic drainage, loculated collections can occur.
   a. Fibrin depositions around bacterial collections bind to collagen, forming walled-off abscesses.
   b. The subsequent inability of neutrophils to penetrate these collections leads to ongoing infection.
   c. Morbidity results not from the abscess directly but from the subsequent inability of the body's defense mechanisms to clear the infection once it has been walled off.

III. Etiology
A. Intraabdominal abscess formation may be secondary to intraabdominal trauma or visceral perforation.
B. Intraabdominal abscess may be a sequela of intraabdominal operation.

IV. Signs and Symptoms

> **In the critically ill patient, intraabdominal abscess may only be suggested by progressive multi–organ system failure.**

A. Persistent or intermittent spiking fevers
B. Leukocytosis
C. Hypotension
D. Tachycardia
E. Metabolic acidosis
F. Abdominal pain or tenderness
G. Anorexia or feeding intolerance

V. Diagnostic Tests
A. **Early diagnostic evaluation is the rule.**
B. **Plain films** may reveal:
1. Right-sided subdiaphragmatic air–fluid levels
2. Free air

3. Displacement of intraabdominal contents or obliteration of the psoas shadows (suggests a large abscess)
C. **CT scan** has become the standard for diagnostic evaluation of potential intraabdominal abscess.
 1. PO and IV (if renal function permits) contrast should be administered.
 2. Postoperative abscesses usually become discrete and well defined by postoperative days 7–10.
 3. Sensitivity and specificity have both been reported at > 90%.

VI. Management
A. Abscess drainage
1. **Percutaneous drainage** (via CT scan or ultrasound) may be done provided the following criteria are met:
 a. Precise anatomic definition of the abscess
 b. Another intraabdominal viscera is not transgressed by drainage
2. **Surgical exploration and drainage** is necessary for:
 a. Multiple loculated collections
 b. Suspected collections not visualized with diagnostic imaging
 c. Ongoing sepsis not responsive to percutaneous drainage

B. Fluid resuscitation
C. Antibiotics
1. Ciprofloxacin and metronidazole
2. Ampicillin and gentamicin and metronidazole
3. Gentamicin and clindamycin
4. Ticarcillin/clavulanate (Timentin)
5. Imipenem or meropenem

PANCREATITIS—ACUTE

I. Etiology
A. Excessive alcohol intake (more common etiology in males)
B. Gallstones (more common etiology in females)
C. Hyperlipidemia
D. Hypercalcemia (resulting from hyperparathyroidism)
E. Trauma (e.g., penetrating, blunt, postoperative, ERCP-induced)
F. Anatomic causes (e.g., pancreatic duct obstruction; tumor of the pancreas, common bile duct, or duodenum; stricture; duodenal diverticula; pancreatic divisum; choledochocele) [Figure 9-4]
G. Ischemia
H. Medications (e.g., azathioprine, estrogens, thiazides, furosemide, sulfonamides, tetracycline, steroids, procainamide, valproic acid, clonidine, pentamidine)
I. Toxins (e.g., methanol, organophosphates, insecticides, scorpion venom)

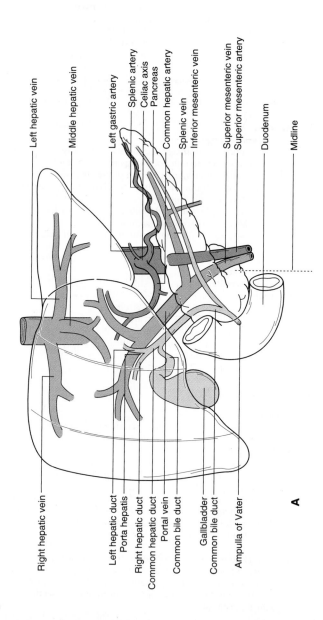

Left hepatic vein

Middle hepatic vein

Left gastric artery

Splenic artery

Celiac axis

Pancreas

Common hepatic artery

Splenic vein

Inferior mesenteric vein

Superior mesenteric vein

Superior mesenteric artery

Duodenum

Midline

Right hepatic vein

Left hepatic duct

Porta hepatis

Right hepatic duct

Common hepatic duct

Portal vein

Common bile duct

Gallbladder

Common bile duct

Ampulla of Vater

A

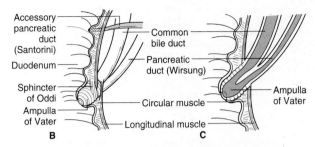

Figure 9-4. (*A*) Biliary and pancreatic anatomy. (*B*) External view of the relationship between the common bile duct and the pancreatic duct. (*C*) Internal view of the relationship between the common bile duct and the pancreatic duct.

    J. Infection (e.g., mumps, Coxsackievirus, hepatitis, cytomegalovirus, mycoplasma, tuberculosis, parasites)

    K. Idiopathic causes [e.g., biliary sludge (the cause in 66%–75% of cases)]

II. Signs and Symptoms

    A. Constant midepigastric pain relieved with sitting or leaning forward (50% radiate to the back)

    B. Nausea and vomiting

    C. Anorexia

    D. Epigastric tenderness (may extend to the RLQ because of inflammation along the paracolic gutter)

    E. Abdominal distention, absent bowel sounds, guarding, and rebound

    F. Fever, tachycardia, hypotension, and shock

    G. Palpable epigastric mass

    H. Jaundice, ascites

    I. Cullen's sign (see Table 9-1)

    J. Grey Turner's sign (see Table 9-1)

III. Diagnostic Tests

    A. Obtain **laboratory tests,** including:

        1. ABG

        2. CBC with differential

        3. Platelet count

        4. Electrolytes

        5. BUN/creatinine

        6. Calcium, magnesium, and phosphorus

        7. Liver function tests: alkaline phosphatase, bilirubin, serum glutamate oxaloacetate transaminase, and serum glutamate pyruvate transaminase

        8. Triglycerides

        9. Amylase and lipase

            a. Serum amylase has a sensitivity of 60%–90% with < 70% specificity.

      b. Lipase is 90%–99% sensitive and specific.

B. Obtain an **ECG.**

C. Obtain a **chest radiograph** to rule out free air.

D. Abdominal films provide nonspecific findings, such as air in the duodenal loop, a dilated proximal jejunal loop (sentinel loop sign), pancreatic calcifications, and distended colon to mid-transverse colon (colon cutoff sign).

E. Ultrasound assesses the presence of gallstones, pseudocysts, calcification, edema, and ductal dilation.

F. Contrast-enhanced CT (pancreatic protocol) is most sensitive and specific for the diagnosis of acute pancreatitis. This dynamic CT scan provides the **Balthazar grade:**
1. Grade A—normal pancreas
2. Grade B—focal or diffuse enlargement
3. Grade C—intrinsic pancreatic abnormalities and peripancreatic inflammation
4. Grade D—single, ill-defined fluid collection or phlegmon
5. Grade E—two or more defined fluid collections or the presence of gas in or adjacent to the pancreas

IV. Management

A. ICU admission is indicated in moderate-to-severe cases or in high-risk patients. This decision can be made based on the hemodynamic status of the patient and the number of Ranson's criteria present on admission (Table 9-4).

B. Use lactated Ringer's solution and normal saline to maintain intravascular volume and urine output at 0.5–1.0 cc/kg/hr.

C. Use a Foley catheter to ensure accurate urine quantification.

D. If ileus or vomiting are present, use a NG tube to decrease the amount of gastric acid entering the duodenum.

E. For analgesia, meperidine hydrochloride is better than morphine because of the possible spasmodic effects on the sphincter of Oddi.

F. If necessary, follow the management protocol for alcohol withdrawal:
1. Thiamine, 100 mg IM/IV qd for 3 days
2. Folate, 1 mg IM/IV qd for 3 days

G. All cases require NPO.
1. In moderate-to-severe cases in which prolonged periods of NPO are expected, parenteral nutrition is indicated and should be started early.
2. Jejunal enteral feeds are indicated when the acute phase of pancreatitis has resolved, yet the patient is unable to tolerate oral feeding. Jejunal feeding does not stimulate exocrine pancreatic secretion.

H. Pharmacologic management includes:
1. Octreotide, 100–200 µg SQ tid
2. H_2 blockers (i.e., one of the following):
    a. Famotidine, 20 mg IV q 12 hr
    b. Ranitidine, 50 mg IV q 8 hr

Table 9-4. Ranson's Criteria for Determining the Prognosis of Acute Pancreatitis

Signs	Nongallstone Pancreatitis	Gallstone Pancreatitis
At admission:		
Age	>55 years	>70 years
WBC count	>16,000 cells/mm^3	>18,000 cells/mm^3
Glucose	>200 mg/dl	>220 mg/dl
LDH	>350 IU/dl	>400 IU/dl
SGOT	>250 IU/dl	>250 IU/dl
After initial 48 hours:		
Hematocrit	Decrease >10%	Decrease >10%
BUN	Increase >5 mg/dl	Increase >5 mg/dl
Serum Ca	<8 mg/dl	<8 mg/dl
Arterial PO$_2$	<60 mm Hg	<60 mm Hg
Base deficit	>4 mEq/L	>5 mEq/L
Fluid sequestration	>6 L	>4 L
Mortality:	<3 signs = 1%	
	3–4 signs = 15%	
	5–6 signs = 50%	
	≥ 7 signs = approximately 100%	

BUN = blood urea nitrogen; LDH = lactate dehydrogenase; SGOT = serum glutamate oxaloacetate transaminase; WBC = white blood cell.

      c. Cimetidine, 300 mg IV q 8 hr
   3. Insulin as needed to maintain normoglycemia
   4. Prophylactic antibiotics
      a. The data are insufficiently strong to mandate prophylaxis or to set it as the standard of care.
      b. If prophylactic antibiotics are used in necrotizing disease, imipenem/cilastatin is the drug of choice.
I. Indications for **operative treatment** include:
   1. Mechanical etiology (e.g., gallstones) [Cholecystectomy is performed after the acute process is resolved.]
   2. Uncertainty of diagnosis or acute abdomen
   3. Local complications or pancreatic necrosis
  J. **Operative procedures** include:
   1. ERCP and possible sphincterotomy
   2. Open or laparoscopic cholecystectomy
   3. Open packing and débridement of infected necrotizing pancreatitis
   4. Drainage (open or percutaneous) of abscess or infected pseudocyst
V. Complications

A. Pancreatic pseudocyst
B. Necrotizing pancreatitis secondary to infection or severe injury
C. Shock
D. ARDS
E. Renal failure

VI. Prognosis (see Table 9-4)

PEPTIC ULCER DISEASE

I. Etiology

A. Aggressive factors promoting ulceration include:
   1. *H. pylori* (present in 95%–100% of duodenal ulcer patients; 60%–80% of gastric ulcer patients; and 20% of young, normal volunteers)
   2. Acid and pepsin
   3. Hypergastrinemia (Zollinger-Ellison syndrome)

B. Impaired mucosal defense may be caused by:
   1. **Drugs**
      a. NSAIDs
      b. Steroids (when used with NSAIDs)
      c. Nicotine (e.g., cigarettes)
   2. **Low bicarbonate production** by the stomach and duodenum
   3. **Gastric stasis**
      a. In gastric stasis there is inadequate clearance of normal amounts of acid.
      b. Duodenal disease may perpetuate itself by duodenal scarring and further delaying gastric emptying.
   4. **Alcohol** (induces gastritis)

II. Signs and Symptoms

A. Recurrent, dull, burning epigastric pain 1–3 hours after a meal
B. Pain that increases after eating (usually indicates a gastric ulcer)
C. Pain that is relieved after eating (usually indicates a duodenal ulcer)

III. Physical Examination. Examination will reveal:

A. Moderate epigastric pain
B. Rebound
C. Rigidity
D. Guarding
E. Occult blood in the stool

IV. Diagnostic Tests

A. General laboratory tests include CBC, chemistry profile, and coagulation parameters.
B. Duodenal ulcers are diagnosed by contrast radiography or endoscopy.
C. Gastric ulcers are diagnosed by endoscopy, and biopsy must be done to rule out malignancy.

D. *H. pylori* infection is detected with:

1. Invasive tests (i.e., endoscopy) [used to evaluate a patient > 50 years of age with GI bleeding or severe pain]
2. Noninvasive tests
   a. Serology for antibodies to *H. pylori* is used for initial screening but not for efficacy of treatment.
   b. Labeled urea breath tests are used to confirm the eradication of *H. pylori* 4 weeks after the end of treatment.
3. Endoscopic tests
   a. Rapid urease test
   b. Histologic examination (biopsy evaluates inflammation and mucosa)
   c. Culture

V. Management

A. Duodenal ulcers

1. First-line therapy is a H_2 antagonist for 8 weeks and evaluation and treatment for *H. pylori*.
2. For recurrent or persistent disease, use omeprazole and repeat the evaluation and treatment for *H. pylori*.

B. Gastric ulcers

1. Discontinue ulcerogenic drugs (e.g., NSAIDs).
2. First-line therapy is a H_2 antagonist.
3. If there is concern for malignancy, a repeat biopsy is indicated. In addition, all gastric ulcers should be biopsied at the time of surgery to rule out malignancy.
4. Screening and treatment for *H. pylori* should be reserved for recurrent or persistent gastric ulcers.
5. It is usually best to resect a perforated gastric ulcer.

C. Acute pharmacologic therapy of peptic ulcer disease

1. H_2 antagonists
   a. Famotidine, 20 mg PO/IV bid
   b. Ranitidine, 150 mg PO bid or 50 mg IV bid
   c. Cimetidine, 400 mg PO bid or 300 mg IV q 8 hr
   d. Nizatidine, 150 mg PO qd/bid
2. Mucosal protectant: sucralfate, 1 g PO before meals and before sleep
3. Proton pump inhibitors
   a. Omeprazole, 20–40 mg PO qd/bid
   b. Lansoprazole, 15 mg PO qam

D. Treatment of *H. pylori* infection

1. Bismuth, metronidazole, tetracycline, and ranitidine (inexpensive) [95% eradication at 6 weeks; 14 days of therapy]
   a. Bismuth, 2 tablets qid
   b. Metronidazole, 250 mg PO qid
   c. Tetracycline, 500 mg PO qid (amoxicillin, 500 mg PO qid in children)
   d. Ranitidine, 150 mg PO bid (continue for a total of 6 weeks)
2. Amoxicillin, omeprazole, and clarithromycin (expensive,

well tolerated) [82% eradication at 6 weeks; 14 days of therapy]
  a. Amoxicillin, 1 g PO bid
  b. Omeprazole, 20 mg PO bid
  c. Clarithromycin, 500 mg PO bid
3. Metronidazole, omeprazole, and clarithromycin (expensive, well tolerated) [10 days of therapy]
  a. Metronidazole, 500 mg PO bid
  b. Omeprazole, 20 mg PO bid (continue 2 weeks after initial 14 days of eradication)
  c. Clarithromycin, 500 mg PO bid
  E. **Operative management** is reserved for persistent ulcers, perforation, or acute hemorrhage.

VI. **Long-term Complications of Peptic Ulcer Surgery**
  A. **Recurrent peptic ulceration**
    1. Recurrent ulcers are usually treated with medical therapy.
    2. Marginal ulceration usually requires reoperation.
  B. **Dumping syndrome**
    1. Dumping syndrome occurs after meals because of a loss of fundic relaxation with a gastric load. Carbohydrate meals exacerbate the syndrome.
    2. It is characterized by tachycardia, diaphoresis, hypotension, and abdominal pain.
    3. It is treated by separating liquid and solid meals, or conversion of Billroth I to II or Billroth II to Roux-en-Y.
  C. **Postvagotomy diarrhea**
    1. Postvagotomy diarrhea is usually characterized by watery diarrhea that occurs 30 minutes after a meal.
    2. The diarrhea improves with time.
  D. **Malabsorption**
    1. Malabsorption results in vitamin B_{12} deficiency caused by a loss of intrinsic factor to bind the vitamin B_{12} in the ileum.
    2. The patient should eat many small meals each day.
  E. **Bile reflux gastritis**
    1. Bile reflux gastritis results from pyloric ablation with bile stasis in the stomach.
    2. It is diagnosed on biopsy with associated bilious vomiting and abdominal pain.
    3. It is treated with conversion to Roux-en-Y gastrojejunostomy.
  F. **Reactive hypoglycemia**
    1. Rapid absorption of glucose results in overproduction of insulin and rebound hypoglycemia.
    2. Hypoglycemia improves with multiple small meals.

VII. **Perforation**
  A. **Types of perforation**
    1. **Free** perforation occurs when duodenal or gastric contents spill freely into the peritoneal cavity.
    2. **Contained** perforation occurs when free spillage is pre-

vented by the formation of a walled-off abscess by adjacent structures.

B. Pathology

  1. Most duodenal ulcer perforations (i.e., 90%) occur in the anterior duodenal bulb.

  2. Many gastric ulcer perforations (i.e., 60%) occur on the lesser curvature at the junction of the parietal and antral cells.

C. Signs and symptoms

  1. Gnawing abdominal pain before perforation (hours, days, or months) that acutely becomes more severe

  2. Tachypnea, tachycardia, and hypotension (associated with acute perforation)

  3. GI bleeding (occasionally a result of perforation or ulceration)

  4. Epigastric pain (becomes more diffuse on perforation)

D. Physical examination

  1. The patient may be febrile.

  2. The patient often lies supine, immobile, and with the knees flexed.

  3. The abdomen is without bowel sounds, is tender, and rebound is often present.

  4. Rectal examination usually reveals heme-positive stool.

E. Diagnostic tests

  1. Blood tests reveal an elevated WBC count.

  2. Free air is seen on plain radiograph (70%) and CT scan.

F. Management

  1. Nonoperative therapy

    a. Indications for nonoperative therapy include:

      (1) Long-standing perforation (> 24 hours) and evidence by water-soluble contrast radiography (Gastrografin, hypaque) that the perforation has sealed

      (2) Perforated duodenal ulcer

      (3) Minimal peritonitis

    b. Contraindications to nonoperative therapy include:

      (1) Perforated gastric ulcer (results in multiple abdominal abscesses)

      (2) Steroids (inhibit healing)

      (3) Continued leak on contrast study

      (4) Patient currently on antiulcer treatment

  2. Operative therapy

    a. Indications for surgery include:

      (1) Perforation

      (2) Bleeding

      (3) Obstruction

      (4) Intractable pain

    b. Operative therapy is often limited to **local treatment or resection** of the ulcer and management of the patient with H_2 antagonists or proton pump inhibitors for life.

(1) This form of management depends on a patient who is reliable, conscientious, and able to afford the medication.

(2) Definitive and selective ulcer operations are for patients who are hemodynamically stable, able to undergo a lengthier operation, and perforated < 24 hours.

(3) Patients who failed medical therapy should undergo a definitive ulcer operation. The more selective the better.

c. **Procedures for peptic ulcer disease**

(1) **Vagotomy and pyloroplasty**

(a) Truncal vagotomy and pyloroplasty is most often used in a patient undergoing surgery for bleeding who is unstable to undergo a more selective antiulcer procedure.

(b) Truncal vagotomy and pyloroplasty is often plagued by postoperative complications, including gastric motility disorders, dumping syndrome, postvagotomy diarrhea, and bile reflux gastritis.

(c) Truncal vagotomy has a short operative time and a short learning curve.

(d) Highly selective vagotomy (parietal cell vagotomy) is a longer procedure and requires more experience. However, it preserves antral and distal gut innervation while sectioning vagal fibers of the fundus and avoids the complications of truncal vagotomy.

(i) Indications include intractable duodenal ulcer disease (elective surgery) and bleeding duodenal ulcer in a stable patient (emergency surgery).

(ii) Contraindications include prepyloric or gastric ulcer and gastric outlet obstruction.

(2) **Resective therapy** (usually not first-line)

(a) Vagotomy and antrectomy with Billroth I or II reconstruction removes gastrin and cholinergic innervation (results in reduced acid secretion), has low mortality and recurrence rates, and results in a 25% incidence of dumping syndrome and diarrhea.

(b) Subtotal gastrectomy

(c) Total gastrectomy

d. **Emergency surgery**

(1) In an **unstable** patient, oversew the ulcer and place an omental patch or perform truncal vagotomy and pyloroplasty.

(2) In a **stable** patient, oversew the ulcer and per-

form a vagotomy and antrectomy or proximal gastric vagotomy.

STRESS ULCERS

I. Pathogenesis

A. The gastric mucosa is covered by a protective layer of mucus that prevents adverse effects from the acidity of the gastric environment.

B. Ischemia to the lining of the stomach induces a loss of this protective layer and enables the formation of stress ulcers.

C. These superficial erosions in the gastric mucosa do not erode to cause perforation.

D. Occult bleeding occurs in 20% of long-term ICU patients but only results in 5% of patients with clinically obvious hemorrhage.

II. Risk Factors for Stress Gastritis

A. Increased acidity

B. Decreased bicarbonate

C. Decreased mucosal blood flow

D. Increased mucosal permeability

III. Indications for Stress Ulcer Prophylaxis

A. Absolute indications

1. Mechanical ventilation (respiratory failure)
2. Coagulopathy (platelet count < 50,000, INR > 1.5, or PTT > 2 minutes)

B. Relative indications

1. Low cardiac output
2. COPD
3. Prolonged bowel rest
4. Steroids, chemotherapy
5. Critically ill, sepsis
6. Trauma (e.g., head injury, multiple trauma, extensive burns)
7. Renal failure

IV. Strategies for Stress Ulcer Prophylaxis

A. Gastric pH control

1. Inhibit gastric acid production with a H_2 antagonist or neutralize intragastric acid with antacids. Both are equally effective in reducing the incidence of bleeding.
2. The pH should be monitored every 2–4 hours.

B. Luminal nutrients

1. The instillation of enteral feedings directly into the stomach has been shown to reduce the incidence of stress ulcers.
2. The theories behind this include an antacid-like effect or the restoration of the protective lining by the stomach after the provision of nutrients and energy.

C. Cytoprotection

1. Cytoprotective agents recreate the protective barrier of the stomach without changing the gastric pH.
2. Sucralfate is the most common agent, has no toxicity, and is relatively inexpensive. Administer 1 g PO qid.

D. Hemodynamic management
1. The goal is to maintain adequate blood flow to the gut.
2. Hemodynamic management prevents areas of localized ischemia.

V. Complications Associated with Stress Ulcer Prophylaxis
A. Aspiration pneumonia
1. There is a high incidence of aspiration in critically ill patients, especially those on ventilators.
2. The reduction of gastric pH allows for bacterial overgrowth in the stomach, which then increases the bacterial load with aspiration.

B. Drug interaction
C. Gastric bezoars secondary to sucralfate
D. Adverse CNS effects of H_2 blockers
E. Thrombocytopenia with H_2 blockers

VI. Management of Stress Ulcers
A. Give enteral feeds if there is adequate gastric emptying.
B. Start one of the following medications:
1. Sucralfate, 1 g PO per NG tube q 6 hr
2. Famotidine, 20 g IV q 12 hr
3. Ranitidine, 50 mg IV q 12 hr or 0.5 mg/kg over 30 minutes, then continuous infusion at 0.25 mg/kg/hr to keep gastric pH > 5

C. Antacids may be added to any of the previous regimens (i.e., enteral feeds, sucralfate, cimetidine, or ranitidine)
1. Give antacids at a dose of 30 ml and check gastric pH after 1 hour.
2. If pH < 5, give 60 ml and repeat until pH > 5.

D. Stop ulcer prophylaxis as early as possible.
E. Occult blood testing should only be done with Gastroccult (Smith, Kline & French). Hemoccult (Smith, Kline & French) has multiple false-positives, including low gastric pH and cimetidine.

10

Hematology and

Coagulation

Management

BLOOD PRODUCTS AND COAGULATION FACTORS

I. Blood Products (Table 10-1)
  A. Whole blood
  B. Packed RBCs
  C. Leukocyte-reduced RBCs
  D. Irradiated RBCs
  E. Washed RBCs
  F. Platelets
  G. Fresh frozen plasma
  H. Cryoprecipitate

II. Coagulation Factors (Table 10-2)
  A. Specific factors
   1. **Factor I** (fibrinogen), an acute phase reactant, whose production is increased in inflammatory conditions
   2. **Factor II** (prothrombin). Its actions include:
     a. Conversion of fibrinogen to fibrin
     b. Conversion of factors V and VIII into activated forms (Va and VIIIa, respectively) [positive feedback]
     c. Conversion of XIII to XIIIa
     d. Binding of prothrombin to endothelial protein thrombomodulin activates protein C and protein S (which degrades factors Va and VIIIa) [negative feedback]
     e. Stimulation of synthesis of endothelin
     f. Stimulation of fibrinolysis by converting pro-tissue plasminogen activator (pro-tPA) into tPA

255

Table 10-1. Blood Products

Component	Content/Preparation	Use	Comments
Whole blood	RBCs, WBCs, platelets, and clotting factors	Rarely used	After 24 hours of collection, platelets and clotting factors function poorly
Packed RBCs	RBCs concentrated to a hematocrit of 60%–80%	Most commonly used product to correct anemia One unit should raise the hematocrit by 3% and the hemoglobin by 1 g/dl	35-day shelf life stored in CPDA-1 42-day shelf life in other storage media
Leukocyte-reduced RBCs	Packed RBCs that are centrifuged and filtered (to decrease the number of WBCs)	Prevent febrile, nonhemolytic, transfusion reactions	
Irradiated RBCs	Packed RBCs to which 25 Gy of gamma radiation has been applied	Prevent GVHD in bone marrow transplant and leukemia patients	
Washed RBCs	RBCs that are washed in normal saline, which reduces protein (i.e. immunoglobulin) content	Prevent allergic transfusion reactions and anaphylaxis in patients with IgA deficiency	

Platelets	Typically, one unit is obtained from one unit of whole blood; platelet transfusion of 6 units of pooled platelets is equivalent to 6 different donors	Thrombocytopenia, acquired platelet defect	Six units of platelets equivalent to about 300 ml of volume; 5-day shelf-life; stored in plasma that contains normal concentrations of clotting factors
Fresh frozen plasma	Whole blood minus RBCs and platelets; contains normal levels of all clotting factors	Prolonged PT	Transfusion of one unit increases circulating clotting factors by 20%–30%; Can be stored for 1 year
Cryoprecipitate	Concentrated factor I (fibrinogen), factor VIII, factor XIII, and von Willebrand factor	Product of choice to correct bleeding secondary to hypofibrinogenemia and hemophilia	

CPDA-1 = citrate-phosphate-dextrose-adenine-1; GVHD = graft-versus-host disease; PT = prothrombin time; RBC = red blood cell; WBC = white blood cell.

Table 10-2. Characteristics of Coagulation Factors

Roman Numeral	Name(s)	Site of Production	Half-life	Comments
I	Fibrinogen	Liver	90 hr	Fibrin monomers formed after thrombin cleavage of peptides A and B from fibrinogen; monomers overlap into a two-stranded fibril
II	Prothrombin	Liver	60 hr	A serine protease, with serine at the active site
III	TF; thromboplastin	—	—	Initiator of all *in vivo* coagulation Constitutively expressed integral membrane protein found on surface of fibroblasts macrophages, and other stromal cells that surround blood vessels Functions as receptor for factor VII
V	Proaccelerin	Liver Megakaryocytes (bone marrow)	25 hr	Va serves as cofactor to Xa
VII	Proconvertin	Liver	6 hr (shortest half-life of vitamin K–dependent factors)	Vitamin K–dependent Binds to TF When phospholipid (i.e., platelets) is present, bound VII becomes VIIa

VIII	Antihemophilic factor	Liver	12 hr when complexed to vWF (2–3 min in absence of vWF)	Circulates in plasma; noncovalently complexed with vWF Factor VIIIa serves as cofactor to IXa
IX	Christmas factor	Liver	12 hr	Vitamin K–dependent Factor IXa (a serine protease) significantly increases conversion of X to Xa
X	Stuart Prower factor	Liver	24 hr	Vitamin K–dependent Factor Xa (a serine protease) converts prothrombin to thrombin
XI	Plasma thromboplastin antecedent	Liver	—	Not involved in *in vivo* coagulation
XII	Hageman factor	Liver	—	Not involved in *in vivo* coagulation
XIII	Fibrin stabilizing factor	Liver Megakaryocytes (bone marrow)	3–5 days	XIIIa covalently cross-links fibrin monomers
—	Protein C	Liver	7 hr	Vitamin K–dependent
—	Protein S (not an enzyme)	Liver	—	Vitamin K–dependent Serves as cofactor to APC

APC = activated protein C; TF = tissue factor; vWF = von Willebrand factor.

g. Promotion of aggregation as a platelet agonist

3. Factor III [tissue factor (TF), thromboplastin], the initiator of all *in vivo* coagulation. Increased expression of TF is associated with several pathologic states.

  a. Disseminated intravascular coagulation (DIC) results from increased TF expression.

  b. Atherosclerosis is associated with increased endothelial and monocyte expression of TF.

  c. Thrombotic complications of malignant disease are secondary to increased TF expression of tumor cells and host cells.

4. Factor V (proaccelerin)

5. Factor VII (proconvertin)

6. Factor VIII (antihemophilic factor). Deficiency results in hemophilia A, an X-linked recessive disorder.

7. Factor IX (Christmas factor). Deficiency results in hemophilia B (Christmas disease), an X-linked recessive disorder.

8. Factor X (Stuart Prower factor). Deficiency results in Stuart disease, an autosomal recessive disorder.

9. Factor XI (plasma thromboplastin antecedent), which is not involved in *in vivo* coagulation. Deficiency does not result in a bleeding disorder. However, deficiency prolongs the partial thromboplastin time (PTT).

10. Factor XII (Hageman factor), which is also not involved in *in vivo* coagulation. Deficiency does not result in a bleeding disorder, but it prolongs the PTT. In fact, factor XII deficiency predisposes to thrombosis. Hageman factor is also intricately involved in the kallekrein–kinin pathway.

11. Factor XIII (fibrin stabilizing factor)

12. Protein C, which regulates coagulation. Deficiency results in a hypercoagulable state. Endothelial cells express thrombomodulin, which binds circulating thrombin. Circulating protein C binds to the thrombin–thrombomodulin complex and forms activated protein C (APC), which is a serine protease that degrades factors Va and VIIIa.

13. Protein S. Deficiency results in a hypercoagulable state.

B. Importance of vitamin K

  1. Six factors (factors II, VII, IX, and X; proteins C and S) produced in the liver require vitamin K for synthesis. It is necessary for γ-carboxylation of selected glutamic acid residues, which bind calcium tightly. Calcium binding is required to bring the clotting factors into close proximity with platelet surfaces.

  2. Vitamin K deficiency (or warfarin anticoagulation) precludes carboxylation, therefore rendering the six clotting factors ineffective.

III. Clotting Cascade. There is only one clotting cascade *in vivo*. The coagulation cascade is presented as two interacting systems—intrinsic and extrinsic.

A. Key components. A deficiency of either of the following factors leads to severe bleeding disorders.
   1. Factor XI (Christmas factor)
   2. Factor VIII (antihemophilic factor)
B. Coagulation cascade (Figure 10-1)
   1. Activated factor IXa substantially increases conversion of X to Xa.
   2. The reactions of the clotting cascade, which require calcium, take place on phospholipid (i.e., platelet) surfaces.
   3. Factor III (TF) is a constitutively expressed, integral membrane protein found on the surface of fibroblasts, macrophages, and other stromal cells that surround blood vessels. It functions as a receptor for factor VII. In the presence of calcium, factor VII binds to the extracellular domain of TF and becomes activated to factor VIIa.

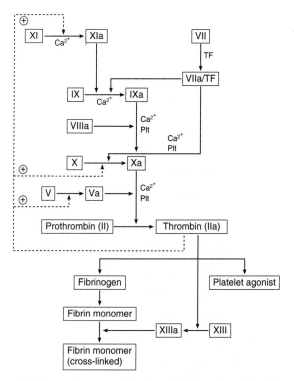

Figure 10-1. Coagulation cascade. Ca^{+2} = calcium ion; plt = platelet; TF = tissue factor; and + = positive feedback of thrombin.

DEEP VENOUS THROMBOSIS (DVT)

I. **Pathogenesis**
   A. **Predisposing factors** (Virchow's triad)
      1. Venous stasis, which impairs clearance of activated co-agulation factors
      2. Endothelial injury, which causes endothelial cells to be activated by cytokines and release tissue factor and plasminogen activator inhibitor 1, leading to the reduction in thrombomodulin
      3. Prothrombotic or hypercoagulable state
   B. **Risk factors**
      1. Age > 40 years
      2. Female sex
      3. Obesity (not a proven risk factor)
      4. Malignancy
      5. Previous thrombosis
      6. Procedures: orthopedic (e.g., hip or knee surgery), neurosurgical, or urologic surgery; any surgery > 2 hours (e.g., extensive pelvic or abdominal surgery for malignancy)
      7. Pregnancy
      8. Oral contraceptives
      9. Nephrotic syndrome
      10. Lupus anticoagulant
      11. Dysfibrogenemia
      12. Sepsis
      13. Deficiencies of proteins C and S, antithrombin III, plasminogen, heparin cofactor II
      14. Acute myocardial infarction (MI)
      15. Stroke
   C. **Anatomic considerations.** Occurrence of DVT in the left leg is more frequent (femoral artery crosses femoral vein).

II. **Clinical Presentation**
   A. **Anatomic site**
      1. **Lower extremity DVT**
         a. Femoral occlusion produces signs below the knee.
         b. Iliac occlusion produces signs below the groin.
      2. **Upper extremity DVT.** This condition is less frequent and usually associated with indwelling catheters (subclavian >> internal jugular) or anatomic abnormalities (e.g., fracture, tumor, aneurysm, injury, thoracic outlet obstruction).
   B. **Signs and symptoms**
      1. Pain
      2. Pitting edema
      3. Cyanosis (phlegmasia cerulea dolens)
      4. Homans' sign (limitation of dorsiflexion of foot) [absent in 55% of cases]
      5. Blanching (phlegmasia alba dolens) secondary to arterial spasm

C. **Imaging**
1. Duplex ultrasound (Doppler and B-mode) [sensitivity = 90%; specificity = 80%]
   a. If this test is negative and there is still clinical suspicion, it should be repeated in 2 days and 5–7 days.
   b. This test is less specific above the inguinal ligament because of inability to compress pelvic veins.
2. Venography
3. Impedance plesmography (rarely used)
   a. This test has 95% accuracy in totally occluded thigh veins.
   b. However, it must be unilaterally abnormal to be diagnostic.

III. **Management**
A. **Bed rest**
1. Elevate limb 8–10 inches and use Trendelenburg position.
2. Ambulate with stockings after 4–5 days.
B. **Heparin.** The goal is rapid achievement of therapeutic levels.
1. **Dosing.** Initial empiric- or weight-based systems may be modified depending on the results of PTTs.
   a. **Empiric therapy** (see MONITORING ANTICOAGULATION: II C 3 c; **Table 10-3**)
   b. **Weight-based formula** (see MONITORING ANTICOAGULATION; II C 3 d; **Table 10-4**)
2. **Dose variations** (see MONITORING ANTICOAGULATION: II C 3)
3. **Duration of treatment** (see MONITORING ANTICOAGULATION: II C 4)
4. **Complications.** These include bleeding, thrombocytopenia, arterial thromboembolism, and osteoporosis.

> **When the platelet count falls by 50% or is < 100,000 cells/µl, discontinue all heparin.**

C. **Low-molecular-weight heparins**
1. **Dosage** for **venous thromboembolism**
   a. Dalteparin, 100 U/kg SQ bid

Table 10-3.	Empiric Therapy Adjustments for Heparin		
PTT	**Bolus (IU)**	**Hold Infusion (min)**	**Rate Change (IU/hr)**
<50	5000	0	↑ by 120
50–59	0	0	↑ by 120
60–85	0	0	No change
86–95	0	0	↓ by 80
96–120	0	30	↓ by 80
> 120	0	60	↓ by 160

PTT = partial thromboplastin time.

Table 10-4.	Weight-Based Adjustments for Heparin			
PTT	**PTT × Control**	**Bolus (IU/kg)**	**Hold Infusion (min)**	**Rate Change (IU/kg/hr)**
< 35	< 1.2	80	0	↑ by 4
35–45	> 1.2–1.5	40	0	↑ by 2
46–70	> 1.5–2.3	0	0	No change
71–90	> 2.3–3.0	0	0	↓ by 2
> 90	> 3.0	0	60	↓ by 3

PTT = partial thromboplastin time.

     b. Enoxaparin, 100 U/kg SQ bid
   2. Dosage for **unstable angina**
     a. Dalteparin, 100 U/kg SQ bid
     b. Enoxaparin, 100 U/kg SQ bid

D. Warfarin
   1. Pharmacology (see MONITORING ANTICOAGULATION: I C 1)
   2. Dosing (see MONITORING ANTICOAGULATION: I C 4)
     a. Dose. Adjust the dose until the INR is stable. (**Table 10-5;** see MONITORING ANTICOAGULATION: I C 4 a).
     b. Duration of therapy (see MONITORING ANTICOAGULATION: I C 4 b)
   3. Complications. These include bleeding, skin necrosis, dermatitis, and painful erythema over subcutaneous fat. Warfarin may be teratogenic. With recurrence on adequate therapy, low-molecular-weight heparin or an inferior vena cava filter may be necessary.

E. Inferior vena cava filter
   1. Absolute indications
     a. Recurrent thromboembolism during anticoagulation
     b. Anticoagulation contraindicated and high risk for DVT or with documented DVT
     c. Anticoagulation not tolerated and high risk for DVT or with documented DVT
     d. Recurrent PE
     e. Pulmonary embolectomy
     f. Device or ligation failure with recurrent PE
   2. Relative indications
     a. 50% pulmonary vascular occlusion
     b. Propagating iliofemoral thrombus despite anticoagulation
     c. Large free-floating iliofemoral thrombus; high-risk patient

F. Fibrinolysis or surgery
   1. Thrombolysis is indicated on a limited basis for patients with low risk of bleeding and extensive iliofemoral thrombosis or pulmonary embolism (PE) and associated hypoxemia, hypotension, syncope, or heart failure.

Table 10-5. Indications for Warfarin Therapy With Appropriate INR Values

Indication	INR value
Treatment of DVT or PE	2.0–3.0
Treatment of antithrombin III, or protein C or S deficiencies	2.0–3.0
DVT prophylaxis	2.0–3.0
Prevention of thromboembolism in patients with atrial fibrillation, acute MI, or valvular heart disease	2.0–3.0
Recurrent systemic emboli	3.0–4.0
Mechanical heart valves (stroke prophylaxis)	3.0–4.0

DVT = deep venous thrombosis; MI = myocardial infarction; PE = pulmonary embolism.

        a. For venous thrombosis: streptokinase, 250,000 U bolus followed by infusion of 100,000 U for up to 72 hours

        b. For PE: tPA, 100 mg IV over 2 hours

   2. Surgery is indicated with chronic thromboembolic pulmonary hypertension and massive PE in patients for whom thrombolysis is contraindicated. It may also be used to reduce venous obstruction rapidly in patients with phlegmasia cerulea dolens and impending gangrene.

IV. Prophylaxis. In practice, a combination of the described methods is utilized.

  A. Intraoperative sequential compression devices

  B. Graded compression [thromboembolic disease (TED)] stockings (low-risk patients)

  C. Heparin (low doses): 5000 IU SQ q 8–12 hr (optimally, the first dose is given at least 1–2 hours before surgery)

  D. Low-molecular-weight heparins

    1. Advantages

        a. Better bioavailability, longer half-life, and dose-independent clearance

        b. Predictable anticoagulation, so monitoring is not required for treatment or prophylaxis unless patient weight is < 50 kg or > 80 kg or renal insufficiency is present

        c. Ability to inactivate platelet-bound Xa (unlike heparin), which increases the anticoagulant effect when compared with unfractionated heparin

    2. Risks (similar to those of unfractionated heparin)

        a. Recurrence of DVT (5%–7%)

        b. Bleeding (1%–2%)

        c. Heparin-induced thrombyctopenia (HIT)

      d. Osteoporosis (lower risk than with unfractionated heparin)

    3. Activity. It is problematic to compare studies using different preparations of low-molecular-weight heparins because they differ in their activity (Xa:IIa activity ratio). Xa activity is thought to be responsible for the anticoagulant effect, whereas IIa activity is responsible for the bleeding side effect.

    4. Dosing (Table 10-6)

  F. Warfarin. Some specialties other than general surgery (e.g., orthopedics) use warfarin for prophylaxis.

  G. HIT. Options for DVT prophylaxis include:

    1. Danaparoid sodium

    2. Hirudin

    3. Bivalirudin

    4. Argatroban

    5. Ancrod (Malayan pit viper venom)

V. Particular Forms of Deep Venous Thrombosis (DVT)

  A. Calf vein thrombosis

    1. It is safe to withhold anticoagulant therapy in patients with suspected calf vein thrombosis and normal results on serial examinations by compression ultrasonography.

    2. In 30% of cases, calf thrombi extend to the iliac veins.

  B. Thrombophilia (increased tendency for thromboembolism)

    1. Indications for investigation of thrombophilia

      a. Single episode of idiopathic thromboembolism (in the absence of recent major surgery, trauma, immobilization, or metastatic cancer) and one or more of the following conditions:

        (1) Patients < 50 years of age with recurrent DVT

        (2) Family history of venous thromboembolism

        (3) Thrombosis in an unusual site (mesenteric or cerebral vein)

        (4) Massive venous thrombosis

      b. Recurrent episodes of venous thromboembolism

    2. Laboratory abnormalities associated with initial and recurrent DVT

      a. Congenital deficiencies of antithrombin III, protein C and S, or plasminogen

      b. Congenital resistance to APC

      c. Hyperhomocystinemia

      d. Elevated levels of antiphospholipid antibodies

  C. Venous thromboembolism in pregnant women

Unfractionated heparin and low-molecular-weight heparin do not cross the placenta.

---

    1. Treat with heparin until the clot resolves and then begin prophylaxis with low-molecular-weight heparin.

    2. Begin warfarin therapy (safe for breastfeeding infant) after delivery.

Table 10-6. Low-Molecular-Weight Heparin Formulations and Dosing

Low-Molecular-Weight Heparins	Uncomplicated Abdominal or Pelvic Surgery*	High-Risk Patient; Abdominal or Pelvic Surgery for Cancer†	Orthopaedic Surgery	Acute Spinal Injury	Multiple Trauma	Medical Conditions
Dalteparin	2500 IU SQ	5000 IU SQ	5000 IU SQ (8–12 hours before surgery)	—	—	2500 IU SQ qd
Enoxaparin	2000 IU SQ	4000 IU SQ	4000 IU SQ (10–12 hours before surgery), then 3000 bid after surgery	3000 IU SQ bid	3000 IU SQ bid	2000 IU SQ qd
Nadroparin	3100 IU SQ	—	40 IU/kg SQ (2 hours before surgery), then qd × 3, then 60 IU/kg	—	—	—
Tinzaparin	3500 IU SQ	—	50 IU/kg SQ (2 hours before surgery), then qd	—	—	—
Ardeparin	—	—	50 IU/kg SQ bid after surgery	—	—	—

*Given 2 hours before surgery.
†Given 10–12 hours before surgery, then every day.

D. Venous thromboembolism in children

1. The condition is usually a complication of a serious disease (e.g., trauma, surgery, cancer, congenital heart disease, prematurity).

2. In 40% of children and 80% in newborns, such thromboembolism occurs in the upper extremity due to indwelling catheters. This may cause superior vena cava syndrome, chylothorax, or even post-thrombotic syndrome (see IV E).

3. **Treatment**

   a. Children. Give heparin, 75 U/kg/hr bolus, then 20 U/kg/hr. Once therapeutic levels have been reached, start warfarin and continue heparin for 4–5 days. See adult protocol and Table 10-3.

   b. Newborns. Give heparin, 75 U/kg bolus, then 28 U/kg/hr for 10–14 days. If thromboembolism is associated with a catheter, give heparin through the catheter for 1–5 days.

E. Post-thrombotic syndrome

1. **Etiology.** Venous hypertension due to recanalization of venous thrombus results in a patent, scarred vein with incompetent valves.

   a. The hypertension leads to increased venous pressure in the legs due to loss of muscular pump mechanism.

   b. The incompetence leads to flow into the superficial veins with muscular contraction, resulting in edema and impaired viability of subcutaneous tissues, and even ulceration.

2. **Incidence.** Post-thrombotic syndrome occurs after DVT 25% of the time. The incidence rate is reduced by the use of compression stockings.

3. **Signs.** Chronic aching and swelling of the calf occur.

F. Recurrent DVT

1. At the end of anticoagulative therapy, it is best to obtain a baseline ultrasound or impedance plethysmograph in case of possible recurrence.

2. Recurrence is a difficult diagnosis to make. The most important mimicking condition is exacerbated post-thrombotic syndrome.

HYPERCOAGULABLE STATES

I. Disseminated Intravascular Coagulation (DIC)

A. Definition. DIC is pathologic activation of coagulation by an underlying disease process with laboratory evidence of:

1. Procoagulant and fibrinolytic activation

2. Reduced protein C or protein S activity

3. Biochemical evidence of end-organ dysfunction (e.g., lungs, liver, kidney)

B. Etiology

1. **Increased exposure to TF**
   a. Injured tissue (from trauma, tissue necrosis, burns)
   b. Malignant cells. Many malignant cells express TF (e.g., leukemia, solid tumors).
   c. Stimulated monocytes or endothelial cells, which enhance TF expression. Endotoxin (gram-negative sepsis), cell wall polysaccharides (gram-positive sepsis), and circulating immune complexes (autoimmune and inflammatory disorders) result in increased TF expression.
   d. Endothelial sloughing, which exposes subendothelial TF, as a result of acidosis. At a pH of 7.2 or less, even fully heparinized blood clots.

2. **Thrombogenic phospholipids** on the inner leaflet of all cell membranes (animal and bacterial). The mechanism of procoagulant activation is unclear.
   a. Obstetric disorders (e.g., abruptio placentae, eclampsia, abortion, amniotic fluid embolism), lead to increased exposure to broken placental cells.
   b. Intravascular hemolysis (e.g., transfusion reactions, some infections) result in broken RBCs.
   c. Ascitic fluid (LeVeen or Denver shunts) introduce broken peritoneal cells into circulation.

C. **Clinical presentation and diagnosis (Table 10-7)**

For diagnosis of DIC, evidence of either hemorrhage, thrombosis, or both *must* be present.

---

1. **Bleeding.** This results from depletion of clotting factors (more pronounced in the setting of liver disease), depletion of platelets, or hyperfibrinolysis.
   a. Wound bleeding, which is common after surgery or trauma
   b. Waterhouse-Friderichsen syndrome, with hemorrhagic necrosis of the adrenals

2. **Thrombosis** (usually microvascular)
   a. Organs at risk include lungs (ARDS), kidneys (acute renal failure), liver (hepatic insufficiency), heart [MI, congestive heart failure (CHF)], and brain (multiple sclerosis changes, stroke).
   b. Purpura fulminans may lead to gangrene of the digits secondary to infarction of skin vessels. This condition is associated with *Neisseria meningitidis* bacteremia, *Streptococcus pneumoniae* bacteremia, and protein C and protein S deficiency.

3. **Compensated ("low-grade") DIC.** Increased production of clotting factors by the liver results in near-normal laboratory tests.
   a. Trousseau's syndrome (migratory deep venous thrombosis) occurs.
   b. Concomitantly, increased fibrin degradation prod-

Table 10-7. Disorders Associated With Disseminated Intravascular Coagulation (DIC)

Infection
- Gram-negative endotoxemia with hypotension or shock
- Severe gram-positive septicemia
- Rocky Mountain spotted fever
- Viral infection (herpes)
- Malaria (*Plasmodium falciparum*)

Complications of pregnancy and delivery
- Gram-negative sepsis
- Abruptio placentae
- Amniotic fluid embolism
- Retained dead fetus
- Toxemia

Pediatric disorders (especially in the newborn)

Malignant diseases
- Metastatic carcinoma (prostate, pancreas, lung, stomach, colon, breast)
- Leukemia (especially acute promyelocytic leukemia)

Liver diseases (cirrhosis)

Complications of surgery: extracorporeal circulation

Critical tissue damage
- Brain tissue destruction
- Massive trauma
- Heat stroke
- Extensive burns

Miscellaneous
- Hemolytic transfusion reactions
- Vasculitis
- Aneurysms
- Giant hemangioma
- Snake bites

(From Ansell JE: Acquired bleeding disorders. In *Irwin* and *Rippe's Intensive Care Medicine*, 4th ed. Edited by Irwin RS, Cerra FB, Rippe JM. Philadelphia, Lippincott Williams & Wilkins, 1999.)

---

ucts may lead to a qualitative platelet defect and subacute bleeding.

    D. Laboratory results (Table 10-8). These are used to support but not make the diagnosis.

        1. Fibrinolysis. Endothelial cells exposed to thrombin, endotoxin, or cytokines release tPA. Fibrin-bound tPA acti-

Table 10-8. Laboratory Findings in Disseminated Intravascular Coagulation (DIC) Compared With the Coagulopathy of Liver Disease

		DIC	
Test	Liver Disease	Low-Grade	Fulminant
PT*	Long	Normal, short	Long
PTT*	Long	Normal, short	Long
Thrombin time*	Long	Normal, short, long	Long
Fibrinogen*	Low	High–normal–low	Low
Factor VIII	Normal–high	Normal–high	Low
Fibrin monomers	±	+	++++
Fibrinopeptide A	±	+	++++
Fibrinogen dedgradation products/D-dimer*	±	++	++++
Euglobin lysis time	Normal	Normal–short	Short
Antithrombin III	Low	Normal	Low
Platelet count*	Mildly low	Normal–mildly low	Low
Blood smear* (microangiopathic	No	±	+

PT = prothrombin time; PTT = partial thromboplastin time; ± = slightly positive; ++++ = strongly positive
*Indicates those tests easily obtained in a short period (e.g., 1–2 hr), which constitute a so-called DIC screen.
(From Ansell JE: Acquired bleeding disorders. In *Irwin* and *Rippe's Intensive Care Medicine*, 4th ed. Edited by Irwin RS, Cerra FB, Rippe JM. Philadelphia, Lippincott Williams & Wilkins, 1999.)

vates fibrin-bound plasminogen to plasmin, which initiates fibrin cleavage. Soluble fibrin increases plasmin formation because platelets (which produce plasminogen activator inhibitor to keep fibrinolysis in check) are absent. In addition, tPA can degrade platelet glycoproteins Ia and IIb/IIIa, which are required for platelet adhesion and aggregation.

    a. Fibrin degradation products test. This assay measures fibrinogen and fibrin (cross-linked and non—cross-linked) degradation products. It is elevated in 85% to 100% of patients with DIC as well as in those with PE, MI, DVT, and renal insufficiency.

    b. D-dimer test. This assay, which is more specific but less sensitive, measures plasmin degradation of cross-linked fibrin only. It is elevated in 90% of patients with DIC.

2. Prothrombin time (PT) [unreliable]. Prolonged in 50% to 75% of patients with DIC, PT is normal in up to 50% of affected patients secondary to increased circulating activated clotting factors.

3. **PTT** (unreliable). PTT is normal in up to 50% of patients with DIC secondary to increased activated clotting factors.

4. **Platelet count** (neither sensitive nor specific). This is usually low in DIC.

5. **Individual clotting factor assays** (including fibrinogen level). These assays are not helpful. Most patients with DIC usually have high fibrinogen levels.

6. **Peripheral blood smear** (may show schistocytes)

E. **Management**

1. Identify and treat the underlying condition.

2. Provide supportive therapy [maintain blood pressure (BP), optimize oxygen delivery].

3. If the underlying condition is rapidly reversible, watch and wait. Use fresh frozen plasma and platelets as needed to correct coagulopathy.

4. Stop microvascular thrombosis. Mortality usually results from respiratory, liver, or kidney failure, not bleeding. Individualize heparin, tPA, or urokinase therapy.

Data support the use of urokinase and tPA in DIC secondary to trauma or sepsis, provided initial clotting parameters are normal.

---

5. Control bleeding. Replace clotting factors with fresh frozen plasma or platelets when levels are abnormal.

6. Consider heparin therapy in the following circumstances:
   a. With a surgically intact vascular system
   b. With actual or potentially serious bleeding or clotting
   c. If the underlying disorder is *not* rapidly reversible

II. **Antiphospholipid Syndrome**

A. **Definition.** This syndrome is an acquired hypercoagulable state resulting from antiphospholipid immunoglobulins. It is seen in 1% to 2% of the population.

B. **Pathophysiology.** The exact mechanism is unclear. Proposed hypotheses include the following:

1. Increased TF expression from endothelial cells

2. Inhibition of protein C activation, which results in a prothrombotic state

3. Impaired prostacyclin I_2 (PGI_2) production. PGI_2 causes local vasodilation, inhibits platelet activation, and promotes tPA release. Decreased PGI_2 production results in increased thrombosis and impaired fibrinolysis.

4. Increased platelet reactivity

C. **Signs and symptoms.** Recurrent vessel thrombosis is involved, and the specific nature of signs and symptoms depends on the affected organ.

Antiphospholipid syndrome affects veins and arteries of all sizes.

---

1. Placenta: recurrent pregnancy losses
2. Heart: MI
3. Brain: stroke
4. Venous system: DVT or PE
5. Skin: gangrene or livedo reticularis
6. Adrenal glands: Addison's disease
7. Small or large bowel infarction

D. Laboratory results

1. Anticardiolipin test. Serum immunoglobulins that bind to cardiolipin result in a positive assay. IgG levels > 40 are specific for antiphospholipid syndrome.
2. Prolonged PTT. Lupus anticoagulants are immunoglobulins that inhibit *in vitro* anticoagulant tests. Therefore, the presence of antiphospholipid antibodies prolongs the PTT (as well as Russell's viper venom time and kaolin clotting time). Although addition of normal sera to the samples normalizes clotting times in patients with clotting deficiencies, times remain abnormal in patients with antiphospholipid antibodies.
3. VDRL (false-positive). Antiphospholipid antibodies bind to phospholipids used in test.
4. Thrombocytopenia. This condition is frequently present but rarely severe enough to cause bleeding.

E. Management

> **Prothrombotic risks should be eliminated.**
> **Patients should stop smoking and take no**
> **estrogen-containing medications.**

1. Warfarin for patients with stroke, DVT, or PE (goal is INR of 2.5–3.0) [see MONITORING ANTICOAGULATION: I C 4, p. 275.]
2. Prednisone and cyclophosphamide for patients with recurrent thrombosis while on adequate warfarin anticoagulation
3. Heparin plus aspirin (heparin 10,000 U SQ bid + aspirin 81 mg) for pregnant women with documented antiphospholipid antibody syndrome and a history of pregnancy losses

III. Other Hypercoagulable States

A. Definition. A hypercoagulable state is an acquired or congenital predisposition to thrombosis in circumstances that would not cause thrombosis in a normal individual.

B. Regulation of coagulation

1. Antithrombin III, which inactivates thrombin (IIa) and Xa. Heparin and endogenous glycosaminoglycans (heparins) serve as catalysts.
2. Heparin cofactor II, which is a heparin-dependent (but antithrombin III–independent) inhibitor of thrombin. It has no effect on other clotting factors.

      3. Protein C and protein S, which are vitamin K–dependent factors that inactivate Va and VIIIa (see BLOOD PRODUCTS AND COAGULATION FACTORS: II A 12, 13 and Table 10-2)

C. Congenital abnormalities resulting in hypercoagulability

    1. Antithrombin III deficiency. This autosomal dominant disorder occurs in about 0.2% to 0.4% of the general population.

    2. Protein C and S deficiency

      a. Homozygous deficiencies result in a profound hypercoagulable state in the neonatal period. DIC (purpura fulminans) and death result from any stimulus that initiates coagulation.

      b. Heterozygous protein C deficiency occurs in about 0.1% to 0.5% of the population, resulting in a hypercoagulable state.

    3. APC resistance (most common hypercoagulable state). Defective factor Va (factor V Leiden) imparts resistance to degradation by APC.

    4. Heparin cofactor II deficiency. This reportedly increases the incidence of venous thrombosis.

D. Acquired abnormalities resulting in hypercoagulability

    1. Antithrombin III deficiency secondary to trauma or medication (oral contraceptives)

    2. Lupus anticoagulant

    3. Heterozygous protein C deficiency plus warfarin administration (rare)

    4. DIC secondary to such conditions as sepsis and malignancy

E. Clinical presentation

    1. In most cases, the initial thrombotic episode appears in early adulthood (< 40 years).

      a. Venous thrombosis and PE

      b. Arterial thrombosis (rare)

    2. For patients > 45 years of age who develop venous thrombosis, an acquired abnormality (especially malignancy) must be ruled out.

F. Diagnostic tests. Laboratory investigation of unexplained venous thrombosis in patients < 45 years should include:

    1. Antithrombin III levels

    2. Protein C and S levels

    3. Screening for APC resistance

    4. Assays for anticardiolipin antibodies and lupus anticoagulant

G. Management

    1. Symptomatic individuals: anticoagulant treatment with heparin, low-molecular-weight heparin, or warfarin

    2. Prophylaxis: anticoagulant treatment (heparin, low-molecular-weight heparin, or warfarin), which is especially important perioperatively

> **In asymptomatic individuals with hypercoagula-
> bility, treatment is controversial. The risk of chronic
> warfarin therapy versus the risk of recurrent thrombosis
> must be considered on an individual basis.**

MONITORING ANTICOAGULATION

I. **Prothrombin Time (PT)**
   A. **Procedure.** Calcium and tissue thromboplastin (TF) are added to citrated plasma. The time it takes for a fibrin clot to form is compared to a control sample. The assay requires normal levels of factor II (prothrombin); factor I (fibrinogen); and factors V, VII, and X. (Factors II, VII, and X are vitamin K–dependent.)

> **Because of the difficulty involved in comparing PTs
> from different laboratories, the World Health Organization
> has established the international normalized ratio, or INR.
> The INR compares the individual laboratory thromboplastin
> to a single, standard, human brain thromboplastin.**

   B. **PT levels.** A normal PT is 11–13 seconds. Prolonged PT may result from the following conditions:
      1. Warfarin administration that leads to inhibition of the vitamin K–dependent clotting factors
      2. Vitamin K deficiency. This condition may be caused by broad-spectrum antibiotics.
      3. Liver disease. The liver is the source of the majority of the clotting factors, and the PT is a very effective measure of liver function.
      4. Hepatocellular disease from suboptimal storage of vitamin K
      5. Obstructive liver disease. Vitamin K requires bile for adequate absorption, and a prolonged PT can also be observed after biliary tract surgery and in patients with common bile duct T tubes.
      6. DIC due to factor consumption
      7. Congenital deficiency of factors I, II, VII, V, or X
   C. **Warfarin use**
      1. **Pharmacology**
         a. Warfarin causes the plasma concentrations of functional factor VII and protein C to fall sharply due to their short half-lives. In contrast, other clotting factors take 24–48 hours to decline.
         b. Initiation of warfarin therapy results in a procoagulant effect that precedes the anticoagulant effect by approximately 24 hours, and therefore, there is a transient hypercoagulable state.

    2. Indications (see Table 10-5). (The table gives appropriate INRs for therapy.)

    3. Contraindications to warfarin anticoagulation
      a. Absolute: pregnancy, active bleeding
      b. Relative: fall risk, alcoholism, history of ulcer disease

    4. Dosage
      a. Initial dose. Begin therapy after the PTT has been stable for 1–2 days [wait 3 days for therapeutic PTT in patients with iliofemoral DVT or PE]. Adjust the dose until the INR is stable (see Table 10-5). Continue heparin until the INR is therapeutic.

**Routinely monitor PT and INR values
during warfarin administration.**

---

      b. Duration of therapy. No definitive results of randomized trials are available. Suggested limits include:
        (1) Thromboembolism in relation to a specific, acute transient event: 3–6 months
        (2) DVT and metastatic cancer: life
        (3) Two episodes of DVT: 1 year
        (4) Three episodes of DVT: life

    5. Drug–drug interactions
      a. Prolonged INR: nonsteroidal anti-inflammatory drugs (NSAIDs), erythromycin, metronidazole, trimethoprim-sulfamethoxazole (TMP-SMX), amiodarone, quinidine, cimetidine, lovastatin, thyroxin
      b. Decreased INR: phenobarbital, rifampin, dietary vitamin K

II. Partial Thromboplastin Time (PTT)

  A. Procedure. Kaolin, glass beads, and phospholipid are added to citrated blood.

**The process that is measured does *not* mimic
physiologic activation of the clotting cascade.**

---

    1. Factor VII is not required for glass beads and kaolin to induce clotting.
    2. Components of the contact-activation system (Hageman factor, factor XI, high-molecular-weight kininogen, and prekallikrein) are also required for a normal PTT. These factors are not required for normal coagulation.

  B. PTT levels. Normal PTT is 28–40 seconds. Prolonged PTT is the result of:
    1. Liver disease
    2. DIC
    3. Antiphospholipid antibody
    4. Any coagulation factor deficiency, except factor VII deficiency

  C. Heparin use
    1. Pharmacology. Heparin, a glycosaminoglycan with a mol-

ecular weight of 5000–50,000, forms complexes with antithrombin III to inhibit clotting factors IIa and Xa (in addition to the contact factors, Hageman factor and factor XI). Heparin also complexes with heparin cofactor II to inhibit thrombin.

2. **Indications**
    a. Treatment of DVT or PE
    b. Treatment of unstable angina, acute MI, or left ventricular mural thrombus. IV heparin is an adjunct to thrombolytic therapy in acute MI (thrombin is released from clot dissolution).
    c. Thromboembolism in pregnancy
    d. Acutely ischemic peripheral vascular disease
    e. Cardiopulmonary bypass

3. **Dosage.** The goal of treatment is rapid achievement of therapeutic levels. Institutional protocols have improved optimal heparin anticoagulation.
    a. Dose: 5000 U IV bolus followed by 1000 U/hr
    b. Maintenance infusion rate: changed according to the PTT

Initially, empiric- or weight-based systems may be used and then modified depending on the PTT.

---

   c. **Empiric therapy** (see Table 10-3)
       (1) Administer 5000 IU IV bolus, then 1280 IU/hr IV infusion.
       (2) Check the PTT 6 hours after each change in dose until it is stable and then daily.
   d. **Weight-based formulation** (see Table 10-4)
       (1) Administer 80 IU/kg IV bolus, then 18 IU/kg/hr IV infusion.
       (2) Check the PTT every 6 hours until it is stable and adjust the dose accordingly.

At first, some patients require large amounts of heparin as a result of a large venous thromboembolism. Once the thromboembolism begins to resolve, the heparin requirements decline.

---

4. **Duration of treatment.** In most patients, 4–5 days of heparin are necessary. Initiate warfarin when heparin levels are therapeutic and when patients are able to use the oral route.

Patients with large iliofemoral DVT or PE are still treated for 7–10 days.

---

5. **Complications**
    a. Bleeding, especially from surgical sites and the retroperitoneum

    b. Hypersensitivity (rare)

    c. Osteoporosis secondary to long-term (> 6 months) heparinization

    d. HIT, which results from the formation of IgG antibodies against heparin. Although the occurrence of this condition is not dose-dependent, the risk increases with the duration of treatment.

        (1) Type I, the benign, reversible, nonimmune form, is characterized by a decreased platelet count from 1–3 days after treatment.

            (a) The platelet count rarely falls below 100,000 cells/μl.

            (b) Incidence is 1% to 10% of patients treated with heparin.

            (c) Thromboembolic complications do not occur.

When the platelet count falls by 50% or is < 100,000 cells/μl, discontinue all heparin.

---

        (2) Type II, the IgG-mediated immune form, is generally seen 5–12 days or more after treatment.

            (a) Formation of antiplatelet IgG. Heparin binds to platelet factor 4, and the complex induces formation.

            (b) Increased risk of thrombotic events. Both venous and arterial [white clot syndrome (clot of platelets)] may occur.

            (c) Immediate onset (if the patient has received heparin in the previous 3 months)

            (d) Decline in platelet count (usually to < 100,000/μl)

            (e) Bleeding (rare)

            (f) Treatment

                (i) Danaparoid is an immediate anticoagulant but cross-reacts with platelet factor 4 in 10% of cases of HIT.

                (ii) Ancrod, a defibrinogenerating enzyme from snake venom, has no cross-reactivity but takes 12 hours to become an effective anticoagulant. It is contraindicated in sepsis and DIC.

D. Problems with heparinization and PTT

    1. The extent of anticoagulation may not be reflected in the PTT.

    2. There is *no* correlation between bleeding complications and the anticoagulant effect.

    3. Tight control of the PTT does not reduce the incidence of bleeding complications.

> **To reverse heparinization, administer protamine sulfate, 1 mg per 100 U heparin. Infusion should be over 5–10 minutes, because rapid infusion may cause dyspnea, bradycardia, hypotension, flushing, and anaphylaxis.**

III. Activated Clotting Time (ACT)
   A. Procedure. Blood is added to tubes containing Celite, a finely divided clay, which shortens the clotting time.
   B. ACT levels. Normal ACT is < 100 seconds. Prolonged ACT occurs with heparinization; the goal is 300–600 seconds.
   C. Advantage over PT and PTT. ACT may be obtained at the bedside. It is useful for guiding heparinization intraoperatively (especially for cardiopulmonary bypass).

TRANSFUSION THERAPY

I. Red Bood Cell (RBC) Transfusion
   A. Goal: to increase oxygen delivery
   1. **Oxygen delivery** (DO_2)

   $$DO_2 = cardiac\ index \times oxygen\ content \times 10$$

   a. Normal values: 520–720 ml/min/m^2
   b. Requires pulmonary artery catheter for accurate measurement
   2. **Oxygen content** (CaO_2)

   $$CaO_2 = [hemoglobin\ (g/dl) \times oxygen\ saturation\ (\%) \times 1.34 + PaO_2 \times 0.0031$$

   where 1.34 = milliliters of oxygen carried by 1 gram of hemoglobin (Hgb) and 0.0031 = plasma diffusion coefficient of oxygen
   B. Properties of RBCs
   1. RBCs are stored in a citrate-phosphate-dextrose-adenine (CPDA) medium.
   2. The shelf life of stored RBCs is 21 days, and when transfused, RBCs have a half-life of 57 days.

> **One unit of transfused RBCs increases Hgb by 1 g/dl (or increases the hematocrit by about 3%).**

   C. Guidelines for RBC transfusion
   1. **"Transfusion trigger."** Use of an Hgb < 10 mg/dl (or a hematocrit < 30%) as the requirement for RBC transfusion is an outdated practice that data do not support.

> **RBC transfusion should be guided by clinical judgment and not by a single laboratory value.**

2. **Perioperative transfusion.** Studies have found that individuals with Hgb levels > 8 g/dl (> 6 g/dl for elective cases) fared as well as those with Hgb levels > 10 g/dl.

3. **Chronic anemia** (secondary to renal failure or other conditions). Affected patients tolerate general anesthesia and surgery without evidence of morbidity or mortality as a result of the anemia.

4. **Comorbid disease.** Consider concomitant conditions when transfusing. Some patients may have increased transfusion requirements as a result of the following:

    a. Coronary artery disease: patients have flow-limited oxygen delivery

    b. Poor nutritional status: decreased erythropoeisis

    c. Coagulopathy: increased incidence of blood loss

5. **Active hemorrhage** (e.g., GI or traumatic origin) [> 500 ml]. Treat with RBC transfusion and crystalloid regardless of the patient's Hgb level.

6. **Critically ill status.** In such cases a pulmonary artery catheter may be extremely useful in directing transfusing practices. Oxygen delivery can be accurately assessed. All patients with decreased oxygen delivery and abnormally low Hgb should be transfused.

Blood should be transfused one unit at a time followed by reassessment of the anemic patient. Document the reason for RBC transfusion in the medical record.

E. **Risks** (infectious and noninfectious) [**Table 10-9**]

F. **Hemolytic transfusion reactions**

1. **Signs and symptoms:** fever, chills, headache, chest pain,

Table 10-9. Risks Associated with Red Blood Cell Transfusion

Infectious Risks	Frequency	Noninfectious Risks	Frequency
Hepatitis A	Rare	Fever (nonhemolytic)	1%–2%
Hepatitis B	1/100,000	Urticaria	1%
Hepatitic C	1/120,000	Hemolytic transfusion reaction	1/6000
HIV	1/1,000,000	Fatal hemolytic transfusion reaction	1/100,000
Creutzfeld-Jacob disease	None reported		
Cytomegalovirus	Variable		
Malaria	1/4,000,000		
Bacterial contamination	1/1,000,000		
Syphilis, babesiosis	Rare		

anxiety, pain at the infusion site, respiratory distress, even shock

2. **Laboratory results**
   a. Free Hgb in plasma
   b. Hemoglobinuria
   c. Decreased haptoglobin and hemopexin levels
   d. Increased creatinine and acute renal failure (secondary to lysed RBC membranes in the golmerulus)

3. **Management**
   a. Stop transfusion immediately when hemolysis is suspected.
   b. Give IV fluids.
   c. Promote osmotic diuresis. Give mannitol, 1 g/min to a total of 50 g.
   d. Give antipyretics.
   e. Alkalinize the urine.

> **Fatal transfusion reactions are usually secondary to clerical error that results in giving the wrong blood to a particular patient.**

II. Platelet Transfusion

A. Indications

1. Platelet count < 25,000 cells/μl
2. Platelet count < 50,000 cells/μl and active bleeding, planned surgical procedure, or bleeding time > 7.5 minutes
3. Platelet count < 100,000 cells/μl and intracerebral hemorrhage or following cardiopulmonary bypass or massive transfusion
4. Documented qualitative platelet defect (aspirin, NSAIDs, clopidogrel), Glanzmann's thrombasthenia, or Bernard-Soulier syndrome) and active bleeding, planned surgical procedure, or bleeding time > 7.5 minutes

B. Risk.
The risk of **infection** associated with platelet transfusion is six times greater than the risk of RBC transfusion (remember that it takes six units of whole blood to make the standard transfusion "six-pack" of platelets).

III. Fresh Frozen Plasma Transfusion

A. Indications

1. PT > 16 seconds or PTT > 55 seconds and active bleeding or planned surgical procedure or following massive transfusion
2. Documented deficiency of factor V and active bleeding or planned surgical procedure
3. Reversal of warfarin anticoagulation and active bleeding or planned surgical procedure
4. Treatment of thrombotic thrombocytopenic purpura or hemolytic uremic syndrome
5. Antithrombin III deficiency

B. Risk.
The risk of **infection** with transfusion of fresh frozen plasma is similar to that associated with whole blood, be-

cause one unit of fresh frozen plasma is derived from one unit of whole blood. However, the standard transfusion of fresh frozen plasma is two units.

IV. Cryoprecipitate Transfusion
A. Indications
1. Fibrinogen level < 100 mg/dl and active bleeding or planned surgical procedure
2. Documented deficiency of factor XIII deficiency and active bleeding or planned surgical procedure
3. Actively bleeding uremic patients after desmopressin acetate (deamino-8-D-argine vasopressin; ddAVP) treatment proves ineffective.

B. Risk.
Factor concentrates (II, VII, VIII, IX, and X) are available for specific factor deficiencies (including hemophilia). Although the risk of **infection** associated with cryoprecipitate is similar to that associated with fresh frozen plasma, the risk with individual component transfusion is slightly less because the solution undergoes a viral inactivation process prior to storage.

V. Massive Transfusion
A. Definition.
Massive transfusion is more than one blood volume of RBCs transfused within 24 hours (i.e., 5000 ml or 20 units in a 70-kg adult).

B. Risk.
Transfused RBCs are deficient in platelets and coagulation factors. Consequently, **bleeding** occurs.

C. Prophylactic measures.
Massive transfusion involves prophylactic administration of **fresh frozen plasma** and **platelets**. This is unwarranted but should be guided by platelet count, PT, and PTT. These three values should be reassessed after every transfusion of four units or RBCs.

VI. Transfusional Adjuncts and Hemostatic Agents
A. ddAVP
1. **Mechanism of action.** The addition of ddAVP causes a release of von Willebrand factor from endothelial cells.
2. **Indications.** Treatment of active bleeding or planned surgical procedure in patients with uremia or von Willebrand's disease warrants use of ddAVP.

B. Aprotinin (Trasylol)
1. **Mechanism of action.** This agent inhibits plasmin (and kallikrein), consequently inhibiting fibrinolysis.
2. **Indications**
   a. Cardiopulmonary bypass. In 20 randomized prospective trials, aprotinin significantly reduced bleeding.
   b. Oral surgery
   c. Orthotopic liver transplantation (OLT)
3. **Adverse reactions**
   a. Anaphylaxis. Aprotinin is a bovine protein, and anaphylaxis can occur after the second exposure with an incidence of < 0.1%.
   b. Renal failure
   c. Graft thrombosis

C. Estrogen.
The mechanism of action is unclear. Estrogen shortens bleeding times in uremic patients.

11

Hepatobiliary Disease

BILIARY INFECTIONS

I. **Anatomic Considerations**
   A. **Gallbladder**
      1. Length: 7–10 cm
      2. Volume: 50–60 ml
   B. **Choledochus** (common bile duct)
      1. Length: 7.5 cm
      2. Diameter: 0.4 cm (patients < 50 years); 0.7 cm (patients > 70 years)
   C. **Papilla of Vater:** controlled by sphincter of Oddi

II. **Cholelithiasis**
   A. **Prevalence.** In the United States, where one million cases of cholelithiasis are diagnosed every year, prevalence is 10% to 15%.
   B. **Risk factors.** These include obesity, diabetes mellitus, cirrhosis, truncal vagotomy, total parenteral nutrition, starvation, age > 40 years, female sex, and multiparity.
   C. **Composition of gallstones**
      1. Cholesterol: golden
      2. Pigment (bilirubin): black
      3. Mixed (cholesterol and pigment): yellow-brown
   D. **Asymptomatic cholelithiasis.** A large majority (80%) of patients with cholelithiasis are asymptomatic. Mortality is < 1%. Indications for cholecystectomy include:
      1. Children < 16 years of age
      2. Sickle cell disease
      3. Nonfunctioning gallbladder
      4. Porcelain gallbladder
      5. Calculi > 2.5 cm
      6. Large gallbladder polyps ≥ 5 mm
   E. **Symptomatic cholelithiasis.** Of cases of asymptomatic disease, 2% per year will become symptomatic. The condition commonly progresses to cholecystitis.

    1. Symptoms include biliary colic, flatulence, eructation, nausea, and emesis.

    2. Symptomatic disease is an indication for elective cholecystectomy.

III. Choledocholithiasis

A. Pathogenesis

1. Primary stones, which are usually pigment stones, form *de novo* in the choledochus. These stones may:

    a. Occur as a result of stasis or infection (brown stones contain bacteria)

    b. Arise after cholecystectomy

2. Secondary stones, which are cholesterol stones, originate from the gallbladder.

B. Clinical presentation: pain, which may be located in the midepigastrum or back; jaundice; elevated transaminases and alkaline phosphatase

IV. Cholecystitis: Cystic Duct Occlusion

A. Etiology. Variations include acalculous and emphysematous types, as well as gangrene, empyema, and perforation.

B. Clinical presentation

1. Right upper quadrant abdominal pain

2. Nausea and vomiting

3. Fever

4. Murphy's sign (tenderness during inspiration in right upper quadrant)

5. Leukocytosis (12,000–15,000 cells/μl)

6. Elevation in bilirubin or transaminases (20% of cases)

C. Diagnostic imaging studies

1. Abdominal radiography

    a. Note that 20% of gallstones are radiopaque.

    b. Air may be visible in the abdomen or in the gallbladder.

2. Right upper quadrant ultrasound. This reveals:

    a. Thickening of the gallbladder wall (> 3 mm)

    b. Pericholecystic fluid

    c. Cholelithiasis or sludge

    d. Porcelain gallbladder

    e. Choledocholithiasis

    f. Common bile duct dilatation

    g. Perforation, empyema, or free fluid

3. Hepatic 2,6-dimethyl-iminodiacetic acid (HIDA) [radionuclide] scan. A HIDA scan, which has a low diagnostic yield in acalculous cholecystitis, may show:

    a. Sequential appearance of tracer in liver, gallbladder, common bile duct, and duodenum (normal)

    b. Decreased tracer uptake in hepatocellular disease

    c. Tracer in liver and gallbladder, which indicates common bile duct obstruction only

    d. Tracer in liver, common bile duct, and duodenum without visualization of the gallbladder, which indicates cystic duct obstruction and cholecystitis

> **In the setting of a nonfilling gallbladder, the administration of cholecystokinin (to empty the gallbladder) or morphine (to constrict the sphincter of Oddi) may help eliminate false-positive results (i.e., diagnosis of cholecystisis).**

   D. Management
      1. Laparoscopic cholecystectomy is the treatment of choice.
      2. Open cholecystectomy may be appropriate for severely inflamed or complicated cases.
      3. Cholecystostomy may be used for unstable or nonoperative patients.
   E. Postoperative cholecystitis
      1. Pathophysiology. Biliary stasis, systemic sepsis, and hypotension may lead to cholecystitis, which is often acalculous in nature.
      2. Diagnosis (high index of suspicion)
         a. Patients are often sedated, intubated, and very ill.
         b. Right upper quadrant tenderness and a palpable mass are often absent.
         c. Once the diagnosis is entertained, a HIDA scan is indicated to visualize the biliary system, with possible false-positive or false-negative results. If the HIDA scan shows a nonfilling gallbladder, cholescystokinin or morphine should be administered.
      3. Management. If cholecystitis is identified, then cholecystectomy is indicated if the patient is suitable to undergo surgery. If not, a cholecystostomy tube may be placed to drain the infection, and surgery may be scheduled at a later time.
V. Cholangitis
   A. Etiology. Possible causes include cholelithiasis, stricture, pancreatitis, external compression, and foreign object.
   B. Clinical presentation
      1. Essential features: bactibilia, stasis, obstruction
      2. Charcot's triad: right upper quadrant pain, fever, jaundice
      3. Reynold's pentad: right upper quadrant pain, fever, jaundice, hypotension, mental status change
   C. Laboratory results. Liver function tests are abnormal, and leukocytosis is present.
   D. Diagnostic imaging studies
      1. Ultrasonography
      2. Percutaneous cholangiography
      3. Endoscopic retrograde cholangiopancreatography (ERCP) [preferred diagnostic modality]. This procedure may be therapeutic.
      4. CT or HIDA scans. These scans may be used to document obstruction of the choledochus.
   E. Management
      1. Fluid resuscitation

  2. Antibiotics
  3. Decompression of the biliary tree
   a. ERCP
   b. Percutaneous transhepatic drainage
   c. Surgery (common bile duct exploration)

VI. Bactibilia

 A. Positive bile culture (incidence)
  1. Cholangitis (> 95%)
  2. Presence of biliary stent (> 95%)
  3. Benign obstruction (85%)
  4. Enteric anastomosis (80%)
  5. Cholecystitis (60%)
  6. Choledocholithiasis (55%)
  7. Malignant obstruction (10%)

 B. Organisms
  1. Common agents: *Klebsiella* species, *Enterococcus*, *Escherichia coli*
  2. Anaerobes (10% of patients): *Clostridium perfringens, Bacteroides*
  3. Resistant gram-negative bacteria: *Pseudomonas aeruginosa, Enterobacter* species
  4. Opportunistic organisms: *Candida albicans, Cryptosporidium,* cytomegalovirus (CMV)
  5. Helminthic species: *Ascaris lumbricoides, Strongyloides stercoralis,* and *Echinococcus* species; the liver flukes *Clonorchis sinensis, Opisthorchis,* and *Fasciola hepatica*

VII. Antibiotic Regimens for Various Procedures and Biliary Tract Conditions

 A. Elective procedures: cefazolin, mezlocillin, or a second-generation cephalosporin
 B. Critically ill patients: penicillin/β-lactamase inhibitor combination agent (consider adding an aminoglycoside and clindamycin or metronidazole)
 C. Other organisms
  1. Resistant organisms: ciprofloxacin, imipenem, vancomycin
  2. Fungi: amphotericin B or fluconazole
  3. CMV: ganciclovir
  4. Helminths: mebendazole, thiabendazole, priziquantel

CIRRHOSIS AND ASCITES

 I. Etiology of Cirrhosis
  A. Ethanol abuse
  B. Viruses [e.g., hepatitis B (HBV), hepatitis C (HBC)]
  C. Autoimmune conditions
  D. Metabolic disorders (e.g., Wilson's disease, hemochromatosis, ($_1$-antitrypsin deficiency)

 II. Complications of Cirrhosis
  A. Ascites (Figure 11-1)
   1. Of all individuals with ascites, 80% have cirrhosis.

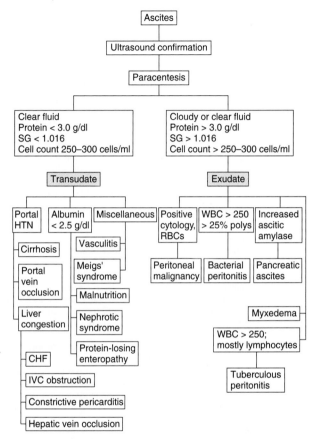

Figure 11-1. Ascitic fluid evaluation algorithm. CHD = congestive heart failure; HTN = hypertension; IVC = inferior vena cava; RBC = red blood cell count; SG = specific gravity; WBC = white blood cell count.

2. **Pathogenesis**
   a. Increased hepatic and splanchnic lymph formation
   b. Hypoalbuminemia
   c. Sinusoidal hypertension
   d. Sodium and water retention by kidneys secondary to decreased hepatic degradation of aldosterone
3. **Laboratory results:** serum albumin—ascites albumin gradient
   a. Difference > 1.1 g/dl: ascites secondary to portal hypertension

   b. Difference < 1.1 g/dl: ascites not secondary to portal hypertension
   4. Infected ascites
      a. Perform paracentesis and obtain WBC and culture fluid.
         (1) A WBC < 300 cells/μl rules out infection.
         (2) If a solitary organism is present in the ascites culture after surgery, this is most often a result of contamination or spontaneous bacterial peritonitis, whereas polymicrobial flora is usually a primary intraabominal process.
      b. Begin IV antibiotics and, in critical patients, peritoneal lavage through a dialysis catheter. Avoid aminoglycosides if possible in patients with cirrhosis.
   B. Other complications
      1. Variceal hemorrhage (see GASTROINTESTINAL HEMORRHAGE in Chapter 9)
      2. Hepatocellular failure
      3. Hepatic encephalopathy
      4. Hypersplenism
III. Management of Ascites in Patients With Cirrhosis
   A. General management

**Ascites is easier to prevent than treat.
Resuscitation should be less vigorous, especially
with respect to crystalloid solutions, but adequate
to reestablish a functional extracellular volume.**

---

   1. Avoid volume loading to treat low urine output. This fluid disproportionately increases ascites. If vital signs are stable with mild oliguria, this situation is seldom serious.
   2. If oliguria persists or recurs, administer colloid or concentrated human albumin to reexpand extracellular volume.
   B. Medical treatment. A combination of diet and dual diuretics is effective in 90% of patients.
      1. Diet
         a. Restrict sodium intake to < 2000 mg/day. Fluid restriction is seldom necessary.
         b. Do not correct hyponatremia unless the patient has symptoms or serum sodium < 120 mg/dl.
      2. Diuretics. The goal of therapy is weight loss of 0.5–1.0 kg/day until symptoms of fluid retention have decreased. Start with a single drug; a two-drug regimen may be necessary.
         a. Start spironolactone at 100 mg/day (maximum 400 mg/day).
         b. Start furosemide at 40 mg/day (maximum 160 mg/day).

**Urinary sodium is a useful parameter to follow during
diuresis. As long as it is > 10 mEq/L, therapy may continue.**

3. **Large-volume paracentesis** (single removal of 4–6 liters of fluid)
   a. This procedure is indicated only for tense ascites.
   b. This procedure should be followed by sodium restriction and dual diuretics.
   c. Postparacentesis albumin infusion is not required.

C. Surgical treatment

1. Child's classification

   a. This classification system combines clinical with biochemical data to predict hepatic functional reserve in patients with cirrhosis (**Table 11-1**).
   b. Operative mortality according to class is as follows:
      (1) Child's A: 0% to 5%
      (2) Child's B: 10% to 15%
      (3) Child's C: > 25%

2. Shunts

   a. **Peritoneovenous shunt (Denver or LeVeen)**
      (1) A peritoneovenous shunt has no survival advantage compared to medical therapy.
      (2) A peritoneovenous shunt should be reserved for the patient with ascites refractory to medical therapy who is not a candidate for hepatic transplantation or serial therapeutic paracentesis.
   b. **Transjugular intrahepatic portosystemic shunt (TIPS)**
      (1) A TIPS is useful for managing a patient with variceal hemorrhage secondary to portal hypertension (see ACUTE VARICEAL HEMORRHAGE in Chapter 9).
      (2) A TIPS is not recommended for treatment of ascites (mortality is higher when compared to medical therapy).

3. Orthotopic liver transplantation (OLT)

   a. Consider this surgical procedure first for acceptable candidates for transplantation.

Table 11-1. Child's Classification: Operative Risk Stratification for Portosystemic Shunts

Criteria	Good Risk (A)	Moderate Risk (B)	Poor Risk (C)
Serum bilirubin	< 2.0 mg/dl	2.0–3.0 mg/dl	> 3.0 mg/dl
Serum albumin	> 3.5 mg/dl	3.0–3.5 mg/dl	< 3.0 mg/dl
Ascites	None	Easily controlled	Not easily controlled
Encephalopathy	None	Minimal	Advanced
Nutrition	Excellent	Good	Poor
PT (seconds above control)	< 4.0	4.0–6.0	> 6.0
Operative mortality	0%–5%	10%–15%	>25%

PT = prothrombin time.

> **Refractory ascites is an inclusion criterion for OLT.**

    b. The 5-year survival is 80%.
  4. Prevention and treatment of peritoneovenous shunt complications
    a. Initial shunt management

> **Peritoneovenous shunts should be avoided in patients with hyperbilirubinemia and prolonged PT.**

      (1) Preoperatively culture the ascitic fluid and provide a short course of antibiotics to prevent shunt infection.
      (2) Prior to the procedure, begin heparin, 5000 U SQ bid, to help prevent the coagulopathy.
      (3) At the time of surgery, drain most of the ascites, and in high-risk patients, irrigate the abdomen with normal saline.

> **Draining the ascites helps avoid volume overload in the immediate postoperative period.**

      (4) Maintain flow through the shunt with an abdominal binder and incentive spirometry.
      (5) Monitor the prothrombin time (PT) during the postoperative period.
        (a) If the PT is prolonged more than a few seconds, or ecchymoses and incisional bleeding occur, minimize autotransfusion of ascites by sitting the patient up, stopping breathing exercises, and releasing the abdominal binder.
        (b) Fresh frozen plasma may help correct the coagulopathy.
        (c) If disseminated intravascular coagulation (DIC) develops, start a heparin infusion and consider ligation of the shunt.
    b. Shunt failure
      (1) Early failure is usually a technical problem with kinking of the catheter or not placing the catheter in the most central position.
      (2) Late failure is often a result of proteinaceous debris in the valve, which responds to valve replacement.
      (3) Excess sodium and fluid ingestion may overwhelm the valve.
      (4) A contrast study of the shunt may reveal the level of obstruction, which is often obvious at reoperation.
    c. Shunt infection

(1) Patients with early shunt infection often develop encephalopathy, systemic sepsis, and bleeding diatheses.

(2) Start broad-spectrum antibiotics immediately.

(3) Remove the shunt if necessary. Such removal is very often appropriate.

FULMINANT HEPATIC FAILURE

I. **Definition.** Fulminant hepatic failure is the appearance of severe acute liver disease with hepatic encephalopathy in a previously healthy person. Diagnosis of encephalopathy within 2 weeks of the onset of jaundice is required. Prolongation of the PT and mental status changes are also prerequisites for diagnosis.

II. **Etiology**

> **Identification of the cause of hepatic failure is necessary because of implications for prognosis, therapy, and prevention.**

A. **Idiopathic disease** (most common; diagnosis is given after identifiable causes are ruled out)

B. **Viral infection:** acute hepatitis A virus (HAV), acute HBV, hepatitis D virus (HDV) superinfection/coinfection with chronic hepatitis B carrier; HBV reactivation, acute hepatitis C virus (HCV), acute hepatitis E virus (HEV), indeterminate viral hepatitis, Epstein-Barr virus (EBV) infection, CMV, herpes simplex, varicella

C. **Hepatotoxic drugs:** acetaminophen, enflurane, erythromycin, halothane, isoflurane, isoniazid, ketoconazole, nonsteroidal anti-inflammatory drugs (NSAIDs), rifampin, sodium valproate, sulphonamides, tetracycline, tricyclic antidepressants

D. **Other hepatotoxic agents:** *Amanita phalloides,* carbon tetrachloride, yellow phosphorus

E. **Metabolic causes:** acute fatty liver of pregnancy, Wilson's disease, galactosemia, Reye's syndrome

F. **Cardiovascular causes:** portal vein thrombosis, Budd-Chiari syndrome, right ventricular failure, cardiac tamponade, heat stroke, circulatory shock

G. **Metastatic tumor**

III. **Diagnostic work-up**

A. **Laboratory tests**

1. **Serum:** CBC with differential, prothrombin time/partial thromboplastin time (PT/PTT), electrolytes, BUN/creatinine, bilirubin, albumin, AST/ALT, alkaline phosphatase, amylase, toxicology, copper, ammonia, ceruloplasmin

2. **Urine:** toxicology, 24-hour copper and penicillamine challenge, if appropriate
3. **Viral serology**
   a. HAV: IgM anti-HAV
   b. HBV: HBsAg, IgM anti-HBc, HBV DNA
   c. HCV: Anti-HCV antibody, HCV mRNA
   d. HDV: IgM anti-HDV
   e. HEV: anti-HEV antibody
   f. Serology for CMV, EBV, herpes
4. **Autoantibodies, immunoglobulins**
B. **Imaging studies**
   1. Chest radiograph
   2. Ultrasound of the liver (for size, texture, and patency of portal and hepatic veins) and spleen (for size)
   3. CT scan of abdomen
C. **Slit lamp examination** for Keyser-Fleischer rings

IV. **Management**
   A. **ICU** (mandatory admission)
   B. **IV hydration**
   C. **Hemodynamic monitoring**
   D. **Prophylaxis for GI bleeding:** H_2 blockers or sucralfate
   E. **Blood products** for coagulation deficit if overt bleeding is evident
   F. **Appropriate therapeutic drugs**
   G. **OLT** (treatment of choice). **Contraindications** include:
      1. Uncontrolled intracranial hypertension
      2. Uncontrolled systemic hypotension
      3. Sepsis
      4. ARDS
      5. Psychiatric and social factors. These must be considered, especially in cases of attempted suicide.

Patients should be listed early for OLT.

V. **Sequelae of Hepatic Failure**
   A. **Hepatic encephalopathy and cerebral edema**
      1. **Clinical presentation**
         a. **Hepatic encephalopathy** is graded on a scale of 0–4 but may fluctuate during the course of disease **(Table 11-2)**.
         b. **Cerebral edema** is present in 80% of patients with grade 4 hepatic encephalopathy.
            (1) This edema is associated with elevated intracranial pressure (ICP) as well as a reduction in cerebral blood flow and cerebral metabolic rate.
            (2) As ICP rises, impairment in cerebral oxygenation results with the development of cerebral ischemia, and tentorial herniation occurs in 25% of cases.
      2. **Management**
         a. **Monitor subdural ICP.**

Table 11-2. Grades of Hepatic Encephalopathy

Grade	Characteristics
0	Normal level of consciousness
	No neurologic abnormalities
1	Mild confusion, euphoria, poor concentration, occasional dysphoria, slurred speech
	Reversed sleep pattern; fully coherent when roused
	Mild tremors
	Normal tone and reflexes
	Symmetric slowing under triphasic waves on EEG
2	Increasing confusion and disorientation but still rousable and rational
	Incontinence
	Asterixis easily elicited; brisk reflexes and increased muscle tone
	Symmetric slowing and triphasic waves on EEG
3	Sleep most of the time but can be roused to commands
	May be markedly agitated, occasionally aggressive, incoherent, or no speech
	Upgoing plantar/clonus, localized/flexion, response to pain
	Triphasic waves on EEG
4	Not rousable to commands but may be responsive to painful stimuli; comatose
	Clinical features of cerebral edema may be present: hyperventilation, pupillary abnormalities, opisthotonus, and extensor plantars
	Abnormal respiratory pattern
	Asterixis absent, sustained clonus, extensor response to pain (decerebrate posturing)
	Delta waves on EEG

    (1) An increase in ICP > 20 mm Hg, if untreated, is associated with the subsequent development of tentorial herniation.

    (2) Attempt to keep the ICP < 15 mm Hg and the cerebral perfusion pressure > 50 mm Hg.

  b. Maintain normothermia.

  c. Keep the head up at approximately 30° to the horizontal.

  d. Administer IV mannitol, 0.5–1 g/kg over 5 minutes. This may be repeated until serum osmolality is 310 mOsm/L.

  e. Administer neomycin and **lactulose** to treat encephalopathy.

  f. Perform neurologic evaluations frequently. Pay specific attention to increased muscle tone, hyperreflexia, and abnormal pupillary reflexes.

> **Mannitol should be used to treat elevated cerebral pressures. It has been shown to increase cerebral blood flow in grade 4 encephalopathy.**

B. Cardiovascular disturbances

1. **Clinical presentation.** These conditions are characterized by marked hemodynamic changes heralded by a **significant reduction in pulmonary and systemic vascular resistance** with **compensatory increases in cardiac output and metabolic rate**.

   a. As many as 50% of patients have episodes of **hypotension** despite elevated cardiac outputs.

   b. Affected patients exhibit a close relationship between oxygen delivery and oxygen extraction by the tissues. The calculation of arterial oxygen content requires co-oximetry rather than a calculated arterial oxygen saturation because of the shift in the oxygen—hemoglobin (Hgb) dissociation curve.

2. **Management**

   a. If hypotension persists in face of optimal volume loading and cardiac output, then **vasopressors** are indicated. Epinephrine and norepinephrine have been shown to be more effective than dobutamine.

   b. In patients with severe liver disease, use of a **peripheral vasodilator** such as prostacyclin or N-acetylcysteine is associated with increased oxygen delivery and oxygen consumption by the tissues. These agents enhance cerebral oxygen delivery and raise the cerebral metabolic rate for oxygen.

> **Hemodynamic goals for maintenance of oxygen delivery are > 700 ml/min/m^2.**

C. Pulmonary disturbances

1. Patients develop low pulmonary vascular resistance, increased alveolar-arterial oxygen difference, and possible hypoxemia.

2. With the onset of grade 3 encephalopathy, patients should be placed on **mechanical ventilation** for both airway protection and treatment of hypoxemia.

D. Electrolyte and renal dysfunction

1. **Clinical presentation**

   a. **Hyponatremia** occurs as a result of water retention and an intracellular sodium shift from inhibition of Na–K ATPase.

   b. **Elevated lactic acid** and **metabolic acidosis** occur in 30% of cases, usually as a result of acetaminophen. This may result from excessive production (tissue hypoxia), impaired hepatic uptake, or impaired hepatic metabolism of lactate. Prognosis is poor.

c. **Renal failure** is defined as urine output < 300 ml/24 hr. This condition results from a functional abnormality in the kidney. Normal kidney function returns with recovery of liver function or liver transplant.

d. **Hypoglycemia.** Blood glucose is generally preserved until there is massive hepatic parenchymal damage. A dextrose infusion of 5% to 50% may be required.

e. **Hepatorenal syndrome** is thought to result from a strong renal vasoconstrictor response to systemic vasodilation that accompanies liver failure. Typical findings include urine specific gravity > 1.010, sodium < 10 mmol/L, and urine:plasma creatinine ratio < 10.

   (1) **Avoid hemodialysis,** because it causes an abrupt increase in ICP and a decrease in cerebral perfusion pressure.

   (2) Given the risk of renal failure in patients with hepatic failure, **avoid nephrotoxic agents** and **maintain renal support.**

2. **Management**

   a. **Avoid saline administration.**

   b. **Administer continuous glucose** to correct hypoglycemia that results from reduced hepatic glycogen stores and hyperinsulinemia.

   c. **Consider dopamine,** 2–4 µg/kg/hr.

   d. **Avoid nephrotoxic agents.**

   e. **Consider a pulmonary artery catheter** to assess fluid status.

   f. Acute tubular necrosis or functional renal failure occurs in more than 50% of cases. **Consider continuous hemofiltration** to avoid large shifts in solute.

E. **Sepsis.** As many as 80% of patients develop bacterial sepsis, and 30% acquire a fungal infection. Sepsis is the most common cause of late death.

   1. **Defects in host defenses** involve impaired opsonization as well as impaired leukocyte chemotaxis and intracellular killing.

   2. **Close antimicrobial surveillance** is more important than prophylactic antibiotics.

F. **Disorders of coagulation and fibrinolysis**

   1. **Hepatocellular necrosis** results in marked impairment in synthesis of clotting factors, consumptive coagulopathy, activation of the fibrinolytic pathway, and platelet abnormalities.

   2. The **coagulopathy should not be treated** unless there is bleeding or an invasive procedure is needed. Fresh frozen plasma should be used to replenish clotting factors.

VI. **Early Predictors of Death**

A. **Acetaminophen poisoning** (see Chapter 24), **with *one* of the following:**

1. pH < 7.3, irrespective of grade of encephalopathy
2. Encephalopathy of grade 3 or 4 with PT > 100 seconds and serum creatinine > 3.4 mg/dl

B. All other causes of disease, with *one* of the following:

1. PT > 100 seconds, irrespective of grade of encephalopathy (see Table 11–2)
2. Any three of the following variables, irrespective of the grade of encephalopathy:
   a. Age < 10 or > 40 years
   b. Etiology other than acetaminophen, HAV, or HBV
   c. Period of jaundice to encephalopathy > 7 days
   d. PT > 50 seconds
   e. Serum bilirubin > 17.5 mg/dl

PORTAL HYPERTENSION

I. Definition. Portal hypertension is abnormal elevation of portal venous pressure (normal pressure is 5–6 mm Hg).

II. Pathophysiology

A. Venous collaterals between the portal system and the systemic vasculature spontaneously develop via the short gastric vein, azygous vein, esophageal and paraesophageal veins, superior middle and inferior rectal veins, and periumbilical veins.

B. As portal pressure rises to > 20 mm Hg, varices develop.

C. Portal systemic shunting results in a hyperdynamic state.

III. Etiology

A. Prehepatic (rare, more common in pediatric population)

1. Extrinsic compression: tumors
2. Portal vein obstruction: congenital atresia, thrombosis, stenosis

B. Intrahepatic (most common)

1. Liver cirrhosis is the cause of 85% of portal hypertension in the United States. It involves:
   a. Regenerative nodules, which cause distortion of anatomy
   b. Progressive narrowing of sinusoidal and postsinusoidal vessels
2. Schistosomiasis, a common cause worldwide, involves a presinusoidal block by parasitic ova.
3. Hemochromatosis, Wilson's disease, and hepatic fibrosis are other causes.

C. Posthepatic (rare)

1. Budd-Chiari syndrome. The characteristics of this idiopathic condition include:
   a. Hepatic vein thrombosis
   b. Hypercoagulable states
   c. Infection
2. Constrictive pericarditis. The characteristics of this condition include:

      a. Marked increase in inferior vena cava pressure

      b. Resistance to hepatic venous outflow

  D. Increased portal venous flow

      1. Found in primary splenic disease

      2. Treated with splenic shunts or arteriovenous fistulae

  E. Splenic vein thrombosis secondary to pancreatitis or pancreatic cancer

IV. Signs and Symptoms

  A. Ascites (see CIRRHOSIS AND ASCITES), with hepatic sinusoidal hypertension, decreased albumin, and hyperaldosteronism

  B. Encephalopathy. With the development of portosystemic collaterals, blood is shunted around the liver; therefore, it is not purified.

  C. Esophageal varices

  D. Malnutrition

  E. Splenomegaly

  F. Collateral venous development (caput medusae, hemorrhoids)

V. Diagnosis

  A. Esophagogastroduodenoscopy

  B. Child's classification to evaluate operative risk (see Table 11-1)

  C. Portal venous anatomy: look for presence of patent portal vein

      1. Noninvasive technique. Doppler ultrasound indicates:

         a. Portal vein and tributaries

         b. Direction of flow

      2. Invasive technique. Angiography, the most accurate imaging modality, shows:

         a. Splenic and superior mesenteric arteriography with delayed venous phase

         b. Portal venous pressure measured by wedge pressure of hepatic vein

VI. Management

  A. Medical treatment (elective)

      1. Varices

         a. TIPS

         b. Sclerosis

            (1) Endoscopic sclerosis of varices

            (2) Initially effective in 80% to 90% of patients

            (3) Often requires repeated treatments

            (4) Complications: esophageal stricture

         c. Maintenance therapy (not in acute situation): β-blockade

            (1) Propranolol, 40 mg PO bid, or

            (2) Nadolol, 40 mg PO qd

      2. Ascites (see CIRRHOSIS AND ASCITES)

      3. Encephalopathy

  B. Surgical treatment (elective)

      1. Prophylactic surgery

         a. Patients with varices prior to any episodes of bleeding (only 40% ultimately bleed from varices)

b. No improvement in survival

> **Prophylactic treatment for portal hypertension, which does not improve survival, is not recommended.**

2. **Therapeutic surgery**
   a. Patients who have had variceal bleeding
   b. Survival related to Child's classification (see Table 11-1)
3. **Nonselective shunts.** These shunts decompress the portal venous system into the inferior vena cava.

> **Nonselective shunts are associated with an increased risk of encephalopathy and hepatic failure.**

   a. **End-to-side portacaval shunt** (most commonly performed nonselective shunt)
      (1) Ligation and closure of hepatic end of portal vein
      (2) Anastomosis of distal end to inferior vena cava
      (3) Rebleeding < 5%
      (4) Portal flow reduced to zero
   b. **Mesocaval shunt**
      (1) Anastomosis of the superior mesenteric vein to the inferior vena cava with a 16- to 18-mm prosthetic vascular graft
      (2) Exposure of the superior mesenteric vein with relative ease
      (3) Complications
         (a) Risk of hepatic failure
         (b) Possible conversion of portal vein into outflow vessel secondary to change in relative pressures
         (c) Prosthetic material–associated problems
            (i) Increased potential for infectious complications
            (ii) Lower long-term patency
   c. **Side-to-side portacaval shunt**
      (1) Technically more difficult secondary to the need to expose a greater portion of veins
      (2) Conversion of portal vein into outflow vessel, thus decompressing the liver
         (a) May be helpful in Budd-Chiari syndrome
         (b) May be helpful in cases with refractory ascites and bleeding from esophageal varices
4. **Selective shunt** (distal splenorenal or Warren shunt). This shunts only gastroesophageal venous blood into the systemic circulation and significantly reduces postoperative encephalopathy.
   a. Anastomosis of distal end of splenic vein to left renal vein
   b. Ligation of proximal splenic vein

    c. Ligation of collaterals between the portal and the systemic venous system around the gastric, pancreatic, and splenic regions (e.g., coronary vein)

    d. Maintenance of portal venous flow, decreasing risk of hepatic failure

    e. No effect on ascites production, because portal sinusoidal pressure is unchanged

5. Nonshunt procedures

    a. Liver transplantation

        (1) Addresses underlying liver disease

        (2) Appropriate for otherwise healthy patients with poor hepatic reserve

    b. Sugiura procedure: paraesophageal devascularization with esophageal transection and reanastomosis

        (1) Highly effective with low mortality rate in Japanese series

        (2) Involves transthoracic esophageal devascularization, transabdominal gastric devascularization, splenectomy, selective vagotomy, and pyloroplasty

12

Infectious Diseases

ANTIBIOTICS AND RESISTANCE

I. **General Principles of Antibiotic Selection**
   A. **Drug selection**
      1. **Organism susceptibility (most important factor;** cultures should be used to guide therapy)
      2. Drug toxicity
      3. Antibacterial effect (i.e., bactericidal versus bacteriostatic)
      4. Renal and hepatic function
      5. Age and gestational status
      6. Site of infection
      7. Mode and frequency of antibiotic administration
      8. Anticipated synergy
      9. Cost
   B. **Number of antibiotic agents required.** Definitive treatment of most organisms requires one antimicrobial drug. The following organisms should be covered by two antibiotics because of the rapid development of resistance, except in UTIs, where there is high antibiotic concentration. (The mnemonic device is **SPACE.**)
      1. *S*erratia
      2. *P*seudomonas, *P*rovidencia
      3. *A*cinetobacter
      4. *C*itrobacter
      5. *E*nterobacter

II. **β-Lactam Antibiotics**
   A. **Mechanism of action.** These drugs, all of which are bactericidal, are inhibitors of cell wall synthesis. They covalently and irreversibly bind to the active site of bacterial transpeptidase, a penicillin-binding protein (PBP) that cross-links cell wall residues.
   B. **Penicillins.** Both natural and synthetic penicillins are available.
      1. **Penicillinase-sensitive (natural) penicillins** (e.g., penicillin V, penicillin G)

    a. Antimicrobial spectrum
- **(1)** Gram-positive cocci (except penicillinase-producing *Staphylococcus* and *Enterococcus*)
- **(2)** Gram-positive bacilli (except *Clostridium difficile*)
- **(3)** *Neisseria* (except penicillinase-producing *Neisseria gonorrhoeae*)
- **(4)** Spirochetes
- **(5)** *Actinomyces*

    b. Adverse reactions
- **(1)** Hypersensitivity (common)

CAUTION: Penicillinase-sensitive penicillin causes 10% of all drug reactions. Allergic reactions may involve urticaria, pruritus, maculopapular rashes, or anaphylaxis.

- **(2)** Seizures (rare)

2. Penicillinase-resistant (semisynthetic) penicillins (e.g., dicloxacillin, methicillin, nafcillin, oxacillin)

    a. Antimicrobial spectrum
- **(1)** These drugs have a narrow spectrum and are clinically useful only for treating penicillinase-producing staphylococci.
- **(2)** These drugs do not inhibit enterococci or gram-negative bacteria.

    b. Adverse reactions
- **(1)** Hypersensitivity
- **(2)** Interstitial nephritis (primarily with methicillin)

3. Aminopenicillins (e.g., ampicillin, amoxicillin)

    a. Antimicrobial spectrum
- **(1)** Enterococci
- **(2)** *Escherichia coli*
- **(3)** *Haemophilus*
- **(4)** *Listeria*
- **(5)** *Proteus mirabilis*
- **(6)** All anaerobes except *C. difficile* [if ampicillin + sulbactam (Unasyn) is used]

    b. Adverse reactions (similar to those of natural penicillins)

CAUTION: Rashes are about twice as common with ampicillin than with any other penicillin.

---

4. Carboxypenicillins (ticarcillin, carbenicillin) and **ureidopenicillins** (mezlocillin, piperacillin) [also called extended-spectrum penicillins]

    a. Antimicrobial spectrum, which is the same as aminopenicillins with the following additions:
- **(1)** Enterobacteriaceae (*E. coli, Enterobacter, Klebsiella, Proteus, Salmonella, Serratia, Shigella*)
- **(2)** *Pseudomonas*
- **(3)** Ticarcillin-clavulanate (Timentin) and pipera-

cillin-tazobactam (Zosyn) have extended spectrums that cover all anaerobes except *C. difficile.*

    b. Adverse reactions (similar to those of natural penicillins)

> **CAUTION: Ticarcillin [both alone and in combination with clavulanate (Timentin)] has a high sodium load and should be used cautiously in patients with CHF.**

C. Cephalosporins

    1. First-generation cephalosporins (e.g., cephalothin, cephalexin, cefazolin)

        a. Antimicrobial spectrum

            (1) Gram-positive bacteria (except anaerobes and enterococci) [excellent activity], including penicillinase-producing staphylococci but not methicillin-resistant *Staphylococcus aureus* (MRSA)

            (2) *E. coli*

            (3) *Klebsiella*

            (4) *P. mirabilis*

        b. Adverse reactions

            (1) Hypersensitivity may be a problem. Cephalosporins exhibit cross-reactivity with penicillins in 5% to 8% of patients.

            (2) Cephalosporins may be safely administered to patients who displayed only a rash or pruritus in reaction to penicillin.

> **CAUTION: *Never* give any cephalosporin to a patient with a history of anaphylaxis to penicillin.**

    2. Second-generation cephalosporins (e.g., cefaclor, cefamandole, cefmetazole, cefonicid, cefotetan, cefoxitin, cefuroxime)

        a. Antimicrobial spectrum

            (1) Gram-positive bacteria: less activity than first-generation agents

            (2) Gram-negative bacteria: extended spectrum that also includes *Haemophilus, Enterobacter,* and *Proteus vulgaris*

            (3) Anaerobic activity: excellent for cefoxitin and cefotetan only

        b. Adverse reactions

            (1) Hypersensitivity

            (2) Hypoprothrombinemia and bleeding (possibly) with agents that have a methylthiotetrazole moiety (cefamandole) [effect reversed by vitamin K]

    3. Third-generation cephalosporins (e.g., cefoperazone, cefotaxime, ceftazidime, ceftizoxime, ceftriaxone)

        a. Antimicrobial spectrum

(1) Gram-positive bacteria: less activity than first-generation drugs

(2) Gram-negative bacteria: extended activity against *Citrobacter, Enterobacter, Proteus, Salmonella, Serratia,* and *Shigella*

(3) *Pseudomonas:* ceftazidime and cefoperazone have extended activity for coverage

(4) Anaerobes: little activity

b. Adverse reactions

(1) Hypersensitivity

(2) Hypoprothrombinemia and bleeding (cefoperazone) [effect reversed by vitamin K]

4. Fourth-generation cephalosporin (e.g., cefepime)

a. Antimicrobial spectrum

(1) Gram-positive bacteria: significant activity (including penicillinase-producing staphylococci)

(2) Gram-negative organisms: extended spectrum, including *Pseudomonas* (same as third-generation drugs)

(3) Anaerobic activity: little

b. Adverse reactions

(1) Hypersensitivity

(2) Hypothrombinemia (rare)

D. Carbapenems and monobactams

1. Carbapenems (e.g., imipenem, meropenem). Carbapenems are **potent inducers of β-lactamase.** Although they are resistant to the enzyme, they render pathogens **resistant to other β-lactam antibiotics.**

a. Antimicrobial spectrum

(1) Gram-positive bacteria (except MRSA)

(2) Gram-negative bacteria (including *Pseudomonas*)

(3) Anaerobes (except *C. difficile*)

(4) *Haemophilus, Morganella, Proteus, Providencia,* and *Pseudomonas* (increased activity by meropenem)

b. Adverse reactions

(1) GI upset, with nausea and vomiting

(2) Seizures (less common with meropenem)

> **In combination with imipenem, cilastatin inhibits renal dipeptidase and prevents the renal metabolism of imipenem.**

2. Monobactams (e.g., aztreonam). These agents are **poor inducers of β-lactamase** and exhibit little cross-sensitivity to penicillins and cephalosporins.

a. Antimicrobial spectrum

(1) Gram-negative bacteria (most species, including *Pseudomonas*)

(2) Gram-positive or anaerobic bacteria: no activity

b. Adverse reactions

(1) Superinfection due to gram-positive agents

(2) Little renal toxicity, which makes aztreonam a good alternative to aminoglycosides in patients with renal insufficiency

III. Inhibitors of Bacterial Protein Synthesis

A. Antimicrobials that inhibit the 50S subunit (all bacteriostatic)

1. **Macrolides** (e.g., erythromycin, azithromycin, clarithromycin)

   a. **Antimicrobial spectrum**
      (1) Organisms covered by the natural penicillins (erythromycin is a good substitute for penicillin V in penicillin-allergic patients) plus
      (2) *Legionella*
      (3) *Campylobacter*
      (4) *Mycoplasma*
      (5) *Bordetella*
      (6) *Chlamydia*
      (7) *Haemophilus*
      (8) *E. coli*
      (9) *Klebsiella*
      (10) *Moraxella*

Clarithromycin is indicated for MAI prophylaxis in HIV infected patients with CD4 counts < 100 cells/mm³.

---

   b. **Adverse reactions**
      (1) GI upset with diarrhea, nausea, and vomiting
      (2) Hepatic P450 inhibition (not seen with azithromycin), leading to drug–drug interactions [e.g., most notable interaction involves terfenadine, leading to torsades de points (fatal arrhythmia)]

2. **Chloramphenicol**

   a. **Antimicrobial spectrum. Chloramphenicol is the drug of choice for typhoid fever,** which is caused by *Salmonella typhi*. This agent is a broad-spectrum antibiotic.
      (1) Gram-positive bacteria
      (2) Gram-negative bacteria
      (3) Anaerobes
      (4) *Rickettsia*

PRECAUTION: Chloramphenicol should be reserved for use with life-threatening pathogens that are not susceptible to other antimicrobial agents.

---

   b. **Adverse reactions.** These effects have limited the use of chloramphenicol.
      (1) Aplastic anemia. An irreversible effect, this anemia is not dose-related. The condition, which occurs in about 1 in 40,000 patients who receive the drug, is characterized by pancytopenia.

(2) Gray syndrome. This dose-related liver toxicity occurs in newborns who receive the drug. The condition is characterized by vomiting, cyanosis, abdominal distention, and shock. It is fatal in 60% of cases.

(3) Bone marrow suppression. This effect is dose-related and reversible.

3. Lincosamides (e.g., clindamycin)

  a. Antimicrobial spectrum

  (1) Most gram-positive organisms (except entero-cocci)

  (2) Most anaerobes (except *C. difficile*); limited coverage against gram-negative aerobes

  b. Adverse reactions

  (1) Diarrhea

  (2) Pseudomembranous colitis (*C. difficile* colitis)

B. Antimicrobials that inhibit the 30S subunit (some bactericidal, some bacteriostatic)

  1. Aminoglycosides (e.g., amikacin, gentamicin, neomycin, streptomycin, tobramycin) [bactericidal]

  a. Antimicrobial spectrum

  (1) Aerobic gram-negative bacteria (including *Pseudomonas*)

  (2) Staphylococci

  (3) Enterococci (some strains)

  (4) No activity against other gram-positive or anaerobic bacteria

---

Aminoglycosides have excellent synergy with β-lactam antibiotics (gram-negative bacteria) and vancomycin (enterococci).

---

  b. Adverse reactions

  (1) Nephrotoxicity secondary to acute tubular necrosis. This condition, which is more common in patients with renal insufficiency, decreases in frequency if serum levels are monitored.

  (2) Ototoxicity [both cochlear (decreased sound perception) and vestibular (nystagmus, vertigo, nausea, and vomiting)]

  (3) Neuromuscular blockade. This condition, which is rare but potentially lethal, results from inhibition of presynaptic acetylcholine release. It can be prevented by infusing aminoglycoside over 20–30 minutes.

  2. Tetracyclines (e.g., minocycline, tetracycline, doxycycline) [bacteriostatic]

  a. Antimicrobial spectrum (broad spectrum, although widespread resistance is prevalent)

  (1) Gram-positive bacteria

  (2) Gram-negative bacteria

        (3) Rickettsiae
        (4) Mycobacteria
        (5) *Chlamydia* and *Mycoplasma*
    b. Adverse reactions
        (1) Superinfection (GI and vaginal)
        (2) GI upset, with nausea and vomiting
        (3) Photosensitivity
        (4) Dental problems (i.e., staining of tooth enamel)

CAUTION: Tetracyclines should *not* be given to pregnant women and children < 10 years of age.

---

  3. Spectinomycin (binds to a different site on the 30S subunit than aminoglycosides) [bacteriostatic]
    a. Antimicrobial spectrum
        (1) Gram-positive bacteria
        (2) Gram-negative bacteria, including *N. gonorrhoeae*

The only use for spectinomycin is for treatment of anogenital gonorrhea.

---

    b. Adverse reactions (similar to those of the aminoglycosides)
IV. Miscellaneous Antibiotics
  A. Quinolones (e.g., ciprofloxacin, ofloxacin, levofloxacin, sparfloxacin)
    1. Mechanism of action
        a. Inhibition of bacterial DNA replication by antagonism of the enzyme topoisomerase II (DNA gyrase)
        b. Bactericidal
    2. Antimicrobial spectrum
        a. Gram-positive cocci: activity against most staphylococci (including some MRSA) but little activity versus streptococci (except sparfloxacin)
        b. Gram-negative bacteria: very good coverage against all gram-negative bacteria including *Neisseria, Moraxella, Pseudomonas,* and the Enterobacteriaceae
        c. Anaerobes: generally poor coverage, except for sparfloxacin, the newest quinolone, which has moderate activity
    3. Adverse reactions
        a. Hypersensitivity reactions
        b. GI upset, with nausea and vomiting
        c. Seizures (rare), dizziness, and headache
        d. Inhibition of hepatic P450 enzymes, leading to increased levels of some medications
        e. Photosensitivity (sparfloxacin)

CAUTION: Currently, quinolones are contraindicated in pregnant females and in children < 17 years of age.

B. Trimethoprim-sulfamethoxazole (TMP-SMX)

  1. Mechanism of action

    a. Two drugs that synergistically inhibit bacterial folic acid synthesis

      (1) Trimethoprim: competitive inhibitor of bacterial dihydrofolate reductase

      (2) Sulfamethoxazole: competitive inhibitor of dihydropteroate synthase

    b. Bacteriostatic (except in the urine, where it is bactericidal)

  2. Antimicrobial spectrum

    a. Gram-positive cocci: good activity against staphylococci (including some MRSA) and streptococci, with only variable activity against enterococci

    b. Gram-negative bacteria: good activity against most gram-negatives (including some *Pseudomonas*)

    c. *Pneumocystis carinii* and other protozoa as well as *Nocardia*

    d. Anaerobes: not useful

  3. Adverse reactions

    a. Hypersensitivity (increased in patients with AIDS)

    b. GI upset, with nausea and vomiting

    c. Erythema multiforme and Stevens-Johnson syndrome

    d. Drug fever

    e. Eosinophilia

    f. Hemolytic anemia in patients with glucose-6-phosphate dehydrogenase (G6PD) deficiency

    g. Displacement of drugs and bilirubin from albumin-binding sites leading to:

      (1) Increased drug levels of warfarin, oral hypoglycemic agents, phenytoin, and nonsteroidal anti-inflammatory drugs (NSAIDs)

      (2) Increased bilirubin levels and jaundice

CAUTION: TMP-SMX should not be used during the last month of pregnancy, because increased fetal unconjugated bilirubin levels might lead to kernicterus.

C. Vancomycin

  1. Mechanism of action

    a. Inhibits cell wall synthesis

    b. Forms complexes with the precursor of the peptidoglycan backbone

  2. Antimicrobial spectrum

    a. Gram-positive organisms (including MRSA and enterococci): excellent coverage of almost all gram-positive organisms [except vancomycin-resistant enterococci (VRE)]

    b. Gram-negative bacteria: no coverage

    c. Anaerobes (mixed coverage): coverage for *Clostridium* (including *C. difficile*) but not for *Bacteroides*

3. **Adverse reactions**
   a. Histamine release, which may lead to flushing ("red-man" syndrome) or anaphylaxis
   b. Ototoxicity and nephrotoxicity (rare, unless in combination with aminoglycoside)
   c. Drug fever
   d. Rash
   D. **Metronidazole**
   1. **Mechanism of action**
      a. Reduction of a nitro group at one end of the molecule inside anaerobic cells, leading to the generation of free radicals that damage the DNA of the target organism
      b. Bactericidal
   2. **Antimicrobial spectrum**
      a. Anaerobes: all species (including *C. difficile*)
      b. Protozoa (*Trichomonas, Giardia,* and *Amoeba*)
      c. Aerobic organisms: no effect
   3. **Adverse effects.** An Antabuse-like reaction occurs with alcohol.
V. **Antibiotic Resistance**
   A. **Mediators of resistance**
   1. **Plasmids:** self-reproducing extrachromosomal bacterial DNA that can be transferred between bacteria via conjugation
   2. **Transposable genetic elements:** transposons and insertion sequences, which cannot self-replicate
   3. **Genetic mutation**
   B. **Mechanisms of resistance**
   1. **β-Lactam antibiotics**
      a. **Bacterial production of the enzyme β-lactamase,** which hydrolyzes the amide bond of the β-lactam ring
         (1) Encoding by chromosomal DNA, plasmids, or transposons
         (2) Production of β-lactamases
            (a) Many different microbes, including staphylococci, enterococci, anaerobes, and gram-negative bacteria, manufacture a wide variety of β-lactamases.
            (b) β-lactamases are active against penicillins, cephalosporins, or both.
         (3) Commercial β-lactamase inhibitors
            (a) Such agents include clavulanic acid, sulbactam, and tazobactam.
            (b) The combination of one of these agents with a penicillin increases the spectrum of activity of the penicillin (especially against gram-negative bacteria and anaerobes).
      b. **Altered PBPs**
         (1) Some alterations lead to penicillin resistance but not cephalosporin resistance.

(2) Some alterations render target organisms resistant to all β-lactam drugs (e.g., MRSA, enterococci).

2. **Aminoglycosides**
   a. **Enzymatic aminoglycoside modification**
   b. **Altered drug uptake**
      (1) Such resistance occurs naturally (enterococci) or by mutation.
      (2) Aminoglycosides must be actively transported into the cell for efficacy. In a low pH, low-oxygen environment, active transport is also decreased, which explains the intrinsic resistance of anaerobes.
   c. **Decreased ribosomal affinity**
3. **Tetracyclines**
   a. **Altered drug uptake**
   b. **Active extrusion** of the drug from the cell (enteric gram-negative organisms)
4. **Erythromycin** (and other macrolides)
   a. **Altered ribosome-binding site**
   b. **Erythromycin esterase,** which hydrolyzes the lactone ring
5. **Quinolones**
   a. **Active extrusion** of the drug from the cell (resistant *E. coli*)
   b. **Mutation in DNA gyrase gene**
   c. **Altered porin molecule in the cell wall,** which ordinarily permits drug entry into the cell
6. **Vancomycin**
   a. Production of ligase enzymes that modifies cell wall peptidoglycans (transposon-mediated) that bind vancomycin with reduced affinity
   b. Sensitivity of VRE to chloramphenicol, quinolones, teicoplanin, or quinupristin-dalfopristin (Synercid)
7. **TMP-SMX**
   a. Inability of the drug to penetrate the cell wall (intrinsic or acquired)
   b. Bypass of the enzymes dihydrofolate reductase and dihydropteroate synthase (especially in a thymidine-rich environment)
   c. Production of dihydropteroate synthase or dihydrofolate reductase that is resistant to TMP-SMX (enteric gram-negative bacteria)
   d. Increased production of *para*-aminobenzoic acid (PABA) [folic acid precursor]
   e. Enzymatic degradation of sulfamethoxazole
8. **Metronidazole** (resistance of anaerobes to metronidazole is rare)

CATHETER MAINTENANCE

I. **Venous Catheters**
   A. **Placement**

1. Catheters should only be placed by individuals who are trained in their use or under the supervision of such individuals.
2. Strict sterile preparation, with drapes, should be practiced, and gloves as well as a gown and mask should be used.
3. Transparent, occlusive, sterile dressings should be placed according to institutional policy.

B. Maintenance

1. Use of an antiseptic or antibiotic under the dressing should be considered.
2. Catheters should be regularly inspected by physicians and nurses to monitor for local inflammation and infection.
3. Catheters should be accessible only to trained individuals who use aseptic technique.
4. Indwelling heparin solution should be used when indicated.
5. Central venous catheters should be removed as soon as peripheral IV catheters can be used to replace them.

Dressing changes should occur under sterile conditions every 1–3 days as directed by hospital policy.

C. Central venous line changes

1. Some centers advocate routine line changes every 3–7 days.
2. Consider changing all catheters placed under outside or unknown conditions over a guidewire (e.g., trauma, outside institution).
3. As soon as safe and convenient, femoral vein catheters should be removed and replaced with jugular or subclavian catheters.
4. Change a line over a guidewire when the patient's temperature $\geq$ 101.5°F (38.6°C).
   a. If the patient continues to have a temperature $\geq$ 101.5°F (38.6°C), consider leaving the fresh catheter placed over a guidewire for 48 hours before replacing.
   b. Send the tip of the catheter and the intradermal portion for culture. If the catheter tip grows > 15 CFU, remove the catheter and place a new line in a new site.
   c. Consider a Gram's stain of the catheter tip for rapid diagnosis.
5. Change a line over a guidewire for bacteremia.
   a. Send the tip of the catheter and the intradermal portion for culture. If the tip grows > 15 CFU, remove the catheter and place a new line in a new site.
   b. Consider a Gram's stain of the tip for rapid diagnosis.

      c. Monitor for endocarditis.

      d. Consider administration of antibiotics.

  6. If the catheter insertion site displays signs of infection, remove the catheter, culture the tip and intradermal portion, and place a fresh catheter in a new site.

      a. Provide local wound care.

      b. Consider administration of antibiotics.

      c. Monitor for suppurative thrombophlebitis, and consider resection of infected veins.

II. Arterial Catheters

A. Placement

  1. Catheters should only be placed by individuals who are trained in their use or under the supervision of such individuals.

  2. Strict sterile preparation, with drapes, should be practiced, and gloves as well as a gown and mask should be used.

  3. Transparent, occlusive, sterile dressings should be placed according to institutional policy.

B. Maintenance

  1. Catheters should be regularly inspected by physicians and nurses to monitor for local inflammation and infection.

  2. Catheters should only be accessed by trained individuals who use aseptic technique.

  3. Pressurized heparin solution (slow infusion) should be used when indicated.

  4. The catheter should be removed as soon as it is no longer indicated. Firm, steady pressure should be applied for a sufficient period of time to prevent hematoma formation after removal. The duration of pressure is:

      a. 15 minutes for a radial artery (longer if hypocoagulable)

      b. 45 minutes for a femoral artery (longer if hypocoagulable)

Dressing changes should occur under sterile conditions every 2 days or as directed by hospital policy.

C. Arterial line changes

  1. Some centers advocate routine arterial line changes every week.

  2. If the insertion site displays signs of infection, remove the catheter, and place a fresh catheter in a new site. Culture the catheter tip.

III. Urinary Catheters

A. Placement

  1. Catheters should only be placed by individuals who are trained in their use or under the supervision of such individuals.

2. Strict sterile preparation, with drapes, should be used.

Indwelling urethral catheters should be removed as soon as conversion to condom sheath drainage or intermittent urethral catheterization is possible.

B. **Maintenance**
   1. The urine and urethral meatus should be regularly inspected by physicians and nurses to monitor for infection.
   2. Closed system sterile drainage should be used.
   3. Urinary drainage tubing should only be handled by trained individuals who use aseptic technique.

C. **Catheter changes**
   1. Culture urine if the patient's temperature is $\geq$ 101.5°F (38.6°C).
      a. If culture grows > 100,000 CFU, remove the catheter, replace only if clinically required, and treat the UTI if clinically indicated.
      b. Consider antifungal bladder irrigation or oral fluconazole for fungal UTIs.
   2. Monitor urine for gross hematuria or thrombus occlusion.
      a. Flush the catheter for oliguria to evaluate for clot or mucous obstruction.
      b. Replace the catheter if unable to flush clots or mucus. Consider using either a larger or three-channel catheter.
      c. For ongoing hematuria causing repeated occlusion, consider continuous bladder irrigation with saline or astringent.
      d. Monitor for anemia.
      e. Obtain urologic consultation or cystoscopy for unexplained hematuria.

CENTRAL NERVOUS SYSTEM (CNS) INFECTIONS

I. **Acute Bacterial Meningitis.** Outcome depends on prompt recognition and treatment.

Treatment of bacterial meningitis should not be delayed for diagnostic tests (e.g., lumbar puncture, brain imaging).

A. **Etiology**
   1. **Community-acquired disease.** Causal microbes by age group are:
      a. < 3 months [*E. coli,* group B streptococcus (*Streptococcus agalactiae*), *Listeria monocytogenes*]
      b. 3 months to 18 years [*Neisseria meningitidis, Streptococ-*

cus pneumoniae, Haemophilus influenzae (occurs less commonly secondary to *H. influenzae* type b vaccine)
  c. 18–50 years (*S. pneumoniae, N. meningitidis*)
  d. > 50 years (*S. pneumoniae, L. monocytogenes*, gram-negative bacilli)
  2. **Hospital-acquired disease.** Up to 40% of cases in large, urban hospitals are nosocomial, and many cases are caused by gram-negative organisms.
  3. **Immunocompromised hosts.** Causes include *L. monocytogenes* and gram-negative bacilli.
  4. **Surgical or traumatic disease.** This type of meningitis is associated with neurosurgery, ventriculoperitoneal shunts, or head trauma. It is caused by staphylococci, gram-negative bacilli, and *S. pneumoniae.*
B. **Clinical presentation**

**A high index of suspicion of disease
is necessary in neonates, elderly individuals,
and ICU patients because of minimal signs at
presentation and inability to attain a good history.**

---

  1. **Fever** [> 101.5°F (38.6°C)]
  2. **Meningeal symptoms and signs**
     a. Headache
     b. Neck stiffness (nuchal rigidity); resistance to forward flexion of neck (may be absent in neonates and elderly patients)
     c. Photophobia
     d. Brudzinski's sign: flexion at hip and knee in response to forward neck flexion
     e. Kernig's sign: inability to completely extend the legs
  3. **Neurologic symptoms and signs** (may be present but not required for diagnosis)
     a. Confusion
     b. Seizures
     c. Focal findings, particularly cranial nerve involvement such as facial weakness or hearing loss
     d. Coma and signs of increased intracranial pressure (ICP) [see HEAD TRAUMA in Chapter 26]
  4. **Other infectious sources,** including lungs, ears, sinuses, and cardiac valves
  5. **Skin lesions in meningococcal infections** such as petechiae, purpura, and ecchymoses
C. **Differential diagnosis**
  1. Other systemic infections, particularly in confused, febrile patients without meningeal signs (e.g., septic encephalopathy)
  2. Viral meningitis
  3. Chronic bacterial meningitis [e.g., tuberculosis (TB), neurosyphilis]
  4. Fungal or protozoal meningoencephalitis

5. Viral or bacterial encephalitis
6. Subarachnoid hemorrhage
7. Chemical meningitis
8. Cerebral abscess, especially if focal signs are present
9. Parameningeal infections
10. Mollaret's meningitis
11. Noninfectious, inflammatory etiologies such as vasculitis, Behçet's disease, sarcoidosis, and postinfectious syndrome (e.g., acute disseminated encephalomyelitis)

D. Diagnostic tests
1. **Blood cultures and other emergent laboratory tests**
   a. **Blood cultures** are positive in 40% to 60% of patients with meningococcal, pneumococcal, or *H. influenzae*-caused meningitis.
   b. **Other necessary laboratory tests** include CBC with differential, coagulation studies, electrolytes, calcium, magnesium, phosphate, renal and liver functions, and urinalysis.

With suspected bacterial meningitis, begin administration of empiric antibiotics following blood cultures.

---

2. **Lumbar puncture (LP)**
   a. Perform brain imaging (CT or MRI) prior to LP if signs of increased ICP (e.g., papilledema, coma, focal neurologic signs) are present. Check coagulation parameters before the procedure.
   b. Send CSF for analysis.
      (1) Cell count
         (a) In bacterial meningitis, the WBC count is usually 1000–10,000 cells/mm^3 with a predominance of neutrophils (> 80%).
         (b) In partially treated meningitis (e.g., treatment for a preexisting sinus, ear, or lung infection), the WBC count is lower and the percentage of lymphocytes is higher.
      (2) Protein (abnormal values > 45 mg/dl; usually 100–400 mg/dl in bacterial meningitis)
      (3) Glucose (abnormal values < 20 mg/dl) [only useful when unequivocally low]
      (4) Gram's stain (positive in 60%–90% of cases)
      (5) Bacterial cultures (positive in 70%–85% of cases)
      (6) Acid-fast bacillus (AFB), cryptococcal antigen, Lyme titer, VDRL, viral cultures, polymerase chain reaction (PCR) for viral detection, fungal cultures
3. **Chest x-ray**
4. **ECG**
5. **CT or MRI of brain**
E. Management
1. **Start empiric antibiotics** following blood cultures.
   a. **Narrowing of antibiotic selection,** depending on the

results of the Gram's stain as well as blood and CSF cultures

    b. Duration of therapy: 7–21 days depending on causal pathogen and clinical course

    c. Antibiotic regimens

      (1) Age of < 3 months or > 50 years: ampicillin + third-generation cephalosporin

      (2) Age of 3 months to 50 years: third-generation cephalosporin ± vancomycin

      (3) Immunocompromised status: vancomycin + ampicillin + ceftazidime

      (4) After neurosurgery, penetrating cranial trauma, or shunt infection: vancomycin + ceftazidime

  2. Consider corticosteroids, which have been shown to benefit pediatric patients with *H. influenzae* meningitis.

    a. The dexamethasone dosage is 0.15 mg/kg q 6 hr for 4 days.

    b. Use of these agents in children with other infectious etiologies and in adults is controversial.

  3. Treat seizures if suspected by history.

  4. Manage severe cerebral edema with evidence of herniation with mannitol and steroids.

  5. Consider infectious disease and neurology consults.

F. Complications

  1. Increased ICP

  2. Syndrome of inappropriate antidiuretic hormone (SIADH)

  3. Coma

  4. Seizures

  5. Hydrocephalus in children

  6. Subdural effusion

  7. Venous and arterial infarcts

  8. Meningococcemia associated with circulatory shock and Waterhouse-Friderichsen syndrome

II. Viral Encephalitis. As with bacterial meningitis, a high index of suspicion is necessary to initiate appropriate treatment.

  A. Etiology

    1. Herpes viruses

      a. Herpes simplex virus (HSV)

        (1) Type 1 (HSV-1): most common sporadic cause of encephalitis in the United States

        (2) Type 2 (HSV-2): less common than HSV-1

      b. Epstein-Barr virus (EBV)

      c. Cytomegalovirus (CMV)

      d. Varicella-zoster virus (VZV)

    2. Arboviruses (transmitted by mosquitoes or ticks)

      a. Alphavirus

        (1) Eastern equine encephalitis: 50% to 75% mortality

        (2) Western equine encephalitis: approximately 10% mortality

        (3) Venezuelan equine encephalitis

    b. Flavivirus: St. Louis encephalitis and Japanese B encephalitis

    c. Bunyavirus

  3. Enteroviruses (occurring in late summer and early fall)

  4. HIV (particularly following initial infection)

  5. Paramyxoviruses (measles and mumps viruses)

  6. Arenaviruses

  7. Rabies

B. Clinical presentation

  1. Signs and symptoms of meningitis, along with altered consciousness, may occur. Neurologic findings can progress rapidly over 24–48 hours.

    a. Confusion

    b. Personality changes

    c. Seizures

    d. Focal findings

      (1) Aphasia, particularly receptive aphasia due to temporal lobe involvement in HSV encephalitis

      (2) Other impairments of cognitive function such as apraxia, visual-spatial difficulties, and acute memory problems

      (3) Hemiparesis

      (4) Ataxia

      (5) Cranial nerve findings: visual field deficit, ophthalmoplegia, nystagmus, facial weakness

    e. Involuntary movements such as myoclonus

    f. Coma and signs of elevated ICP [see HEAD TRAUMA in Chapter 26]

  2. Fever is present.

C. Differential diagnosis

> **Viral encephalitis may be difficult to distinguish from bacterial meningitis.**

---

  1. Fever in the setting of delirium, acute stroke, postictal state, withdrawal state (e.g., alcohol withdrawal), or systemic infection (e.g., aspiration pneumonia or subacute bacterial endocarditis)

  2. Bacterial and viral meningitis

  3. Bacterial encephalitis

    a. *Mycoplasma* infection

    b. Lyme meningoencephalitis

    c. Neurosyphilis

    d. Rickettsiae

  4. Fungal or protozoal meningoencephalitis (cryptococcosis, toxoplasmosis)

  5. Subarachnoid hemorrhage

  6. Subdural hematoma

  7. Cerebral abscess (especially if focal signs are present)

  8. Parameningeal infections

9. Noninfectious, inflammatory etiologies
   a. Vasculitis
   b. Behçet's disease
   c. Sarcoidosis
   d. Postinfectious conditions (e.g., acute cerebellitis of childhood, acute disseminated encephalomyeltis)
   e. Paraneoplastic syndromes (e.g., limbic or brain stem encephalitis)
D. **Diagnostic tests**
   1. **Blood cultures**
   2. **Laboratory tests:** CBC with differential, coagulation studies, electrolytes, calcium, magnesium, phosphate, renal and liver functions, and urinalysis

---

> **When treating suspected viral encephalitis, start empiric antivirals and antibiotics following blood cultures.**

---

   3. **LP**
      a. Perform brain imaging (CT or MRI) and check coagulation parameters before the procedure.
      b. Send CSF for analysis.
         (1) Cell count
             (a) Viral encephalitis: usually 10–500 cells/mm^3 with a predominance of lymphocytes
             (b) HSV encephalitis: xanthochromic or containing RBCs
         (2) Protein (usually > 45 mg/dl)
         (3) Glucose (usually normal but may be slightly decreased)
         (4) Gram's stain
         (5) Bacterial cultures
         (6) PCR for viral detection
         (7) Viral cultures (do not aid with management but are useful epidemiologically, particularly in seasonal outbreaks)
         (8) AFB, cryptococcal antigen, Lyme titer, VDRL, fungal cultures (if appropriate)
   4. Chest x-ray
   5. ECG
   6. CT or MRI of brain with and without contrast
   7. EEG (once patient is stable)
E. **Management**
   1. **Ensure airway management.** Patients with encephalitis may present in stupor or coma or in status epilepticus.
   2. **Provide supportive care** [e.g., nutritional status, deep venous thrombosis (DVT) prophylaxis, physical therapy]. Patients with encephalitis may require prolonged ICU admission.
   3. **Manage severe cerebral edema** with mannitol and steroids.
   4. **Administer antibiotics.**

> **Initial empiric pharmacologic treatment of viral encephalitis frequently requires coverage for acute bacterial meningitis as well.**

    a. If encephalitis is suspected, start acyclovir, 10 mg/kg q 8 hr IV.
        (1) Maintain adequate IV hydration for patients on acyclovir.
        (2) Continue acyclovir for 14 days.
    b. Start empiric antibiotics for bacterial meningitis (see I E 1 c) [usually].
        (1) It is very difficult to differentiate a partially treated bacterial meningitis (e.g., outpatients on oral antibiotics or inpatients on antibiotics for systemic infections) from viral encephalitis on the initial presentation.
        (2) Reevaluate need for antibiotics on the first day following admission.
  5. Treat seizures if suspected by history.
  6. Consider infectious disease and neurology consults.

> **The use of corticosteroids is controversial and is not routinely recommended.**

  7. Perform a brain biopsy only if other treatable conditions (e.g., vasculitis or acute disseminated encephalomyelitis) are possibilities.
E. Complications
  1. Increased ICP
  2. Coma
  3. Seizures
  4. Residual neurologic deficits such as amnesia or other cognitive dysfunction (frequent in HSV encephalitis, where survival is approximately 90% if treatment started within 4 days of onset)

FEVER OF UNKNOWN ORIGIN (FUO)

  I. Definition. FUO is an illness of more than 3 weeks' duration with a fever of > 101°F (38.3°C) on multiple occasions and an uncertain diagnosis after 1 week of intensive investigation.
  II. Etiology. In the ICU, sources of fever may be either noninfectious **(Table 12-1)** or infectious **(Table 12-2)**. The **causes** of FUO number more than 200.
  III. History
    A. Fever
    B. Previous medical problems and dental history
    C. Medications
    D. Surgical history
    E. Exposure to animals and TB

Table 12-1. Noninfectious Sources of Fever in the Intensive Care Unit

Inflammatory conditions
- Reaction to medications
- Reaction to blood products
- Collagen vascular diseases (SLE, rheumatoid arthritis, temporal arthritis, polyarteritis nodosa)
- Vasculitis
    (hypersensitivity, Henoch-Schönlein purpurea, Wegener's granulomatosis, giant cell arteritis)
- Microcrystalline arthritis (gout, pseudogout)
- Postpericardiotomy syndrome
- Pancreatitis
- Reaction to IM injections

Vascular conditions
- Deep venous thrombophlebitis
- Pulmonary embolism
- Dissecting aortic aneurysm
- Bowel ischemia
- Hemorrhage (into CNS, retroperitoneum, joint, lung, or adrenals)

Metabolic conditions
- Heat stroke
- Malignant hyperthermia secondary to anesthesia or medications
- Adrenal insufficiency/hemorrhage
- Alcohol withdrawal
- Seizures
- Neuroleptic malignant syndrome
- Subacute thyroiditis

Neoplasia
- Lymphoma
- Renal cell carcinoma
- Hepatoma
- Malignancy metastatic to liver
- Colon carcinoma
- Atrial myxoma

SLE = systemic lupus erythematosus; IM = intramuscular; CNS = central nervous system.
(Reprinted with permission from George MH, Glew RH: Infectious disease problems in the intensive care unit. In *Irwin and Rippe's Intensive Care Medicine,* 4th ed. Edited by Irwin RS, Cerra FB, Rippe JM. Philadelphia, Lippincott Williams & Wilkins, 1999.)

Table 12-2.   Infectious Sources of Fever in the Intensive Care Unit

Urinary tract conditions
- Pyelonephritis
- Prostatitis, prostatic abscess

Vascular devices
- IV access site
  (phlebitis, bacteremia or fungemia, cellulitis)
- Intra-arterial access site (bacteremia, fungemia)

Respiratory conditions
- Tracheobronchitis
- Pneumonia
- Sinusitis
- Empyema
- Lung abscess

Surgery-related wounds
- Wound infection (superficial or deep)
- Deep-seated abscess
  (liver, spleen, kidney, brain, subphrenic, bowel)

Skin/soft tissue conditions
- Decubitus ulcer
- Cellulitis

Gastrointestinal disorders
- Antibiotic-associated colitis/*Clostridium difficile* colitis
- Ischemic colitis (mesenteric infarction)
- Biliary conditions
  [cholecystitis (including acalculous), cholangitis]
- Hepatitis (transfusion-related) [CMV, HBV, HCV]
- Intraabdominal abscess
- Diverticulitis

Prosthetic device infections
- Cardiac valve/pacemaker
- Joint replacement prosthesis
- Peritoneal dialysis catheter
- CNS intraventricular shunt

Miscellaneous conditions
- Pyarthrosis
- Osteomyelitis
- Meningitis

IV = intravenous; CMV = cytomegalovirus; HBV = hepatitis B virus; HCV = hepatitis C virus; CNS = central nervous system.
(Reprinted with permission from George MH, Glew RH: Infectious disease problems in the intensive care unit. In *Irwin and Rippe's Intensive Care Medicine,* 4th ed. Edited by Irwin RS, Cerra FB, Rippe JM. Philadelphia, Lippincott Williams & Wilkins, 1999.)

   F. Travel history
   G. Trauma history
   H. Family history, social history, and occupational history
IV. Physical Examination

With suspected FUO, a very detailed and thorough head-to-toe examination is of paramount importance.

   A. Eyes
      1. Conjunctiva (conjunctivitis, petechiae as in endocarditis)
      2. Sclera (scleritis in rheumatologic disorders)
      3. Anterior chamber (uveitis)
      4. Pupil dilatation to look for Roth's spot (endocarditis), retinal hemorrhage, vasculitis, retinitis (CMV, toxoplasmosis)
   B. Lymph nodes (especially in the cervical region)
   C. Skin and oral mucous membranes (careful inspection and palpation)
      1. Osler's nodes (red or painful nodules with a whitish center)
      2. Janeway's lesions (nontender red macules on the palms and soles)
      3. Petechiae on the palate
      4. Splinter hemorrhage in the nailbed in infectious endocarditis
      5. Rose spots (blanching pink papules on the trunk) in salmonellosis
      6. Cutaneous hyperpigmentation in Whipple's disease
      7. Cutaneous metastases, leukemic skin changes, or palpable purpura in cutaneous vasculitis
   D. Heart (auscultation for murmurs) [endocarditis or myxoma]
   E. Abdomen (to rule out hepatomegaly or splenomegaly) and rectum
   F. Extremities and joints
   G. Neurologic examination
V. Diagnostic Work-up
   A. Laboratory tests
      1. CBC with differential and platelet count
      2. Electrolytes, liver function tests, lactate dehydrogenase (LDH)
      3. Urinalysis
      4. Erythrocyte sedimentation rate and C-reactive protein
      5. Antinuclear antibodies
      6. Rheumatoid factor
      7. Blood cultures
      8. CMV antibodies
      9. TB skin test
      10. Heterophile antibody
      11. HIV test
      12. Hepatitis screen
      13. Protein electrophoresis

B. **Imaging**
1. Chest radiograph
2. CT scan of head, chest, abdomen, and pelvis
3. Radionuclide scans (gallium 67, indium 111)
4. Echocardiography (transthoracic or transesophageal)
5. Bone scan

C. **Invasive procedures**
1. Biopsy
   a. Skin
   b. Lymph node
   c. Liver
   d. Bone marrow
   e. Temporal artery
2. Laparascopy or laparotomy

VI. **Management**
A. Until the diagnosis is established, antipyretics for symptomatic relief are indicated.
B. Therapy should be directed at the cause. Culture-documented infections are treated with the appropriate antibiotics.

Empiric antibiotic administration (with the exception of culture-negative endocarditis) is not indicated.

C. Presumed temporal arteritis may be managed with low-dose empiric steroids for both diagnostic and therapeutic purposes.
D. An empiric trial with antituberculous drugs is justified in elderly patients in the appropriate clinical setting for TB.

FUNGAL INFECTIONS

I. **Classification**
A. **Pathogenic fungi** (e.g., *Histoplasma, Blastomyces, Coccidioides*)
1. Usually occur in endemic areas
2. Cause infection in hosts with intact immune responses
B. **Opportunistic fungi** (e.g., *Candida, Torulopsis,* Mucoraceae, Phycomycetes, *Aspergillus, Cryptococcus*). Infected patients have:
1. Impaired immune function
2. Loss of normal epithelial barriers

II. **Definitions**
A. **Fungemia:** isolation of a fungal species from one blood culture
B. **Invasive fungal disease:** access of fungus to otherwise sterile tissue and recognition (usually) by pathology or by quantitation ($> 100,000$ isolates per gram of tissue)
C. **Disseminated fungal disease:** noncontiguous invasion of organs with the same fungal isolate resulting from hematogenous spread

III. **Predisposing Factors**

A. **Medications**
   1. Broad-spectrum antibiotics (especially if more than three antibiotics or duration > 7 days)
   2. Steroids

B. **Chronic conditions**
   1. Acute renal failure
   2. Malnutrition
   3. Diabetes mellitus

C. **Altered host defenses**
   1. Trauma
   2. Burns (second- or third-degree)
   3. Indwelling central access catheters
   4. Immunosuppression (including HIV)
   5. APACHE score > 10
   6. Ventilator > 48 hours

D. **Age > 40 years**

E. **Parenteral nutrition**

F. **Peritonitis or intraabdominal access**

IV. **Cryptococcosis**

A. **Epidemiology and etiology**
   1. This opportunistic fungal infection has a worldwide distribution.
   2. The causal pathogen is the encapsulated yeast *Cryptococcus neoformans.*

B. **Clinical presentation**
   1. Meningitis (most common initial manifestation) with fever, headache, neck stiffness, and changes in mental status
   2. Pulmonary disease, either diffuse or focal, with fever, cough, dyspnea, pleuritic chest pain, and hemoptysis
   3. Skin lesions on the face, neck, scalp, or trunk in the form of erythematous papules or pustules
   4. Endopthalmitis with blurred vision and pain, although sometimes asymptomatic
   5. Dissemination (perhaps), with infection of essentially all organs

C. **Diagnostic tests**
   1. **Definitive diagnosis** is culture of the organism from biopsy specimens or body fluids.
   2. Cryptococcal polysaccharide capsular antigen in CSF or other body fluids is both sensitive and specific.
   3. LP shows elevated opening pressure (sometimes), decreased glucose, elevated protein, and lymphocytic pleiocytosis.

**Specimens from lumbar puncture examined
in an Indian ink preparation reveal the
presence of yeast cells with capsules.**

---

   4. CT scan or MRI: in patients with neurologic symptoms (recommended)

V. Candidiasis

A. Epidemiology and etiology

1. Candidiasis, the most commonly occurring fungal infection, is caused by a ubiquitous yeast that colonizes mucosal surfaces.

2. *Candida albicans* is the most common species, with other species of *Candida,* including *C. krusei, C. tropicalis,* and *C. parapsilosis. Torulopsis glabrata,* although usually regarded as a species of *Candida,* is a separate yeast form.

B. Clinical presentation

1. Oral candidiasis may be asymptomatic or with a burning sensation, dry mouth, or taste disturbances. Various manifestations occur.

   a. Pseudomembranous form (white, elevated, removable plaques with a cottage cheese-like appearance)

   b. Erythematous form (flat red patches on the hard or soft palate)

   c. Hyperplastic form (partially removable white plaques)

2. Esophageal candidiasis may manifest as dysphagia, odynophagia, or retrosternal pain. Diagnosis involves endoscopy and mucosal biopsy.

3. Vaginal candidiasis, minor cutaneous candidal infections (paronychia and onychomycosis), and invasive or disseminating candidiasis may also occur. Definitive diagnosis requires identification of pseudohyphae on a KOH preparation or Gram's stain of a specimen from an oral lesion.

VI. Histoplasmosis

A. Epidemiology and etiology

1. Histoplasmosis is the most common endemic mycosis in patients with AIDS. It may be the first manifestation of AIDS in up to 75% of endemic areas.

2. *Histoplasma capsulatum,* the causal agent, is an airborne pathogen that most commonly causes acute pulmonary infection.

B. Clinical presentation

1. **Systemic signs:** fever, weight loss

2. **Respiratory problems:** cough, dyspnea

3. **CNS:** fever; headache; mental status changes; seizures; focal neurologic deficits; CSF findings, including elevated protein; decreased glucose; lymphocytic pleiocytosis

4. **Skin lesions:** erythema multiforme, papules, ulcerative plaques, maculopapules, eczematous lesions, erythematous papules with papulonecrotic centers, lymphadenitis

5. **GI manifestations:** diarrhea, abdominal pain, hepatosplenomegaly, intestinal obstruction, perforation, peritonitis or bleeding

6. Uncommon manifestations: adrenalitis with adrenal insufficiency, pancreatitis, pericarditis, prostatic abscess, septic shock

C. Diagnostic tests

1. **Chest x-ray findings** (related to the stage of the disease process): hilar adenopathy, discrete infiltrates, pleural effusion, diffuse interstitial or reticulonodular infiltrates
2. **Cultures:** fungal isolates from blood, pulmonary secretions, CSF, bone marrow, colon, lymph nodes, brain, liver, urine, peritoneal fluid
3. **Stains** [Gomori's or periodic acid–Schiff (PAS)] (more rapid diagnosis): positive in 50% to 70% of cases (*H. capsulatum* antibodies)

Polysaccharide antigen detection in body fluids by radioimunoassay permits a rapid diagnosis.

VII. **Coccidioidomycosis**

In healthy individuals, coccidioidomycosis may cause mild respiratory illness, but in HIV-infected patients, it may be fatal.

A. **Epidemiology and etiology**
   1. This disease is endemic to central America, Argentina, and the southwestern United States (Arizona, Texas, New Mexico).
   2. The causal pathogen is *Coccidioides immitis,* a soil fungus.
B. **Clinical presentation**
   1. **Pulmonary disease,** with either focal (discrete lung nodules, hilar adenopathy, focal alveolar infiltrates, pleural effusions, or lung cavities) or diffuse findings, that resembles *P. carinii* pneumonia (PCP)
   2. **Meningitis,** with CSF findings, including low glucose, increased protein, lymphocytic pleiocytosis, positive complement-fixation antibody titer
   3. **Cutaneous disease,** with papules, pustules, ulcers, and subcutaneous abscesses
   4. **Dissemination,** with hepatic involvement or localized extrathoracic lymphadenopathy (or other visceral organ involvement such as the heart, pancreas, esophagus, and adrenal glands)
   5. **Positive anticoccidioidal serology** without clinical evidence of infection
C. **Diagnostic tests**
   1. **Culture** of sputum, bronchoalveolar lavage blood, or tissue (positive)
   2. **Coccidioidal tube–precipitin and complement-fixing IgG antibody** (positive in ~90% of HIV-infected patients with active disease)
VIII. **Blastomycosis**
   A. **Etiology**
      1. The causal pathogen is *Blastomyces dermatitis* (a dimorphic fungus), which is found in humid areas with soil of high organic content and acid pH.

        2. Infection is acquired by inhalation of conidia.

B. Clinical presentation

    1. Localized disease

    2. Pulmonary involvement, with fever, cough, dyspnea, and weight loss

    3. Disseminated disease, with weight loss, cough, dyspnea, meningitis, or fulminant sepsis syndrome

C. Diagnostic tests

    1. Chest radiography: demonstration of pleural effusion, bilateral nodules, focal lobar disease, or diffuse interstitial disease

    2. Blood, CSF, or bronchoscopic specimen (positive)

    3. Histopathologic identification (90% of patients)

IX. Aspergillosis

A. Epidemiology and etiology

    1. The causal organisms are *Aspergillus fumigatus* and *Aspergillus flavus,* which are filamentous fungi found in soil, water, and decaying vegetation.

    2. These airborne pathogens have low virulence.

B. Clinical presentation

    1. Pulmonary manifestations (portal of entry: respiratory tract)

        a. Allergic bronchopulmonary aspergillosis

        b. Invasive aspergillosis

        c. Pseudomembranous necrotizing bronchial aspergillosis

        d. Chronic necrotizing aspergillosis

        e. Ulcerative and plaque-like tracheobronchitis

    2. Brain involvement, with symptoms and signs of an abscess

    3. Sinus or orbit disease

        a. Acute, invasive sinusitis (usually)

        b. Otomastoiditis: secondary involvement of temporal lobes (possibly)

    4. Myocardial abscesses, endocarditis with large friable vegetations, pericardial disease

    5. Renal aspergillomas, which can cause fever, low back pain, and hematuria

C. Diagnostic tests

    1. Blood

        a. CBC with differential

        b. Electrolytes

        c. Renal and liver function tests

    2. Cultures

        a. Blood (at least two peripheral) [rarely positive]

        b. Oropharynx, sputum, sputum aspirates

        c. All drain sites, gastric aspirate, wounds

        d. Skin insertion site and tips of vascular catheters

---

Demonstration of *Aspergillus* by both culture and microscopic examination of tissue is necessary for diagnosis.

   3. Urinalysis and urine culture
   4. Stool culture
   5. LP, if neurologic symptoms or signs are present
   6. Chest radiograph
X. Management
   A. Types of treatment. Four broad categories have been identified for the use of antifungal treatment of patients in ICU and surgical patients.
      1. Prophylaxis is the use of an antifungal prior to colonization. It is not routinely indicated.
      2. Preemptive therapy is the initiation of therapy in colonized or high-risk patients to prevent invasion or dissemination. No definite data support this approach, except in high-risk neutropenic patients.
      3. Empiric therapy involves the treatment of patients believed to have deep candidiasis without microbiologic, serologic, or histologic confirmation. Clinical indications for empirical treatment include:
         a. Unstable or deteriorating premature neonates with any skin breaks from which *Candida* has been grown, positive urine microscopy, or positive yeast culture
         b. Candiduria in high-risk patients with deteriorating clinical status
      4. Treatment. Indications include:
         a. Positive blood culture in high-risk patients
         b. Isolation of a fungus from any sterile site (except urine)
         c. Positive microscopy for a yeast from a sterile specimen prior to culture confirmation
         d. Histologic evidence of yeast or mycelial forms in tissue from at-risk patients
   B. Treatment measures for specific fungal diseases
      1. Oral candidiasis. Clotrimazole troches or nystatin suspension should be used.
      2. Positive intravascular catheter tips (> 15 CFU). Changing of the catheter site is necessary.
      3. Severe *Candida* infections. Fluconazole and amphotericin B are currently the only available parenteral antifungal agents. Various studies have reported similar effectiveness of fluconazole when compared to amphotericin B, which has been the gold standard in the past. Indications for amphotericin B include:
         a. Hemodynamic instability
         b. *Candida* endopthalmitis
         c. High-grade candidemia
         d. *C. krusei* and *T. glabrata* infections (organisms resistant to fluconazole)
         e. Cryptococcosis (amphotericin B with or without flucytosine)
         f. Initial treatment of histoplasmosis, blastomycosis, and invasive aspergillosis

    4. Meningitis (with high ICP or hydrocephalus)
        a. Ventricular shunting, high-dose steroids, or frequent lumbar punctures to remove CSF (all possibly necessary)
        b. Suppressive therapy with either fluconazole or amphotericin B
    5. Histoplasmosis
        a. Acute treatment with amphotericin B
        b. Lifelong maintenance (to prevent relapse) with either itraconazole, fluconazole, or amphotericin B
    6. Coccidioidomycosis (in patients with AIDS). Treatment results in a response of < 50%.
        a. Acute treatment: amphotericin B
        b. Long-term maintenance: itraconazole or fluconazole
    7. Blastomycosis
        a. Initial therapy: amphotericin B
        b. Maintenance therapy: itraconazole
    8. Invasive aspergillosis: IV amphotericin B with rifampin or flucytosine for critically ill patients, along with appropriate surgical intervention and lifelong suppression with either amphotericin B or itraconazole

NECROTIZING SOFT TISSUE INFECTIONS

I. Definitions
    A. Necrotizing fasciitis: subcutaneous infection resulting in fascial necrosis and widespread undermining of the skin
    B. Fournier's gangrene: necrotizing fasciitis involving the male genital organs
    C. Clostridial myonecrosis (gas gangrene): fulminant skeletal muscle infection caused by *Clostridium* species
II. Bacteriology of Necrotizing Fasciitis
    A. Polymicrobial (75%) [mixed anaerobes and aerobes]
    B. *Streptococcus* (group A)
    C. *Staphylococcus aureus*
    D. Gram-negative species (*E. coli, Proteus* species)
    E. *Bacillus* species
III. Predisposing Factors
    A. To bacterial inoculation
        1. IV drug abuse (or "skin popping")
        2. Burns
        3. Trauma (blunt or penetrating)
        4. Animal bites
        5. Surgery (wound infection)
        6. Perforated viscus
        7. Skin infections (e.g., varicella)
    B. To spread of infection
        1. IV drug abuse
        2. Diabetes mellitus
        3. Obesity
        4. Malnutrition

5. Advanced age
6. Peripheral vascular disease
7. Immunosuppression (positive HIV status, use of cortico-steroids, chemotherapy)

IV. **Clinical Presentation**

A. **Location of involved sites**
1. Extremity (50%)
2. Perineum or buttock (20%)
3. Trunk (20%)
4. Head or neck (10%)

B. **Skin changes** such as edema, erythema, vesicles, bullae, necrosis

C. **Soft tissue crepitus** (on physical examination)

D. **Local pain at anatomic site**

E. **Fever**

F. **Diabetic ketoacidosis**

G. **Systemic toxicity** manifested by hypotension, tachycardia, tachypnea, acidosis

V. **Laboratory results** (nonspecific)

A. **Leukocytosis** [WBC frequently > 20,000 cells/mm^3]

B. **Hypocalcemia** (secondary to saponification with necrotic fat)

C. **Anemia** (secondary to hemolysis)

D. **Creatine phosphokinase (CPK)** [sensitive but not specific; a normal CPK essentially excludes the diagnosis of muscle necrosis]

VI. **Diagnosis**

A. **Clinical aspects.** The primary basis of diagnosis is history and physical examination.

B. **Radiography**
1. Plain films: unreliable (presence of soft tissue gas, a late finding, in 25%–75% of cases)
2. MRI: sensitive for evaluation of soft tissue processes
3. CT: very sensitive for soft tissue gas (may be performed in patients with history and physical examination inconsistent with necrotizing soft tissue infection)

C. **Bedside procedures** (in patients with equivocal history and physical examination)
1. **Fine-needle aspiration**
   a. This procedure identifies gross pus or bacteria on Gram's stain in 58% of patients with necrotizing soft tissue infections.
   b. The classic Gram's stain for clostridial myonecrosis is abundant gram-positive bacilli but absence of leuko-cytes.
2. Incisional biopsy and frozen section staining
3. Fascial inspection when necrotizing fasciitis is suspected
   a. An incision should be made over the area in question and carried down to the fascia.
   b. Attempts to pass a probe along the fascial plane should be met with resistance.

c. If no resistance is encountered, the diagnosis of necrotizing fasciitis is confirmed.

VII. Management

A. Surgical treatment

1. Immediate and aggressive débridement is critical to successful management of necrotizing soft tissue infections.

> **Surgery should not be delayed for any reason. The time that elapses between diagnosis and initial operation directly influences patient morbidity and mortality.**

2. Objectives of initial operation include:
   a. Thorough wound inspection to determine the extent of soft tissue involvement
   b. Aggressive débridement of all necrotic tissue
   c. Examination of frozen sections to determine the extent of débridement when the border of normal tissue is not obvious
   d. Sampling of wound tissue or exudate for culture and sensitivity

> **Routine reexploration should be performed no later than 24 hours after the initial operation.**

3. Objectives of routine reexploration include:
   a. Ensuring that all necrotic tissue has been débrided, and repeating débridement where necessary
   b. Amputation in the following situations:
      (1) Persistent fulminant infection despite multiple débridements
      (2) Nonfunctional extremity secondary to extensive muscle necrosis
      (3) Circumferential necrotizing fasciitis
4. Diverting colostomy should be performed for patients with necrotizing fasciitis of the perineum.

B. Medical treatment

1. Use of IV antibiotics
   a. Initial (empiric) therapy should cover streptococci, staphylococci, anaerobes, and gram-negative bacteria.
   b. Antibiotics should be changed when necessary according to Gram's stain and culture of the infected tissue.
   c. Antibiotics should be continued until all signs of local wound infection and systemic toxicity have resolved.
   d. Specific regimens include:
      (1) Penicillin + metronidazole + aminoglycoside
      (2) Clindamycin + aminoglycoside
      (3) Ampicillin-sulbactam (Unasyn), ticarcillin-clavulanate (Timentin), or piperacillin-tazobactam (Zosyn)

           (4) Imipenem-cilistatin
      2. Administration of IV fluids
      3. Correction of electrolyte deficits
      4. Use of aggressive nutritional support (enteral whenever
         possible)
      5. Hyperbaric oxygen (HBO) [controversial; no prospec-
         tive study has proven HBO to be useful in necrotizing soft
         tissue infections]
VIII. Prognosis
   A. Mortality (25% overall)
   B. Factors that influence mortality
      1. Systolic blood pressure (BP) on admission
      2. Size of infection (as determined by the initial débride-
         ment)
      3. Time from diagnosis to operation
      4. Disease location (higher mortality in perineal disease)

PNEUMONIA

   I. Aspiration Pneumonia. See ASPIRATION SYNDROMES in Chapter
      19.
  II. Community-Acquired Pneumonia (CAP)
   A. Epidemiology
      1. An estimated 4 million cases of CAP, with 600,000 hospi-
         talizations, occur annually in the United States, at a cost
         of $23 billion.
      2. Pneumonia, the sixth leading cause of death in the
         United States, is the most common cause of death from
         infectious diseases.
   B. Risk factors
      1. Congestive heart failure (CHF)
      2. Age > 65 years
      3. Previous viral respiratory tract infection
      4. HIV infection or immunosuppression secondary to med-
         ication or other disease
      5. Aspiration
      6. Underlying lung disease
   C. Etiology. Generally, pathogenic organisms can be classified
      into two groups: (1) microbes that are inherently virulent
      and cause pneumonia in normal and immunocompromised
      hosts, and (2) agents of lower virulence that are pathogenic
      because of impaired immune defenses.
      1. Bacteria
         a. *S. pneumoniae* (20%–60%)
         b. *H. influenzae* (3%–10%)
         c. *S. aureus* (3%–5%)
         d. Gram-negative bacteria (3%–5%)
         e. Atypical agents (10%–20%)
            (1) *Legionella* (2%–8%)
            (2) *Mycoplasma pneumoniae* (1%–6%)

        (3) *Chlamydia pneumoniae* (4%–6%)
- **2.** Viruses (2%–15%)

D. Clinical presentation
- **1.** Fever [< 101.5°F (38.6°C)]
- **2.** Cough, sputum production
- **3.** Dyspnea
- **4.** Pleurisy
- **5.** Tachypnea
- **6.** Tachycardia
- **7.** Specific findings on physical examination
  - **a.** Crackles on auscultation
  - **b.** Rash or petechiae
  - **c.** Heart murmurs or friction rubs

E. Diagnostic tests
- **1. Laboratory tests**
  - **a. All patients**
    - **(1)** WBC count with differential
    - **(2)** Sputum Gram's stain and culture
  - **b. Seriously ill patients**
    - **(1)** Electrolytes and renal and liver function tests
    - **(2)** ABG analysis
    - **(3)** Blood cultures
    - **(4)** Mycoplasma IgM
  - **c. Pleural fluid analysis** (if available)
    - **(1)** WBC and differential
    - **(2)** LDH
    - **(3)** pH
    - **(4)** Protein
    - **(5)** Glucose
    - **(6)** Gram's stains, including stains for AFB
    - **(7)** Culture for bacteria and mycobacteria
- **2. Chest radiography**
  - **a.** Lobar or segmental consolidation
  - **b.** Bronchopneumonia
  - **c.** Interstitial infiltrates
  - **d.** Cavitary lesions
- **3. CT scan** (more sensitive)
  - **a.** Interstitial disease
  - **b.** Empyema
  - **c.** Cavitation
  - **d.** Adenopathy
  - **e.** Multifocal disease

F. Management
- **1. Antibiotics.** All patients with CAP should receive antibiotics directed against the identified pathogens from the sputum and blood cultures (Table 12-3).
  - **a. Empiric antibiotics**
    - **(1) Outpatients (adults):** oral macrolide, doxycycline, amoxicillin, or cephalosporin
    - **(2) Inpatients:** IV second- or third- generation cephalosporin with or without erythromycin un-

Table 12-3. Antibiotic Agents in the Treatment of Community-Acquired Pneumonia

Pathogen	Preferred Antibiotic(s)	Alternative Antibiotic(s)
Streptococcus pneumoniae	Penicillin	Cephalosporin (first- or second-generation), macrolide, or doxycycline
Haemophilus influenzae	Ampicillin, cefuroxime, or TMP-SMX	Fluoroquinolone or doxycycline
Staphylococcus aureus	Oxacillin or nafcillin with or without gentamicin	Cefuroxime, ceftriaxone, or vancomycin
Moraxella catarrhalis	Cephalosporin (second- or third-generation) or TMP-SMX	Macrolide, fluoroquinolone, or doxycycline
Anaerobes	Clindamycin	Penicillin with metronidazole
Gram-negative bacteria	Cephalosporin (second- or third-generation) with or without an aminoglycoside	Fluoroquinolone or imipenem
Legionella	Erythromycin or ciprofloxacin	Clarithromycin
Mycoplasma pneumoniae	Doxycycline or erythromycin	Clarithromycin or fluoroquinolone
Chlamydia pneumoniae	Doxycycline or erythromycin	Clarithromycin or fluoroquinolone
Nocardia	Sulfonamide or TMP-SMX	Doxycycline or imipenem
Chlamydia psittaci	Doxycycline	Chloramphenicol
Coxilla burnetii	Doxycycline	Chloramphenicol
Influenza A virus	Amantadine or rimantadine	
Hantavirus	Supportive care and inotropes	Ribavirin (experimental)

TMP-SMX = trimethoprim-sulfamethoxazole.

til patients are afebrile for > 24 hours and oxygen saturation $> 95\%$, when they can begin receiving the oral form

  (3) Oral fluoroquinolones: acceptable alternatives for Legionnaires' disease, mycoplasma pneumonia, and chlamydia pneumonia

  b. **Duration of therapy** (arbitrary)

  (1) Common bacterial pneumonia: 5–10 days
  (2) Mycoplasma pneumonia: 10–14 days
  (3) Legionnaires' disease: 14–21 days

2. **Follow-up.** Radiography should be used to document pulmonary clearance for patients with delayed responses, recurrent pneumonia, or with suspected bronchogenic neoplasm or underlying lung disease.

H. **Prognosis**

  1. **Mortality rate** is low for outpatients with CAP, and it is 10% to 25% for hospitalized patients with the disease.

  2. **Prognosis** is poor with the following factors:

  a. Age > 65 years

  b. Comorbidity, including diabetes, renal failure, heart failure, chronic disease, alcoholism, immunosuppression, and neoplasm

  c. Respiratory rate > 30 breaths/min, systolic BP < 90 mm Hg, diastolic BP < 60 mm Hg, $PO_2 < 60$ mm Hg on room air

  d. Extrapulmonary site of infection (meningitis, septic arthritis)

  e. WBC < 4000 cells/mm^3 or $> 30,000$/mm^3

  f. Altered mental status

  g. Hematocrit $< 30\%$

  h. Chest x-ray showing multiple lobe involvement, rapid spread, or pleural effusion

  i. Pathogens such as *S. pneumoniae*, *Legionella*, or *S. aureus*

I. **Prevention**

  1. Identification of high-risk populations

  2. Administration of influenza vaccine and pneumococcal vaccine

III. **Hospital-Acquired Pneumonia (HAP)**

  A. **Definition.** HAP is **any pneumonia that occurs > 48 hours after admission** to the hospital, excluding any infection that is incubating at the time of admission.

  B. **Epidemiology**

  1. The **incidence** is 5–10 cases per 1000 admissions, which may increase by a factor of as much as 6 to 20 in patients on ventilators.

  2. Currently the **second most common nosocomial infection** in the United States, HAP has the **highest morbidity and mortality.**

  3. HAP results in **increased hospital stays** (average of 7–9 days per patient).

C. Risk factors
1. Patient-related factors
  a. Coma
  b. Advanced age (> 70 years)
  c. Malnutrition
  d. Prolonged hospitalization
  e. Hypotension
  f. Cigarette smoking
  g. Metabolic acidosis
  h. Severe acute or chronic illness (e.g., COPD, diabetes mellitus, renal failure, respiratory failure)
2. Infection control and intervention-related factors
  a. No washing of hands or changing of gloves between patients
  b. Use of contaminated respiratory therapy devices and equipment
  c. Prolonged or complicated thoracoabdominal procedures
  d. Medications [e.g., sedatives, corticosteroids, cytotoxic agents, antacids, histamine (H_2) blockers, antibiotics (prolonged and inappropriate use)]
  e. Nasogastric or endotracheal tubes
D. Etiology and Pathogenesis
1. Essential requirements (at least one)
  a. Impaired host defenses
  b. Presence of a virulent pathogen
  c. Sufficient number of causal organisms in the lower respiratory tract
2. Improper infection control
  a. Aspiration of esophageal or gastric contents
  b. Hematogenous spread from a distant site
  c. Exogenous penetrations from an infected site (pleural space)
  d. Microaspiration of oropharyngeal flora colonized with pathogenic bacteria
  e. Direct inoculation into the airways of intubated patients
3. Causal pathogens
  a. Enteric gram-negative bacteria (*Enterobacter* species, *E. coli*, *Klebsiella* species, *Proteus* species, *Serratia marcesens*, *H. influenzae*)
  b. *S. aureus,* including MRSA [most commonly seen in patients with head trauma, coma, renal failure, diabetes mellitus]
  c. Polymicrobial etiology (50% of patients on mechanical ventilators)
  d. Anaerobes (recent abdominal surgery, witnessed aspiration)
  e. *Legionella* (high-dose steroids)
  f. *Pseudomonas aeruginosa* (prolonged ICU stay, antibiotics, steroids, structural lung disease)

F. Clinical presentation
   1. Fever, chills
   2. Dyspnea
   3. Purulent sputum
   4. Tachypnea
   5. Tachycardia
   6. Changes in mental status
G. Diagnostic tests
   1. CBC with differential
   2. Sputum culture and Gram's stain
   3. Blood culture
   4. Chest radiograph (new pulmonary infiltrate)
   5. Bronchoscopy or bronchoalveolar lavage (BAL) [see Chapter 30]
H. Management

Begin empiric treatment of HAP when the presumptive diagnosis is made.

---

   1. **Empiric treatment**
      a. Sputum with gram-positive organisms: oxacillin or vancomycin
      b. Sputum with gram-negative organisms
         (1) Nonintubated patients: third-generation cephalosporin
         (2) Ventilator-dependent patients: aminoglycoside plus extended-spectrum penicillin, fluoroquinolone, third-generation cephalosporin, extended-spectrum penicillin with β-lactamase inhibitor or imipenem
      c. Postaspiration pneumonia: clindamycin

Tailor therapy based on organism identification and sensitivity.

---

   2. **Duration of therapy**
      a. Gram-positive infections (except MRSA): 5 days
      b. MRSA: 3 weeks
      c. Gram-negative infections: 7–10 days
IV. Ventilator-Associated Pneumonia (VAP)
   A. Definition and background
      1. VAP is a **parenchymal pulmonary infection that occurs in patients with respiratory failure who have required mechanical ventilation for at least 48 hours** prior to the onset of the infection.
      2. The **development of multiple infections** is frequent in patients with suspected VAP.
      3. Only 30% of ventilated patients with chest x-rays suggestive of pneumonia have histologically defined infections. **Noninfectious causes of pulmonary infiltrates** include:
         a. Aspiration pneumonitis

    b. ARDS
    c. Pulmonary contusion
    d. Atelectasis
    e. CHF
    f. Tumor

> **Injudicious use of antibiotics in VAP leads to colonization of the upper and lower airways with resistant organisms. Superinfections by these organisms increase mortality.**

B. Etiology and pathogenesis
  1. Colonization of the oropharynx, which is usually free of pathogenic organisms
    a. Transcolonization from contiguous structures (sinuses, tooth plaque, GI tract)
    b. Gram-negative oropharyngeal colonization in critically ill patients (often)
  2. Aspiration of oropharyngeal or GI contents into the lower airways
    a. Secretions that pool above the cuff of the endotracheal tube can be easily aspirated when the cuff pressure decreases.
    b. Gastric contents can be similarly aspirated.
    c. Suction catheters, positioned above the cuff of the endotracheal tube, reduce the incidence of pneumonia.
    d. Bacterial "coating" of the endotracheal tube occurs after the tube has been in place for more than 24 hours. Positive pressure ventilation or frequent suctioning may disperse the bacteria more distally.
  3. Causal organisms
    a. Frequently isolated organisms
      (1) *P. aeruginosa*
      (2) *S. aureus*
      (3) *Enterobacter*
      (4) *Klebsiella*
      (5) *E. coli*
    b. Infrequently isolated organisms
      (1) Anaerobes
      (2) *S. pneumoniae*
      (3) *Moraxella*
      (4) *Legionella*
C. Clinical presentation
  1. Fever
  2. Leukocytosis
  3. Purulent tracheal secretions
  4. New or progressive pulmonary infiltrate
D. Diagnostic procedures

> **Antibiotic therapy affects the sensitivity and specificity of any microbial culture.**

1. **Open lung biopsy**
   a. This diagnostic standard requires an invasive procedure.
   b. Histopathologic evidence of infection includes bacteria, neutrophils, and cellular debris within the terminal bronchioles.
2. **Endotracheal aspirate cultures**
   a. Unreliable for diagnosis of VAP
   b. Positive aspirate cultures in most patients with an endotracheal tube
   c. Sensitivity = 80%; specificity = 25% (many false-positives)
3. **Bronchoscopic-guided protected sampling brush (PSB) culture**
   a. Quantitative culture of brush tip samples
   b. Growth rate considered significant: $> 10^3$ CFU/ml
   c. Sensitivity = 40%; specificity = 80% (only 40% in patients on antibiotics)
4. **Bronchoalveolar lavage** (BAL)
   a. Quantitative culture of BAL fluid (see Chapter 30)
   b. Growth rate considered significant: $> 10^4$ CFU/ml
   c. Sensitivity = 65%; specificity = 65%
   d. Presence of $< 50\%$ neutrophils: closely correlates with the absence of pneumonia

E. **Management**
   1. **Antibiotics**
      a. Once pneumonia is suspected based on clinical criteria, antibiotics can be started empirically. However, VAP is caused by a wide variety of organisms, making it difficult to select empiric therapy.
      b. The choice of antibiotics may be guided by tracheal aspirate cultures. Antibiotic therapy depends on the organism isolated by quantitative culture.
      c. UTI, line infection, sinusitis, wound infection, and DVT should be ruled out. Then PSB or BAL should be performed on all patients with no other apparent source of infection. If a patient is not responding adequately or the clinical picture is more complex, PSB or BAL may guide therapy.
   2. **Therapeutic bronchoscopy**
      a. This procedure should be performed immediately following an episode of frank aspiration.
      b. This treatment is appropriate for patients with lobar or complete lung collapse.
   3. **Tracheostomy** in ventilator-dependent patients
      a. **Indications**
         (1) Patients who are ventilator-dependent for > 2 weeks and not actively weaning
         (2) Patients expected to be ventilator-dependent for > 2 weeks [e.g., traumatic brain injury (TBI)]

    b. Timing
- **(1)** Tracheostomy should occur as soon as one of the above indications is met.
- **(2)** In patients with TBI, early tracheostomy (before the seventh hospital day) requires significantly fewer days of mechanical ventilation, has fewer severe respiratory tract infections, and necessitates shorter courses of IV antibiotics.

F. Mortality rate
1. ICU patients: 50% to 70%
2. Similarly ill patients without VAP: 25%
3. ARDS + VAP: > 70%

V. *Pneumocystis carinii* Pneumonia (PCP)

A. Etiology and pathogenesis
1. *Pneumocystis carinii,* the causal pathogen, is a unicellular eukaryote with a ubiquitous geographic distribution. Although *P. carinii* was traditionally considered a protozoan, it has recently been identified as a fungus based on ultrastructural and staining characteristics.
2. *P. carinii* exists in two forms:
   - **a.** Trophozoite
   - **b.** Cyst
3. The presumed method of natural acquisition is via an airborne route. After *P. carinii* enters the respiratory tract, it causes a mild subclinical infection in immunocompetent hosts and then remains as a lung saprophyte that may be reactivated during immunosuppression.

B. Risk factors. The primary predisposing factor for the proliferation of *P. carinii* is impaired cellular immunity. Conditions that put patients at risk include:
1. AIDS
2. Bone marrow transplantation
3. High-dose chemotherapy
4. Hodgkin's disease
5. Acute lymphocytic leukemia
6. Protein malnutrition

C. PCP in patients with AIDS
1. The incidence of PCP in patients with AIDS is decreasing.
2. Of the HIV-infected patients who receive primary prophylaxis for PCP, 28% develop the pneumonia at some time during their illness, despite prophylaxis; 15% develop PCP as the initial AIDS-defining illness.
3. Of the HIV-infected patients who do *not* receive primary prophylaxis for PCP, 46% of patients develop PCP as the initial AIDS-defining illness.

D. Clinical presentation
1. Fever, chills
2. Dyspnea, chest pain
3. Cough, sputum production
4. Tachypnea
5. Tachycardia

  6. Rales
  7. Spontaneous pneumothorax or acute bronchospasm
  8. Extrapulmonary manifestations (rare) [e.g., manifestations in the lymph nodes, bone marrow, liver, or spleen]
E. **Radiographic findings: chest x-ray**
  1. Diffuse or interstitial pulmonary infiltrates
  2. Upper lobe disease, cyst formation (multiple, thin-walled, subpleural cysts), or pneumothorax
  3. Blebs, bullae, cavitation, and nodular infiltrates (occasionally)
  4. Normal appearance (10%–30% of cases)
F. **Diagnostic tests**
  1. **Laboratory results**
     a. CBC with differential: elevated WBC count
     b. CD4 count: patients with CD4 count < 200 cells/mm^3 are at high risk
     c. ABG: hypoxemia, increased alveolar-arterial gradient, or hypocarbia
     d. Serum LDH: elevated in 90% of patients
  2. **Other tests**
     a. Bronchoscopic BAL with or without transbronchial biopsy (to establish PCP)
     b. Sputum induction (very sensitive in HIV-infected patients but not in others)
G. **Management**
  1. TMP-SMX (first-line drug) for 21 days
  2. Pentamidine (second-line drug) for 21 days
  3. Alternative therapies such as trimethoprim and dapsone, clindamycin, and primaquine or trimetrexate for 21 days
  4. Adjunctive steroids [required in patients with moderate-to-severe PCP (defined as PO$_2$ < 70 mm Hg or alveolar-arterial gradient > 35 mm Hg)]
     a. Administration: at the onset or within the first 72 hours of antimicrobial therapy
     b. Prednisone dosage: 80 mg a day for 5 days, then 40 mg a day for 5 days, then 20 mg a day until completion of PCP therapy
H. **PCP prophylaxis**
  1. **Indications**
     a. CD4 count < 200 cells/mm^3
     b. Prior episode of PCP
     c. History of oropharyngeal candidiasis
     d. Unexplained fever [$> 100°$F ($37.8°$C)] for > 2 weeks
  2. **Drug regimens**
     a. TMP-SMX: 1 double-strength tablet daily
     b. Dapsone: 100 mg PO daily
     c. Aerosolized pentamidine
I. **Prognosis**
  1. The mortality rate from PCP varies from 5% to 43%.
  2. Patients who require mechanical ventilation have a median survival time of 1.65 years.

URINARY TRACT INFECTIONS (UTIs)

I. **Definitions**
  A. **UTI:** presence of microorganisms in the urinary tract, including the kidneys, collecting system, bladder, and prostate
  B. **Bacteriuria:** presence of bacteria in the urine, which usually occurs as a result of infection or contamination

II. **Pathogenesis**
  A. **Types or methods of spread**
    1. **Non–hospital-acquired UTI**
        a. This condition results from the entry of bacteria into the bladder that colonize the vaginal introitus or the anterior urethra.
        b. In the female, the short urethra and the proximity of urethral meatus to the rectum facilitate the colonization and entrance of bacteria into the bladder.
    2. **Hematogenous spread**
    3. **Lymphatic spread**
    4. **Colovesicle fistula**
  B. **Causal pathogens** (> 95% of UTIs are caused by a single species)
    1. *E. coli*
    2. *Staphylococcus saprophyticus*
    3. *P. mirabilis*
    4. *Klebsiella pneumoniae*
    5. Enterococci
    6. *Pseudomonas* species
    7. Yeast

III. **Clinical Presentation**
  A. Dysuria, urgency, frequency
  B. Fever, chills
  C. Flank pain, low back pain, low abdominal heaviness
  D. Costovertebral tenderness or hypogastric tenderness (possible)

IV. **Diagnostic Tests**
  A. Urinalysis (centrifuged midstream urine sample)
    1. WBC > 5–10 cells per high-power field or presence of bacteria (possible)
    2. Positive leukocyte esterase or positive nitrites on urine dipstick (possible)
    3. Urine culture with more than 100,000 CFU/ml of urine
  B. CBC with differential: possible leukocytosis with left shift
  C. Other diagnostic tests (see VI A–G)

V. **Management.** Therapeutic decisions are usually dictated by various factors, including sex, primary infection versus recurrence, and the nature of the UTI (e.g., complicated versus uncomplicated, catheter-associated).

VI. **Specific Types of UTIs**
  A. **Acute uncomplicated cystitis in women**
    1. **Pathogens:** *E. coli* (80%), *S. saprophyticus* (5%–15%), oc-

casionally *Klebsiella* species, *P. mirabilis,* or other microorganisms

2. **Predisposing factors:** sexual intercourse, use of diaphragm and spermicide, delayed postcoital micturition; history of recent UTI, diabetes, pregnancy

3. **Clinical presentation:** abrupt onset of severe dysuria, increased frequency, suprapubic pain or low back pain, suprapubic tenderness on examination

4. **Diagnostic tests:** urinalysis revealing pyuria

5. **Treatment:** two options
   a. TMP-SMX or ciprofloxacin for 3 days (empiric regimen)
   b. TMP-SMX or ciprofloxacin for 7 days (women > 75 years; those with diabetes, recent UTI, diaphragm use, duration of symptoms > 7 days)

B. **Recurrent infections in women**

1. **Cause:** primarily from reinfection but occasionally from noneradicated focus of infection

2. **Predisposing factors:** use of diaphragm and spermicide, genetic predisposition, postmenopausal status, and (rarely) anatomic or functional abnormalities of the urinary tract

3. **Diagnosis:** documentation by at least one urine culture

4. **Treatment:** several options
   a. Postcoital prophylaxis, continuous prophylaxis, or therapy initiated by the patient
   b. Estradiol cream (topical) in postmenopausal women

C. **Acute uncomplicated pyelonephritis in young women**

1. **Pathogens:** *E. coli, P. mirabilis, K. pneumoniae, S. saprophyticus*

2. **Clinical presentation:** severity varies from mild to moderate illness to urosepsis, with nausea, vomiting, fevers, chills, flank pain, and costovertebral tenderness

3. **Laboratory diagnosis**
   a. CBC with differential (increased WBC count with left shift) [perhaps], electrolytes, and BUN/creatinine
   b. Blood cultures
   c. Urinalysis as well as urine culture and sensitivity

4. **Treatment:** varies according to severity of illness
   a. For **illness that is not severe** and for reliable patients who have no nausea or vomiting, consider TMP-SMX or ciprofloxacin for 10–14 days.
   b. For **severe illness, urosepsis, or pregnancy,** treatment is more complex.
      (1) Admit for hydration and IV antibiotics such as ceftriaxone, ciprofloxacin, or gentamicin until fever has subsided, and then give ciprofloxacin for a total of 14 days.
      (2) If the patient does not improve in 72 hours, repeat cultures and consider ultrasound or CT to rule out perinephric or intrarenal abscess or ob-

struction and other unknown urologic abnormalities.

c. Obtain a follow-up urine culture in 2 weeks after the completion of treatment.

D. Complicated UTIs

1. **Causes:** anatomic, functional, or metabolic abnormalities of the urinary tract or by organisms that are resistant to antibiotics

2. **Severity:** ranges from mild cystitis to frank urosepsis

3. **Pathogens:** *E. coli, Proteus* species, *Klebsiella* species, *Pseudomonas* species, *Serratia* species, enterococci, staphylococci

4. **Diagnostic tests:** urinalysis and urine culture and sensitivity; consider radiologic investigation of the urinary tract

5. **Treatment:** varies according to severity of illness

   a. For empiric therapy in patients with **mild-to-moderate illness,** give oral ciprofloxacin for 10–14 days.

   b. For patients who are **critically ill,** consider IV ampicillin and gentamicin or imipenem for 10–14 days (may change to oral treatment after clinical improvement).

   c. Modify treatment when identification and susceptibilities are known.

   d. Identify and correct the underlying urinary tract abnormality.

   e. Obtain urine culture 2 weeks after the completion of the therapy.

E. UTIs in young men

1. **Pathogenesis:** usually an indication of an underlying urologic abnormality (men < 50 years of age)

2. **Risk factors:** homosexuality, lack of circumcision, sexual partner with a vaginal colonization by uropathogens, HIV infection with a CD4 count < 400 cells/mm^3

3. **Diagnostic tests:** urinalysis and urine culture and sensitivity

> **If young men with UTIs respond to therapy, further work-up is usually noncontributory.**

4. **Treatment:** TMP-SMX or a fluoroquinolone for 7 days

F. Catheter-associated UTIs

1. **Epidemiology**

   a. More than 1 million catheter-associated UTIs occur in the United States every year.

   b. Catheter-associated UTIs are probably the most common cause of gram-negative sepsis in hospitalized patients. Almost all patients who are catheterized for more than 4 weeks develop bacteriuria.

2. **Prevention**

   a. Sterile insertion and care of catheters, prompt removal, and use of closed collecting systems

      b. Replacement of catheters that have been in place for more than 2 weeks when treating UTI

> **Urinary catheters should be removed as soon as they have served their purpose.**

   3. Treatment. Symptomatic bacterial infections should be treated as complicated UTIs on the basis of antimicrobial sensitivities.
     a. Consider changing the catheter.
     b. If the isolate is a yeast (*Candida* or *Torulopsis*), consider fluconazole or amphotericin B bladder irrigation.

G. Asymptomatic bacteriuria in patients without catheters
   1. Diagnostic test. The **criterion for infection is > 100,000 CFU/ml** on two consecutive cultures.
   2. Screening. Pregnant women in the first trimester should be screened for bacteriuria, and **patients scheduled for urologic surgery** should be screened for asymptomatic bacteriuria.
   3. Treatment. Children and pregnant women with asymptomatic bacteriuria should receive treatment. A 3-day regimen of oral TMP-SMX or cephalosporin is usually sufficient.

WOUND INFECTIONS: ANTIBIOTIC PROPHYLAXIS AND MANAGEMENT

I. Classification of Operative Wounds
  A. Types of wounds. Operative wounds may generally be grouped in **four ways (Table 12-4).**
    1. Clean wounds
    2. Clean contaminated wounds
    3. Contaminated wounds
    4. Dirty wounds
  B. General risks of wound infection. The **risk of infection** for each type of operative wound is presented in Table 12-4. Each institution should further define these risks based on the particular frequency of wound infections for each type of operative procedure.

II. Factors Associated With Postoperative Infection
  A. Patient Factors
    1. Adults
     a. Malnutrition
     b. Obesity
     c. Diabetes mellitus, peripheral vascular disease
     d. Hypoxemia
     e. Hypovolemia
     f. Immunocompromised status
     g. High ASA classification (i.e., IV or V)

Table 12-4. Classification of Operative Wounds

Type of Wound	Risk of Infection*	Characteristics
Clean	2.1%–2.6%	Elective procedure
		Primarily closed and undrained
		No inflammation
		No transection of GI, GU, oral, biliary, or tracheo-bronchial systems
		No break in sterile technique
Clean contaminated	3.3%–8.0%	Emergency clean case
		Controlled opening of GI, GU, oral, biliary, or tracheo-bronchial systems
		Reoperation via clean incision within 7 days
		Blunt trauma
		Minimal spillage from hollow organ
		Minor break in sterile technique
Contaminated	6.4%–28%	Chronic open wound to be grafted
		Penetrating trauma less than 4 hours old
		Acute, nonpurulent inflammation
		Major spillage from hollow organ
		Major break in sterile technique
Dirty	7.1%–41.2%	Purulence or abscess
		Preoperative perforation of GI, GU, biliary, or tracheo-bronchial systems
		Penetrating trauma more than 4 hours old

GI = gastrointestinal; GU = genitourinary.
*The information in this table is only a general guideline. The risk of wound infection must be defined by prevalence according to type of case in each institution.

    h. Elderly status (age > 70)
       (1) Decreased immune function
       (2) Decreased healing of skin wounds
       (3) Chronic disease (e.g., diabetes mellitus, periph-

eral vascular disease, coronary artery disease, renal failure, COPD)

(4) High incidence of asymptomatic bacteremia

B. **Operative Factors**

1. **Perioperative factors**

   a. Long preoperative hospitalization
   b. No preoperative shower
   c. Early shaving of site
   d. Hair removal
   e. Prior antibiotic therapy

2. **General**

   a. Intraoperative contamination
   b. Lengthy operation
   c. Hypotension
   d. Massive transfusion

3. **Vascular surgery–related**

   a. Surgery on the lower extremity
   b. Delayed surgery
   c. Diabetes mellitus
   d. Past history of vascular surgery
   e. Short (8-hour) antimicrobial prophylaxis

III. **Causal Pathogens (Table 12-5)**

IV. **Methods for Prevention of Wound Infections.** Important perioperative concerns are vigilance regarding aseptic techniques and antimicrobial prophylaxis.

A. **Preoperative**

1. Antimicrobial shower
2. Hair removal by clipping in incision area

B. **Intraoperative**

1. Gentle manipulation of the tissues
2. Minimal use of foreign bodies (e.g., mesh implants, sutures)
3. Obliterating dead space
4. Strict hemostasis

C. **Postoperative**

1. Closed suction
2. Wound surveillance

V. **Prophylactic Antibiotics**

A. **Administration.** These agents should initially be given 30 minutes prior to the incision and again during the procedure if time requires (see Table 12-5).

B. **Usefulness.** Prophylaxis is not effective beyond the operating room.

VI. **Management of Postoperative Wound Infections**

A. **Extent of infection**

1. **Contamination**

   a. Involves the presence of bacteria in normally sterile tissue
   b. Removal of minimal bacteria and adjuncts of infections effected by host defenses
   c. Examples: perforated appendicitis, duodenal ulcer

Table 12-5. Pathogens Responsible for Operative Wound Infections and Suggested Prophylactic Antibiotics

Type of Procedure	Pathogens	Suggested Antibiotics for Prophylaxis
Skin and soft tissue	*Streptococcus* sp, *Staphylococcus* sp	Oxacillin, penicillin, cefazolin
Colorectal	*Enterococcus* sp, *Bacteroides* sp, *Enterobacter* sp	Cefotetan; cefoxitin; cefotaxime; ampicillin or vancomycin + gentamicin or aztreonam + metronidazole
Gastroduodenal	*Streptococcus viridans, Staphylococcus aureus, Escherichia coli, Candida* sp, anaerobes, enteric gram-negative bacilli	Cefazolin or vancomycin
Vascular	*S. aureus, Staphylococcus epidermidis,* enteric gram-negative bacilli	Cefazolin or vancomycin
Cardiac	*S. aureus, S. epidermidis,* enteric gram-negative bacilli	Cefazolin or vancomycin
Head and neck	*S. aureus, Streptococcus* sp, oral anaerobes	Clindamycin, cefazolin, penicillin
Biliary	*S. aureus, S. epidermidis, E. coli, Klebsiella* sp, *Proteus* sp, *Enterobacter* sp, *Entercoccus* sp, *Clostridium* sp	Mezlocillin; ampicillin + sulbactam
Obstetrics and gynecology	Group B streptococcus, anaerobes, *Enterococcus* sp, enteric gram-negative bacilli	Cefazolin or vancomycin

Contamination does not warrant use of postoperative antibiotics, because the infectious source is dealt with at the time of surgery.

2. **Resectable infection**
   a. Involves infectious processes contained within the involved organ
   b. Treatment by excision
   c. Examples: appendicitis, cholecystitis
3. **Frank infection**
   a. Stratification according to severity

        b. Example: frank peritonitis (does not require a post-operative antibiotic course beyond 5 days)
- **4. Complex infection**
  - **a.** Severe infection where source cannot be readily removed
  - **b.** Example: infected pancreatic necrosis where nidus is not removed

B. Diagnosis of wound infection
1. High index of suspicion
2. Careful observation on a daily basis
3. Evidence of erythema, warmth, tenderness, discharge, or fluctuance in or around the wound

> **If signs of a wound infection appear within 24 hours of surgery, streptococcal or clostridial infection should be considered.**

C. Treatment
1. Open, culture, and débride wound.
2. Pack wound twice daily with wet-to-dry dressings.
3. Examine wound daily for signs of progression or dehiscence.
4. Do not administer antibiotics for a wound infection unless systemic manifestations are present (e.g., sepsis, cellulitis).
5. The **presence of fever and leukocytosis at the end of antibiotic therapy** usually represents **sterile peritonitis** or **a systemic inflammatory response.** This is **an indication to look for another source** (i.e., abscess).
6. The phase when infection is cured but severe peritoneal and systemic inflammation exists is called **tertiary peritonitis.** Further antimicrobial administration is unnecessary unless a proven source of infection is present.

D. Duration of antibiotic therapy for some common operative conditions
1. **Appendicitis** (nonperforated appendicitis: single dose; perforated appendicitis: 3 days)
2. **Ulcer perforation** (< 12 hours: single dose; > 12 hours: 4 days)
3. **Colonic injury** (< 12 hours: single dose; > 12 hours: 3.5 days)
4. **Diverticulitis** (local peritonitis: 4.5 days; diffuse peritonitis: 5 days)
5. **Intestinal ischemia** (1 day)

VII. Disorders of Wound Healing
- **A. Abdominal wound dehiscence**
  - **1. Causes**
    - **a.** Imperfect technical closure
    - **b.** Increased intraabdominal pressure (bowel distention, ascites, coughing, vomiting, straining)
    - **c.** Hematoma with or without infection

  d. Wound infection
  e. Comorbidity (e.g., diabetes mellitus, uremia, malignancy)
  f. Tissue inadequate for strong closure
  g. Malnutrition
  h. Age (> 70 years)
  i. Respiratory failure
2. Diagnosis
  a. High degree of suspicion
  b. Inspection of wound for infection, necrosis or breakdown of fascia, clear fluid discharge from wound, laxity of sutures, or evisceration of abdominal contents

---

If wound dehiscence is a possibility, the wound should be probed with a sterile finger, and fascia and suture integrity should be assessed.

---

3. Treatment
  a. Débride the wound operatively.
  b. Consider fascial biopsies for infection.
  c. Reclose the wound operatively.
  d. Consider use of retention sutures.
  e. Leave the skin open to close by secondary intention if infection is possible. Otherwise, consider closure with strict surveillance of the wound.
B. Anastomostic leaks
  1. Causes
    a. Ischemia
    b. Imperfect technical anastomosis
    c. Tension across the anastomosis
    d. Contamination (localized or gross)
    e. Distal obstruction
  2. Diagnosis
    a. High degree of suspicion
    b. Elevated WBC, fever, abdominal tenderness, sepsis or hemodynamic instability
    c. CT scan (or upper and lower GI study) with water-soluble contrast showing leakage of contrast into the abdomen or an abscess cavity near the anastomosis
  3. Treatment. Operative revision or resection of anastomosis with or without diversion is necessary.

13

Multiorgan Failure

I. **Definitions**
   A. **Systemic inflammatory response syndrome (SIRS)** is characterized by two or more of the following conditions:
      1. Temperature > 100.4°F (38°C) or < 96.8°F (36°C)
      2. Heart rate > 90 beats/min
      3. Respiratory rate > 20 breaths/min or PCO_2 < 32 mm Hg
      4. WBC count > 12,000 cells/mm^3 or < 4000 cells/mm^3
      5. WBC bands > 10%
   B. **Bacteremia** is the presence of bacteria in the blood confirmed by positive blood culture.
   C. **Sepsis** consists of SIRS with confirmed infection.
   D. **Septic shock** consists of hypotension and evidence of end-organ hypoperfusion secondary to sepsis.
   E. **Multiple organ dysfunction syndrome (MODS)** involves a continuum of potentially reversible changes that occur in more than one organ system following an insult (e.g., hemorrhage, trauma, infection). Changes may be subtle, and laboratory findings are not specific. Types of MODS are:
      1. **Pulmonary:** ARDS, hypoxemia, hypercapnia
      2. **Hepatic:** hyperbilirubinemia or prolonged prothrombin time (PT)
      3. **Renal:** oliguria, anuria, increased creatinine
      4. **Cardiac:** decreased CO [or normal CO in a hyperdynamic state]
      5. **Neurologic:** altered mental status (septic encephalopathy), polyneuropathy, myopathy
      6. **Hematologic:** disseminated intravascular coagulation (DIC)
      7. **GI:** upper GI bleed, acalculous cholecystitis, ileus, pancreatitis, ischemic colitis
II. **Mediators of Inflammation and Organ Dysfunction**
   A. **Cytokines**
      1. **Initiatory cytokines**
         a. **Tumor necrosis factor-α (TNF-α)**

(1) **Synthesis.** TNF-α, the first cytokine released after endotoxin challenge, is produced predominantly by monocytes and macrophages.

(2) **Function.** TNF-α serves to:

(a) Activate polymorphonuclear cells (PMNs)

(b) Promote PMN egress from bone marrow

(c) Stimulate PMN demargination

(d) Stimulate B- and T-cell action

(e) Stimulate maturation and migration of monocytes and macrophages

(f) Stimulate redistribution of protein from the skeletal muscle to the liver

(g) Act at the hypothalamus [anterior hypothalamic preoptic area (AH-POA)] and induce fever (endogenous pyrogen)

(h) Act as a procoagulant by upregulating tissue factor (TF) and downregulating thrombomodulin (predisposes to DIC)

(i) Cause anorexia and cachexia

(j) Promote hypotension and increased capillary permeability (at high systemic levels)

b. **Interleukin-1 (IL-1)**

(1) **Synthesis.** IL-1 is produced in membrane bound (IL-1a) and secretory (IL-1b) forms by a wide variety of cells (mainly macrophages).

(2) **Release.** The release of IL-1 is stimulated by endotoxin, TNF-α, or IL-1 itself.

(3) **Function.** IL-1 serves to:

(a) Stimulate release of TNF-α, IL-1, IL-6, IL-8, interferon-γ (IFN-γ), platelet-activating factor (PAF)

(b) Stimulate maturation and release of PMNs and lymphocytes from bone marrow

(c) Act at the AH-POA to induce fever (endogenous pyrogen)

(d) Act as a procoagulant by upregulating TF and downregulating thrombomodulin

(e) Stimulate the release of the hormones adrenocorticotropic hormone (ACTH), thyroid-stimulating hormone (TSH), adrenal corticosteroids, insulin, and glucagon

(f) Stimulate osteoclasts (bone resorption)

(g) Cause anorexia and cachexia

2. **Proinflammatory cytokines induced by IL-1 and TNF-α**

a. **IL-6**

(1) **Synthesis.** IL-6 is produced by fibroblasts, monocytes, and macrophages (especially Kuppfer cells).

(2) **Function.** IL-6 serves to:

(a) Increase hepatic synthesis of acute-phase proteins (e.g., fibrinogen, serum amyloid A,

C-reactive protein, ceruloplasmin, α_1-antitrypsin)

   (b) Decrease hepatic synthesis of albumin and transferrin (negative acute-phase reactants)

   (c) Stimulate B cells to differentiate into plasma cells and secrete antibody

   (d) Stimulate T-cell proliferation and differentiation

  b. IL-8 (chemokine)

   (1) Synthesis. IL-8 is produced by fibroblasts, endothelial cells, T cells, monocytes, and macrophages.

   (2) Functions. IL-8 serves to:

    (a) Act as a chemoattractant for PMNs

    (b) Promote PMN enzyme release

  c. IL-12

   (1) Synthesis. IL-12 is produced by monocytes and B cells.

   (2) Function. IL-12 serves to:

    (a) Act as a T-cell growth factor

    (b) Enhance B-cell proliferation

    (c) Stimulate natural killer (NK) cells

    (d) Stimulate the production of IL-8, IL-10, TNF-α, and IFN-γ

3. Anti-inflammatory cytokines

  a. IL-4

   (1) Synthesis. IL-4 is produced by helper T cells (T_H cells).

   (2) Function. IL-4 serves to:

    (a) Inhibit synthesis and release of IL-1, IL-6, IL-8, IL-10, and TNF-α

    (b) Stimulate production of an IL-1 receptor antagonist

    (c) Stimulate production of anti-inflammatory leukotrienes

    (d) Stimulate B- and T-cell growth and differentiation

  b. IL-10

   (1) Synthesis. IL-10 is produced by T_H cells, B cells, monocytes, and macrophages.

   (2) Function. IL-10 serves to:

    (a) Inhibit the effects of IFN-γ on macrophages

    (b) Inhibit synthesis and release of IL-1, IL-6, IL-8, and TNF-α

    (c) Stimulate production of IL-1 receptor antagonist

B. Miscellaneous inflammatory mediators

  1. IFN-γ

   a. Synthesis. IFN-γ is produced by T cells.

   b. Function. IFN-γ serves to:

        (1) Stimulate B cells to differentiate and produce antibody

        (2) Activate PMNs

        (3) Enhance PMN phagocytosis

        (4) Stimulate proinflammatory cytokine release from monocytes and macrophages

        (5) Increase monocyte–endothelial and leukocyte–endothelial adhesion

2. Platelet-activating factor (PAF)

  a. Synthesis. PAF is produced by PMNs, NK cells, endothelial cells, platelets, monocytes, and macrophages.

  b. Function. PAF causes:

    (1) Platelet aggregation

    (2) Hypotension and increased vascular permeability (proximal mediator of septic shock)

    (3) Bronchoconstriction

    (4) Decreased cardiac inotropy

    (5) PMN activation

3. Monocyte chemotactic protein 1

  a. Synthesis. This chemotactic protein is produced by lymphocytes and fibroblasts.

  b. Function. This chemotactic protein stimulates monocyte chemotaxis and activation.

4. Eicosanoids

  a. Eicosanoids, which are metabolites of arachidonic acid, are synthesized and released in response to a stimulus; they are not stored.

  b. Prostaglandins (PGs) and **thromboxanes** are products of cyclooxygenase, which is synthesized by all nucleated cells.

    (1) Synthesis. PGE_2 synthesis is induced by IL-1, IL-6, and TNF-α.

    (2) Function. PGE_2 serves to:

      (a) Inhibit production of IL-1, IL-6, and TNF-α

      (b) Inhibit B- and T-cell proliferation

      (c) Inhibit macrophage antigen presentation

  c. Leukotrienes are products of lipoxygenase, which is synthesized only by myeloid cells.

    (1) Synthesis. Leukotriene B4 (LTB4) is produced by PMNs and macrophages after endotoxin exposure.

    (2) Function. LTB4 serves to:

      (a) Act as a chemoattractant for PMNs

      (b) Stimulate leukocyte–endothelial adhesion

      (c) Increase vascular permeability

      (d) Stimulate IL-1 and IL-6 production

C. Neutrophil–endothelial interactions

  1. PMNs rapidly respond to chemoattractants [C3a, C5a, IL-8, and reactive oxygen metabolites (ROMs)] produced during inflammation.

2. Surface integrin (especially leukocyte-functional antigen) expression is upregulated after IL-1 and TNF-α exposure. Endothelial integrin counterreceptors (intercellular adhesion molecule 1) are similarly upregulated.
3. The result is increased neutrophil–endothelial adhesion and neutrophil transmigration toward the chemoattractant.
4. Cytokines, PAF, and neutrophil adhesion stimulate neutrophil degranulation and formation and ROMs.

III. **Pathogenesis of Systemic Inflammatory Response Syndrome (SIRS), Sepsis, and Multiple Organ Dysfunction Syndrome (MODS)**
   A. **Initial insult**
      1. **Causes**
         a. Trauma (e.g., blunt or penetrating injury, surgery, burn)
         b. Infection
         c. Tissue ischemia
         d. Hemorrhage
      2. **Results**
         a. Localized accumulation of PMNs and macrophages
         b. Production of inflammatory mediators
   B. **Systemic response.** The goal is to recruit T cells, B cells, platelets, and coagulation factors to the site of injury.
      1. In the **"one-hit" model,** the systemic response is a result of a systemic spillover from the areas of compartmentalized inflammation.
      2. In the **"two-hit" model,** low-level inflammatory insults "prime" the PMNs, macrophages, and endothelial cells, so that any subsequent inflammation (even minor) will prompt a systemic response.
   C. **Effect.** Organ dysfunction results from a culmination of theses changes.
      1. **Endothelial damage** (secondary to PMN reactive oxygen metabolites) leads to fluid transudation.
      2. **Excessive platelet aggregation** leads to maldistribution of peripheral blood flow and ischemia.
      3. **Vasomotor dysregulation** (secondary to inflammatory mediators) further impairs organ oxygen delivery.
   D. **Immunosuppression**
      1. Proinflammatory mediators stimulate the compensatory anti-inflammatory response (production of IL-4, IL-10, soluble IL-1 receptor antagonist, soluble TNF-α receptors).
      2. Immune suppression may occur if the anti-inflammatory response is excessive. This phenomenon is termed compensatory anti-inflammatory response syndrome (CARS), which accounts for the increased susceptibility to infection seen after traumatic injury, burns, and hemorrhage.
   E. **Hypercatabolism**
      1. Adrenal corticosteroids, catecholamines, and glucagon

increase glucose turnover and create a state of insulin resistance.

2. IL-1, IL-6, and TNF-α stimulate skeletal muscle proteolysis for hepatic gluconeogenesis.

3. Proteolysis progresses to include visceral muscle.

4. Glutamine and alanine represent more than 50% of amino acids derived from proteolysis. Glutamine is the primary enterocyte fuel, and glutamine depletion may result in bacterial translocation and infection.

5. Early enteral nutrition in affected patients reduces septic complications in burns, head injuries, and trauma.

IV. **Prognosis in Multiorgan Failure** (**Table 13-1**)

V. **Reperfusion Injury**

   A. **Definition.** Reperfusion injury is organ damage caused by the resumption of blood flow after a period of organ ischemia.

   B. **Most affected organ.** The **intestine is most prone to ischemia** secondary to profound splanchnic vasoconstriction that occurs following trauma or burns. The **mechanism of reperfusion injury in the intestine** involves several processes.

   1. Catabolism of ATP during ischemia leads to an increase in purine metabolites, hypoxanthine, and xanthine.

   2. Under normal circumstances, xanthine oxidase (dehydrogenase) converts hypoxanthine and subsequently xanthine into urate. The dehydrogenase form utilizes NAD as the electron receptor during the reaction.

   3. Ischemia mediates the conversion of xanthine dehydrogenase to xanthine oxidase, which utilizes oxygen as the electron receptor. During this reaction, oxygen is converted to the superoxide radical.

   4. Oxygen, which is deficient during ischemia, is reintroduced suddenly at reperfusion, and superoxide is generated. The superoxide radical leads to a free radical chain reaction that ultimately results in tissue injury (the hydroxyl radical is usually the most proximal mediator of injury).

   5. In response to ROMs, PMNs accumulate at the site of injury. These PMNs degranulate and produce ROMs, which amplify tissue injury.

Table 13-1. Mortality in Multiorgan Failure

Number of Organ Systems Affected	Mortality Rate
0	3%
1	30%
2	50%
3	80%
4	90%
5	100%

6. A systemic response may result from the reperfusion injury. An increased number of primed PMNs and their metabolites may get trapped in the pulmonary capillaries and initiate ARDS and subsequent MODS (i.e., "gut as the motor of MODS").

C. **Reperfusion injury in other organs**

1. **Stomach:** hemorrhagic necrosis or gastritis that follows hypotension or severe stress

2. **Liver:** hyperbilirubinemia that follows shock or liver transplantation

3. **Pancreas:** ischemic pancreatitis that follows shock or cardiopulmonary bypass

4. **Heart:** global or regional cardiac dysfunction that follows reperfusion status post–myocardial infarction (MI)

5. **Kidney:** acute tubular necrosis

6. **Brain:** global or regional CNS dysfunction that follows reperfusion status post-stroke

7. **Peripheral vascular system:** compartment syndrome that follows peripheral vascular bypass

D. **Prevention.** Pharmacologic antioxidants and free radical scavengers can prevent reperfusion injury if administered after the ischemic period but before reperfusion.

1. **Allopurinol:** inhibits xanthine oxidase and therefore the initial superoxide generation

2. **Mannitol:** scavenges the hydroxyl radical

3. **Superoxide dismutase:** converts the superoxide anion to hydrogen peroxide

4. **Catalase:** converts hydrogen peroxide to oxygen and water

14

Neurologic Disorders

ALTERED LEVEL OF CONSCIOUSNESS IN THE ICU

I. **Definitions**
  A. **Consciousness** is the patient's awareness of self and the environment. Alterations in consciousness should be differentiated from changes in mental status and should be clearly defined.
  B. **Stupor** is a condition in which the patient can only be aroused by repeated painful stimuli.
  C. **Coma** is a state in which only brainstem and spinal cord reflexes are present (i.e., the patient is unresponsive and cannot be aroused). Coma requires either bilateral hemispheric or thalamic impairment or a single brainstem lesion.
  D. **Lethargy** is an imprecise term that necessitates a detailed description.

II. **Differential Diagnosis**
  A. **Broad differential diagnosis** (Table 14-1)
  B. **Differential diagnosis based on examination findings**
    1. The absence of focal neurologic signs suggests:
       a. Toxic or metabolic etiology
       b. Subarachnoid hemorrhage
       c. Nondominant hemispheric stroke
       d. Complex partial seizures
       e. Encephalitis
    2. The presence of focal neurologic signs, which usually have a primary neurologic process, suggests:
       a. Ischemic or hemorrhagic stroke
       b. Mass lesion
       c. Focal seizure disorder

III. **Physical Examination**
  A. The goal of the physical examination is to categorize the presentation in **functional** and **structural** terms.
    1. Determine whether focal neurologic findings are present

Table 14-1. Broad Differential Diagnosis of Altered Levels of Consciousness

Supratentorial Lesions
Thalamic lesions and infarcts
Mass lesions
   Intracerebral lesions or hemorrhage
   Subdural or epidural hemorrhage
   Infarction
   Primary or metastatic tumors
   Abscess or closed head injury

Subtentorial Lesions
Compressive lesions
   Cerebellar hemorrhage, abscess, or infarct
   Cerebellar tumor
   Infarct or abscess
   Basilar aneurysm
   Posterior fossa subdural or extradural hemorrhage
Destructive or ischemic lesions
   Pontine hemorrhage
   Brainstem infarct or demyelination

Diffuse and Metabolic Disorders
Diffuse Intrinsic disorders
   Encephalitis
   Subarachnoid hemorrhage
   Concussion or postictal states
   Primary neuronal disorders
Extrinsic or metabolic disorders
   Anoxia or ischemia
   Hypoglycemia
   Nutritional deficiencies
   Hepatic encephalopathy
   Uremia
   Drug poisons
   Acid–base disorders
   Temperature regulation
   Endocrine disorders

or absent. Focal findings suggest a primary neurologic event rather than a systemic cause.

2. If focal findings are present, determine whether the lesion is supratentorial (i.e., located in the cortex and diencephalon) or infratentorial (i.e., located in the brainstem and cerebellum).

3. Determine whether the patient's condition is traumatic or nontraumatic in nature. The management and prog-

nosis of traumatic and nontraumatic neurologic conditions differ. This chapter focuses primarily on nontraumatic neurologic conditions. Refer to Chapter 26 for a discussion of head trauma.

B. General physical evaluation should focus on possible etiologies.

1. Check the patient's vital signs, which may reveal evidence of shock or cardiac arrhythmia.

2. Evaluate the patient for hypothermia or hyperthermia.

3. Look for signs of meningitis (e.g., Brudzinski's sign, Kernig's sign).

4. Check the odor of the patient's breath, which may indicate intoxication, uremia, or diabetic coma.

5. Look for signs of trauma, such as Battle's sign (i.e., blood behind the ears), raccoon eyes, and skin rashes (e.g., purpura in meningococcemia).

6. Check the patient's respiratory patterns to determine if the patient has sufficient respiratory drive to "breathe over" the ventilator.

C. Perform a **detailed neurologic examination** and search for asymmetry in function at any level. This basic "coma examination" should be performed on daily ICU rounds and after changes in the patient's neurologic status. Recent intake of paralytic agents or heavy sedation will invalidate the examination.

The most important diagnostic and prognostic study in the comatose patient is serial neurologic examinations.

---

1. **Observation**

   a. Observe the patient for any spontaneous movement or vocalization.

   b. Observe the patient's response (e.g., eye opening, facial expressions, motor localization, withdrawal, posturing) to increasing levels of stimuli. This is designed to determine the minimum stimuli to which the patient is capable of responding.

      (1) Start by asking the patient to respond to vocal stimuli and to obey motor commands.

      (2) If the patient does not respond, use louder noise and more noxious stimuli (e.g., supraorbital nerve compression, sternal rub, pressure applied to the nail bed).

2. **Detailed cranial nerve examination**

   a. Evaluate the patient's response to visual threat to determine if there is any asymmetry suggestive of a visual field cut.

   b. Examine the pupils for size, symmetry, and light reactivity.

   c. Using a sterile piece of gauze, check the corneal reflex for reactivity and asymmetry.

    d. Examine the oculocephalic reflex (Doll's eyes).

    e. If the pupillary and corneal reflexes are absent, determine oculovestibular response using the ice water caloric test.

  3. Sensory testing (Figure 14-1)

  4. Motor testing

    a. Motor testing is a continuation of the initial examination.

    b. Stimulate each extremity by applying pressure to the nail bed. Note the patient's response (e.g., localization, generalized withdrawal, extensor or flexor posturing, no response).

  5. Reflex testing

    a. Test the deep tendon reflexes and the plantar responses.

    b. Bilaterally upgoing toes in an acutely unresponsive patient suggest a brain herniation syndrome.

  6. Glasgow coma scale (GCS) [Table 14-2]

    a. Record the GCS score with each set of vital signs.

    b. The GCS aids with prognostic determinations.

IV. Diagnostic Tests

  A. Laboratory tests

    1. Blood glucose

    2. Electrolytes, BUN/creatinine

    3. Liver and thyroid function tests

    4. Cardiac enzymes

    5. CBC and platelet count

    6. Prothrombin time (PT) and partial thromboplastin time (PTT)

    7. ABG

    8. Drug levels in the blood

    9. Ammonia level

    10. Urine toxicology screen

    11. Cultures of blood, sputum, and urine

  B. Chest radiograph and **ECG** are also required in the diagnostic work-up of patients with an altered level of consciousness.

  C. Unless the etiology of coma is clearly nonneurologic in origin (e.g., asystolic episode), perform an emergent **CT scan** of the head without contrast after the patient has been stabilized. The CT scan can be used to rule out a mass lesion.

  D. Perform a **lumbar puncture** after a CT scan of the head in cases of suspected meningitis or encephalitis.

  E. Perform an emergent bedside **electroencephalogram (EEG)** in cases of suspected status epilepticus.

V. Management of Acute Changes in Consciousness

  A. Rapidly assess and stabilize the patient's airway, breathing, and circulation.

  B. Administer $D_{50}W$, naloxone, and thiamine if indicated (e.g., diabetes, suspected narcotic overdose, severe alcohol abuse).

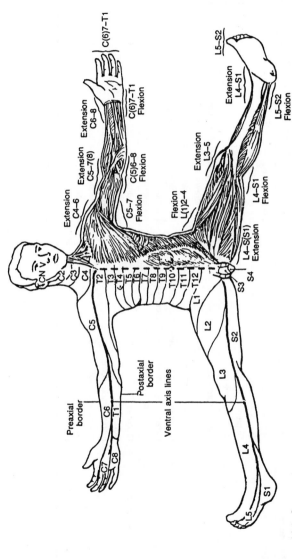

Figure 14-1. Sensory dermatomes and muscular innervation. (Reprinted with permission from April AW: *NMS Clinical Anatomy*, 3rd ed. Baltimore, Williams & Wilkins, 1997, p 28.)

Table 14-2. Glasgow Coma Scale

Parameter	Adult/Child	Infant	Score*
Eye opening	Spontaneous	Spontaneous	4
	To voice stimulus	To voice stimulus	3
	To pain	To pain	2
	No eye opening	No eye opening	1
Motor response	Follows commands	Moves spontaneously/purposely	6
	Localizes a pain stimulus	Withdraws to touch	5
	Withdraws from pain	Withdraws from pain	4
	Flexor posturing from pain (decorticate)	Flexor posturing from pain (decorticate)	3
	Extensor posturing to pain (decerebrate)	Extensor posturing to pain (decerebrate)	4
	No response to pain	No response to pain	1
Verbal response	Oriented	Coos and babbles	5
	Confused	Irritable cries	4
	Inappropriate words	Cries in response to pain	3
	Incomprehensible sounds	Moans in response to pain	2
	No sounds	No response	1
	Intubated	Intubated	T

*The score is arrived at by adding the scores from each of the three parameters. The highest possible score is 15, and the lowest possible score is 3 or 2T.

VI. Prognosis
  A. Determination of neurologic prognosis is crucial to the patient's long-term management and to the family's questions concerning end-of-life issues.
  B. Prognosis is based on serial neurologic examinations during the first 7 days.
   1. Poor prognostic signs include:
     a. Absent brainstem reflexes in a euthermic patient at admission in the absence of a drug overdose or intoxication (continues through the first 3 days)
     b. No eye opening in response to pain (at 7 days)
   2. Good prognostic signs include:
     a. Early verbalization
     b. Motor localization

BRAIN DEATH

  I. Definition. Brain death is the absence of brain function when the proximate cause is known and irreversible.

> **Each state has its own set of legal guidelines
> for the certification of brain death. The treatment
> team must be aware of these regulations.**

 II. Cardinal Findings in Brain Death
  A. Coma or unresponsiveness
    1. Apply nail-bed and supraorbital pressure.
    2. A patient who is comatose or unresponsive will have no cerebral motor response to pain in all extremities.
  B. Absence of brainstem reflexes
    1. In the absence of brainstem reflexes, the **pupils** will show no response to light, will be in midposition, and will be 4–9 mm in size.
    2. Any ocular movement excludes brain death. Two **ocular reflexes** should be tested to determine the absence of brainstem reflexes.
      a. The **oculocephalic reflex** is evaluated with the Doll's eye test.
        (1) With the head tilted at 30°, turn the head from side to side.
        (2) The eyes will not deviate in brain death.
        (3) The cervical spine must be stable to perform this test.
      b. The **oculovestibular reflex** is evaluated with the cold caloric reflex test.
        (1) Irrigate the ear canals with 50 ml of cold water.
        (2) Allow 1 minute after injection and 5 minutes between each ear.
        (3) No deviation of the eyes indicates absence of brainstem reflexes.

3. **Facial sensation** and **motor response** are also tested to evaluate the brainstem reflexes. Absence of these reflexes is indicated by:
   a. No corneal reflex to touch with a cotton wisp
   b. No jaw reflex
   c. No grimacing to deep pressure on the nail beds, supraorbital ridge, or temporomandibular joint
4. **Pharyngeal** and **tracheal** reflexes can also be used to evaluate for brain death, which is indicated by the absence of:
   a. Gag reflex
   b. Cough response to bronchial suctioning

C. **Apnea**
   1. The patient needs to be supervised closely during apnea testing.
   2. Prerequisites for apnea testing include:
      a. Core temperature $\geq 97°F$ ($\geq 36.5°C$)
      b. Systolic blood pressure ≥ 90 mm Hg
      c. Euvolemia (i.e., positive fluid balance in the last 6 hours)
      d. Normal P_{CO_2} (i.e., arterial $P_{CO_2} \geq 40$ mm Hg)
      e. Normal P_{O_2} (may preoxygenate to obtain arterial $P_{O_2} \geq 200$ mm Hg)
   3. The following is the procedure for apnea testing.
      a. Connect a pulse oximeter and disconnect the ventilator.
      b. Deliver 100% oxygen at 6 L/min into the trachea.
      c. Look for respiratory movements (i.e., abdominal or chest excursions producing adequate tidal volumes). After 8 minutes, measure arterial P_{O_2}, P_{CO_2}, and pH and reconnect the ventilator.
         (1) If respiratory movements are absent and arterial P_{CO_2} is ≥ 60 mm Hg (i.e., 20 mm Hg increase over normal baseline), then the test is positive and supports brain death.
         (2) If respiratory movements are observed, then the test is negative and does not support brain death.
         (3) If the P_{CO_2} is < 60 mm Hg or the P_{CO_2} increase is < 20 mm Hg over baseline, the apnea test is indeterminate and another confirmatory test is required (see IV).
      d. If during the apnea test the systolic blood pressure falls below 90 mm Hg or the patient has significant desaturation and cardiac arrhythmias are present, reconnect the ventilator and obtain an immediate ABG.

III. **Clinical Diagnosis of Brain Death**

**The diagnosis of brain death is clinical in nature.
After the initial declaration, a repeat clinical
evaluation is necessary (arbitrarily done 6 hours later).**

A. Diagnostic criteria for clinical diagnosis of brain death include:
  1. Exclusion of coexisting medical conditions that may complicate clinical assessment (e.g., paralytics, electrolyte disturbances, acid–base abnormalities)
  2. No drug intoxication or poisoning
  3. Core temperature $\geq 90°F$ ($\geq 32°C$)

B. Situations that make clinical diagnosis impossible include:
  1. Severe facial trauma
  2. Preexisting pupillary abnormalities
  3. Toxic levels of sedative drugs (e.g., tricyclic antidepressants, aminoglycosides, anticholinergics, antiepileptics, chemotherapeutic or neuromuscular blocking agents)
  4. Sleep apnea or severe pulmonary disease with chronic carbon dioxide retention

C. Clinical observations that may coexist with brain death include:
  1. Spontaneous movements of limbs other than pathologic flexion or extension response
  2. Respiratory-like movements (e.g., shoulder elevation and adduction, back arching, intercostal expansion without significant tidal volume)
  3. Sweating, blushing, and tachycardia
  4. Normal blood pressure or sudden increases in blood pressure
  5. Absence of diabetes insipidus
  6. Deep tendon reflexes, superficial abdominal reflexes, Babinski reflex

IV. Confirmatory Tests. Confirmatory tests are not required but may be used in patients when clinical testing cannot be reliably performed. Any of the suggested confirmatory tests may produce similar results in patients with catastrophic brain damage who do not meet the clinical diagnosis of brain death.

A. Conventional **angiography** is the most sensitive test. Brain death is confirmed if there is no intracerebral filling at the carotid bifurcation or circle of Willis. In addition, the external carotid circulation is patent and filling of the superior longitudinal sinus may be delayed.

B. EEG confirms brain death if there is no electrical activity during 30 minutes of recording.

C. Transcranial Doppler ultrasonography
  1. Brain death is indicated by small systolic peaks in early systole without diastolic flow or reverberating flow, indicating very high vascular resistance, and therefore, greatly increased intracranial pressure.
  2. The initial absence of signals cannot be interpreted as brain death because 10% of patients may not have insonation windows.

D. Technetium-99m (^{99m}Tc) hexamethylpropyleneamine oxime brain scan is the least sensitive test and indicates brain death if there is no isotope uptake in brain parenchyma.

DELIRIUM

I. Definitions

    A. Delirium is the acute presentation of impaired attention usually associated with an altered level of consciousness. It is the most common neurologic problem in the ICU and is synonymous with the term "acute confusional state."

    B. Dementia is a chronic disorder of memory with attention problems occurring only in the later stages.

II. Etiology

    A. Drug use (e.g., sedatives, narcotics, anticholinergics, corticosteroids)

    B. Metabolic encephalopathies

    C. Anoxic-ischemic encephalopathy

    D. Systemic infections (e.g., UTI, pneumonia)

    E. Withdrawal from drugs (e.g., alcohol)

III. Differential Diagnosis

    A. Neurologic disorders (e.g., dementia, stroke, seizure, head injury)

    B. Cardiopulmonary disorders [e.g., myocardial infarction (MI), congestive heart failure, pulmonary embolus, hypoxia, pneumonia, COPD]

    C. GI disorders (e.g., hepatic encephalopathy, severe fecal impaction)

    D. GU disorders (e.g., uremia, UTI, urinary retention)

    E. Infections or vasculitis

    F. Metabolic disorders (e.g., electrolyte disturbance, hyperglycemia, hypoglycemia, hyperthyroid, hypothyroid, malnutrition)

    G. Drugs (e.g., alcohol, sedatives, hypnotics, anticholinergics, immunosuppressive agents, opioids)

IV. Diagnostic Work-up

    A. Perform thorough **general and neurologic examinations.**

        1. According to the DSM-IV, the following diagnostic criteria must be present to make the diagnosis of dementia:

            a. Disturbance of consciousness with reduced ability to focus, sustain, or shift attention

            b. Change in cognition (e.g., memory deficit, disorientation, language disturbance) or development of perpetual disturbance that is not accounted for by preexisting, established, or evolving dementia

            c. Disturbance develops over a short period of time (i.e., hours or days) and tends to fluctuate during the course of the day

            d. Evidence that the disturbance is caused by the direct physiologic consequences of a general medical condition

        2. The diagnosis of delirium does not require hyperalertness or agitation; the hypoalert patient with impaired attention also should be diagnosed with delirium.

    B. Review the patient's **medications.**

C. Conduct **laboratory and diagnostic studies.**
1. **Initial studies** include electrolytes, renal and liver function tests, blood glucose, divalent cations, CBC and coagulation parameters, urinalysis, ECG, and chest radigraph.
2. As **additional studies,** consider urine toxicology screen, cardiac enzymes, drug levels (e.g., antiepileptic drugs), thyroid function test, ABG, blood cultures, lumbar puncture, VDRL, and assessment of HIV status.
3. Perform a bedside **EEG** after the patient has been stabilized to assess the level of encephalopathy and to rule out subclinical seizures.
4. A **CT scan** of the head without contrast is sufficient to rule out hemorrhagic stroke and subdural hematoma and to identify early changes in large ischemic hemispheric infarcts.
5. A **MRI** of the brain with and without contrast is the preferred study for a suspected mass lesion and for evaluation of HIV-positive patients.

V. **Management**

> **Appropriate diagnosis and management is imperative because of the increased mortality associated with delirium.**

A. Continue to conduct and record **neurologic evaluations.**
1. A brief neurologic evaluation should be performed with each set of vital signs by the nursing staff.
2. A daily, more detailed neurologic examination should be performed by a physician.
B. Provide the appropriate **pharmacotherapy.**

> **Use caution in sedating a delirious patient, particularly if the cause remains unknown. If the patient is oversedated, it may become impossible to follow neurologic status on the basis of serial examinations and to provide prognosis.**

1. Use benzodiazepines (e.g., midazolam, lorazepam) and thiamine in patients suspected of narcotic or alcohol withdrawal.
2. Benzodiazepines are the drug of choice in benzodiazepine withdrawal, alcohol withdrawal, and hepatic failure. A short-acting benzodiazepine (e.g., midazolam) may be needed initially in severely agitated ICU patients.
3. With the exception of benzodiazepine withdrawal, alcohol withdrawal, and hepatic failure, haloperidol remains the drug of choice for the chemical restraint of a delirious patient.
   a. Moderate-to-severe agitation
      (1) Give an initial dose of 2–10 mg IM.
      (2) A maintenance dose of 2–5 mg q 6–8 hr controls most patients.

      (3) In some young patients, doses of up to 5 mg/hr have been used for short periods of time. If this schedule or other high-dose regimen is required, the treatment team should consult the neurology or psychiatry service.

  b. Mild agitation

      (1) Give 5–10 mg PO bid.

      (2) Elderly patients may not be able to tolerate this dose and should be started at half the dose (i.e., 2.5–5.0 mg PO bid).

ISCHEMIC STROKE

I. Etiology

  A. Embolic

  B. Thrombotic

  C. Lacunar

  D. Arterial dissection (especially in trauma patients)

  E. Vasculitis

  F. Hypotension

    1. In an ICU patient, a hypotensive event can lead to a classic cerebral arterial distribution stroke in the presence of a fixed arterial stenosis or to a watershed distribution infarct in the setting of more severe, global cerebral ischemia.

    2. Watershed refers to the brain regions supplied by the most distal regions of the major cerebral vessels (i.e., the anterior, middle, and posterior cerebral arteries).

    3. Watershed infarcts occur between the distributions of the anterior and middle cerebral arteries and between the middle and posterior branches.

II. Signs and Symptoms

  A. Focal neurologic signs that are difficult to identify include:

    1. Hemiparesis

    2. Aphasia

  B. The initial presentation of an acute stroke can be accompanied by:

    1. Stupor

    2. Coma

    3. Delirium

    4. Seizures

  C. Common patterns of deficits in various stroke syndromes are shown in Figure 14-2.

Consider stroke in the differential diagnosis of any focal or diffuse neurologic deterioration in an ICU patient.

III. Diagnostic Tests

  A. Laboratory studies include:

    1. CBC

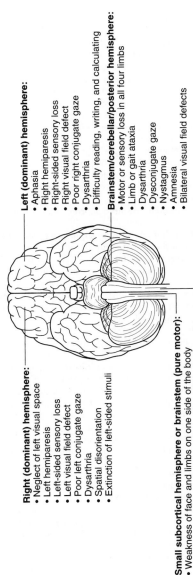

Right (dominant) hemisphere:
- Neglect of left visual space
- Left hemiparesis
- Left-sided sensory loss
- Left visual field defect
- Poor left conjugate gaze
- Dysarthria
- Spatial disorientation
- Extinction of left-sided stimuli

Left (dominant) hemisphere:
- Aphasia
- Right hemiparesis
- Right-sided sensory loss
- Right visual field defect
- Poor right conjugate gaze
- Dysarthria
- Difficulty reading, writing, and calculating

Brainstem/cerebellar/posterior hemisphere:
- Motor or sensory loss in all four limbs
- Limb or gait ataxia
- Dysarthria
- Dysconjugate gaze
- Nystagmus
- Amnesia
- Bilateral visual field defects

Small subcortical hemisphere or brainstem (pure motor):
- Weakness of face and limbs on one side of the body
- No abnormalities of higher brain function, sensation, or vision

Small subcortical hemisphere or brainstem (pure sensory):
- Decreased sensation of face and limbs on one side of the body
- No abnormalities of higher brain function, motor function, or vision

Figure 14-2. Common patterns of deficits based on location of stroke.

2. Platelets
3. PT and PTT
4. Serum electrolytes
5. Blood glucose
6. Cardiac enzymes
7. Renal and liver function tests

B. Obtain an **ECG** and **chest radiograph.**

C. Perform an emergent **CT scan of the head** without contrast to rule out intracranial or subarachnoid hemorrhage, hemorrhagic infarcts, and mass lesions.

D. Despite a negative head CT scan, perform a **lumbar puncture** in patients suspected of meningoencephalitis or subarachnoid hemorrhage.

E. If seizures are suspected, perform an **EEG.** However, an EEG usually does not have to be performed acutely.

F. If carotid dissection is suspected in a trauma patient, perform an emergent **carotid arteriogram** or **magnetic resonance angiogram.**

G. Perform a **carotid ultrasound** to rule out critical carotid stenosis.

H. Perform a **transthoracic or transesophageal echocardiogram** to rule out a cardioembolic source.

I. Perform **emergent brain imaging** by CT scan or MRI after any neurologic decline to rule out mass effect and hemorrhagic transformation. Additional imaging in the stable patient is not necessary for long-term management; however, it can document the anatomic location of the infarct and aid secondary treatment decisions (e.g., aspirin versus long-term anticoagulation with warfarin).

J. Perform multiple **blood cultures** in patients with suspected endocarditis.

K. For suspected connective tissue disorders, particularly in younger patients, obtain erythrocyte sedimentation rate, antinuclear antibodies, rheumatoid factor, and VDRL.

L. For suspected hypercoagulable state, obtain antiphospholipid antibodies, protein C and S, activated protein C, and antithrombin III levels.

IV. **Acute Management.** The management of an acute ischemic stroke remains controversial. The following guidelines are based on current practice.

A. Stabilize the patient medically. Patients in stupor or coma need to be **intubated** for airway protection, and all patients should be **well oxygenated.**

B. All ischemic stroke patients should receive **deep venous thrombosis (DVT) prophylaxis** (i.e., heparin, 5000 U SQ q 12 hr), unless medically contraindicated, and **sequential compression devices.**

C. Nutritional status should be maintained with **nasogastric feeding,** if necessary. If the patient is alert and not intubated, a bedside swallowing evaluation can determine aspiration risk.

D. **Anticoagulation and antiplatelet therapy** includes heparin and aspirin.
 1. **Heparin**
    a. Start heparin at 800–1000 U IV q 1 hr without a bolus. The systolic blood pressure should be kept < 180 mm Hg to avoid hemorrhagic transformation and the PTT should be kept between 50 and 70.
    b. Multiple clinical trials have not demonstrated a clear benefit in the use of IV heparinization in ischemic stroke.
    c. Patients with a stroke after coronary bypass surgery do not benefit from anticoagulation.
    d. Patients with cardioembolic etiology (e.g., atrial fibrillation) or severe cardiomyopathy may benefit from anticoagulation.
    e. The risk of bleeding from heparinization increases with larger infarcts, severely elevated blood pressure, and advancing age of the patient.
 2. **Aspirin.** Unless medically contraindicated, all patients that are not systemically heparinized should be given aspirin, 325 mg PO/PR once a day, and heparin, 5000 U SQ q 12 hr.
E. **Thrombolysis** is beneficial in an ischemic stroke if given within 3 hours of symptom onset.
 1. Administer **tissue plasminogen activator (tPA),** 0.9 mg/kg IV to a maximum of 90 mg. Give 10% as an initial bolus and the remainder over 60 minutes. tPA should only be administered by personnel familiar with acute stroke management.
 2. Contraindications to tPA administration include:
    a. Major surgery within previous 14 days
    b. Recent MI
    c. Recent use of PO or IV anticoagulation
    d. Stroke or head injury within previous 3 months
    e. Rapidly improving neurologic signs
    f. GI or urinary bleeding within previous 21 days
F. Treat potential **complications.**
 1. Treat **fever** with antipyretics to lower body temperature and prevent enlargement of the infarct.
 2. Control **hyperglycemia.**
 3. Control **blood pressure.**
    a. The type of stroke determines how blood pressure is regulated.
       (1) After an **acute stroke,** brain autoregulation of blood flow fails, and perfusion becomes directly dependent on systemic blood pressure.
       (2) According to AHA guidelines, blood pressure after an **ischemic stroke** should not be treated unless mean blood pressure is > 130 mm Hg or systolic blood pressure is > 220 mm Hg.
       (3) In contrast to ischemic stroke, **hemorrhagic**

stroke does not allow blood pressure to rise to relatively high levels to maintain cerebral perfusion.

b. Both oral and parenteral medications can be used in the regulation of blood pressure.

   (1) Oral medications (e.g., captopril) should be used as first-line agents, if possible. SL medications are contraindicated because of their rapid onset of action and sudden lowering of blood pressure, which can increase infarct size.

   (2) If parenteral medications are required, IV labetalol should be attempted first. IV nicardipine and nitroprusside are second-line agents.

Rising blood pressure associated with bradycardia may indicate increasing intracranial pressure (Cushing phenomenon), which requires emergent evaluation.

   (a) Diastolic blood pressure > 140 mm Hg: start infusion of sodium nitroprusside.

   (b) Systolic blood pressure > 230 mm Hg and/or diastolic blood pressure 121–140 mm Hg:

   (i) Administer labetalol, 20 mg IV over 1–2 minutes.

   (ii) Dose may be repeated or doubled q 10 min up to 150 mg total.

   (iii) If response is not satisfactory, start sodium nitroprusside.

   (c) Systolic blood pressure 180–230 mm Hg and/or diastolic blood pressure 105–120 mm Hg (make two readings 5–10 minutes apart):

   (i) Administer labetalol, 10 mg IV over 1–2 minutes.

   (ii) Dose may be repeated or doubled q 10–20 min up to 150 mg total.

4. Treat **edema.** Peak swelling of an acute infarct occurs approximately 96 hours after the onset of symptoms. If the initial head CT scan demonstrates early signs of edema (i.e., sulcal effacement and loss of distinction of the gray–white junction), the patient is at risk for brain herniation.

   a. Keep the head of the bed elevated at a 20°–30° angle.

   b. Use isotonic fluids for gentle hydration in ischemic stroke patients. Avoid hypotonic fluids because of their effect on intracranial pressure.

   c. In patients with deteriorating clinical status due to worsening edema, more aggressive interventions include hyperventilation, osmotic diuresis, and surgical decompression. However, these patients generally have a poor outcome if signs of early herniation develop before the peak swelling period.

    d. There is no indication for the use of corticosteroids to reduce brain edema after a stroke or for the prophylactic use of antiepileptic medications in ischemic stroke. When seizures do occur, they should be treated aggressively.

NEUROMUSCULAR WEAKNESS

I. Guillain-Barré Syndrome

A. Definition. Guillain-Barré syndrome (GBS) is thought to be an immunologically mediated postinfectious disorder. It is also called acute inflammatory demyelinating polyneuropathy and is currently the most common cause of acute-onset neuromuscular weakness.

B. Predisposing factors

1. Most patients have a preceding upper respiratory tract infection; a small percentage have an enteritis.
2. Possible viral triggers include cytomegalovirus, Epstein-Barr virus, hepatitis viruses, HIV, varicella-zoster virus, mumps, and measles.
3. *Campylobacter* enteritis can precede an axonal variant of GBS and is associated with anti-GM1 antibodies. Prognosis is worse when GBS is associated with axonal damage.
4. Mycoplasma infection may be present.
5. Predisposing systemic diseases include systemic lupus erythematosus, Hodgkin's lymphoma, sarcoidosis, and AIDS.
6. Surgical patients may have a slightly increased risk of GBS 2–3 weeks postoperatively.

C. Signs and symptoms

1. Initial symptoms in many patients include **distal paresthesias** in the extremities and **musculoskeletal pain,** particularly in the back.
2. **Weakness** can have a symmetric or asymmetric onset.
    a. In cases of symmetric onset, although weakness can begin either distally or proximally, it usually starts proximally in the lower extremities and progresses to the upper extremities over a few days.
    b. Asymmetric weakness requires a search for a central cause or a mononeuropathy (e.g., compressive neuropathy after trauma or prolonged surgical positioning, mononeuropathy multiplex).
    c. Rapid progression of weakness or early onset of neuromuscular weakness are associated with a prolonged hospital course requiring ICU care.
3. **Areflexia or hyporeflexia** is present in the majority of patients. If the deep tendon reflexes are preserved after several days of weakness, the diagnosis becomes less likely.
4. In the presence of **ophthalmoplegia and ataxia** (Miller-Fisher variant of GBS) it is necessary to differentiate between GBS and a brainstem lesion.

   5. **Autonomic disturbances** include cardiac arrhythmias, orthostatic hypotension, hypertension, paralytic ileus, and altered sweating.
D. Differential diagnosis
   1. Spinal cord compression
      a. Compression of the spinal cord can present initially as a flaccid paraparesis or quadriparesis with hyporeflexia. It may be difficult to identify a spinal cord level.
      b. A defined sensory level or bowel and bladder symptoms suggest a spinal cord lesion rather than GBS.
   2. Acute infection (e.g., Lyme disease, syphilis, viral and bacterial meningitis), particularly if the cell count in the CSF is > 50 cells/μl
   3. Toxins (e.g., botulism, diphtheria) and heavy metal poisoning
   4. Myasthenia gravis and other disorders of the neuromuscular junction
   5. Carcinomatous meningitis with invasion of nerve roots
   6. Electrolyte disorders (e.g., hypophosphatemia, hypokalemia)
   7. ICU-specific disorders (e.g., critical illness polyneuropathy, acute quadriplegic myopathy, necrotizing myopathy of critical care), usually associated with prolonged ICU hospitalization, multiorgan failure, and sepsis
   8. Mononeuritis multiplex
   9. Myopathy
   10. Acute porphyria
   11. Tick paralysis
E. Diagnostic work-up
   1. Perform **general and neurologic examinations.** It is important to grade the strength in each muscle group.
   2. Perform bedside **pulmonary function tests** to assess vital capacity (VC) and negative inspiratory force (NIF).
   3. Obtain the following **laboratory tests:**
      a. Electrolytes
      b. Calcium, magnesium, and phosphate
      c. BUN/creatinine
      d. Liver function tests
      e. PT and PTT
      f. CBC, platelet count, and ABG
      g. Creatine kinase (CK)
      h. Erythrocyte sedimentation rate
      i. Antinuclear antibody
      j. Rheumatoid factor
      k. Appropriate viral and bacterial serologies (especially HIV in patients at risk)
      l. Anti-GM1 antibodies
      m. IgA level (stat if IV Ig is to be administered)
   4. Perform a **lumbar puncture** in all patients with suspected GBS.
      a. Albuminocytologic dissociation with elevated CSF

protein and < 10 mononuclear cells/μl is a hallmark of GBS; however, it may take > 7 days after the onset of weakness to develop.

   b. The presence of granulocytes or > 50 mononuclear cells/μl suggests a primary infectious process.

5. Obtain a **chest radiograph** and **ECG.**

6. **Nerve conduction studies** are required for diagnosis and prognosis.

7. Obtain a **MRI of the cervical spine** in patients with acute-onset quadriparesis. Consider **total spine imaging** in patients with acute-onset paraparesis dependent on presentation.

F. **Management**

In cases of GBS, the quality of supportive care determines outcome because recovery occurs in most patients.

---

1. Treatment modalities for **pulmonary complications** associated with GBS include:

   a. **Ventilatory support**

      (1) Indications for mechanical ventilation include:

         (a) VC < 12 ml/kg

         (b) Rapidly decreasing VC (elective intubation for VC 12–20 ml/kg)

         (c) Inability to protect airway (e.g., severe dysphagia)

      (2) Do not wait for the PCO_2 to rise as an indication for intubation.

   b. **Pulmonary toilet**

   c. **Incentive spirometry** for patients not intubated

   d. **Observation of VC and NIF** as weaning parameters

   e. **Tracheostomy** in patients intubated for > 2 weeks

2. Treat any **dysautonomias** (i.e., autonomic neuropathy) that develop.

   a. **Sinus tachycardia** can alternate with bradycardia. If possible, avoid pharmacologic intervention because of heart rate lability.

   b. **Orthostatic hypotension** should be treated with fluids.

   c. **Severe hypertension** can alternate with hypotension. Treat severe hypertension with nitroprusside, if necessary. Avoid β-blockers and calcium channel blockers because of cardiac effects and long-term action.

   d. **Urinary retention** may require continuous or intermittent bladder catheterization.

   e. Treat **constipation** with the appropriate bowel regimen.

   f. When treating **ileus,** keep patient NPO and provide IV fluids. If distention, nausea, and vomiting develop, a nasogastric tube may be necessary.

3. Administer **DVT prophylaxis.**

4. Early recognition and treatment of **infectious complications** is important.

5. Send the patient for **physical therapy.**
6. Maintain **nutritional status.**
7. Provide **skin care** to avoid pressure sores.
8. All patients who have difficulty ambulating should receive **immunotherapy** (i.e., plasmapheresis or IV Ig).
   a. **Plasmapheresis** usually requires central access.
      (1) Exchange a total volume of 200 ml/kg body weight over 7–14 days (i.e., 4–5 exchanges of 3.5–4.0 L for a 70-kg person spaced over 7–14 days).
      (2) Contraindications to plasmapheresis include recent MI, arrhythmias, and hypotension.
   b. **Human Ig** is easier to administer than plasmapheresis but may be in short supply.
      (1) Dose 0.4 g/kg body weight/day for 5 days.
      (2) IgA deficiency is an absolute contraindication and renal disease is a relative contraindication.

G. **Prognosis**
   1. GBS has a mortality rate of 2%–5%, usually from complications (e.g., infections, pulmonary embolus, dysautonomias).
   2. Long-term marked neurologic disability occurs in 5%–10% of patients; only 15% have no residual deficit.
   3. Poor prognostic signs include:
      a. Older age
      b. Fulminant presentation
      c. Rapid progression to ventilatory status
      d. Prolonged requirement for mechanical ventilation (i.e., > 1 month)
      e. Severely reduced compound muscle action potential amplitudes by electromyogram (EMG)

II. **Myasthenic Crisis**
   A. **Definitions**
      1. **Myasthenia gravis** is a disease of the neuromuscular junction due to IgG antibodies targeted to the nicotinic acetylcholine receptor. It tends to be a disease of younger women and older men. In younger patients it may coexist with other autoimmune conditions (e.g., thyroid disease, rheumatoid arthritis, lupus, polymyositis). It can be associated with thymic hyperplasia or thymoma.
      2. **Myasthenic crisis** is an exacerbation of weakness sufficient to lead to respiratory compromise. It is usually a combination of respiratory muscle insufficiency and an inability to handle oral secretions. In the majority of cases, patients experiencing a myasthenic crisis have been previously diagnosed with myasthenia gravis. However, a small percentage may present initially in myasthenic crisis after an obstetric or general surgical procedure or the administration of neuromuscular blockers.
   B. **Predisposing factors**
      1. Infection (e.g., UTI, pneumonia)
      2. Recent initiation of corticosteroids

3. Selected surgical procedures

4. Drugs

    a. Never use penicillamine in patients with myasthenia gravis.

    b. Medications that may worsen the symptoms of myasthenia gravis include succinylcholine, neuromuscular blocking agents, quinine, quinidine, procainamide, aminoglycosides, propanolol, timolol eyedrops, and calcium channel blockers.

C. Signs and symptoms

    1. Bulbar symptoms (e.g., dysphagia, ptosis, diplopia) [most common presentation]

    2. Facial weakness

    3. Dyspnea and progressive respiratory compromise

    4. Generalized weakness

D. Differential diagnosis

    1. Lambert-Eaton syndrome (particularly in older patients with a suspected neoplasm)

    2. Myopathies (including mitochondrial diseases)

    3. Thyroid disease (i.e., hypothyroidism and hyperthyroidism)

    4. Polyneuropathies (e.g., GBS in previously undiagnosed patients, chronic inflammatory demyelinating polyradiculoneuropathy)

    5. Organophosphate poisoning and botulism

    6. Drugs (especially neuromuscular blockers)

    7. Motor neuron disease

    8. Brainstem lesion

E. Diagnostic work-up

    1. Perform **general and neurologic examinations.** Grade the strength in each muscle group with attention to cranial nerves and proximal muscle groups.

    2. Perform bedside **pulmonary function tests** to assess VC and NIF. If the patient has severe lower facial weakness it may be difficult to assess true VC because of inability to create a good seal.

    3. Obtain the necessary **laboratory tests.**

        a. In previously diagnosed patients, obtain:

            (1) Electrolytes

            (2) Calcium, magnesium, and phosphate

            (3) Renal and liver function tests

            (4) CBC, platelet count, PT, and PTT

            (5) ABG

        b. In previously undiagnosed patients, consider adding:

            (1) Creatine phosphokinase

            (2) Thyroid function tests

            (3) Antithyroid antigens

            (4) Antinuclear antibody

            (5) Rheumatoid factor

            (6) Cultures (urine, sputum, and blood) to identify intercurrent infection

(7) Acetylcholine receptor antibodies (AChRAb)
   (a) Titers of AChRAb also can be followed in previously diagnosed patients to assess relative severity of autoimmune response.
   (b) AChRAb is a highly specific marker of disease, but may be absent in 10% of patients with generalized myasthenia gravis.

4. Perform a **lumbar puncture** only if an alternative diagnosis, such as GBS, is being considered.
5. Obtain a **chest radiograph** and **ECG.**
6. Obtain an **EMG** and perform **nerve conduction studies** in previously undiagnosed patients.
7. Obtain a **CT scan of the chest** if it was not previously performed.
8. Pursue **brain imaging** only if a brainstem lesion is suspected.

F. Management
1. Management of **pulmonary complications** is similar to that for GBS (see p 373). Follow forced vital capacity and maximal inspiratory and expiratory pressures.
2. Rule out **cholinergic crisis** if the patient is on anticholinesterase medication.
   a. In comparison to myasthenic crisis, true cholinergic crisis is very rare.
   b. Consider edrophonium or neostigmine tests only if cholinergic crisis is suspected. These tests should be performed by an experienced physician in a monitored setting.
   c. In patients with myasthenic crisis with respiratory failure, the usual standard of care is to discontinue all cholinergic medications. Restart cholinergic medications at half the usual dose when the patient is ready for weaning.
3. Administer **DVT prophylaxis.**
4. Strive for early recognition and treatment of **intercurrent infections** (e.g., UTI, pneumonia).
5. Send the patient to **physical therapy.**
6. Maintain **nutritional status.**
7. **Therapeutics** include plasmapheresis, prednisone, and pyridostigmine.
   a. **Plasmapheresis** is effective in myasthenic crisis. Perform 5–8 exchanges of 1.5–2.0 L/exchange. IV Ig may have similar efficacy, but no comparative trial has been performed.
   b. Consider initiation of **prednisone,** 1 mg/kg PO once a day while the patient is hospitalized.
      (1) Up to 50% of patients worsen in the first few days of initiation, but approximately 80% will have long-term benefit.
      (2) Although prednisone is efficacious in the long-

term treatment of poorly controlled myasthenia gravis, patients frequently worsen acutely.

   c. Pyridostigmine is a cholinesterase inhibitor that can be used to help alleviate weakness.

     (1) The common dose is 60 mg PO q 4–6 hr.

     (2) The maximal dose is 120 mg PO q 3 hr (comparable to neostigmine, 1 mg IV).

8. Thymectomy results in a clinical response in the majority of patients; however, no randomized trial has been performed comparing efficacy of thymectomy versus immunosuppressive treatment alone.

   a. Indications for thymectomy include:

     (1) All patients with thymoma (unless surgery is medically contraindicated)

     (2) Patients with generalized myasthenia gravis who are responding poorly to cholinergic medications

   b. If preoperative pulmonary function tests are $< 80\%$ of predicted, consider preoperative plasmapheresis. If pulmonary function is not optimal after plasmapheresis and optimization of oral medications, the patient will probably have prolonged postoperative course and will require tracheostomy.

   c. Avoid all drugs operatively and postoperatively, because they may cause a clinical exacerbation.

   d. If intubation is required postoperatively, it may be necessary to hold cholinergic medications. If intubation is not required, restart cholinergic medications at 50% of preoperative dose and slowly increase as needed and tolerated.

III. Neuromuscular Weakness Associated with Critical Illness

  A. Risk factors

    1. Sepsis

    2. Multiorgan failure

    3. Neuromuscular blockers (particularly for myopathies)

  B. Differential diagnosis

    1. Consider the following diagnoses in all patients who develop neuromuscular weakness after prolonged ICU care:

      a. Critical illness polyneuropathy (e.g., axonal neuropathy, noninflammatory CSF)

      b. Acute quadriplegic myopathy

      c. Necrotizing myopathy of critical care

      d. Postoperative GBS

      e. New-onset myasthenia gravis or other neuromuscular junction disorders

      f. Spinal cord disease

      g. Electrolyte abnormality

    2. These diagnoses tend to be identified in ICU patients who become difficult to wean from mechanical ventilation for unclear reasons.

C. **Diagnostic work-up**
   1. Perform **general and neurologic examinations.**
   2. Obtain the following **laboratory tests:**
      a. CK
      b. Electrolytes
      c. Calcium, magnesium, and phosphate
      d. Renal and liver function tests
      e. CBC, platelet count, PT, and PTT
      f. ABG
   3. Perform a **lumbar puncture** to differentiate inflammatory and infectious etiologies from noninflammatory conditions (e.g., critical illness polyneuropathy).
   4. Obtain a **MRI of the spine** in all patients with acute-onset quadriparesis or paraparesis.
   5. Obtain an **EMG** and perform **nerve conduction studies.**

D. **Management** is supportive, as in severe cases of GBS and myasthenic crisis.

SEIZURES IN THE ICU

I. **Classification**
   A. **Primary generalized** seizures are characterized by bilateral symmetric onset.
      1. **Tonic–clonic** seizures were previously referred to as grand mal seizures. It is necessary to differentiate tonic–clonic seizures from secondary generalized seizures with subtle focal onset.
      2. **Absence** seizures were previously referred to as petit mal seizures. An absence seizure results in a brief loss of consciousness frequently associated with eye blinking. Absence seizures are most common in the pediatric population and can be confused with complex partial seizures in adults.
      3. Less common types of primary generalized seizures include:
         a. Tonic
         b. Clonic
         c. Myoclonic epilepsy
   B. **Partial** seizures are characterized by focal onset.
      1. **Simple partial** seizures are characterized by:
         a. Focal motor or sensory symptoms associated with preservation of consciousness
         b. Motor symptoms characterized by clonic movements of a foot or arm or, more subtly, facial twitching
         c. The aura phenomenon (e.g., sense of impending doom, unusual sensory symptoms, olfactory or gustatory hallucinations) not followed by loss of consciousness
      2. **Complex partial** seizures are also referred to as psychomotor seizures or temporal lobe epilepsy, although

they can arise from any cortical area (e.g., frontal lobe seizures). Complex partial seizures are characterized by:
  a. Loss of consciousness
  b. Aura phenomenon and automatisms (e.g., lip smacking, eyelid blinking)
  c. Paucity of focal motor activity
  d. Delirium, stupor, or coma

  C. Status epilepticus is continuous seizure activity for > 30 minutes or, more commonly, multiple seizures of short duration between which the patient does not recover consciousness.
   1. Convulsive status epilepticus is the most frequent type.
   2. Any seizure type can present as status, including simple and complex partial seizures.

II. Predisposing Factors

  A. Metabolic derangements (particularly hyponatremia, uremia, hypoglycemia, hyperglycemia, and hepatic failure)
  B. Alcohol and drug withdrawal (includes patients given benzodiazepines and narcotics as inpatients only)
  C. Meningoencephalitis or systemic infection
  D. Drug side effects (especially effects of cyclosporine, cyclophosphamide, lidocaine, tricyclic antidepressants, imipenem, penicillins, and ciprofloxacin)
  E. Acute stroke or an old infarct
  F. Space-occupying lesion (e.g., tumor, abscess)
  G. Fat emboli in trauma patients
  H. Postoperative transplant patients

III. Differential Diagnosis

  A. Myoclonus is a brief shock-like movement due to muscle contraction. It can be segmental or generalized. Postanoxic myoclonus can occur after cardiac resuscitation.
  B. Extensor and flexor posturing in comatose patients can be difficult to distinguish from seizure activity.
  C. Dystonia is a sustained muscle contraction that can be manifested as posturing (e.g., torticollis). It is frequently due to a drug reaction (e.g., haloperidol, metoclopramide).

IV. Diagnostic Work-up

  A. Perform **general and neurologic examinations.** Note any focality.
  B. Review **medications.**
  C. Obtain the following **laboratory tests:**
   1. Blood glucose
   2. Serum electrolytes, BUN/creatinine
   3. CBC and platelet count
   4. PT and PTT
   5. Calcium, magnesium, and phosphate
   6. Liver function tests and ammonia level
   7. Antiepileptic drug levels
   8. Cardiac enzymes
   9. Urine toxicology
   10. Appropriate cultures if encephalitis or meningitis is suspected

D. Obtain an **ECG** to rule out arrhythmia or acute ischemia.

E. Obtain a **chest radiograph** to assess for aspiration or pneumonia.

F. Obtain a **CT scan of the head** without contrast after the patient has been stabilized to rule out a hemorrhage or large space-occupying lesion. If a tumor or abscess is suspected, consider a **MRI of the brain** with and without contrast because of greater sensitivity.

G. A **bedside EEG** can demonstrate focal slowing in the absence of an acute seizure. If subclinical status epilepticus is suspected, consider continuous EEG monitoring.

H. Consider a **lumbar puncture** in patients suspected of meningitis or encephalitis.

V. Management

A. Non–status epilepticus seizures

1. Correct underlying **metabolic disorders** or other predisposing factors.

2. Unless medically contraindicated, administer **phenytoin,** which is the most effective, parenterally administered antiepileptic in the ICU.

a. Loading dose: 15 mg/kg IV, administered no faster than 50 mg/min

b. Maintenance dose: 5 mg/kg/day IV/PO divided bid–tid

3. **Follow phenytoin levels** closely.

a. Drug interactions (especially with cyclosporine) can cause phenytoin toxicity (ataxia, nystagmus, diplopia, nausea, vomiting) or result in undertreatment.

b. Hypoalbuminemia in ICU patients with poor nutritional status can cause increased free phenytoin levels with apparently normal serum levels.

4. If necessary, use **phenobarbital** as an alternative to phenytoin; however, it can cause excessive sedation.

5. Address the need for long-term oral **antiepileptic therapy** before transfer from the ICU.

B. Status epilepticus

1. **Status epilepticus is a medical emergency.**

2. Management is determined by the time since recognition of status epilepticus.

a. 0–2 minutes: assess airway, breathing, vital signs, and oxygen saturation.

b. 2–10 minutes

(1) Obtain an ECG.

(2) Assess IV access.

(3) Obtain the following laboratory tests:

(a) Electrolytes

(b) Glucose

(c) Calcium, magnesium, and phosphate

(d) CBC

(e) Renal and liver function tests

(f) Drug levels

          (g) Toxicology screen
- **(4)** Give thiamine, 100 mg IV, and 1 ampule of $D_{50}W$ IV.

c. 10–30 minutes
- **(1)** Administer lorazepam, 2-mg IV boluses given no faster than 2 mg/min to a total of 0.1 mg/kg. An alternative is diazepam, 2-mg IV boluses given no faster than 5 mg/min to a total of 0.25 mg/kg.
- **(2)** Administer phenytoin concurrently with lorazepam. The load dose is 15 mg/kg IV at a rate of up to 50 mg/kg. Monitor the ECG and check blood pressure every minute with phenytoin load.
- **(3)** Obtain history and examination after treatment has been initiated. Request emergent neurology consult.
- **(4)** Schedule an emergent CT scan of the head.
- **(5)** If patient continues to seize or remains unresponsive, perform emergent bedside EEG monitoring.
- **(6)** Consider antibiotics and lumbar puncture if patient is febrile or meningoencephalitis is suspected.

d. 30–40 minutes
- **(1)** Administer an additional 7 mg/kg IV of phenytoin. Continue monitoring and check phenytoin level 20 minutes after the initial load.
- **(2)** Intubate if not done previously.
- **(3)** If seizures do not respond to additional phenytoin, load with phenobarbital, 20 mg/kg IV given no faster than 100 mg/min.

Phenobarbital and benzodiazepines given together severely depress respiration.

---

e. > 50 minutes
- **(1)** With the appropriate consultants, consider continuous anesthesia with pentobarbital or midazolam in patients not responding to treatment. The dose is titrated to achieve a burst–suppression pattern on EEG.
- **(2)** Even in patients responsive to benzodiazepines and phenytoin, a prolonged postictal period characterized by unresponsiveness usually follows. A bedside EEG can differentiate a postictal state from continuous seizures.
- **(3)** Remember that paralytic agents given for intubation mask any motor seizure activity.
- **(4)** Check laboratory tests previously sent, review predisposing factors to search for etiology, and obtain a CT scan of the head without contrast if the patient is stable.

15

Nutrition

I. **Malnutrition**
   A. **Risk factors**
      1. Recent surgery or trauma
      2. Sepsis
      3. Chronic illness
      4. Eating disorders (e.g., anorexia)
      5. Dysphagia
      6. Recurrent nausea, vomiting, or diarrhea
      7. Pancreatitis
      8. Inflammatory bowel disease
      9. GI fistulas
      10. Cancer, chemotherapy, or radiation
      11. Diet
   B. **Complications**
      1. Impaired wound healing
      2. Anemia
      3. Impaired GI tract, cardiac, and respiratory function
      4. Muscle atrophy
      5. Brain dysfunction
      6. Hypothermia
      7. Reduced basal metabolism
   C. **Classification of protein-calorie malnutrition**
      1. Mild: loss of 10% of usual body mass
      2. Moderate: loss of 10%–20% of usual body mass
      3. Severe: loss of > 20% of usual body mass

II. **Calorie Requirements**
   A. **Daily calorie requirements** vary according to the state of the patient (Table 15-1).
   B. **Determining calorie requirements**
      1. The **Harris-Benedict equation** is used to calculate **basal energy expenditure** (BEE; kcal/day):

Males: BEE = 66 + (13.7 × W) + (5 × H) − (6.7 × A)

Females: BEE = 655 + (9.6 × W) + (1.8 × H) − (4.7 × A)

Table 15-1. Daily Calorie Requirements for Adults With Various Stresses

Condition of Patient	Calories (kcal/kg/day)	Calories (kcal/day; 70–kg person)	Percentage of Normal (%)
Normal adult	20–25	1400–1750	100
Mild stress	25–30	1750–2100	120–125
Major stress	30–35	2100–2450	120–140
Burn/sepsis	> 40	> 2800	> 200
Starvation	17–25	1190–1750	85–100
Postoperative	20–26	1400–1820	100–105
Cancer	22–36	1540–2520	110–145
Peritonitis	21–32	1470–2240	105–125
Infection/ Trauma	26–40	1820–2800	130–155
Weight gain	—	—	(Add 1000 kcal/day to normal requirement)

$W = $ *weight (kg)*, $H = $ *height (cm)*, $A = $ *age (years)*

2. **Daily calories** required can be calculated as:

$$BEE = 25 \times W$$

3. **Total energy expenditure (TEE)** can be calculated as:

$$TEE = BEE \times \text{activity factor} \times \text{stress factor}$$

   a. The **activity factor** is defined according to the patient's status.
      (1) Ventilator support = 1.10
      (2) Bedridden = 1.15
      (3) Normal = 1.25
   b. The **stress factor** varies according to the circumstances (Table 15-2).
   c. The best way to determine TEE in critically ill patients is **indirect calorimetry,** which measures oxygen consumption and carbon dioxide production.
4. The **oxygen consumption index** is the best single measurement of hypermetabolism and can be calculated as:

$$\text{Oxygen consumption} = \frac{\text{metabolic rate}}{4.3}$$

III. Caloric Sources and Supplements
   ### A. Carbohydrates
   1. **Caloric value** = 3.4 kcal/g
   2. Carbohydrates stimulate insulin release, which inhibits the mobilization of free fatty acids from adipose.

Table 15-2. Increased Metabolic Activity by Patient Status

Patient Status	Increased Metabolic Activity (%)	Stress Factor
Elective operation	0–5	1.00–1.05
Peritonitis	5–25	1.05–1.25
Long bone fracture	15–30	1.15–1.30
Multiple trauma	30–55	1.30–1.55
Severe head injury	30–50	1.30–1.50
Sepsis	50–75	1.50–1.75
Burns		
10%	25	1.25
20%	50	1.50
30%	70	1.70
40%	85	1.85
50%	100	2.0
75%	100–110	2.1

3. Carbohydrate metabolism produces an abundance of carbon dioxide, which can be detrimental to patients with compromised lung function.
4. Excess carbohydrates can lead to fatty infiltration of the liver.
5. The body's use of carbohydrates may be impaired in sepsis and other stress states, resulting in hyperglycemia.
6. The **respiratory quotient (RQ)** is the ratio of carbon dioxide production to oxygen consumption and is expressed as:

$$RQ = \frac{V_{CO_2}}{V_{O_2}}$$

The RQ of carbohydrates is 1. An overall RQ > 0.9 indicates excess carbohydrate calories or fatty acid synthesis, in which case the total carbohydrate calories should be reduced by 40%.

B. Lipids
1. **Caloric value** = 9 kcal/g
2. In hospitalized patients, lipids provide 30%–50% of ingested calories.
3. Total fat delivery should not exceed 1.0–1.5 g/kg/day in an adult hospitalized patient.
4. The RQ for lipogenesis is 8.67. For oxidation of fats, the RQ is 0.7.
5. Linoleic and linolenic acids are the essential fatty acids and are components of IV fat emulsions. In patients with some fat intolerance, a minimum of 2%–4% of the daily calorie requirement should be essential fatty acids to meet the essential fatty acid requirements.

C. **Protein**
   1. **Caloric value** = 4.0 kcal/g
   2. **Recommended intake** is as follows:
      a. Normal states: 1.0–1.5 g/kg/day
      b. Catabolic states (e.g., sepsis, trauma): 1.5–2.0 g/kg/day
      c. Severe stress states (e.g., burns): 2–3 g/kg/day
   3. The RQ for protein is 0.8.
   4. **Nitrogen balance (NB)**
      a. Evaluate NB with the following equation:

$$NB \ (g) = \frac{protein \ intake \ (g)}{6.25 \ g} - (24\text{-}hour \ urinary \ nitrogen \ + \ 4)$$

$$6.25 \ g \ protein = 1 \ g \ nitrogen$$

   b. The NB should be 2–4 g daily. If it is negative, there is excessive catabolism, and the patient requires more protein.
   5. **Nonprotein-calorie:nitrogen ratio**
      a. Evaluate the nonprotein-calorie:nitrogen ratio.
         (1) A **normal** ratio is **150–250:1.**
         (2) A ratio of 125:1 is equivalent to 20% of calories supplied as protein.
         (3) The ratio should decrease with increasing stress.
      b. If protein is increased without an increase in calories (i.e., decrease in nonprotein-calorie:nitrogen ratio), protein will be broken down for energy.

D. **Elemental needs**
   1. **Chromium** is a cofactor for the action of insulin.
   2. **Selenium** is a cofactor for enzymes. It limits formation of the hydroxyl ion.
   3. **Zinc** is involved in nucleic acid synthesis. Deficiency increases the risk of infection. The normal dose is 4 mg daily.
   4. **Copper** deficiency leads to pancytopenia. The normal dose is 0.5–1.5 mg/day.
   5. **Glutamine** provides energy for intestinal mucosa during fasting. The normal dose is 0.5 g/kg/day.
   6. **Branched-chain amino acids** (e.g., leucine, isoleucine, valine) are required for protein synthesis. The normal dose is 0.5–1.2 g/kg/day.

IV. **Dietary Modifications in Disease States**
A. **Diabetes**
   1. Maintain serum glucose at 100–180 mg/dl.
   2. Use insulin in total parenteral nutrition (TPN) formulations to control hyperglycemia.
   3. Insulin drip is another option for aggressive glucose control and is ideal for critically ill patients with significant fluctuations in glucose levels.

B. **Acute renal failure (ARF)**
   1. ARF patients require 0.5–1.0 g/kg/day of protein. When

dialysis is used, protein can be increased to 1.2 g/kg/day for hemodialysis patients and 1.5–2.5 g/kg/day for peritoneal dialysis patients.
   2. Concentrated formulas provide adequate nutrition in limited volumes.
   3. Patients receiving peritoneal dialysis may absorb dextrose from the dialysate. The amount absorbed can be calculated as:

Dextrose from dialysate (kcal) = glucose concentration (g/L)
$$\times\ 3.4\ kcal/g \times 0.8 \times volume\ (L)$$

   4. Vitamin requirements for ARF patients are as follows.
      a. Patients on hemodialysis should be given 8.2 mg/day of pyridoxine to prevent deficiency.
      b. Ascorbic acid, 60–100 mg/day, should be provided to avoid increased serum oxalate levels.
      c. Folate should be supplemented at 1 mg/day.
      d. Trace elements should be given only three times per week.
      e. Vitamin D and calcium should be dosed based on calcium levels.

C. **Respiratory disease**
   1. Patients with respiratory disease require 1.5–2.0 g/kg/day of protein. If fatigue is a concern, decrease protein intake to 1.2 g/kg/day.
   2. Limit carbohydrates to 4 mg/kg/day to prevent lipogenesis.
   3. Restrict fluid to 1.0–1.5 L/day. Restrict sodium if hypernatremia develops.
   4. Aspiration precautions must be instituted.

D. **Hepatic disease**
   1. Start with 1.5 g/kg/day of protein. If hepatic encephalopathy develops, decrease protein to 0.7 g/kg/day, and then increase as tolerated.
   2. Hepatic disease is associated with defective lipid clearance, decreased lipolytic activity, decreased removal of free fatty acids, glucose intolerance, and insulin resistance.

V. **Enteral Nutrition**

Feed the gut whenever possible!

A. **Indications**
   1. **Routine indications**
      a. Protein-calorie malnutrition with inadequate oral intake of nutrients for ≥ 5 days
      b. Normal nutritional status but half of required oral intake for 7–10 days
      c. Severe dysphagia
      d. Major full-thickness burns
      e. Massive small bowel resection in combination with TPN
      f. Low-output enterocutaneous fistula

    2. Absolute indications
- **a.** Major trauma
- **b.** Radiation therapy
- **c.** Mild chemotherapy
- **d.** Liver failure and severe renal dysfunction

    3. Relative indications
- **a.** Intensive chemotherapy
- **b.** Immediate postoperative or stress period
- **c.** Acute enteritis
- **d.** Resection of small bowel ($> 90\%$)

B. Contraindications

    1. Absolute contraindications
- **a.** Shock (hemodynamic instability)
- **b.** Bowel obstruction
- **c.** Intestinal ischemia
- **d.** Ileus
- **e.** Profuse vomiting

    2. Relative contraindications
- **a.** Partial obstruction
- **b.** Severe diarrhea
- **c.** Severe pancreatitis
- **d.** Intraabdominal infection
- **e.** High-output fistula

C. Guidelines for enteral formula selection

    1. General considerations
- **a.** Select a product that is lactose free in the critically ill patient.
- **b.** Higher amounts of fat delivered into the stomach may result in slower gastric emptying.
- **c.** Fat provided as medium-chain triglycerides may result in less GI intolerance. However, long-chain fatty acids are also needed to provide essential fatty acids.
- **d.** Most critically ill patients have increased protein requirements. A product with a nonprotein-calorie:nitrogen ratio $< 125{:}1$ will better meet these protein requirements.

    2. Standard isotonic formulas
- **a.** An isotonic formula is a low-residue, balanced mixture of carbohydrate, protein, and fat.
- **b.** The nonprotein-calorie:nitrogen ratio is $150{:}1$.
- **c.** Macronutrients are in an intact state.
- **d.** The typical caloric density is 1.0 kcal/ml.
- **e.** Isotonic formulas are generally not appropriate for critically ill patients.

    3. Standard fiber-containing formulas
- **a.** Fiber-containing formulas are identical to isotonic formulas except for the presence of fiber, usually in the form of a soy polysaccharide.
- **b.** Fiber prolongs gut transit time, increases short-chain fatty acid availability, and improves intestinal architecture.

    4. High-density formulas
        a. Patients who are fluid restricted or who have high calorie and protein requirements benefit from higher nutrient density.
        b. These patients should receive 1.5–2.0 kcal/ml of high-density formula.
    5. High-protein formulas
        a. High-protein formulas are able to meet higher protein requirements without excessive caloric intake.
        b. The nonprotein-calorie:nitrogen ratio is $< 125:1$.
    6. Elemental peptide–based formulas
        a. Macronutrients are in simpler forms.
        b. Protein is in the form of dipeptides, tripeptides, or free amino acids.
        c. Fat is made up of varying proportions of medium- and long-chain triglycerides.
        d. Fat content is usually low (i.e., $\leq 10\%$ of total calories).
  D. Common enteral formulas (Table 15-3)
  E. Sites of feeding
    1. Stomach
        a. Advantage. The stomach acts as a reservoir and tolerates high osmolar loads. It may accept bolus feeds.
        b. Disadvantage. There is a high risk of aspiration. The patient should have intact mental status, a gag reflex, and no gastric atony.
    2. Small bowel
        a. Advantage. There is a reduced risk of aspiration, and the patient may be fed distal to atony or fistula.
        b. Disadvantage. Low tolerance to high osmolar load and bolus feedings; requires a low-viscosity formula and continuous irrigation of the tube to maintain patency.
  F. Placement of a feeding tube
    1. A nasogastric tube may be used to feed the stomach, although a **soft tube with a stylet and a radiopaque stripe is preferred.** The soft tube may also be placed into the small bowel.
    2. Specific steps should be followed when placing a feeding tube for short-term enteral therapy (see Chapter 34).
    3. If long-term enteral therapy is indicated in patients unable to take nutrients by mouth, there are two options for tube placement.
        a. Long-term **gastric tubes** may be placed operatively or endoscopically.
        b. Jejunostomy tubes may be used to feed the gut distal to the stomach. They may be placed operatively without risk of aspiration or they may be placed through a special gastric tube, which has a higher risk of aspiration.
VI. Parenteral Nutrition

Table 15-3. Common Enteral Formulas

Formula	Volume (kcal/ml)	Volume (mOsm/L)	Protein (g/L)	Fat (g/L)	Carbohydrates (g/L)
Amin-Aid	1.9	1095	19	19	366
Citrotein	0.6	—	40	1.7	121
Ensure	1.0	450	37	35	144
Ensure Hipro	1.0	610	50	25	128
Ensure Plus	1.5	650	63	50	200
Hepatic Aid	1.7	360	43	36	289
Impact	—	375	56	28	130
Isocal	1.0	300	34	44	132
Isocal HN	1.0	300	44	45	113
Isosource VHN	1.0	300	62	29	130
Jevity	1.0	310	44	37	133
Magnacal	1.9	590	70	76	250
Nepro	2.0	635	70	96	215
Osmolite	1.06	300	44	35	144
Osmolite HN	1.06	310	44	37	149
Promote (fiber)	1.0	370	63	28	139
Pulmocare	1.5	490	62	92	115
Replenia	1.0	615	30	95.6	—
Stresstein	1.2	910	37	27	173
Sustacal	1.0	675	61	58	—

continued

Table 15-3. Common Enteral Formulas

Formula	Volume (kcal/ml)	Volume (mOsm/L)	Protein (g/L)	Fat (g/L)	Carbohydrates (g/L)
Sustacal HN	1.5	700	61	58	130
TraumaAid	1.0	—	28	12	166
Travasorb H	1.1	600	29	15	210
Travasorb R	1.3	590	23	18	274
Two-Cal HN	2.0	665	70	91	217
Vivonex	1.0	550	21	1	226
Vivonex HN	1.0	810	43	1	211
Vivonex Plus	1.0	650	45	6.7	190
Vivonex T.E.N.	1.0	630	38	3	206

A. Indications

1. **Preoperative indications**

   a. Preoperatively, TPN is reserved for **severely malnourished** patients (i.e., weight loss > 10% and serum albumin < 2.5, or weight loss > 20%).

   b. For maximum benefit, maintain the patient on TPN for **5–7 days before surgery.**

2. **Absolute indications**

   a. Malabsorption (e.g., massive small bowel resection, radiation enteritis, protracted diarrhea)

   b. High-dose chemotherapy or radiation

   c. Moderate-to-severe pancreatitis

   d. Loss of > 10% of usual body weight

   e. Catabolic state and NPO for 5–7 days

3. **Relative indications**

   a. After major surgery when regular enteral diet will not be resumed for 10 days

   b. After stresses such as moderate trauma or burns (30%–50% total body surface area) when enteral diet will not be resumed for 7–10 days

   c. Enterocutaneous fistula

   d. Inflammatory bowel disease

   e. Hyperemesis gravidarum

   f. Enteral nutrition will not be started within 7–10 days of hospitalization

   g. Enteral feeds cannot meet nutritional requirements

B. Composition of parenteral formulas

1. There is a standard **solution content** for each type of parenteral formula (i.e., peripheral and central) [Table 15-4].

2. The **lipid formulation** may be dosed on a twice weekly schedule or, in some institutions, may be combined in TPN formulation and given continuously.

   a. For 500 kcal/day, give 10% lipids at 20 ml/hr IV.

   b. For 1000 kcal/day, give 20% lipids at 20 ml/hr IV.

3. Table 15-5 lists **daily additives** for central parenteral nutrition formulas.

C. Creating a TPN formula

1. Determine daily fluid, calorie, and protein requirements.

2. Choose an amino acid solution and calculate volume needed for protein.

Table 15-4. Solution Content of Parenteral Formulas

Parenteral Nutrition	Dextrose (%)	Amino Acid (%)	Fat (%)
Peripheral*	5–10	3.00–4.25	20
Central†	15–30	3.5–10.0	10–20

*The peripheral formula is a total of 600–900 mOsm/L (or 0.3–0.6 kcal/ml).
†The central formula is ≥ 1900 mOsm/L (or 0.6–1.2 kcal/ml).

Table 15-5. Daily Additives for Central Parenteral Nutrition Formulas

Nutrient	Standard Content	Customary Range
Sodium	130 mEq	0–150 mEq
Phosphate	2 mmol	0–20 mmol
Magnesium	5 mEq	0–15 mEq
Chloride	50 mEq	0–150 mEq
Potassium	30 mEq	0–80 mEq
Calcium	4.7 mEq	0–10 mEq
Acetate	90 mEq	70–220 mEq
Vitamin K	1 mg	
Multivitamins (10-ml formulation)		
Vitamin A	3300 IU	—
Vitamin D	200 IU	—
Vitamin E	10 mg	—
Vitamin C	100 mg	—
Vitamin B_1 (thiamine)	3 mg	—
Vitamin B_2 (riboflavin)	3.6 mg	—
Vitamin B_6 (pyridoxine)	4 mg	—
Vitamin B_{12}	5 μg	—
Niacin	40 mg	—
Pantothenic acid	15 mg	—
Folic acid	0.4 mg	—
Biotin	60 μg	—
Trace elements (3-ml formulation)		
Zinc	5 mg	—
Copper	1 mg	—
Manganese	0.5 mg	—
Chromium	—	—
Selenium	—	—

3. Determine the dextrose solution and number of calories.
4. Determine volume of lipid infusion and dosing schedule.
5. Check the patient's electrolytes and determine electrolyte composition of TPN.
6. Add daily vitamins and essential elements (e.g., vitamin K, cimetidine).
7. Determine insulin needs. Most patients require insulin while on TPN.

D. **Stepwise approach to TPN ordering**
   1. Calculate total **daily caloric needs:**

Daily caloric needs = BEE × activity factor × stress factor

Amino Acids (%)	Protein (g)	Nitrogen (g)	Calories
1.0	10	1.6	40
1.5	15	2.4	60
2.0	20	3.2	80
2.5	25	4.0	100
3.0	30	4.8	120
3.5	35	5.6	140
4.0	40	6.4	160
4.5	45	7.2	180
5.0	50	8.0	200
5.5	55	8.8	220
6.0	60	9.6	240
6.5	65	10.4	260
7.0	70	11.2	280

Table 15-6. Contents of Amino Acid Solutions*

*These measurements are per liter of solution.

2. Determine **amino acid component** (Table 15-6) using the following equations:

$$Protein\ (g/day) = 1.5\ g \times body\ weight\ (kg)$$

$$Amount\ of\ kcal\ from\ protein = protein\ (g/day) \times 4\ kcal/g$$

$$Volume\ of\ amino\ acids\ from\ 15\%\ stock = \frac{total\ daily\ protein\ (g)}{15\ g/100\ ml}$$

3. Determine the **lipid component** using the following equations:

$$Calories\ from\ fat\ (should\ be\ \textbf{25\%}\ of\ total\ nonprotein\ calories) = \textbf{0.25} \times (total\ BEE - protein\ calories)$$

$$Grams\ of\ fat\ necessary = \frac{total\ calories\ from\ fat}{9\ kcal/g}$$

4. Determine the **volume of fat solution** using the following equations:

$$Volume\ of\ 20\%\ fat\ solution\ for\ a\ 3\ in\ 1\ solution = \frac{total\ daily\ fat\ (g)}{20\ g/100\ ml}$$

$$Volume\ of\ 10\%\ fat\ solution\ for\ a\ 2\ in\ 1\ solution$$
$$(piggyback) = \frac{fat\ (kcal)}{1.1\ kcal/ml}$$

5. Determine the **carbohydrate component** using the following equations:

$$Calories\ from\ dextrose = total\ calories - [protein\ (kcal) + fat\ (kcal)]$$

$$Grams\ of\ dextrose = \frac{calories\ from\ dextrose}{3.4\ kcal/g}$$

$$Volume\ of\ 70\%\ dextrose\ solution = \frac{dextrose\ (g/day)}{70\ g/100\ ml}$$

6. **Characteristics of final solution**
   a. 3 in 1 solution = glucose + protein + lipid
   b. 2 in 1 solution = glucose + protein (lipid is infused separately)

E. **Central line placement for TPN** (see Chapter 49)

F. **Peripheral parenteral nutrition** is an option for short-term therapy. It requires:
   1. Large volumes (formulas are dilute for peripheral use)
   2. Separate infusion of lipids
   3. Frequent peripheral IV placements

VII. **Monitoring Enteral and Parenteral Nutrition**
   A. After confirmation of placement of the feeding tube or central line, start the infusion at a low rate and plan to increase progressively every 6–8 hours. This allows the patient's system to adjust to the new calories.
   B. Check fingersticks for glucose during the first 1–2 days of TPN, or until the patient is stable on an hourly rate.
   C. With tube feeding, check residual volume every 2–4 hours for gastric retention.
   D. Add methylene blue to tube feeds to aid in surveillance for possible aspiration or fistula.
   E. Evaluate electrolytes, liver function, BUN/creatinine, and RQ. Monitor urine for glucose spillage.
   F. Obtain body weight, total protein, albumin, transferrin, and prealbumin before starting TPN.
   G. On a weekly basis, obtain electrolytes, BUN/creatinine, liver function tests, bilirubin, albumin, total protein, and triglycerides. Continue checking daily weights and monitor prealbumin and transferrin weekly to determine nutritional status.
      1. Prealbumin has a half-life of 2–3 days. Prealbumin should increase as the correct nutritional regimen is given. If there is no increase, the regimen must be altered.
      2. Albumin has a half-life of 18–20 days.
      3. Transferrin has a half-life of 5–7 days.

VIII. **Pediatric Nutrition**
   A. **General guidelines**
      1. Children have less body fat than adults and therefore less energy reserves when unable to eat. TPN must be started earlier in children. The schedules suggested in the following guidelines are shortened during hypermetabolic states and preexisting malnutrition.
         a. Premature infant: 1–2 days after NPO status
         b. Term neonates: 3–4 days after NPO status

Table 15-7. Guidelines for Nutrients in Total Parenteral Nutrition Formulas for Children

Nutrient	Amount Required for Term Infants (< 1 Year Or Up To 10 kg)	Amount Required for Older Children (> 1 Year)
Carbohydrate	7%–18% of total calories	25% of total calories
Amino acids	2–3 g/kg/day	1.5–2.5 g/kg/day
Fat (10%–20% emulsion)	4 g/kg/day (maximum)	2–4 g/kg/day
Electrolytes		
Na^+	2–4 mEq/kg/day	2–4 mEq/kg/day
K^+	1–2 mEq/kg/day	1–2 mEq/kg/day
Ca^{+2}	500–600 mg/L	200–400 mg/L
Mg^{+2}	50–70 mg/L	20–40 mg/L
PO_4	400–450 mg/L	150–300 mg/L

  c. Children: 4–6 days after NPO status
  d. Adolescents: 7–10 days after NPO status
 2. Follow the guidelines for **standard TPN formulas** in children of different ages (Table 15-7).
 3. In the **postoperative period,** for advancement of enteral feeds, use low osmolar formulas and feed with small volumes at frequent intervals, checking gastric residuals.
B. Nutritional requirements
 1. Calorie requirements for adequate growth
  a. Newborn or premature: 120 kcal/kg/day
  b. Infant: caloric needs determined by weight. (Most infant formulas contain 20 calories per ounce, usually divided as 50% carbohydrates, 35% fat, and 15% protein.)
   (1) Give 100 kcal/kg/day for the first 10 kg of weight.
   (2) For the next 10 kg of weight, add 50 kcal/kg/day.
   (3) For weight > 20 kg, add 20 kcal/kg/day.
   (4) For example, for a 25-kg child:

$$
\begin{aligned}
10\ kg \times 100\ kcal/kg/day &= 1000\ kcal \\
10\ kg \times \ 50\ kcal/kg/day &= \ 500\ kcal \\
\underline{\ 5\ kg \times \ 20\ kcal/kg/day} &= \underline{\ 100\ kcal} \\
25\ kg \qquad\qquad\qquad\quad\ &= 1600\ kcal/day
\end{aligned}
$$

 2. Protein requirements
  a. 0–6 months: 2.5–3.0 g/kg/day
  b. 6–12 months: 2.0–2.5 g/kg/day
  c. School age: 1.75 g/kg/day
  d. Adolescent: 1.2 g/kg/day
 3. Lipid requirements. Of the total daily calories, 35% should be fat, up to a maximum of 3.5 g/kg/day.

C. Peripheral parenteral nutrition
1. The limiting factor is the osmolality of the solution.
2. To achieve adequate calories, it is essential to use maximum doses of fat and fluid volumes above maintenance. For example:
   a. 20% fat: 4.0 g/kg/day × 9 kcal/g = **36 kcal/kg/day**
   b. 12.5% dextrose (100 ml): 12.5 g/kg/day × 3.7 kcal/g = **46 kcal/kg/day**
   c. 20 g/L protein (100 ml): 2.0 g/kg/day × 4.0 kcal/g = **8 kcal/kg/day**

Obstetrical Disorders

....

HEMORRHAGE

I. **Antepartum Hemorrhage**
  A. **Benign causes of vaginal spotting or bleeding**
    1. **Recent intercourse.** Cervical irritation with intercourse may lead to self-limited vaginal spotting.
    2. **Passage of the cervical mucus plug**
      a. The self-limited discharge of thick mucus is mixed with varying amounts of dark blood.
      b. Passage is spontaneous and usually occurs independently of uterine contractions several weeks prior to the onset of labor.
    3. **Progression of normal labor**
      a. Labor is associated with modest amounts of blood passed per vagina ("bloody show").
      b. Diagnosis requires documented cervical change in the presence of frequent uterine contractions, and it is best accomplished by an obstetrician.
  B. **Pathologic causes of third-trimester bleeding**

> **The onset of bleeding during the third trimester of pregnancy is potentially life-threatening for both the fetus and the mother. It is important to distinguish between benign and pathologic etiologies.**

    1. **Abruptio placentae**
      a. **Definition.** Abruptio placentae is a phenomenon in which the placenta prematurely separates from its site of implantation. This separation leads to intrauterine pooling of maternal blood, which usually drains through the uterine cervix.
      b. **Incidence.** Abruptio placentae complicates approximately 1 in 86 to 120 births. Eighty percent of recognized cases occur prior to the onset of labor.
      c. **Etiology** (as yet unknown)

    (1) Bleeding is initiated in the decidua basalis.

    (2) With progression, the pooling blood creates a plane of separation within the placenta and shears it from the myometrium.

d. Risk factors

    (1) Maternal hypertension (> 140/90 mm Hg)

    (2) Abdominal trauma

    (3) Cocaine use

    (4) History of abruptio placentae

    (5) Rapid decompression of the overdistended uterus (i.e., rupture of membranes in women with polyhydramnios or after delivery of the first fetus in a twin gestation)

e. Other identified associations (controversial)

    (1) Male fetus

    (2) Diabetes mellitus

    (3) Poor weight gain

    (4) Multiparity

    (5) Fetal anomalies

    (6) Tobacco use

    (7) Ethanol consumption

f. Clinical presentation (often a classic symptom triad)

    (1) **Vaginal bleeding.** The single most reliable physical sign of abruptio placentae, vaginal bleeding is present in > 80% of cases.

    (2) **Increased uterine tone or tenderness.** This condition is often a sign of more serious abruptio placentae. Increased tone in the absence of clinical hypovolemia is present in only 17% of cases.

    (3) **Fetal distress or death.** Fetal distress develops in > 60% of all patients with a live fetus. Abruptio placentae is associated with a perinatal mortality rate of 25% to 50%.

g. Precipitation of disseminated intravascular coagulation (DIC). This condition occurs in 30% of severe cases of abruptio placentae. Release of placental thromboplastins may precipitate intravascular or retroplacental coagulation.

    (1) Normal maternal fibrinogen is approximately 450 mg/dl.

    (2) Circulating fibrinogen < 300 mg/dl has been correlated with significant coagulopathy. A fibrinogen level < 150 mg/dl is strongly suggestive of blood loss greater than 2 L. Nearly all gravidas ultimately require transfusion.

h. Types of abruptio placentae

    (1) **Concealed abruptio placentae.** This may occur without appreciable vaginal bleeding.

        (a) Maternal blood, which is walled off from the uterine cervix by portions of the placenta or membranes that remain adherent, pools behind the placenta.

   (b) This condition is most commonly manifested as premature labor. A less frequent symptom is low back pain.

(2) Low-grade abruptio placentae may persist clinically undetected for long periods (e.g., days to weeks).

(3) Chronic abruptio placentae may be manifested as the leakage of dark, flocculent material similar in appearance to prune juice.

2. Placenta previa

a. Definitions. Placenta previa is a condition in which the implantation site of the placenta includes the internal cervical os.

   (1) Placenta previa may be characterized as either **partial or complete,** depending on the degree to which the placenta covers the os.

   (2) Marginal placenta previa describes a condition in which the edge of the placenta approaches but does not cover the os.

   (3) Vasa previa, a related condition, occurs when placental vessels feeding the umbilical cord are closely approximated to the cervical os.

b. Incidence

   (1) Placenta previa occurs less often with increasing gestational age. It complicates as many as 6% of pregnancies at 16–18 weeks' gestation but only 0.6% of term deliveries.

   (2) Expansion of the lower uterine segment with fetal growth is thought to account for the decreased incidence of placenta previa with gestational maturity.

c. Risk factors

   (1) Previous cesarean sections

   (2) High parity

   (3) Advanced maternal age

   (4) Prior pregnancy terminations

   (5) Tobacco use

   (6) Placenta accreta

d. Etiology. Placenta previa may relate to defective decidual vascularization, leading to abnormal attachment of the placenta to the uterine wall.

e. Symptoms

   (1) Acute, painless vaginal bleeding (70% of cases). Vaginal bleeding results from disruption of placental implantation.

     (a) Normal thinning of the lower uterine segment late in gestation may predispose the patient to bleeding.

     (b) Cervical trauma, including intercourse, often leads to the onset of bleeding.

        (2) Uterine contractions (20% of cases)

  3. Fetal hemorrhage

    a. A rare complication of pregnancy, fetal hemorrhage may result from **rupture of a placental vessel** in conditions such as vasa previa.

    b. The **Apt test** can differentiate fetal and maternal sources of vaginal bleeding.

      (1) One part vaginal blood (5–10 ml) is mixed with 5 parts tap water and centrifuged for 2 minutes. Then five parts of the resultant supernatant are mixed with 1 part 0.25 N NaOH solution.

      (2) A pink color in the final supernatant indicates the presence of fetal hemoglobin (Hgb), which is resistant to denaturation. Maternal blood turns yellow-brown.

C. Diagnostic work-up

  1. CBC

  2. Platelet count

  3. Fibrinogen level

  4. Coagulation studies [prothrombin time (PT), partial thromboplastin time (PTT)]

  5. Blood type and antibody screening

D. Management

  1. Amount of blood lost (relative volume) should be assessed initially.

    a. Careful attention should be paid to subtle signs of circulatory insufficiency.

    b. Continuous fetal monitoring should be initiated. The fetus is particularly sensitive to relative placental hypoperfusion, which can occur even in an apparently normotensive gravida.

  2. As with all surgical hemorrhages, **two large-bore IV lines** should be maintained at all times.

    a. Fluid resuscitation should be initiated early to ensure fetal well-being.

    b. Nasal oxygen supplementation should be initiated to further facilitate fetal well-being.

  3. Transabdominal ultrasound should be performed to establish the location of the placenta.

    a. Digital vaginal examination is contraindicated until placenta previa or vasa previa is excluded. If placenta previa cannot be excluded sonographically, a vaginal examination should be performed only by a qualified obstetrician. The physician should be prepared for immediate cesarean section and blood transfusion if necessary.

    b. Ultrasonography allows for diagnosis of fewer than 2% of cases of abruptio placentae. However, ultrasonographic visualization of retroplacental hemorrhage can establish the diagnosis.

  4. Continuous assessment of fetal well-being should be an early part of the evaluation. Either **ultrasonography** or **nonstress testing (NST)** may be used.

   a. **Ultrasonography.** A **biophysical profile** can be performed to assess fetal well-being. For reassurance of fetal well-being, the following conditions should be present.

   (1) Fetal movements (at least 2 movements within 30 minutes)

   (2) Continuous fetal breathing (30 seconds)

   (3) Fetal tone (one extension and flexion motion of a fetal extremity in a 30-minute interval)

   (4) Adequate amniotic fluid

   b. **NST**

   (1) NST is performed by continuously evaluating fetal heart rate by external Doppler monitor for at least 30 minutes.

   (2) A **reassuring NST** includes both adequate long-term variability and reactivity.

   (a) **Reactivity** is defined as a minimum of two increases in the fetal heart rate over baseline of more than 15 beats/min lasting at least 15 seconds during 20 minutes of monitoring.

   (b) **Variability (long-term)** is best defined as changes in the baseline fetal heart rate of at least 5 beats/min.

A sinusoidal pattern of the fetal heart pattern on NST denotes severe fetal anemia and is an ominous finding, often dictating emergent delivery. A sinusoidal fetal heart rate is characterized by regular swings in the baseline heart rate of 5–20 beats/min with a periodicity of 3–5 beats/min.

---

5. Appropriate **blood products** should be transfused for severe anemia or coagulopathies. Maternal hematocrit should be maintained above 30%.

6. **Emergent or induced delivery** may be necessary regardless of fetal maturity, if obstetrical hemorrhage compromises fetal or maternal well-being.

   a. Fetal viability begins at approximately 24 weeks' estimated gestational age. Fetal morbidity and mortality decline significantly after 34 weeks' gestation.

   b. Delivery permits more efficacious control of hemorrhage, removes precipitants of DIC that may occur with abruptio placentae, and results in more rapid correction of coagulopathies.

   c. Vaginal delivery may be successful in cases of marginal placenta previa or stable, low-grade abruptio placentae.

   d. The onset of labor with partial or complete placenta previa requires cesarean section.

7. **Expectant management** is preferred for patients with documented placenta previa early in the third trimester (24–36 weeks).
   a. Tocolysis may be necessary to terminate contractions in these cases.
   b. Magnesium sulfate or calcium channel blockers are the preferred tocolytic agents, because β-adrenergic agents may mask signs of hypovolemia.

II. Postpartum Hemorrhage

A. **Normal discharge.** A serosanguinous discharge, known as **lochia,** is a normal postpartum event.
   1. Most women describe the flow of lochia as similar or less than that of normal menses.
   2. Subjectively greater bleeding should raise concern of postpartum hemorrhage.

B. **Immediate postpartum hemorrhage**
   1. **Definition.** Immediate postpartum hemorrhage, which complicates approximately 5% of deliveries, is defined as the loss of more than 500 ml of blood during the first 24 hours following delivery.
   2. **Etiology** (decreasing order of frequency)
      a. **Uterine atony**
         (1) Adequate contraction of the myometrium is critical for postpartum hemostasis. Poor myometrial tone results in inadequate postpartum tamponade of the spiral arteries.
         (2) **Risk factors**
            (a) Grand multiparity (> 5 deliveries)
            (b) Chorioamnionitis
            (c) Uterine overdistension (e.g., possible with multiple gestations or polyhydramnios)
            (d) General anesthesia
            (e) IV therapy with magnesium sulfate
            (f) Precipitous labor
            (g) Markedly prolonged labor
            (h) Induction or augmentation of labor with pitocin
      b. Unappreciated **pelvic** or **cervical lacerations**
         (1) Bleeding in the presence of a firmly contracted uterus suggests an unappreciated genital tract laceration.
         (2) Such a laceration occurs more frequently following rapid labor or an instrumental delivery.

Blood loss from an episiotomy rarely exceeds 200 ml.

---

      c. **Retained products of conception.** Although this is a relatively rare cause of immediate postpartum hemorrhage, portions of placenta retained after delivery may prevent adequate myometrial contraction and result in significant bleeding.

(1) **Incidence.** This condition occurs significantly more often when the third stage of labor (delivery of the placenta) lasts longer than 30 minutes. **Preterm delivery** is a risk factor associated with retained products of conception.

(2) **Etiology. Placenta accreta,** a frequent cause of retained products of conception, is the abnormal placentation in which trophoblastic tissue penetrates the uterine wall beyond Nitabuch's layer.

   (a) Placenta accreta **prevents complete expulsion of the placenta** with the third stage of labor, and delivery of a placenta accreta may be complicated by uterine inversion. This condition complicates approximately 1 in 7000 pregnancies.

   (b) **Risk factors** include previous cesarean section, pregnancy termination, or implantation of the placenta over the site of a uterine scar.

C. Late postpartum hemorrhage

  1. Incidence. Serious hemorrhage more than 24 hours following delivery complicates < 1% of all deliveries.

  2. Etiology. Causes include **subinvolution of the former placental site** and **retained products of conception.** In addition, **endomyometritis** may precipitate late postpartum bleeding by lysing clots in the spiral arteries.

D. Management. Primary goals are rapid identification of the cause of hemorrhage and minimization of blood loss.

  1. Manual exploration of the uterus should be performed.

    a. The presence of retained products should be ruled out, and uterine tone should be assessed.

    b. Bimanual massage may increase myometrial tone and provide a potential means to tamponade acute bleeding.

  2. Fluid resuscitation should be initiated early to prevent hypovolemia.

  3. Careful inspection of the cervix and vaginal sidewalls should be performed to identify lacerations.

> **Unappreciated cervical or vaginal sidewall lacerations are associated with instrumental deliveries and rapid labor.**

    a. Genital tract lacerations should be suspected when bleeding persists with adequate uterine tone. Cervical lacerations bleed most often from vessels at or above their apex.

    b. Lacerations should be repaired with hemostatic sutures started superior to the apex.

  4. Medical treatment of uterine atony using pharmacologic agents may be necessary.

    a. Pitocin, 20–40 U (diluted in 1000 ml of crystalloid) IV (125–200 ml/hr)

    b. Ergot derivatives such as methylergonovine (Methergine), which are usually administered either IM or PO
      (1) Primary use: only if pitocin is ineffective
      (2) Dose (IM or PO only): 200 μg IM followed by 200 μg PO q 4 hr × 5
      (3) Primary side effect: severe hypertension

Methylergonovine should be avoided in patients with pregnancy-associated hypertension.

---

    c. Carboprost [prostaglandin (PG) F_2 alpha analogue], 250 μg IM repeated q 15–90 min × 8 if necessary
  5. Uterine curettage may be necessary to remove retained products of conception. **Emergent hysterectomy** is frequently required to treat placenta accreta.
  6. Medical management of uterine inversion may be necessary.
    a. If the placenta is separated, an **attempt should be made to replace the uterus** with gentle fundal pressure directed upward through the vagina and the cervix.
    b. Use of **inhalational anesthetics** for pelvic relaxation and reversal may be necessary.
  7. In cases of late hemorrhage, **endometritis** and **IV antibiotics** should be considered.
  8. For severe or protracted hemorrhage, **hypogastric artery ligation, percutaneous uterine artery embolization,** or **hysterectomy** may be necessary.
  9. Management of pelvic hematomas is conservative if the patient is clinically stable and no ongoing bleeding is evident.

HYPERTENSIVE DISORDERS OF PREGNANCY

  I. Definitions. Hypertension, which occurs in 6% to 8% of pregnancies, causes approximately 15% of maternal mortality. There are two distinct types of elevated blood pressure in pregnancy.
    A. Chronic hypertension is manifested by elevated blood pressure before 20 weeks' gestation or persisting after 42 days postpartum.
    B. Pregnancy-induced hypertension (PIH) develops after 20 weeks' gestation. This condition may develop in patients with underlying chronic hypertension. It may be further divided into subcategories based on end-organ involvement.
      1. Preeclampsia, which represents involvement of the renal system, is manifested by proteinuria.
      2. Eclampsia, which involves the central nervous system (CNS), is hallmarked by seizures.

       3. Hemolysis, elevated liver enzymes, and low platelets (HELLP) syndrome involves the hematologic and hepatic systems.

II. Risk factors (Table 16–1)

III. Diagnosis

  A. Chronic hypertension

    1. The **incidence** of chronic hypertension is increased in older, obese African-American patients. It is present in approximately 1% to 5% of pregnancies.

    2. Chronic hypertension may be categorized as either **mild or severe.**

      a. Mild hypertension is characterized by sustained blood pressure elevations > 140/90 mm Hg.

      b. Severe hypertension is characterized by diastolic blood pressures > 110 mm Hg.

  B. PIH. This condition is characterized by sustained blood pressure elevation to levels of 140 mm Hg systolic or 90 mm Hg diastolic, measured in a uniform manner in a sitting position.

    1. Preeclampsia

      a. Mild preeclampsia. Signs and symptoms include:

        (1) Sustained hypertension (see *B–PIH* above)

        (2) Proteinuria (≥ 300 mg per 24-hour urine collection). Urinary dipstick values correlate poorly with 24-hour values; however, values > 1+ on separate occasions more than 4–6 hours apart support the diagnosis.

        (3) Edema (nondependent). This condition may also manifest as rapid increases in maternal weight gain.

        (4) Laboratory results that increase the index of suspicion for preeclampsia:

          (a) Rising Hgb/hematocrit, representing hemoconcentration

          (b) Elevated uric acid > 5.4 mg/dl

          (c) Platelet count < 100,000/μl

Table 16-1.   Risk Factors for Pregnancy-induced Hypertension (PIH)

Risk Factor	Risk Ratio
Nulliparity	3:1
Age > 40 years	3:1
African-American race	1.5:1
Family history of PIH	5:1
Chronic hypertension	10:1
Chronic renal disease	20:1
Antiphospholipid syndrome	10:1
Diabetes mellitus	2:1
Twin gestation	4:1

        (d) Elevated liver enzymes (AST/ALT)
        (e) Rising BUN > 14 mg/dl
        (f) Creatinine > 0.8 mg/dl
  b. Severe preeclampsia. Signs and symptoms include:
    (1) Sustained blood pressure (> 160–180 mm Hg systolic or > 110 mm Hg diastolic) **or**
    (2) Blood pressure criteria for mild preeclampsia (see *a–Mild preeclampsia* above) **and** any of the following characteristics:
      (a) Proteinuria (> 5 g/24-hr urine) [or persistent $3+$ to $4+$ on serial urine dipsticks]
      (b) Oliguria (< 400 ml of urine in 24 hours)
      (c) Intrauterine growth restriction (IUGR) or oligohydramnios
      (d) Pulmonary edema
      (e) CNS symptoms, including visual disturbances, headache unresponsive to conventional therapy, and seizures (eclampsia)
      (f) Epigastric or right upper quadrant pain, indicating liver involvement
      (g) HELLP syndrome
2. Eclampsia. This condition occurs in 0.2% to 0.3% of patients with preeclampsia. Eclampsia is marked by **CNS involvement,** which leads to generalized **seizures.**
  a. The majority of seizures occur before and during birth.
    (1) Antepartum period: 50%
    (2) Intrapartum period: 25%
    (3) Postpartum period: 25%
  b. Headache is the most common complaint prior to the development of seizures. Hyperreflexia and ankle clonus are frequently seen in patients who seize.
3. HELLP syndrome. Approximately one-third of cases develop postpartum.
  a. Affected patients may present with the absence of blood pressure elevation in approximately 10% to 20% of cases.
  b. Diagnosis is made on the basis of the presence of hemolysis, elevated transaminases, and thrombocytopenia.
4. Chronic hypertension with superimposed preeclampsia-eclampsia. Patients with chronic hypertension during the second to third trimester may develop signs and symptoms of preeclampsia or eclampsia.

IV. Management
  A. Chronic hypertension
    1. Patients with mild chronic hypertension should be followed expectantly without medical treatment. Therapy does not improve neonatal or maternal outcome.
    2. Treatment is instituted for persistent diastolic blood pressure elevations > 110 mm Hg.

    a. α-methyldopa, 250 mg PO qid, has been extensively studied in pregnancy and deemed safe.

    b. Labetalol and nifedipine are acceptable alternatives.

Angiotensin-converting enzyme (ACE) inhibitors are not safe for use in pregnancy.

---

3. Patients with chronic hypertension are at increased risk for having a fetus with IUGR. Clinical assessment should guide the antenatal testing based on severity of hypertension.

    a. Antepartum fetal testing should be undertaken after 32 weeks with weekly NSTs when indicated.

    b. Ultrasound assessment for fetal growth is frequently undertaken after 32 weeks.

4. Chronic hypertension is associated with an increased risk of abruptio placentae and superimposed preeclampsia.

B. PIH

The definitive treatment for PIH is delivery. Patients who present with PIH at 37 weeks or more should be delivered.

---

1. Treatment for elevated blood pressure should be started when the systolic blood pressure rises above 180 mm Hg or the diastolic blood pressure rises above 110 mm Hg. The goal is reduction in maternal morbidity, with the diastolic blood pressure between 90 and 105 mm Hg.

    a. First-line agents for blood pressure control

      (1) Hydralazine, 5–10 mg slow IV push, repeated q 10–20 min as needed (up to 30 mg)

      (2) Labetalol, 10–20 mg slow IV push, followed by 20–80 mg IV push q 10 min to a total dose of 300 mg

    b. Agents for severe unresponsive hypertension

      (1) Nitroglycerin, IV, may be necessary.

      (2) Nitroprusside, IV, should be reserved for postpartum patients because of the accumulation of the thiocyanide metabolite and its effects on the fetus.

2. Treatment and prophylaxis for seizures

    a. Magnesium sulfate is the drug of choice. The **goal of therapy** is a magnesium level of 4–8 mEq/L.

      (1) Dose (prophylaxis): loading bolus of 4 g IV over 5 minutes, followed by a continuous infusion of 1–2 g/hr

      (2) Dose (treatment): loading bolus of 6 g IV, followed by a continuous infusion of 2 g/hr

      (3) Duration of therapy: 24 hours postpartum (routinely)

      (4) Conditions that require dose alterations

        (a) Impaired renal function: lower doses

            (b) Increased volume of distribution: higher doses
- **b.** Monitoring of magnesium levels is not mandatory.
  - **(1)** Clinical correlation with magnesium levels involves assessment of respiratory rate, mental status, and deep tendon reflexes.
    - **(a)** 4–8 mEq/L (therapeutic levels): loss of hyperreflexia
    - **(b)** 10 mEq/L: loss of deep tendon reflexes
    - **(c)** 15 mEq/L: respiratory depression
    - **(d)** > 25 mEq/L: cardiac arrest
  - **(2)** In patients who display evidence of magnesium toxicity, magnesium levels help direct treatment.

Treatment of suspected magnesium toxicity involves administration of 10% calcium gluconate, 10 ml IV over 2–3 minutes.

---

3. **Mild preeclampsia remote from term**
   - **a. Conservative management** is appropriate. Whether inpatient or outpatient treatment should be used is controversial.
     - **(1)** Patients should initially be hospitalized for 24 hours for urine collection, blood pressure monitoring, laboratory evaluation, and fetal monitoring. Those who respond to bed rest may be managed as outpatients with daily blood pressure measurements, symptom checks, and frequent laboratory evaluation.
     - **(2)** Patients who are not candidates for outpatient therapy should be followed as inpatients.
   - **b. Delivery is indicated** once patients reach term.
   - **c. Patients who develop worsening symptoms should be treated as for severe preeclampsia** (see HYPERTENSIVE DISORDERS OF PREGNANCY: IV B 4).
4. **Severe preeclampsia remote from term (Figure 16–1)**
   - **a. Magnesium sulfate and antihypertensive therapy** should be initiated as indicated.
   - **b. Fluid restriction** to 2400 ml/24 hr should occur secondary to the increased risk of pulmonary edema. If pulmonary edema is present, furosemide is the treatment of choice.
   - **c. Corticosteroids** are beneficial at less than 34 weeks' gestation. However, delivery should not be delayed if maternal or fetal testing deteriorates.
5. **HELLP syndrome**
   - **a. Antepartum therapy:** dexamethasone, 10 mg IV q 12 hr for 36 hours
   - **b. Postpartum therapy:** dexamethasone, 10 mg IV, followed by 10 mg IV, 5 mg IV, and 5 mg IV at 12-hour intervals

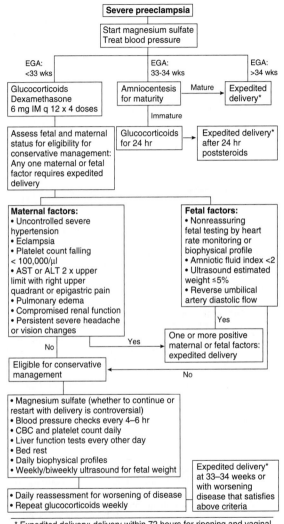

Figure 16–1. Algorithm for the management of severe preeclampsia. Expedited delivery is delivery within 72 hours (for ripening and vaginal delivery) unless the clinical situation dictates faster delivery. AST = aspartate aminotransferase; ALT = alanine aminotransferase; EGA = estimated gestational age.

17

Oncologic Emergencies

HYPERCALCEMIA OF MALIGNANCY. See Chapter
7 regarding the evaluation of hypercalcemia.

   I. **Definition:** Serum calcium levels > 13 mg/dl with associated
      malignancy. Hypercalcemia of malignancy must be thought of
      as a spectrum of disease depending on the type of malignancy
      and the degree of bone involvement.
  II. **Epidemiology.** This condition develops in 10% to 20% of pa-
      tients with malignancies.
 III. **Etiology**
      A. **Pathophysiology**
         1. The primary cause of the disease is increased osteoclastic
            bone resorption, which is due to mediators produced by
            the tumor or host cells. In solid tumors, parathyroid
            hormone–related protein (PTHrP) is the major mediator.
         2. PTHrP stimulates adenylate cyclase in renal and bone sys-
            tems, increases renal tubular reabsorption of calcium
            and osteoclastic bone resorption, and decreases renal
            phosphate uptake.
         3. There is usually a concomitant impairment of the renal
            mechanisms for clearing the increased calcium load.
         4. Parathyroid hormone (PTH), which normally regulates
            calcium homeostasis, also plays a role. PTH:
            a. Increases serum calcium
            b. Increases serum chloride level secondary to PTH-
               induced bicarbonate loss
            c. Decreases serum phosphate as the result of reduced
               renal absorption (if this is present, coexisting hyper-
               parathyroidism should be sought)
      B. **Differential diagnosis**
         1. **Neoplastic disease** is the most common cause of hyper-
            calcemia in hospitalized patients.
         2. **Solid tumors** (primarily breast, renal, and lung) account
            for 80% of malignancy-associated hypercalcemia.

3. **Hematologic malignancies** (e.g., lymphoma, multiple myeloma) account for the remaining 20% of cases.
4. Other diseases that may cause hypercalcemia include sarcoid, renal failure, thyrotoxicosis, vitamin D or A intoxication, milk alkali syndrome, adrenal insufficiency, and familial hypocalciuric hypercalcemia.

IV. **Classification**
   A. **Solid tumors with lytic bony metastases:** breast, lung, kidney, esophagus, thyroid, multiple myeloma, lymphoma
   B. **Humoral hypercalcemia of malignancy (HHM)**
      1. PTHrP: squamous cell carcinoma of the lung, cervix, esophagus; adenocarcinomas of the kidney, breast, bladder
      2. PTH: lung, liver, ovary
      3. Cytokines
      4. Vitamin D: lymphoma

V. **Presentation**
   A. **Impaired renal concentration** leads to polydipsia and polyuria.
   B. **Contraction alkalosis** and **dehydration** lead to further renal damage and even failure.
   C. Associated nephrocalcinosis or nephrolithiasis is rare.
   D. Many features may **resemble signs of the malignant disease being treated.** However, coma, stupor, neurologic localizing signs, hyporeflexia, and visual disturbances may improve with treatment of hypercalcemia.
   E. Certain **ECG changes** are associated with hypercalcemia. These include:
      1. Shortening of the QT interval
      2. Bradycardia
      3. T-wave changes
      4. Increased automaticity and arrhythmia
   F. **Hypercalcemic crisis** involves somnolence, lethargy, general weakness, nausea and vomiting, abdominal pain, and renal failure.

> **In critically ill patients with altered albumin, the levels of ionized calcium correlate better with signs and symptoms.**

VI. **Diagnostic Work-up**
   A. **Serum phosphorus, chloride, and PTH levels should be checked.**
      1. If serum phosphorus is normal or high and the serum PTH and chloride are low (< 100 mmol/L), malignancy should be suspected (PTHrP levels should be checked).
      2. If serum phosphorus is low and serum chloride and PTH levels are high, primary hyperparathyroidism should be suspected.
      3. In patients with known malignancy or low PTH levels, serum PTHrP should be checked. (It is elevated in some forms of HHM.)

B. PTH levels
   1. Immunoreactive PTH levels are suppressed in hypercalcemia of malignancy. Use of an immunoradiometric assay for PTH, the best method in patients without renal failure, has made the diagnosis easier. This assay uses antibodies directed at two sites on the PTH molecule to measure intact PTH.
   2. Three precautions must be taken to avoid misinterpretation and, therefore, misdiagnosis.
      a. In cases of hypercalcemia of malignancy where PTH is the mediator, PTH levels are elevated, not suppressed.
      b. In all patients with increased or inappropriately normal PTH, coexisting primary hyperparathyroidism should be considered.
      c. In patients with increased PTH levels without renal failure, primary hyperparathyroidism must be considered.

C. Chloride:phosphorus ratio
   1. Values > 33 in 96% patients with hyperparathyroidism
   2. Values < 30 in 92% of patients with hypercalcemia from other causes

VII. Management
   A. Normal saline should be administered IV. This replenishes volume and increases urinary calcium excretion by 100–300 mg/day.
   B. Loop diuretics such as furosemide should be administered to promote calciuresis. These agents should be avoided in hypovolemic patients.
   C. Replenishment of electrolytes should proceed carefully.
   D. Discontinuation of agents capable of producing hypercalcemic crisis such as vitamins A and D, thiazide diuretics, and estrogens or antiestrogens should occur.
   E. Calcitonin and corticosteroids are a useful combination in patients with renal failure. This combination is also useful in conjunction with hydration.
   F. Corticosteroids may be effective in hypercalcemia of hematologic malignancies and breast cancer.
   G. Correction of bone resorption
      1. Bisphosphonates (first-line therapy)
         a. Mechanism. Bisphosphonates inhibit osteoclastic bone resorption.
         b. Dosage
            (1) The dosage of pamidronate is 60 mg IV over 4–6 hr. When the corrected calcium level exceeds 13.5 mg/dl, the dose can be increased to 90 mg.
            (2) Some clinical studies found that achievement of normocalcemia required 4 days of therapy. Administration of 60 mg IV every 2 weeks maintained normocalcemia.

> **Pamidronate and calcitonin given in combination
> rapidly reduce serum calcium levels.**

  c. **Effectiveness.** An increase in the plasma PTH and 1,25-
     dihydroxyvitamin D_3 and a decrease in biochemical
     markers of bone resorption herald successful therapy.
2. **Plicamycin**
   a. **Mechanism.** Plicamycin acts directly on osteoclasts to
      reduce bone resorption. This agent lowers serum cal-
      cium in 48 hours or less; the effect lasts up to 4–6 days.
   b. **Dosage.** The dosage is 25 μg/kg IV over 4–12 hr.
   c. **Adverse effects (reversible)** include mild thrombocy-
      topenia.
3. **Calcitonin**
   a. **Indications.** Calcitonin is useful in patients with con-
      gestive heart failure (CHF) or renal failure who can-
      not tolerate saline or diuresis. It has a rapid but tran-
      sient effect.
   b. **Dosage.** For a mild reduction in serum calcium, 8–16
      IU/kg IV/IM q 12 hr should be given.
   c. **Effectiveness.** Calcitonin may be used with pami-
      dronate to achieve more rapid reduction. When cal-
      citonin is nontherapeutic, the pamidronate is thera-
      peutic.
4. **Gallium nitrate**
   a. **Function.** Gallium nitrate inhibits bone resorption
      and increases the calcium content of bone. It lowers
      serum calcium to normal levels in 85% of patients
      with cancer.
   b. **Dosage.** A dose of 200 mg/m^2 is given once daily for
      5 days.

> **The only long-term means of reducing malignancy-
> associated hypercalcemia is by reducing tumor burden.**

ACUTE TUMOR LYSIS SYNDROME

 I. **Definition.** This syndrome is characterized by renal and meta-
    bolic complications from acute destruction of tumor cells sensi-
    tive to radiation or chemotherapy.
 II. **Pathophysiology**
    A. When intracellular electrolytes and products of metabolism
       are rapidly released into the systemic circulation, they can
       produce life-threatening hyperkalemia, hyperuricemia, hy-
       perphosphatemia, and hypocalcemia.
    B. Severity is dependent on renal function.
 III. **Presentation.** Acute tumor lysis syndrome is classically seen in
     patients with Burkitt's lymphoma, lymphoma, and acute and
     chronic leukemia. Clinical manifestations depend on specific
     electrolyte imbalances.

IV. Management

    A. Certain patients require close monitoring and renal protection during the initiation of antineoplastic therapy.

        1. Bulky abdominal disease

        2. Markedly elevated plasma lactate dehydrogenase (LDH)

        3. Renal dysfunction

        4. Metabolic alterations

    B. Prophylaxis against acute renal failure

        1. Vigorous hydration and maintenance of urine output at 2 ml/kg/hr are necessary.

        2. If diuresis cannot be achieved with hydration, dopamine should be administered at 1.5 μg/kg/min.

        3. If diuresis is still poor, furosemide, 40–120 mg IV bolus, or mannitol, 12.5 g of 25% solution, should be started.

        4. Diuresis may be maintained with continuous infusion of furosemide, 3–5 mg/kg/day, or mannitol, 5 g/hr.

    C. A pulmonary artery catheter may be placed to help guide therapy.

    D. Allopurinol, 10 mg/kg IV/PO, is given to control hyperuricemia.

    E. When hyperuricemia exists, urine is alkalinized with sodium bicarbonate infusion or acetazolamide, 250–500 mg IV q 6–8 hr, to prevent the formation of urate stones. Closely follow the urinary pH to determine dosing. The alkalosis aids in preventing the hyperkalemia by causing intracellular shift.

    F. Calcium should be replaced in symptomatic patients (i.e., with positive Chvostek's or Trousseau's sign, impending tetany, or ECG changes).

Avoid administering calcium if the product of calcium multiplied by phosphorus is greater than 60.

SUPERIOR VENA CAVA SYNDROME

I. Etiology

    A. Malignant disease (small cell carcinoma, lymphoma, breast, germ cell, metastatic cancer)

    B. Iatrogenic (e.g., indwelling catheter)

    C. Mediastinal fibrosis

    D. Goiter, aortic aneurysm

II. Presentation

Superior vena cava syndrome is not a life-threatening condition unless airway compromise or respiratory failure occurs.

    A. Cyanosis or swellings of the head, neck, upper thorax, and extremities

    B. Edematous conjunctiva

   C. Jugular venous distention and engorged venous collaterals above the obstruction

   D. Possible associated Horner's syndrome, recurrent laryngeal nerve palsy, or airway obstruction (depending on the location of the tumor)

III. Diagnosis

   A. Clinical suspicion

   B. Radiography: superior mediastinal mass or widening on posterior-anterior and lateral chest x-ray

   C. CT scan: confirmation of diagnosis and determination of the extent of disease

IV. Management

   A. IV access

   B. Positioning, with patient's head above 45° to minimize pressure on the posterior mediastinum and to promote gravity drainage of the head

   C. High-dose corticosteroids

   D. Radiation therapy to shrink tumor

SPINAL CORD COMPRESSION

I. Epidemiology

   A. This condition occurs in 5% of patients with malignant disease.

   B. Any tumor that metastasizes may lead to this complication. It is most often found with lung cancer, myeloma, lymphoma, prostate cancer, breast cancer, and melanoma (10%–15% of cases).

II. Etiology

   A. Epidural metastases in which the tumor involves vertebral body and compresses anterior surface of cord

   B. Direct extension of lymphomatous lymph nodes into the intravertebral space

   C. Vertebral subluxation or spinal subdural hematoma

   D. Pressure on the cord, which leads to hypoperfusion, edema, occlusion, and stasis of the epidural venous plexus, as well as distortion of neural tissues

III. Presentation

   A. Pain (axial in 95% of patients)

      1. Location: close to site of lesions (usually) but sometimes at other sites of disease within the vertebral column

         a. Neck flexion often reproduces symptoms, especially in the thoracic region. Straight leg raises and radicular pain herald lumbosacral disease.

         b. Patients experience more discomfort when they are lying down.

      2. Frequency: usually constant but may be exacerbated by movement, coughing, Valsalva maneuver

   B. Muscle weakness or paralysis (85%)

   C. Sensory loss (75%)

    D. Bowel and bladder dysfunction
    E. Ataxia
IV. Radiologic Evaluation
    A. MRI (diagnostic imaging modality of choice) to determine bone, soft tissue, and cord involvement, as well as delineate the extent of the tumor
    B. Plain radiographs of spine to identify fractures and metastases
    C. Bone scan to identify metastases to bone
    D. Myelography: extradural block of 80% confirms diagnosis of cord compression
V. Management
    A. Dexamethasone, 100 mg IV, then 24 mg IV q 6 hr for 72 hours, and then tapered over 2 weeks, should be administered.
    B. Radiation therapy to attempt shrinkage of tumor improves symptoms in 30% to 50% of patients.
    C. Surgical treatment (i.e., operative cord decompression). Indications for surgery include:
        1. Failure of radiation therapy
        2. Radioresistant tumor
        3. Cervical spine compression
        4. Spinal instability
        5. Diagnosis in doubt

Surgery should not be considered if a patient presents with paraplegia. This approach has no benefit over external beam radiation.

CARDIAC TAMPONADE

I. Predisposing Conditions. Pericardial metastases are possible with many malignancies but are most common with lung and breast cancer, lymphoma, and leukemia.
II. Etiology (Differential Diagnosis of Nontraumatic Tamponade)
    A. Malignancy (50%)
    B. Idiopathic or radiation associated pericarditis or constriction
    C. Hemorrhagic or purulent pericarditis
    D. Cardiomyopathies
III. Presentation
    A. Effusions may become large and remain hemodynamically asymptomatic.
    B. The enlarged sac may produce local symptoms as a result of compression of certain structures.
        1. Coughing
        2. Fullness in the head and neck
        3. Vague GI distress due to visceral engorgement
    C. Signs of hemodynamic impairment may develop.

      1. Tachycardia
      2. Narrow pulse pressure
      3. Pulsus paradoxus
      4. Hypotension

IV. Radiographic Evaluation

    A. Chest radiography may reveal an enlarged cardiac silhouette without signs of pulmonary congestion.

    B. Echocardiography can detect effusions of 20 ml.

V. Management. Drainage of pericardial fluid via a pericardial window is the best option to prevent recurrence of tamponade. Percutaneously placed catheters are less desirable because they are likely to become clogged or infected.

    A. Creation of the **pericardial window** may be approached in three ways: by the subxiphoid route, via left anterior thoracotomy, or thoracoscopically.

    B. Fluid should be drained slowly and sent for cell count and cytology.

NEUTROPENIC ENTEROCOLITIS

I. Predisposing Conditions. Neutropenic enterocolitis is most commonly seen in leukemia or other hematologic malignancies. It affects oncologic patients during periods of neutropenia.

II. Etiology

    A. Pathophysiology

      1. Bacterial infection of the wall of large or small bowel occurs.

      2. Enterocolitis may be exacerbated by bowel mucosa involvement by lymphoma or leukemia cells, which leads to ulceration or mucosal injury secondary to cytotoxic drugs.

      3. Previous administration of antibiotics may lead to bacterial overgrowth.

      4. Ileus may lead to distention, increased transmural pressure, and ischemia.

    B. Differential diagnosis

      1. Appendicitis

      2. *Clostridium difficile* colitis

      3. Ischemic colitis

      4. Pseudoacute abdomen associated with leukemia

      5. Abdominal pain and diarrhea associated with chemotherapeutic agents

III. Presentation. Affected patients present with fever, diarrhea, and abdominal pain and distention. The enterocolitis is characterized by mucosal inflammation of the ileum, cecum, or ascending colon.

IV. Diagnostic Tests

    A. Abdominal radiography (to rule out free air)

    B. CT scan of abdomen

> **Barium enemas or colonoscopy should be
> avoided because of the high risk of infarction.**

V. **Management**
   A. **Medical treatment** involves IV antibiotics, nasogastric suction, and parenteral nutrition.
   B. **Surgical treatment** may be necessary in cases with free air, peritoneal signs, or clinical deterioration.

18

Orthopaedic

Management

I. **Definitions**
   A. A **cast** is a hard-shell, circumferential dressing meant to hold a fracture reduced or immobilize a bone or joint.
      1. **Casting materials**
         a. Plaster is heavy, easily molded, and generally used in acute settings to maintain reduction of a fracture.
         b. Fiberglass is lightweight, stiff, and generally used to maintain immobilization when reduction or alignment is secure.
      2. **Types of casts** (Table 18-1)
   B. A **splint** is an immobilization dressing with a hard shell on one or two surfaces of the extremity (Table 18-2).
   C. **Braces** are removable appliances meant to immobilize or restrict motion (Table 18-3).
   D. **Traction** is an in-line force that pulls along the long axis of an extremity or extremity segment to regain length. It is used to combat muscle forces that cause shortening and malalignment.
      1. **Skeletal traction** uses traction attached to a pin that has been inserted directly into a more distal, uninjured segment of the skeleton. Traction pulls directly on bone via the pin.
      2. **Skin traction** uses axial traction via an appliance applied to the outside surface of an extremity. For example, Buck's traction is a soft boot about the leg and foot, usually applied for pain relief and the maintenance of length in hip fractures before repair.
   E. **Reduction** is the realignment of a bone or joint to restore normal anatomic relationships after fracture or dislocation.
II. **General Orthopaedic Management in the ICU**

Table 18–1. Classification of Casts

Type of Cast	Placement of Cast	Area Immobilized
Short arm cast	Olecranon to palm, with the metacarpal-phalangeal joints and elbow free	Wrist (in flexion/extension plane)
Long arm cast	Upper humerus to palm, with the elbow flexed	Elbow, forearms, wrist
Thumb spica cast	Similar to placement of short or long arm cast, but incorporates the thumb	Thumb
Short leg cast	Tibial tubercle to toes, with the ankle usually at a 90° angle	Foot, ankle (in the plantar/dorsiflexion plane)
Long leg cast	High thigh to toes, with the knee extended or flexed	Knee, tibia, ankle, foot
Hip spica cast	Lower thorax to tibia	Hip, femur

Table 18–2. Classification of Splints

Type of Splint	Description of Splint	Area Immobilized
Coaptation splint	A posterior splint from the proximal humerus to wrist with a U-shaped splint from the axilla to trapezius	Humerus
Sugar-tong splint	Any U-shaped splint meant to cover two sides of long bones with a connection at one end	Wrist, forearm
Posterior splint	A single slab along any posterior surface; may be used in the leg in conjunction with a stirrup-type slab to form a posterior and U-shaped splint	Ankle, foot
Ulnar/radial gutter splint	A single slab on either side of the forearm, wrist, or hand consisting of a U shape based radially or ulnarly	Forearm, wrist, hand

A. **Goals of orthopaedic management in the ICU**
   1. **Restoration of maximum function** and the **earliest safe mobilization** of the patient are the ultimate objectives of all orthopaedic treatment and can be best achieved by focusing on the following four goals.
      a. **Preservation of soft tissues**
         (1) Maintenance of the soft-tissue envelope, with its skin, muscle, and tendon gliding planes, should be of higher priority than eventual bony union in any orthopaedic setting.
         (2) The loss of soft tissue leads to the greatest loss of function and a much more challenging surgical salvage problem than almost any osseous dysfunction.
      b. **Joint congruity and mobility**
         (1) The reestablishment of perfect joint congruity is critical to reduction and the prevention of post-traumatic degenerative joint disease (i.e., arthritis) and is the primary reason for operative treatment of intra-articular fractures.
         (2) Joint mobility is crucial to function. The early achievement of joint mobility after injury avoids the stiffness and dysfunction associated with prolonged joint immobilization.

Table 18–3.	Classification of Braces	
Type of Brace	**Description of Brace**	**Function**
Functional brace	A circumferential, hard-sided dressing around the diaphysis of a long bone	Maintains alignment during healing
Thoracolumbosacral orthosis (TLSO)	Turtle-shell brace	Restricts motion of the thoracolumbar spine
Spinal extension (Jewett) brace	Hyperextension brace	Maintains sagittal alignment during healing of a thoracolumbar fracture
Ankle-foot orthosis	Posterior brace	Resists plantar flexion of the ankle
Short leg walking brace		Provides some protection to tibia and ankle while allowing ankle motion in the plantarflexion and dorsiflexion plane within an adjustable range
Figure-of-eight strap	Appears like the straps of a knapsack without the sack	Provides comfort and stability to middle and proximal clavicle fractures by pulling the distal clavicle posteriorly

      (3) Joint congruity and mobility also affect the treatment of extra-articular fractures because the goal is to secure the diaphyseal or metaphyseal fracture fixation as early as possible to mobilize adjacent joints.

    c. Alignment

      (1) Both axial and rotational alignment must be maintained or restored within certain limits.

      (2) The limits on tolerance of deformity are based on age, skeletal maturity, bony segment involved, distance from joint, plane of injury, fracture pattern, bone quality, and anticipated patient demand.

    d. Skeletal stability. Stable union for weight bearing and function is central to the objectives of all orthopaedic treatment, whether bony or ligamentous.

  2. Conservative, nonoperative treatment should be the goal of any surgeon; surgery should not be considered until the risks of not operating outweigh the potential morbidity of the procedure.

B. Overview of orthopaedic management in the ICU. Before evaluation by an orthopaedic surgeon, triage and initial physician care of a patient with a history of trauma and a suspected orthopaedic problem should be undertaken following a simple protocol.

1. Perform a **complete physical examination,** including motor, sensory, and vascular examinations; inspection of the skin and wounds; and inspection for any deformity.
2. Perform **manual traction** of the extremity to grossly realign it, and then **stabilize** it temporarily. Repeat and document the neurovascular examination after any manipulation.

> **Splint all fractures before mobilization
> of the patient for tests.**

---

3. **Elevate and ice** the extremity. Elevation of the limb should be high enough to provide dependent drainage of swelling at the injury site. This step is not applicable in compartment syndrome.
4. **Immobilize** the fracture with a cast or external fixation frame.
   a. Use external fixation frames for:
      (1) Stable fixation of extremities with extensive soft-tissue injuries
      (2) Rapid stabilization of fractures in the hemodynamically unstable patient
      (3) Patients who require a highly mobile method of skeletal traction
      (4) Movement, elevation, and suspension of injured extremities
   b. In the acute setting, temporary splinting of most fractures or extremity deformities is adequate.
   c. Proper immobilization of a long-bone fracture necessitates immobilization of the joints proximal and distal to the fracture.
   d. Dress open wounds sterilely before immobilization, with or without a bacteriostatic solution.
   e. Before application of a cast, evaluate the time since injury, severity of injury, position of extremity, and degree of manipulation in an attempt to anticipate further swelling. If necessary, a cast may be valved and spread or a splint applied in the short term.
   f. Add generous padding about areas of existing or anticipated swelling.
   g. Assess and dress pin sites daily. Avoid fixation-pin injuries to the contralateral extremity or adjacent thorax, especially in agitated patients.
   h. Monitor circumferential skin integrity at the proximal and distal margins of the cast daily to ensure against breakdown or loss of adequate padding.
   i. Perform neurovascular examinations at the distal end of splinted and casted extremities to monitor for pos-

sible compression injury, compartment syndrome, and skin problems. The potential neurovascular complications of circumferential compressive dressings and casts are too grave to be ignored.

C. Indications for operative orthopaedic management. Operative intervention is undertaken when the following objectives can no longer be met in a closed fashion:

1. Preservation of function and mobility of the soft tissues (e.g., joint capsule, muscle, tendon, ligament) around a joint or extremity

2. Preservation or restoration of absolute congruity and functional mobility of articular surfaces

3. Establishment or reestablishment of skeletal stability and alignment of the spine and extremities

4. Treatment in a manner that minimizes the total time of immobilization and the pursuant complications (acute and chronic)

D. Orthopaedic ward care

1. **Postoperative orthopaedic orders** do not deviate significantly from standard surgical postoperative protocols. However, the following points should be included:

   a. Restrictions on elevating, icing, and positioning the affected extremity

   b. Weight-bearing status and physical and occupational therapy orders

   c. Deep venous thrombosis prophylaxis

   d. Prophylactic antibiotics (particularly if implants or prostheses are placed)

   e. Postoperative radiographs

   f. Pain control medications

2. **Special precautions are often necessary after total joint arthroplasty** to minimize the risk of infection and dislocation.

   a. Fresh postoperative total joint replacement patients should not share a ward room with any patient being treated for or thought to have any kind of infection.

   b. After total hip arthroplasty, depending on the approach, patients may have explicit restrictions on hip range of motion.

   c. After total hip arthroplasty approached posteriorly, patients are allowed only limited hip flexion, adduction, and internal rotation. This may be enforced with an "abduction pillow."

3. **Continuous passive motion (CPM)** is an electrical appliance designed to establish early range of motion in a controlled fashion in an effort to avoid stiffness secondary to postoperative immobilization.

   a. CPM may be applied to a variety of joints and set to the desired range of motion and speed.

   b. The machine should be applied in correct rotation,

with movement at the joint rather than proximal or distal to the joint.

c. Vigilance must be maintained to avoid skin problems secondary to constant or repeated pressure of the machine parts against the operative extremity, particularly in diabetics and patients with indwelling epidural catheters.

4. **Traction** is meant to counteract muscle forces across a joint or along an axial limb segment and should be placed in direct opposition to the combination of forces it is meant to counterbalance. It is a temporizing measure between acute trauma and definitive treatment and is used until achievement of fixation that allows more mobility.

   a. Be careful not to place nerves, vessels, or skin under excessive stretch.

   b. Do not overdistract fractures and joint spaces.

   c. Monitor and protect the health of the soft tissues and skin with regular assessment of dependent surfaces.

   d. Hang the weights free, not resting on the bed frame, trapeze, or floor.

   e. For the patient's comfort, remove and replace traction in a gradual fashion.

   f. Assess and dress entrance and exit sites of skeletal traction pins daily.

III. Orthopaedic Emergencies

A. Hypotensive patient with an unstable pelvis

1. Differential diagnosis. According to advanced trauma life support (ATLS) protocol, in any patient who has experienced high-velocity trauma, intrapelvic bleeding must be included in the differential diagnosis for hypotension.

2. **Diagnostic tests.** An anteroposterior (AP) radiograph of the pelvis should always be immediately obtained along with chest and lateral cervical spine films.

3. **Management**

   a. Follow ATLS protocols for evaluation and management.

   b. Stabilize the bony pelvis and reduce the potential intrapelvic volume, because increased tissue pressure that occurs by maintaining or reestablishing a normal pelvic diameter rapidly leads to tamponade of venous bleeding. For speed and ease of fixation, this is usually accomplished with external fixation.

      (1) For immediate, temporary reduction of pelvic volume before operative intervention, a sheet may be wrapped once around the pelvis and an attempt made to achieve compression by tightening the wrap manually.

      (2) At some trauma centers, pelvic arteriography with or without embolic therapy may be at-

tempted to achieve hemostasis before external fixation.

4. Complications. Discontinuity of the skeletal pelvic ring may cause disruption of the venous plexus and arterial tree posteriorly, leading to a life-threatening intrapelvic exsanguination.

B. Hip dislocation

1. Signs and symptoms. A posteriorly dislocated native hip presents with the hip flexed, adducted, and internally rotated.

2. Physical examination. Complete neurologic and vascular examinations distal to the injury are the first priorities.

3. Diagnostic tests. Physical examination should be followed by AP and lateral radiographs, which must be scrutinized for acetabular, femoral head, and femoral neck fractures.

4. Management

a. Manual reduction must be performed after obtaining radiographs to exclude fracture or fracture-dislocation. Reduction is usually performed with the aid of IV analgesia and sedation or general anesthesia.

(1) After reduction of the femoral head to the acetabulum, test range of motion for stability and crepitus, and repeat the neurovascular examination.

(2) After reduction of a posterior dislocation, immobilize the hip in a position of abduction, external rotation, and neutral extension.

b. Operative intervention

(1) Anything less than a perfectly symmetrical reduction on postreduction radiographs indicates fracture fragments within the joint space and a need for operative intervention.

(2) The **inability to achieve stable reduction in a closed fashion** is an operative emergency because of the risk of avascular necrosis and neurologic compromise.

5. Complications. With posterior dislocation of the hip, urgency emerges from two fronts.

a. In a dislocated position, the medial and lateral femoral circumflex vessels may be compromised. A prolonged period of dislocation correlates directly with risk of post-traumatic avascular necrosis of the femoral head.

b. Hip dislocation stretches the sciatic nerve or directly compresses it, raising the threat of neurapraxia and long-term palsy.

C. Hip fracture

1. Classification

a. Femoral neck fractures represent a threat to the blood supply to the femoral head and the subsequent risk of avascular necrosis of the femoral head.

b. Intertrochanteric fractures span the area from the tip of the greater trochanter to the inferior aspect of the lesser trochanter. These fractures are classified based on the fracture pattern and the number of fragments present.

2. Management

a. General management

(1) **Operative fixation** is indicated in hip fractures to maximize function, increase speed of mobilization, and avoid the complications associated with long-term, bed-bound immobilization.

(2) In the acute phase, most hip fractures (except nondisplaced femoral neck fractures) may be placed in **Buck's traction** for comfort until operative fixation can be performed.

b. Management of femoral neck fractures

(1) Nondisplaced fractures (Garden I and II) may be internally fixed *in situ.*

(2) Displaced fractures may be reduced and fixed, or the head and neck may be replaced with a hemiarthroplasty or total hip replacement.

(3) In younger patients, all efforts are made to anatomically reduce the fracture as soon as possible.

(4) In older patients, the choice of procedure is based on a combination of factors (e.g., age, anticipated demand, degree of displacement).

c. Management of intertrochanteric fractures. There are a variety of operative options for these fractures, including sliding hip screw constructs, fixed-angle blade plates, and intramedullary devices.

D. Knee dislocation

1. Signs and symptoms. A dislocated knee presents obviously deformed, unless it spontaneously reduces in the field, in which case it presents as a large, swollen knee that is unstable in all directions.

2. Physical examination. Complete initial and sequential neurologic and vascular examinations distal to the injury are the first priorities.

3. Diagnostic tests. Physical examination should be followed by AP and lateral radiographs to rule out periarticular fractures.

4. Management

a. Perform **gentle manipulation and reduction** with the aid of IV sedation and analgesia.

b. Repeat the **neurovascular examination,** which should be improved.

c. Examine **radiographs** to rule out periarticular fractures.

d. Obtain a **popliteal angiogram** to rule out possible intimal injury or thrombosis of the popliteal artery.

(1) If there is no vascular injury, the knee may be **im-**

> **mobilized in mild knee flexion** with a dressing designed to accommodate substantial swelling.
>
> (2) If there is vascular injury, consult a vascular surgeon to determine **operative repair versus anticoagulation.**
>
> 5. **Complications** include neurologic and vascular compromise.

E. Open fracture

1. **Physical examination**

   a. Examine the wound, taking special note of **bony stripping** and any **gross contamination.**

   b. Perform focused **distal motor and sensory examinations.**

2. **Management**

   a. **Irrigate** and **loosely dress** the wound.

   b. **Grossly align** and **splint** the extremity.

   c. Administer appropriate **tetanus prophylaxis.**

   d. Administer **IV antibiotics** immediately.

      (1) The accepted routine includes a first-generation cephalosporin (1 g).

      (2) More controversial is the immediate administration of gram-negative coverage, which depends on the type and degree of contamination.

      (3) With gross soil contamination, administer penicillin (4–6 million IU IV) immediately for clostridial coverage, except in allergic patients.

   e. Open fractures must undergo **operative irrigation and débridement within 6 hours** of the injury to accurately assess the level of contamination and significantly reduce the risk of deep infection and subsequent long-term disability.

3. **Complications** include loss of soft tissue and infection.

F. Open or septic joint

1. **Etiology.** *Staphylococcus aureus* is the leading infectious agent, followed by group B streptococci and gram-negative bacteria.

2. **Signs and symptoms.** The primary sign associated with an open or septic joint is a large effusion that may be warm or erythematous and is exquisitely tender to range of motion. The diagnosis may be complicated in neuropathic patients (e.g., diabetics) or confused by overlying cellulitis.

3. **Diagnostic tests.** If a patient's physical examination is consistent with septic joint, aspirate synovial fluid, with care taken not to pass through any potentially cellulitic areas of the subcutaneous tissues. In this case, perform **arthrocentesis.**

   a. Position the patient comfortably at an adequate height and in a position that makes the joint accessible.

   b. Plan the site of puncture where there is the greatest amount of fluid and at an angle that directly leads to the joint space.

    c. Infiltrate the overlying skin and soft tissues with 1% lidocaine through a 25-gauge needle.

    d. Raise a wheal at the arthrocentesis site and penetrate the wheal centrally in a direct line to the joint capsule.

    e. Enter the joint space with an 18- or 20-gauge needle, aspirating gently as it proceeds. Aspirating too aggressively will suction the soft tissue against the needle bevel, obscuring the cannula. Also make sure that the articular surface is not contacted during this process.

    f. When the joint fluid is encountered, hold the needle still and aspirate all of the fluid.

    g. Send the fluid for cell count and differential, crystals, glucose, stat Gram's stain, and culture. Indications of a septic joint include:

        (1) Aspiration of frank pus

        (2) Bacteria by stat Gram's stain

        (3) Cell count of > 100,000 cells/mm^3. (Cell counts of 50,000–100,000 cells/mm^3 are ambiguous and require reliance on other signs for diagnosis.)

    h. Serum CBC with differential and erythrocyte sedimentation rate or C-reactive protein should also be evaluated.

4. Management

    a. In the case of traumatic wounding near a joint without obvious joint involvement, **inject the joint.** This will determine whether the joint is involved.

        (1) The capsule may be sterilely injected at a site not immediately adjacent to the wound. Inject the capsule with an aseptic **clear or colored saline solution.**

        (2) If the fluid extravasates from the wound, this is evidence of joint involvement.

    b. **Open joint** injuries require **immediate operative irrigation.**

    c. **Septic joints** require **immediate operative irrigation and drainage** at most institutions; however, some institutions maintain that serial aspiration is acceptable therapy if diagnosed promptly.

5. Complications include degradation and erosion of otherwise healthy articular cartilage by the immune response to joint space infection.

G. Compartment syndrome

1. Pathogenesis

    a. Pressure in a closed body compartment exceeds perfusion pressure, leading to ischemia of that compartment's vital structures.

    b. This process is usually the result of soft-tissue reperfusion injury after an ischemic period or high-energy trauma and is mediated by the local release of inflammatory cytokines and the subsequent swelling.

c. Although this may occur in any extremity segment, it is most common in the compartments of the leg (Table 18-4).

2. **Risk factors.** The intubated or noncommunicative trauma patient is at increased risk for undiagnosed compartment syndrome.

3. **Signs and symptoms** (the "five Ps")
   a. Poikilothermia (i.e., coolness of the involved extremity)
   b. Paresthesias
   c. Pain (at rest and with passive stretch of the muscles in the compartment involved)
   d. Pulselessness
   e. Pallor

In a patient at high risk for compartment syndrome, the diagnosis should be made long before all signs develop. By the time pulselessness and pallor develop, irreversible damage has occurred.

---

4. **Diagnostic work-up**
   a. Regular **examinations of the soft tissues** of all extremities must be performed as long as the patient is incapable of communication. Any soft-tissue tenseness or rigidity requires further evaluation.
   b. If cooperative examination with a conscious patient is unattainable, **compartment pressure readings** must be taken.
      (1) **Procedure** for compartment pressure measurement
         (a) Compartment pressures may be measured with specially designed needle manometers or by using an IV catheter and a sterile saline bag hooked to a pressure bag and monitor.

Table 18–4. Compartments of the Leg

Compartment	Muscles	Sensory Nerve	Provocative Passive Movement
Anterior	Tibialis anterior, toe extensors	Deep peroneal (dorsal foot)	Toe flexion
Lateral	Peroneals	Superficial peroneal (first web space)	Ankle inversion
Deep posterior	Tibialis posterior, toe flexors	Posterior tibial (plantar foot)	Toe extension
Superficial posterior	Gastrocnemius/ soleus	No sensory nerves	Ankle dorsiflexion

Arterial pressure lines and transducers can also be used to measure compartment pressures.

(b) Prepare the extremity with povidone-iodine solution and drape it in sterile fashion.

(c) For a solitary measurement, use an 18-gauge needle. If continuous monitoring is indicated, insert a small transducer or insert a plastic catheter over a needle and connect it to an extremely low pressure column.

(d) Insert the needle or catheter in the compartment and connect it to a water column manometer or a pressure transducer. Pressure transducers should be zeroed at the level of the compartment.

(e) After measurement, apply a dressing.

(f) If there is any doubt after obtaining compartment pressure readings, serial measurements may be taken or a continuous monitoring catheter may be placed.

(2) **Normal values** for compartment pressures are 10–20 mm Hg. If variation in the equipment or the patient is of concern, values may be compared to pressure readings taken from the same compartments on the contralateral, unaffected side.

(3) If the compartments are palpable, they may be palpated directly to assess the degree of firmness and swelling.

5. **Management.** In a patient with appropriate clinical history, pain on passive stretch or out of proportion with injury, and elevated pressures, **emergent fasciotomy** is indicated.

a. In a multiply injured patient, a brain-injured patient, or a patient with a confusing or equivocal examination, objective data must be collected before deciding to undergo operative fasciotomy.

b. Guidelines for fasciotomy are the subject of vigorous debate. Among the accepted guidelines are a **pressure limit of 40 mm Hg** or any **pressure value within 20 mm Hg of the diastolic blood pressure.** A lower threshold is acceptable in either case if values are accompanied by a convincing clinical presentation.

H. **Spinal injuries** (see Chapter 26)

I. **Cauda equina syndrome**

1. **Definition.** Cauda equina syndrome is an acute compressive injury to the spinal cord distal to the cona medullaris.

2. **Risk factors**
   a. Spinal stenosis
   b. Certain forms of achondroplasia
   c. An acute precipitating event (commonly present)

3. **Signs and symptoms**

      a. Bowel or bladder dysfunction

      b. Saddle-shaped proximal inner thigh and perineum anesthesia or paresthesia

      c. A variable lower extremity neurologic examination

    4. Diagnostic tests. Obtain an emergent MRI of the lumbar spine.

    5. Management. Emergent decompression should be done if indicated by clinical examination and MRI findings.

J. Radial artery cannulation injury

    1. Radial artery cannulation injury is the most common iatrogenic musculoskeletal insult in the ICU setting, usually resulting from the creation and distribution of a thrombus.

    2. Diagnostic work-up

      a. Assess digital vascularity and swelling regularly after insertion of the catheter, for the entire period of cannulation, and for 24 hours after removal of the catheter. The majority of thrombi are discovered after removal of the catheter.

      b. Do not perform Allen's test because it is not predictive of cannulation injury.

    3. Management

      a. The following factors have been shown to reduce the incidence of cannulation injuries:

        (1) Pretreatment with aspirin

        (2) Use of a small-gauge catheter

        (3) Short duration of cannulation

        (4) Removal of catheter with aspiration

      b. If cannulation injury is identified, the patient may require:

        (1) Angiogram

        (2) Chemical or operative thrombolysis with or without digital fasciotomy

K. Long-bone fracture in the multiply injured patient

    1. Studies clearly demonstrate more rapid recovery and fewer immobilization complications (e.g., pulmonary and soft-tissue problems) in multitrauma patients who underwent **immediate (i.e., < 24 hours after injury) operative fixation** of long-bone fractures.

    2. Operative fixation of long-bone fractures in the setting of head injury is more controversial, with no conclusive studies in favor of immediate or delayed fixation.

19

Pulmonary Disorders

ADULT RESPIRATORY DISTRESS SYNDROME (ARDS)

I. Definition. This condition is characterized by severe hypoxemia. All three of the following criteria must be satisfied.
   A. $Pao_2/Fio_2 < 200$
   B. Bilateral infiltrates on chest radiograph
   C. PCWP $\leq$ 18 mm Hg

II. Predisposing Factors
   A. Shock (e.g., cardiogenic, septic, hemorrhagic, anaphylactic)
   B. Recent trauma (e.g., burns, near drowning) **or surgery**
   C. Pulmonary conditions
      1. Pulmonary contusion
      2. Amniotic fluid or fat embolism
      3. Pulmonary embolism (PE)
      4. Aspiration
   D. Inhalation of toxic gases (e.g., oxygen, smoke, ammonia)
   E. Sepsis [e.g., pneumonia-related (most common), intraabdominal, catheter-related]
   F. Metabolic
      1. Uremia
      2. Blood products (e.g., massive transfusion)
   G. GI conditions
      1. Pancreatitis
      2. Bacterial translocation
      3. Aspiration of gastric contents
   H. Drugs
   I. Cardiopulmonary bypass
   J. Disseminated intravascular coagulation (DIC)

III. Pathogenesis and Pathophysiology
   A. Pathogenesis. Development is complex.
      1. Activated complement, as well as endotoxin, attracts neutrophils to the pulmonary microvasculature.
      2. Neutrophils attach to the pulmonary endothelium and release toxic substances that damage the endothelium.

435

B. **Decreased respiratory compliance**
1. Reduction in respiratory compliance is related to the amount of residually inflated lung. The smaller the portion of lung open to gas, the lower the compliance.
2. Impairment of gas exchange is related to the amount of noninflated tissue mass.

C. **Hypoxemia.** The shunt fraction resulting from perfusion of noninflated tissue is probably the primary cause of hypoxemia.

IV. **Clinical Presentation**
A. **Onset.** The clinical syndrome begins within hours of the inciting event. The change from edema to fibrosis can occur as early as 36 hours later.
B. **Early features.** Severe hypoxemia, which is refractory to oxygen therapy, develops, and the FIO_2 is increased to maintain oxygenation.
C. **Radiographic evidence.** The chest radiograph begins to show diffuse infiltration. Over the next 24 hours, it reveals patchy infiltrates, perihilar prominences, and obscured lung fields.

V. **Diagnostic Tests**
A. A **chest radiograph** reveals diffuse alveolar infiltrates. Evaluate this radiograph to differentiate between ARDS and cardiogenic edema.

> **In early ARDS, the hypoxemia is more pronounced than the chest radiograph indicates, whereas in cardiogenic edema, the radiographic abnormalities are more pronounced than the hypoxemia.**

1. In **ARDS,** there is a diffuse bilateral pattern of infiltrates with peripheral predominance and clear lung bases. Usually no cardiomegaly is evident.
2. In **cardiogenic edema,** there is perihilar predominance, Kerley's B lines, and obscured lung bases from effusions and cardiomegaly.

B. In **invasive hemodynamics,** a pulmonary artery catheter determines the pulmonary arterial wedge pressure.
C. A **radionuclide scan** can assess ventilation.
D. **Thoracentesis** can be used to determine if a pleural effusion is exudative (i.e., ARDS) or transudative.
1. Fluid protein/serum protein > 0.5: exudative (ARDS)
2. Fluid protein/serum protein < 0.5: transudative

VI. **Management**
A. **Correct** (or remove) **the underlying cause.**
B. **Reduce edema and lung fluid.**
1. An increase in capillary permeability magnifies the effect of capillary hydrostatic pressure on fluid accumulation.
2. The PCWP should be decreased to the lowest level without compromising left ventricular (LV) function.
3. During the first few days of ARDS, a strategy of fluid re-

striction and diuresis should be pursued while perfusion is carefully supported.

C. Maintain tissue oxygenation.

1. Peripheral oxygen uptake (oxygen consumption per unit time [V_{O_2}]) varies directly with changes in oxygen delivery (D_{O_2}). Oxygen delivery can be manipulated to improve survival.

2. CI is usually elevated in ARDS, but if it is still low (CI < 2), dobutamine may be used (5–15 μg/kg/min).

Avoid vasodilators, because they increase pulmonary shunt, as well as high-dose dopamine, because it constricts the pulmonary veins.

---

3. Keep hemoglobin (Hgb) > 10 g/dl.

D. Ventilator management [see MECHANICAL VENTILATION, p. 451]

1. **Goal of mechanical ventilation.** Ventilator parameters are manipulated so that the patient receives effective gas exchange at the lowest FI_{O_2}.

   a. Keep arterial oxygen saturation > 90%.

   b. Keep the FI_{O_2} < 60% to minimize the risk of oxygen toxicity. If the FI_{O_2} cannot be decreased, increase the positive end-expiratory pressure (PEEP) to decrease the FI_{O_2}.

2. **Maintenance of end-expiratory lung volume**

   a. In the early phases, the adhered walls of collapsed bronchi require higher pressures to open, but once they are open, they need less pressure to remain patent.

   b. Failure to maintain minimum alveolar volume in the early phase of acute lung injury may induce or accentuate the damage.

   c. The efficacy of PEEP in improving oxygen exchange relates directly to its effect on reversal of atelectasis and the redistribution of lung water. This benefit declines as time passes.

   d. In early-stage ARDS, sufficient PEEP mitigates the severity of the stretch injury to keep the alveoli open.

   e. In late-stage ARDS, PEEP may just increase the risk of air space or lung rupture.

3. **Permissive hypercapnia**

Maintaining normocapnia may not be appropriate if the cost is impaired lung healing and a heightened risk of extending tissue damage.

---

   a. Studies suggest that by allowing alveolar volume and peak ventilatory pressures to fall and Pa_{CO_2} to rise, there may be a reduction in barotrauma and enhanced survival in acute lung injury.

b. Physiologic effects of carbon dioxide retention are functions of the severity of hypercapnia and its rate of buildup.

(1) Acute problems

(a) Intracellular acidosis

(b) Nervous system dysfunction

(c) Increased intracranial pressure (ICP)

(d) Muscle weakness

(e) Cardiovascular dysfunction

(2) Chronic problems (e.g., depressed ventilatory drive due to compensatory metabolic alkalosis)

c. Permissive hypercapnia is not indicated in patients with acute head injury, recent cerebrovascular accident (CVA), significant cardiovascular dysfunction, or coexistent metabolic acidosis.

d. Effects of increased $Paco_2$ include:

(1) Increased sympathetic activity

(2) Increased cardiac output

(3) Heightened pulmonary vascular resistance

(4) Altered bronchomotor tone

(5) Impaired skeletal muscle function

(6) Dilation of cerebral vessels

(7) Impaired CNS function

(8) Movement of the Hgb–oxygen disassociation curve to the right. This shift favors an increased unloading of oxygen in the tissues.

4. Strategies for ventilating patients with acute lung injury

a. Tailor the ventilatory strategy to the phase (i.e., apply PEEP in early stages and withdraw in later stages).

After the first 3–5 days, begin to reduce PEEP as oxygenation permits.

---

b. Minimize oxygen demands.

c. Minimize pulmonary vascular pressures.

d. Control alveolar plateau pressure, not $Paco_2$.

(1) Keep alveolar plateau pressures < 35 cm H_2O.

(2) Keep tidal volumes to no more than 6 ml/kg to control alveolar pressures.

(3) As the PEEP increases, slowly decrease tidal volume to keep airway pressure constant.

e. When hypercapnia is not contraindicated, it should be accepted at the onset.

f. The use of low tidal volumes may lead to hypercapnia.

(1) Attention is being focused on recruitment and then maintenance of as many alveolar units as possible. This often requires levels of PEEP in excess of that needed only to lower the FIO_2.

(2) To normalize the pH and PCO_2, ventilator rates of 70–75 breaths/min are often necessary to maintain an adequate minute volume.

      g. Consider the prone position.
        (1) Improves oxygenation in 75% of patients
        (2) Improves Pao_2 significantly during the early phase in 60% to 70% of patients

ASPIRATION SYNDROMES

I. Definitions. Pulmonary aspiration of stomach contents may produce one of the following syndromes:
   A. Chemical tracheobronchitis-pneumonitis from aspiration of sterile gastric contents
   B. Pleuropulmonary infections from aspiration of bacterial pathogens
   C. Airway obstruction from aspiration of solid material

II. Incidence. The actual incidence is unknown but reports range from 0.1% to 76%. However, these numbers refer to any episode of aspiration, and 45% of normal individuals experience aspiration during sleep or anesthesia.

III. Etiology. Causes of aspiration include:
   A. Impaired glottic closure
     1. Neurologic disability
       a. Head injury
       b. Seizures
       c. Cerebral infarct or hemorrhage
     2. Anatomically altered laryngeal competence
       a. Tracheostomy
       b. Endotracheal intubation
       c. Tracheoesophageal fistula
       d. Tumors of the larynx, pharynx, or esophagus
     3. Drugs
       a. Alcohol
       b. General anesthetics
       c. Sedatives
   B. Increased regurgitation
     1. Hiatal hernia or gastroesophageal reflux disease
     2. Nasogastric tubes
     3. Achalasia
     4. Esophageal stricture
     5. Esophageal dysmotility or dysphagia
   C. Increased intragastric pressure
     1. Jejunostomy or gastrostomy
     2. Enteral feeding
     3. Small bowel obstruction
     4. Gastric atony
     5. Supine positioning

IV. Pathology and Pathophysiology
   A. Pathology. The aspiration of stomach contents results in inflammatory lung injury, which is primarily hemorrhagic, granulocytic, and necrotizing when the aspirate is acidic, and mononuclear and granulomatous when the aspirate contains food.

1. **Severity.** The severity of injury depends on the following factors:
   a. pH of the gastric contents (< 2.5, more severe)
   b. Volume (> 25 ml, more severe)
   c. Quality (large particles cause obstruction, small nonobstructing food particles cause prolonged inflammation)
2. **Aspiration pneumonia.** Pneumonia occurs when the aspirate contains pathogenic bacteria from the oropharynx or from colonized gastric contents.
   a. Anaerobic organisms include *Bacteroides melaninogenicus, Fusobacterium, Bacteroides fragilis, Peptostreptococcus,* and microaerophilic streptococci.
   b. Aerobic organisms include *Haemophilus influenzae,* methicillin-resistant *Staphylococcus aureus,* gram-negative enteric bacilli, *Pseudomonas pneumoniae,* and *Serratia marcescens.*

Pneumonia develops in 50% of patients who aspirate, and the mortality is 50%.

B. **Pathophysiology.** The chemical burn causes loss of the alveolar-capillary integrity, which results in exudation of fluid and protein into the interstitial space, alveoli, and bronchi.
   1. Consequences of the initial reaction include decreased pulmonary compliance, vasoconstriction, intrapulmonary shunting, pulmonary edema, increased pulmonary vascular resistance, decreased intravascular volume, or hypotension.
   2. Resulting conditions include hypoxemia, hypercarbia, and acidosis, culminating in ARDS.

V. **Diagnostic Work-up**
   A. **Physical examination**
      1. Tachypnea, tachycardia, cyanosis, apnea, fever, and hypotension are evident.
      2. Adventitial respiratory sounds are audible on chest examination.
   B. **Laboratory studies**
      1. WBC count may be increased, with left shift.
      2. Blood or sputum cultures may be positive.
   C. **Chest radiography**
      1. The radiograph may be normal.
      2. Liquid aspirate seeks the most dependent portion of tracheobronchial tree under the force of gravity (i.e., posterior in a supine patient in the ICU).
      3. If infection occurs, especially with anaerobes, it could produce infiltrate, with or without cavitation, lung abscess, pleural effusion, or bronchopleural fistula.
   D. **Lower respiratory studies**
      1. Expectorated samples
      2. Transtracheal aspiration

      3. Protected specimen with quantitative cultures

      4. Bronchoalveolar lavage (BAL)

      5. Lung biopsy

  E. Upper GI studies

      1. Contrast films

      2. Endoscopy

      3. Gastric emptying study

      4. 24-hour esophageal pH monitoring

VI. Management

  A. Mechanical ventilation with PEEP/continuous positive airway pressure (CPAP) is optimal if infection progresses to respiratory failure.

  B. Bronchoscopy may be performed for diagnostic and therapeutic purposes, especially if the aspirate is large particulate matter and there is clinical and radiologic evidence of volume loss.

  C. Antibiotics are indicated if BAL reveals > 10,000 CFU/ml of pathogenic bacteria. (Cultures of the sputum are less helpful because they may be contaminated by oropharyngeal flora.)

  D. The **underlying pathology should be corrected.**

No conclusive or experimental data document that steroids are beneficial. In fact, they may interfere with normal healing of the lung.

CHRONIC OBSTRUCTIVE PULMONARY DISEASE (COPD)

I. Definition. COPD is a slowly progressive, chronic disorder. It is characterized primarily by airflow obstruction that is not entirely reversible. Airflow is limited, and gas exchange is impaired. The condition does not change markedly over several months.

II. Risk Factors

  A. Cigarette smoking (most important causative agent)

The greater the total tobacco exposure, the greater the risk for development of COPD.

  B. Environmental exposure (dust)

  C. Air pollution

  D. α_1-Antitrypsin deficiency

  E. Poor nutrition *in utero*

  F. Preexisting bronchial hyperresponsiveness

III. Pathology and Pathophysiology

  A. Pathology

      1. Emphysema is an anatomic diagnosis characterized by permanent enlargement of the air spaces distal to the terminal bronchioles accompanied by destruction of their walls and overinflation. Three types are defined according to the distribution of the enlarged air spaces in the lobule and acinus.

  a. Centriacinar (centrilobular) emphysema

  b. Panacinar (panlobular) emphysema

  c. Distal acinar (paraseptal) emphysema

  2. Chronic bronchitis is a clinical diagnosis characterized by a persistent productive cough for at least three consecutive months in at least two consecutive years. Diagnostic features include:

  a. Hypertrophy of the mucous glands in trachea and larger bronchi

  b. Hypersecretion of mucus and metaplastic formation of the mucin goblet cells in the surface epithelium of the bronchi

B. Pathophysiology (airway obstruction)

  1. Reduced lung elasticity (as it occurs in emphysema) decreases the maximum expiratory flow and increases airway resistance.

  2. Stimulation of cholinergic receptors by inhaled irritants or inflammation produces bronchoconstriction.

  3. Inhaled pollutants, recurrent infections, or chronic immunologic stimulation leads to chronic inflammation.

C. Physiologic derangements

  1. Reduced flow rates that limit minute ventilation

  2. Maldistributed ventilation, resulting in both wasted ventilation and impaired gas exchange

  3. Increased airway resistance (increased work of breathing)

  4. Air trapping and hyperinflation

  5. Blunted respiratory center drive in some patients

IV. Clinical Presentation

A. Signs and symptoms

  1. Cough. A morning cough, with sputum production in cases of respiratory infections, occurs. Patients may be thin and, in advanced cases, wasted.

  2. Dyspnea. An increase in the work of breathing through obstructed airways may be present on exertion or at rest. When dyspnea is marked, affected patients sit leaning forward (to gain some mechanical advantage for their accessory muscles).

B. Clinical spectrum. Most patients fall somewhere along a continuum between these two extremes.

  1. Type A ("pink puffers," emphysematous type). Patients exhibit cyanosis, clubbing, increased anteroposterior diameter of the thorax, hyperresonance, decreased breath sounds, and decreased heart sounds.

  2. Type B ("blue bloaters," chronic bronchitis type). Patients have a history of recurrent respiratory tract infections, sputum production, cough, and effort dyspnea, which tends to be episodic. They are rather obese and cyanotic, with prolongation of expiration, diffuse expiratory and inspiratory rhonchi, peripheral edema with hepatomegaly, dilated neck veins, and cor pulmonale. Cardiac examination reveals right ventricular (RV) S_3, loud pulmonary second heart sound, tricuspid regurgitation, RV heave, and increased jugular venous pressure with pulmonary hypertension.

V. Laboratory Work-up

   A. CBC with differential and **sputum cultures.** These tests should be performed if there is any possibility of respiratory tract infection.

   B. Chest radiography. Imaging may reveal increased radiolucency of the lung fields, low and flattened hemidiaphragms, a normal or decreased cardiac silhouette, or emphysematous bullae. (It may also exclude any other underlying pathologies such as lung cancer.)

   C. ECG. This tracing may reveal P pulmonale, right-axis deviation, RV hypertrophy, or any evidence of ischemic heart disease.

   D. ABG. This measurement may reveal hypoxemia (low Po_2) and various degrees of hypercarbia (elevated Pco_2).

   E. Spirometry. These tests represent the primary diagnostic tool for confirming the diagnosis, planning appropriate treatment, and assessing response to treatment.

   1. Diagnosis of COPD is certain if:

      a. The forced expiratory volume in 1 second (FEV_1) is decreased. Hypercapnic respiratory failure from COPD is unlikely unless FEV_1 is < 1.3 L, and it is usually not observed unless FEV_1 is < 1 L.

      b. The forced vital capacity (FVC) is normal or increased.

      c. The FEV_1:FVC ratio is decreased.

   2. COPD may be classified on the basis of these spirometry measurements (Table 19–1).

   F. Chest CT may be used to quantify the extent and the distribution of emphysema.

VI. Management

   A. Smoking cessation

The single most important factor that affects outcome at all stages of COPD is smoking cessation.

   B. Bronchodilators. These agents represent the mainstay of symptomatic treatment for the reversible component of airway obstruction.

   1. β_2-Adrenergic agonists

   2. Anticholinergic drugs (e.g., ipratropium)

   3. Theophylline (disadvantage: narrow therapeutic index and variable interactions with several other drugs)

   C. Corticosteroids. Inhaled or oral agents are justified only in patients who display substantial responses to a steroid trial.

Table 19-1. Classification of Chronic Obstructive Pulmonary Disease (COPD)

Type of COPD	Signs and Symptoms	FEV_1	Other Respiratory Indicators
Mild	Minimal if any shortness of breath, smoker's cough, no abnormal signs	60%–79% of predicted	FEV_1/vital capacity and other indices of expiratory flow mildly reduced
Moderate	Shortness of breath ($\pm$ wheezes) on exertion, cough ($\pm$ sputum), some abnormal signs	40%–59% of predicted	Increased FRC, reduced TLC. Some degree of hypoxemia but no hypercapnia
Severe	Shortness of breath with minimal exertion, wheezing, prominent cough, with cyanosis and peripheral edema	< 40% of predicted	Hypoxemia with hypercarbia

FEV_1 = forced expiratory volume in 1 second; FRC = forced residual capacity; TLC = total lung capacity.

D. Exercise conditioning. An exercise program decreases ventilation and heart rate for a given workload.

E. Nutrition. Weight reduction in obese patients and nutritional support may help malnourished and wasted patients.

F. Immunization. All individuals with COPD should have the following vaccinations:
1. Influenza vaccination every year
2. Pneumococcal vaccination every 6 years

G. Appropriate antibiotics for respiratory tract infections

H. Psychosocial rehabilitation. This treatment aims to prevent deconditioning and allows patients to cope with their disease.

I. Long-term oxygen therapy (LTOT). Clinical trials have demonstrated that in patients with COPD and chronic hypoxemia, LTOT improves survival, decreases secondary polycythemia, prevents the progression of pulmonary hypertension, and improves neuropsychologic health.

> **Supplemental oxygen therapy should be administered to all hypoxemic patients with COPD who present with acute exacerbations. They should *not* be kept hypoxemic for fear of carbon dioxide retention.**

J. **Surgery**
 1. Removal or ablation of a large expanding bullae
 2. Lung volume reduction surgery (for patients with markedly increased functional residual capacity)
 3. Lung transplantation

K. **Ventilatory support**
 1. Use noninvasive intermittent positive-pressure ventilation when it is appropriate.
 2. Intubate for a pH < 7.25 and worsening PCO_2 in a patient who fails to respond to supportive treatment and controlled oxygen therapy.
 3. Although it is prudent to avoid intubating a patient with COPD, the development of stupor or coma may necessitate emergency intubation, a potentially disastrous complication.
 4. The objectives of ventilation are to support gas exchange while resting the muscle of respiration.
 5. Development of auto-PEEP is a concern in patients with airflow obstruction. Auto-PEEP may cause elevation of peak inspiratory and plateau pressures, hypotension, and increased work of breathing. To avoid this, PEEP must be set equivalent to or slightly below the auto-PEEP.
 6. Ventilatory rate and tidal volume should be regulated on mechanical ventilation to return pH toward baseline.
    a. In patients with severe airflow obstruction, attempting to normalize pH may result in elevated plateau pressures and auto-PEEP.
    b. In this situation, reduction of ventilation rate and controlled hypoventilation reduces barotrauma. Adequate oxygenation must be maintained, but the PCO_2 may rise.

VII. **Prognosis.** Three-year survival is inversely related to patient age and directly related to FEV_1.
 A. Age < 60 years and FEV_1 > 50% predicted: 90%
 B. Age > 60 years and FEV_1 > 50% predicted: 80%
 C. Age > 60 years and FEV_1 40% to 49% predicted: 75%

EMBOLIC SYNDROMES

I. **Venous Air Embolism**
 A. **Etiology.** Causes may be traumatic or iatrogenic.
    1. Catheterization (central venous catheter, epidural catheter)
    2. Surgery (neurosurgery, transplant surgery, cryosurgery)

   3. Arthroscopy, endoscopy, laparoscopy, hysteroscopy, thoracoscopy
   4. Contrast injection
   5. Trauma to head, neck, thorax, abdomen
   6. Shunt placement, cardiopulmonary bypass, or pacemaker insertion
   7. Hemodialysis
 B. Signs and symptoms (mimic those of PE)
   1. Dyspnea, tachypnea
   2. Cough, chest pain
   3. Dizziness, confusion
   4. Wheezing, "mill wheel" murmur or hard systolic murmur, tachycardia, tachypnea, hypotension
 C. Diagnostic tests
   1. Swan-Ganz catheter: acute increase in central venous pressure and PCWP without elevation in pulmonary artery occlusion pressure
   2. ECG: tachycardia, right heart strain, myocardial ischemia
   3. Chest radiograph: air fluid level in main pulmonary artery, pulmonary edema, intracardiac air
   4. Precordial Doppler ultrasound or transesophageal echocardiogram
 D. Management
   1. When a venous air embolism is suspected, place a central venous catheter with the patient in a Trendelenburg position with left lateral decubitus tilt.
   2. Attempt to aspirate from the catheter if it is in the right atrium. This might remove the air.
   3. Optimize intravascular volume.
   4. Support circulation.
   5. Administer 100% oxygen.
   6. Discontinue nitrous oxide anesthetics.
   7. Administer hyperbaric oxygen (HBO) therapy if readily available.
II. Cholesterol Embolism
 A. Definition and pathophysiology. A cholesterol embolism is a well-known complication of generalized atherosclerotic disease that occurs spontaneously or after an invasive procedure. Complications include:
   1. Renal failure
   2. Lower extremity ischemia
   3. Bowel infarction or hemorrhage
   4. Ischemic cholecystitis
   5. CVA
 B. Management. Provide supportive therapy depending on the vascular bed embolized.
III. Fat Embolism
 A. Risk factors (trauma-related)
   1. Fractures (closed bone type or involving multiple long bones)
   2. Shock

      3. Absent or improper immobilization as well as delayed operative stabilization

      4. Coexisting pulmonary contusion

B. Etiology

      1. Fractures (long bone or pelvic bone)

      2. Total knee or hip arthroplasty

      3. Burns

      4. Liposuction

      5. Pancreatitis

      6. Bone marrow harvesting and transplantation

      7. Cardiopulmonary bypass

      8. Blood transfusions

      9. Sternotomy

     10. Osteomyelitis

     11. Steroid therapy

C. Pathogenesis. Fat cells and tissue factor (TF) released from the marrow stimulate intravascular coagulation as well as platelet, leukocyte, and endothelial cell activation. The result is endothelial damage and increased capillary permeability, predominantly in the lung.

D. Clinical presentation (onset between 24 and 72 hours after the inciting event)

      1. Pulmonary factors

         a. Subclinical: mild desaturation without clinical symptoms

         b. Subacute: dyspnea and tachypnea with hypoxemia and hypocapnia

         c. Fulminant: severe hypoxemia (ARDS) with decreased cardiac output and increased pulmonary artery pressure from massive embolization and obstruction of a pulmonary artery

      2. Fever

      3. Tachycardia

      4. Petechial rash of anterior chest, sclera, and neck

      5. Ocular features

         a. Conjunctival petechiae

         b. Retinal lesions (visualization of the fat, followed by fluffy exudates, hemorrhage, and macular edema)

      6. CNS features (irritability, confusion, seizures, focal defects, rarely coma)

E. Diagnosis

      1. Laboratory work-up

         a. CBC, prothrombin time/partial thromboplastin time (PT/PTT), DIC profile (i.e., fibrinogen, fibrin split products, D-dimers)

         b. BUN, creatinine, electrolytes

         c. Urinalysis (lipuria)

         d. Blood lipase

         e. Sputum fat content

         f. CSF fat

      2. ECG: sinus tachycardia and right heart strain

       3. ABG: hypoxemia, hypocapnia, and respiratory alkalosis
       4. Imaging
         a. Chest radiography: diffuse bilateral alveolar or interstitial infiltrates
         b. MRI: identifies cerebral fat emboli
       5. Funduscopic examination

  F. Management
     1. Identify and eliminate risk factors.
     2. Aggressively resuscitate.
     3. Administer aggressive pulmonary care.
     4. Consider steroids.

IV. Amniotic Fluid Embolism
  A. Definitions
     1. This syndrome is characterized by cardiovascular collapse, respiratory insufficiency, neurologic defects, and coagulation abnormalities in the peri- or postpartum period.
     2. This type of embolism may be seen in several circumstances, including:
       a. First-trimester abortion (with curettage) or a second-trimester abortion (with saline, prostaglandin, and urea)
       b. Hysterectomy
       c. Amniocentesis
       d. Cesarean section
       e. Abdominal trauma
  B. Incidence. This syndrome occurs in 1:8000 to 1:80,000 births with fetal mortality of 40% and maternal mortality of 80%. It accounts for 10% of maternal deaths.
  C. Pathophysiology
     1. Amniotic fluid enters the venous circulation through endocervical, placental, or uterine veins that have become lacerated. Broken fetal cells or TF induces DIC.
     2. The amniotic fluid then produces pulmonary vasospasm with severe pulmonary hypertension, hypoxemia, and hypotension.
     3. Anaphylactoid reaction occurs, and vasoactive substances such as leukotrienes, prostaglandins, and complement trigger pulmonary vasoconstriction or obstruction.
     4. Pulmonary edema and LV failure with depressed contractility finally occur.
  D. Signs and symptoms
     1. Anxiety, coughing, vomiting, shivering, bad taste in the mouth (initially)
     2. Abrupt onset of dyspnea and hypotension
     3. Rapid progression to cardiopulmonary arrest, hypoxemia, cyanosis, convulsions, profound acidosis, or coma
     4. Pulmonary edema
  E. Diagnostic tests
     1. ECG (ischemia and right heart strain)
     2. ABG

  3. Elevated PT/PTT, decreased platelets and fibrinogen, increased fibrin split products
F. **Management**
  1. Provide immediate cardiopulmonary support for possible amniotic fluid embolism. However, 50% of patients die in the first hour.
  2. Administer CPR, with the patient tilted to the left.
  3. Intubate and use mechanical ventilation.
  4. Administer vasopressors for persistent hypotension.
  5. If there is no response after 5 minutes of advanced cardiac life support (ACLS), deliver the fetus surgically.

EXTRACORPOREAL MEMBRANE OXYGENATION (ECMO)

I. **Definitions**
  A. Extracorporeal membrane oxygenation (ECMO) or extracorporeal life support (ECLS) is the use of extracorporeal circulation and gas exchange to provide temporary life support to patients with cardiac or pulmonary failure.
  B. **Circuit components** (Figure 19–1)
    1. Roller or centrifugal blood pump
    2. Gas exchange membrane with user-controlled variable oxygen and carbon dioxide delivery
    3. Heat exchanger and line pressure monitors
  C. **Cannulation sites** (options)
    1. Femoral vessels (artery and vein)
    2. Superior vena cava (SVC) and aorta
    3. SVC and femoral artery
II. **Indications** (non-neonatal ECLS)
  A. **Adult pulmonary failure**
    1. Graft failure after pulmonary transplantation
    2. ARDS
    3. Bacterial and viral pneumonia
    4. Other lung injury with failure of mechanical ventilation
  B. **Specific criteria**
    1. Peak airway pressure > 45 cm H_2O
    2. PEEP > 10 cm H_2O
    3. $FIO_2 = 100\%$ for > 30 hours with $Pao_2 < 55$ mm Hg
III. **Contraindications**
  A. Any contraindication to full anticoagulation
  B. Prolonged mechanical ventilatory support with irreversible pulmonary fibrosis
IV. **Physiology**
  A. **Venoarterial bypass** with 10% to 50% native CO provides pulsatile flow. Blood bypasses the pulmonary vascular bed. **Systemic oxygen saturation** is a combination of native lung function and membrane oxygenation.
  B. **Veno-veno bypass** where flow is supplied solely by native CO is the alternative route. The amount of systemic venous re-

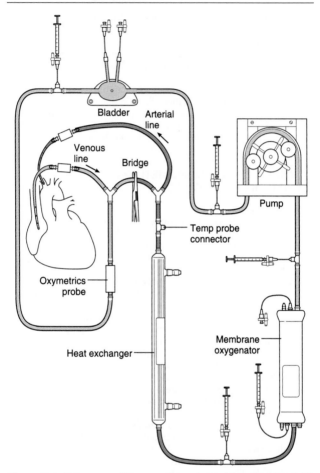

Figure 19-1. Extracorporeal life support in respiratory failure. (Reprinted with permission from Cilley RE and Bartlett RH: Extracorporeal life support for respiratory failure. In *Cardiopulmonary Bypass Principles and Practice*. Edited by Gravlee GP, Davis RF, and Utley JR. Baltimore, Williams & Wilkins, 1993, p 675.)

　　　turn that can be "captured" by the ECMO circuit limits the flow.
　　C. As native lung function recovers, mixed venous saturation improves without increases in circuit oxygenation.
V. Management: Anticoagulation

A. Patients must be maintained with an activated clotting time (ACT) of about 200 seconds.

B. Anticoagulation should be maintained with heparin alone. Platelets or fresh frozen plasma may be used to correct the platelet count or normalize the PT.

C. Modification of the regimen may involve increasing flow rates and allowing the ACT to fall to 160–180 seconds if serious bleeding complications arise.

MECHANICAL VENTILATION

I. Conditions That Initiate Respiratory Failure (Table 19–2)

   A. Airway-related causes

     1. Aspiration

     2. Oxygen toxicity

     3. Inhalation injury

     4. Diffuse pneumonia

     5. Pulmonary contusion

     6. ARDS

   B. Blood-borne causes

     1. Sepsis

     2. Transfusion reaction

     3. Pulmonary embolism

     4. Acute pancreatitis

   C. Respiratory muscle dysfunction

Table 19-2. Causes of Respiratory Failure

Oxygenation Failure ($Pao_2 < 50$ mm Hg)	Ventilatory Failure ($Paco_2 > 50$ mm Hg)
V-Q mismatch	**Defective respiratory control**
Pulmonary embolus	Elimination of hypoxemic drive
Asthma/COPD	Stroke
Interstitial lung disease	
	Impaired respiratory muscle function
Shunt with normal CXR	
Intracardiac right-to-left shunt	Airflow obstruction
Pulmonary AV fistula	(e.g., asthma, COPD)
Microatelectasis	Myasthenia gravis, Guillain-Barré syndrome
Shunt with abnormal CXR	
Pneumonia	**Mechanical abnormalities**
Atelectasis	Trauma/flail chest
Pulmonary edema, CHF, ARDS	Pneumothorax
Pulmonary contusion	

ARDS = adult respiratory distress syndrome; AV = atrioventricular; CHF = congestive heart failure; COPD = chronic obstructive pulmonary disease; CXR = chest x-ray; V-Q = ventilation–perfusion.

        1. Myasthenia gravis

        2. Guillain-Barré syndrome

    D. Other conditions

        1. Malignancy

        2. Massive trauma

        3. Radiation use

  II. Indications for Intubation (Figure 19-2 and Table 19–3)

  III. Types of Ventilators

    A. Volume-cycled

        1. These ventilators deliver a fixed volume of air.

        2. The system develops a peak inspiratory pressure (PIP) necessary to deliver the set volume.

        3. Most ventilators have a pop-off valve if the PIP surpasses the set limits.

    B. Pressure-cycled

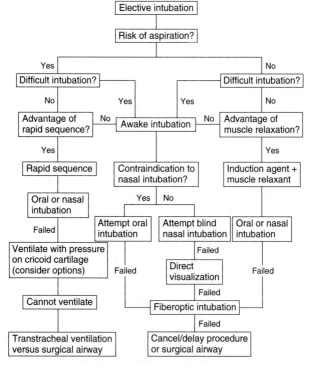

Figure 19-2. Algorithm for elective intubation. (Adapted with permission from Hee MKJ, Plevak DJ, Peters SG: Intubation of critically ill patients. *Mayo Clin Proc* 67:574; 1992.)

Table 19-3. Indications for Intubation*

- Respiratory rate > 35–40 breaths/min
- $Paco_2$ > 55 mm Hg (acute retention with respiratory acidosis)
- Pao_2 < 70 mm Hg on 100% O_2 nonrebreather face mask (check baseline)
- A-a gradient > 400 mm Hg on 100% O_2 face mask
- Need for aggressive bronchopulmonary toilet
- ARDS
- Need for airway protection
- Severe head injury
- High spinal cord trauma/injury
- Uncompensated metabolic acidosis with clinical deterioration

ARDS = adult respiratory distress syndrome.
*Note: These are only relative reasons for intubation. Each patient must be evaluated, taking into consideration individual pathophysiology. **When in doubt, INTUBATE!**

1. These ventilators deliver air at predetermined pressure. The clinician sets the maximal pressure, frequency, and inspiratory time (usually a percentage of the entire cycle).
2. The compliance of the patient's lung determines the resulting tidal volume. As the compliance falls, the lungs become stiffer and more resistant to stretching and the tidal volume decreases.

IV. Patterns of Ventilation Delivery

A. Controlled ventilation

1. The **volume-controlled mode** delivers the chosen tidal volume or pressure at a set respiratory rate.
2. The **pressure-controlled mode** delivers a set pressure, and the resulting tidal volume is dependent on the lung compliance. Often, patients need to be sedated or sedated and paralyzed.

B. Assisted ventilation

1. The ventilator cycles and delivers a breath each time the patient is able to generate some negative pressure. Therefore, the patient signals the ventilator when he or she wants to breathe.
2. The delivered breaths are synchronous with the patient's own attempts.

V. Methods of Ventilation

A. Assist/control ventilation (A/C)

1. This standard method of positive-pressure mechanical ventilation involves volume-cycled lung inflation. It delivers a set rate of breaths and a predetermined volume.
2. The patient has the opportunity to initiate the breaths that the machine delivers. Each breath over the set rate is delivered at a full tidal volume.
3. If the patient does not attempt any breaths, the ventilator

delivers a minimum number of breaths according to the rate set by the operator. This mode protects the patient from apnea.

> **In patients with a high respiratory rate, the increased frequency of machine breaths in A/C ventilation may lead to overventilation and severe respiratory alkalosis as well as hyperinflation.**

B. Intermittent mandatory ventilation (IMV)

1. IMV, like A/C ventilation, delivers a set breath as determined by the operator. Between these predetermined breaths, the patient can breathe spontaneously at his or her own rate and tidal volume.

2. The resultant increased work of breathing can lead to respiratory muscle fatigue. To reduce the work of breathing, pressure support may be added to overcome the resistance of the ventilation circuit.

3. By increasing the work of breathing rather than decreasing alveolar ventilation, IMV can correct respiratory alkalosis.

4. The IMV rate can be slowly decreased so the patient can begin to do more of the work of breathing (IMV weaning) [see XVI B].

C. Synchronized intermittent mandatory ventilation (SIMV)

1. SIMV combines assisted ventilation and spontaneous ventilation to synchronize the machine breath to the patient's spontaneous breathing efforts.

2. At an SIMV rate of 6/min, the ventilator senses a breath attempt from the patient approximately every 10 seconds and delivers a positive-pressure breath. For each additional breath ($> 6/min$), the patient breathes spontaneously. The spontaneous tidal volume achieved depends on the strength of the patient and the compliance of the lungs.

D. High-frequency or jet ventilation

1. This mode uses a **very small tidal volume** (e.g., 100–150 ml or less) and **extremely rapid rates** (e.g., 100–1000 breaths/min).

2. **Indications** include neonatal status, bronchopleural fistula, and intratracheal or intrabronchial surgery.

E. Pressure-support ventilation

1. Each time the patient initiates a breath, the ventilator supplies pressure to assist inspiration.

2. This mode, which is often used as a method of weaning, allows the patient to dictate both the duration of lung inflation and the inflation volume.

   a. It increases the tidal volume and decreases the work of breathing.

   b. It helps overcome the resistance of breathing through ventilator circuits.

3. The pressure support should be set to ensure a spontaneous tidal volume $> 5–6$ ml/kg. Furthermore, 5 cm H_2O is often used initially to overcome the resistance of the endotracheal tube.

VI. **Modification of End-Expiratory Pressure**

A. **CPAP**

1. CPAP involves maintaining a pressure greater than the atmospheric level in a patient who is breathing spontaneously, resulting in a larger functional reserve capacity and better oxygenation.

2. CPAP is present during inspiration and expiration.

B. **PEEP**

1. **Definition.** PEEP refers to positive-pressure ventilation where the equilibrium pressure reached at the end of expiration is not atmospheric pressure but is some small pressure greater than the atmospheric level. A PEEP of 5 cm H_2O is considered physiologic.

2. **Oxygenation.** Increasing PEEP improves oxygenation. This continues until the pressure begins to interfere with venous return by increasing intrathoracic pressure.

   a. Patients with high degrees of shunt or venous admixture are relatively refractory to oxygen and require PEEP to avoid oxygen toxicity from high FIO_2.

   b. In localized lung disease, PEEP can worsen the hypoxemia by overdistending the normal lung and directing flow to the diseased lung.

There is no evidence that the routine use of PEEP is beneficial in all patients.

---

   c. In patients who require an $FIO_2 > 60\%$ to maintain adequate oxygenation, the addition of PEEP can increase arterial oxygenation and allow the FIO_2 to be decreased.

3. **ARDS.** In ARDS, PEEP increases lung compliance and decreases intrapulmonary shunt fraction.

   a. This increases PO_2 and allows the amount of inspired oxygen to be decreased.

   b. In patients at risk for ARDS, PEEP does not appear to reduce the incidence of disease.

4. **Cardiac effects.** In normal lungs, PEEP increases the CO. In stiff lungs, the CO is decreased.

5. **Complications**

   a. Decreased CO

   b. Barotrauma

      (1) When air spaces rupture, air can dissect along tissue planes (interstitial emphysema) or can travel along the bronchovascular bundles into the mediastinum (pneumomediastinum) and up to the neck (subcutaneous emphysema). The air can also

rupture the visceral pleura (pneumothorax) or enter the peritoneal cavity (pneumoperitoneum).

(2) Risk factors include excessive inflation volume and high intrathoracic pressures.

(3) Diagnosis is based on subcutaneous air, chest radiograph, and interstitial air.

(4) Treatment involves a chest tube thoracostomy.

c. Fluid retention

d. Intracranial hypertension

C. Auto-PEEP

1. Development involves obstructed airways. Exhalation is not complete, and there is airflow at the end of expiration. (In a normal lung, when expiration is complete, there is no airflow.)

a. The pressure of the airflow creates a pressure difference between the alveoli and the proximal airways. The elasticity of the alveoli pushing against the resistance of the terminal bronchioles accounts for this pressure.

b. Because alveolar pressure is positive, it is called auto-PEEP.

2. Causes include increased volume, increase in airway resistance, and decreased time for exhalation.

3. Measurement involves occlusion of the expiratory port of the ventilator immediately before a breath. The pressure in the lungs and ventilator circuit equilibrates, and the level of auto-PEEP is displayed on a manometer.

4. Effects include:

a. Auto-PEEP may lead to false elevation of PCWP.

b. Auto-PEEP increases the work of breathing. Hyperinflation puts patients on the flat portion of the pressure–volume curve, and they need higher pressures to move a given volume. The auto-PEEP must be overcome before the patients can take a breath, which decreases the volume of each breath.

5. Management involves:

a. Decreasing the tidal volume

b. Raising the inspiratory flow rate to increase the time for exhalation

c. Decreasing the respiratory rate

VII. Other Ventilator Parameters

A. Inspiratory:expiratory (I:E) ratio

1. In normal individuals who are breathing spontaneously, expiration is twice as long as inspiration. In adults, the I:E ratio should usually be at least 1:2.

2. In special circumstances, alteration in the I:E ratio is necessary.

a. If auto-PEEP is present, the I:E ratio should be increased to provide a longer exhalation time.

b. Bronchospastic patients require a longer expiration time. The I:E ratio should be adjusted to 1:4 or 1:5.

    c. In patients with severe hypoxemia (i.e., ARDS), the I:E ratio should be decreased to allow for increased gas exchange. This is uncomfortable for most patients and usually requires sedation and paralysis.

  B. Compliance

    1. Compliance = tidal volume ÷ plateau airway pressure.

    2. To measure compliance, select inspiratory hold on the ventilator and measure the plateau airway pressure. Then subtract the PEEP. Determine compliance only during passive ventilation, because chest wall muscle contraction can reduce it.

    3. Compliance correlates with the elasticity and distensibility of the lung.

  C. Patient positioning

    1. In unilateral lung disease, the lateral decubitus position, with the less diseased lung down, can improve oxygenation by increasing perfusion and ventilation.

    2. In the early, edematous phase of ARDS, the prone position has proved helpful. This position may be beneficial for 8–12 hours.

VIII. Patient Placement on a Ventilator

  A. Set the mode of ventilation. Usually, A/C is a good way to begin. This is difficult in the patient with a high respiratory rate who may be creating auto-PEEP. In this situation, change to IMV or sedate the patient.

  B. Set the tidal volume. Use 6–12 ml/kg. On the ventilator, it is desirable to have a larger tidal volume to ensure that alveolar collapse does not occur. (For patients not on mechanical ventilation, the normal tidal volume is 5–6 ml/kg.)

  C. Set the respiratory rate. Usually, the machine rate is set at 10–14 breaths/min. This can be adjusted according to each individual patient and the desired minute ventilation.

  D. Set the inspired oxygen. It is usually set at 80% to 100% initially and then adjusted downward by 10% to 20% based on the results of an ABG. An $FIO_2 < 60\%$ is desirable to avoid oxygen toxicity.

IX. Effects of Mechanical Ventilation on Cardiac Performance

  A. Preload. Mechanical ventilation leads to reduced ventricular filling.

    1. An increase in positive (intrathoracic) pressure reduces ventricular distensibility and ventricular filling during diastole.

    2. Compression of pulmonary vasculature decreases LV filling by decreasing venous return or by reducing the right heart ejection fraction.

    3. Decreased RV ejection can lead to RV dilation and can push the interventricular septum into the left chamber and alter LV size.

  B. Afterload. The increased transmural pressure facilitates ventricular emptying during systole.

  C. CO

1. When ventricular filling is reduced, CO is decreased.
2. If ventricular filling is normal, CO is increased.

X. Mechanical Ventilation in the Newborn

A. Endotracheal intubation

1. The oral route is better than the nasal approach.
2. The endotracheal tube should be without a cuff.

B. IMV (standard method) [SIMV in some facilities]. It is more physiologic to allow infants to determine their own minute ventilation.

> **Neonates often have a higher-than-expected saturation rate for a given Pao$_2$ because they have a high proportion of fetal Hgb and an oxyhemoglobin curve that is shifted to the left.**

1. Maintain oxygen saturation levels between 85% and 97%.
2. Ensure adequate removal of carbon dioxide.
   a. Adjust PIP to 4–5 ml/kg. The concept of permissive hypercapnia has been used for many years in the neonatal ICU. Alveolar development is incomplete in newborns.
   b. Consider surfactant administration.

C. High-frequency ventilation (HFV). In extremely small, compressible lungs, HFV may be more efficient in gas exchange.

1. **Types of HFV**
   a. High-frequency positive-pressure ventilation. This form of HFV makes use of regular IMV ventilators, with an increase in frequency to 60–150 breaths/min.

> **High-frequency positive-pressure ventilation must be closely monitored, because these ventilators were not designed for this purpose.**

   b. High-frequency jet ventilation
      (1) Delivers short pulses of pressurized gas directly into the upper airway
      (2) Operates effectively at rates of 150–600 breaths/min
   c. High-frequency oscillation ventilation
      (1) Moves small quantities of air back and forth at rates up to 1000 breaths/min
      (2) Relies on diffusion of gas rather than bulk flow

2. **Uses of HFV**
   a. Optimize adequate ventilation
      (1) Preexisting air leak syndromes or pulmonary hypoplasia
      (2) Obstructive lung disorders (e.g., meconium aspiration, persistence of fetal circulation)
   b. Optimize lung volume

D. ECMO (see EXTRACORPOREAL MEMBRANE OXYGENATION, p. 449)

1. **Use.** ECMO is an alternate method to oxygenate and ventilate a patient. For oxygenation by artificial lung, a circuit of veno-veno or veno-arterial bypass is required.

2. **Indications**
   a. Meconium aspiration syndrome
   b. Congenital diaphragmatic hernia
   c. Persistent pulmonary hypertension
   d. Respiratory distress syndrome
   e. Cardiac failure
   f. Sepsis
   g. Barotrauma

3. **Patient selection**
   a. Reversible respiratory failure
   b. Predicted mortality $> 80\%$
   c. Weight > 2 kg or gestation > 34 weeks
   d. Arterial-alveolar gradient > 610 mm Hg for more than 8–12 hours on 100% FIO_2
   e. $Pao_2 < 50$ mm Hg for 4 hours or < 40 mm Hg for 2 hours
   f. pH < 7.15 for < 2 hours
   g. Severe barotrauma and air leak

XI. **Monitoring During Mechanical Ventilation**

A. **ABG.** Determination should be obtained 10–15 minutes after initiation of ventilation or adjustment of ventilator settings.

B. **Pulse oximetry**
   1. Ear probes are more sensitive to sudden changes than finger probes.
   2. Use is limited in situations where carboxyhemoglobin is present; readings are falsely elevated.

> **Pulse oximetry readings vary with skin pigmentation, which determines the cutoff point for the lowest accurate reading.**

C. **End-tidal carbon dioxide**
   1. **Significance.** End-tidal carbon dioxide provides continuous indirect measurement of $Paco_2$. Alterations result from changes in carbon dioxide delivery to the lungs, alveolar ventilation, or equipment malfunction. **Absence** of end-tidal carbon dioxide occurs as a consequence of esophageal intubation.
   2. **Increases**
      a. Sudden rises reflect precipitous increases in CO or release of a tourniquet, bicarbonate administration, or equipment malfunction.
      b. Gradual rises are due to hypoventilation.
   3. **Decreases**
      a. Sudden declines result from sudden hyperventilation, cardiac arrest, massive PE, air embolism, disconnection from ventilator, and obstruction of the endotracheal tube.

  b. Gradual declines reflect hyperventilation, hypothermia, or pulmonary hypoperfusion.

Avoid alkalosis in patients with COPD. Return their Pco_2 to their normally elevated baseline and not to a normal level (e.g., 40 mm Hg). Hyperventilation in the presence of an elevated HCO_3 can cause seizures and death.

D. Monitoring lung mechanics

  1. Peak airway pressure (PAP). This value is a function of the inflation volume, the airway resistance, and the compliance of the lungs and chest wall. At a constant volume, the PAP is directly proportional to the airway resistance and inversely proportional to the lung compliance.

  a. PAP should be maintained < 50 mm H_2O.

  b. If the PAP is too high and threatening pneumothorax, it can be decreased by reducing the tidal volume, PEEP, or peak flow. The choice depends on the clinical situation.

  2. Compliance. It is more accurate to look at changes in respiratory compliance rather than at a single value. In normal individuals, the static compliance is 90 ml/cm H_2O. In intubated patients with no lung disease, it is 50–70 ml/cm H_2O.

  3. Changes in peak airway pressures. Some changes include:

  a. Increase in peak pressure, with constant plateau airway pressure

   (1) This change results in an increase in airway resistance.

   (2) This change may be a sign of aspiration, bronchospasm, increased secretions, endotracheal tube obstruction, or airway obstruction.

   (3) Treatment involves suctioning, giving bronchodilator medications, and checking the endotracheal tube.

  b. Increase in both the peak and plateau airway pressures. This change may be a sign of pneumothorax, acute lobar atelectasis, acute pulmonary edema, or ARDS or pneumonia. It may also result in asynchronous breathing or COPD with tachypnea and developing auto-PEEP.

  c. Decrease in peak pressure. This results from an air leak or severe hyperventilation where the patient is drawing air into the lungs.

E. Tidal volumes. Monitor to ensure that patients are receiving adequate tidal volumes. Causes of decreased tidal volume include:

  1. Increased inspiratory or expiratory resistance

  2. Bronchospasm

> **Pressure-cycled ventilators are usually not used in patients with COPD or asthma because variable bronchospasm can result in an inconsistent minute ventilation.**

    3. Secretions
    4. Decreased compliance
    5. Pneumothorax
    6. Auto-PEEP
    7. Decreased expiratory time
    8. Decreased set pressure

XII. Adjusting Ventilator Settings
    A. The respiratory rate and the tidal volume are determinants of ventilation (carbon dioxide), whereas FIO_2 and PEEP are determinants of oxygenation (oxygen).
        1. Adjust the respiratory rate (RR) for a desired $Paco_2$. [Use the equation $Paco_2$ (measured) $\times$ RR (measured) $=$ $Paco_2$ (desired) $\times$ RR (desired).]
        2. Patients are more comfortable with larger tidal volumes. Usually the recommended tidal volume of 6–12 ml/kg is adequate and initially chosen until the parameters are adjusted based on an ABG.
    B. Information about ventilator settings and their adjustment is presented in Table 19–4.

> **In patients with severe metabolic disease (acidotic, septic) and poor ventilation, consider sedation and paralysis. This minimizes nonessential metabolic functioning and allows direction of energy to combat the severe disease.**

XIII. Permissive Hypercapnia and Hypoxemia
    A. Permissive hypercapnia. This is the purposeful act of allowing the $Paco_2$ to increase beyond 50 mm Hg.
        1. An acute $Paco_2$ increase to 60 mm Hg is not life-threatening if the pH $\geq$ 7.25, cardiovascular function is adequate, and increasing the tidal volume or pressure limit risks lung injury.
        2. For a $Paco_2 > 60$ mm Hg and pH < 7.25, the clinician must weigh the risks of tissue acidosis and lung injury.
    B. Permissive hypoxemia
        1. In patients who are critically ill, an arterial $Po_2 > 60$ mm Hg is usually acceptable.
        2. If cardiovascular function is adequate and increasing FIO_2 or PEEP is a greater risk with lung injury, a PO_2 level of 50 mm Hg is acceptable.

XIV. Complications of Mechanical Ventilation
    A. Patient agitation (Table 19–5)
    B. Hypotension
        1. Impeded venous return
            a. PEEP
            b. Increased intrathoracic pressure

Table 19-4. Adjusting Ventilator Settings

Situation	Action	Comments
Arterial saturation $\geq$ 94% $PO_2 > 100$ mm Hg	Reduce FIO_2	Once $FIO_2 < 50\%$, PEEP may be reduced by increments of 2.5 cm H_2O per 12 hours until physiologic level is reached Maintain oxygen saturation > 90% ($PO_2 > 60$ mm Hg)
Arterial saturation < 90% $PO_2 < 60$ mm Hg	Increase FIO_2 up to 60%–100%, then consider increasing PEEP by increments of 2.5 cm H_2O until oxygenation improves or CO_2 falls	Consider switching to pressure control mode (remember to sedate with or without paralysis) Add additional PEEP until oxygen saturation is acceptable, with an $FIO_2 < 60\%$
Excessively low pH (< 7.33 due to respiratory acidosis/hypercapnia)	Increase rate or tidal volume to blow off CO_2 Keep peak airway pressure < 40 cm H_2O	—
High pH (> 7.48 due to respiratory alkalosis/hypocapnia)	Reduce rate or tidal volume If the patient is breathing rapidly above the ventilator, it may be necessary to change to IMV mode or sedate the patient	—

CO = cardiac output; FIO_2 = fraction of inspired oxygen; IMV = intermittent mandatory ventilation; PEEP = positive end-expiratory pressure.

  c. Hyperinflation
2. Cardiac dysfunction
3. Systemic inflammatory response syndrome (SIRS)
    a. Fever
    b. Low mean arterial pressure
    c. Tachycardia

Table 19-5. Complications of Mechanical Ventilation

Patient-related Causes	Ventilator-related Causes
Anxiety	Ventilator disconnection
Artificial airway problems	System leak
Pain	Circuit malfunction
Secretions	Inadequate F_{IO_2}
Bronchospasm	Inadequate ventilator support
Pneumothorax	
Pulmonary edema	
Pulmonary embolism	
Hypoxemia, acidosis	
Drug-induced (sedation, allergy)	
Abdominal distention	

F_{IO_2} = fraction of inspired oxygen.

      d. Mental status changes
      e. Leukocytosis
   4. Effects of medications (e.g., sedatives, anxiolytics, narcotics, paralytics)
  C. Acute respiratory distress. Management steps are:
   1. Remove the patient from the ventilator and begin to ventilate manually with 100% oxygen. If no improvement occurs, then there is a possible problem with the endotracheal or tracheostomy tube.
   2. Perform a physical examination, concentrating on cardiopulmonary issues. Obtain vital signs and look at trends.
      a. Auscultate the chest, and check endotracheal tube placement to rule out right mainstem bronchus intubation.
      b. Consider the presence of a ruptured cuff (low delivered tidal volume, inability to maintain PEEP, decreased cuff air, or inability to inflate the cuff).
   3. Assess the patency of the airway, and suction to rule out obstruction.
      a. Thick secretions
        (1) This discharge can plug the tube and result in atelectasis.
        (2) Treatment involves suctioning, physiotherapy, or even repeated bronchoscopy.
      b. Auto-PEEP
   4. Perform necessary assessments to **stabilize airway and ventilation.**
   5. Obtain a chest radiograph. (Confirm endotracheal tube placement and rule out pneumothorax.)
   6. Evaluate compliance.

D. Increased airway pressures

1. **Increased airway resistance.** This may result from:

   a. Narrowing of inspiratory passages (e.g., kinked tube, small endotracheal tube, fluid in the ventilatory circuit, neoplasm, foreign body)

   b. Secretions that can occlude the endotracheal tube or airways

   c. Bronchospasm (treat with nebulized bronchodilators)

2. **Decreased pulmonary compliance** (i.e., a change in pressure for a given change in volume). Causes may include ARDS, pulmonary edema, auto-PEEP, and pneumonia.

   a. Volume-cycled ventilation. Lower compliance means that a higher pressure is needed for delivery of a set volume.

   b. Pressure-cycled ventilation. Lower compliance translates to a low volume delivered for a set pressure.

3. **External lung compression**

   a. Barotrauma/pneumothorax

      (1) Clinical change in patient's status (e.g., increased peak airway pressure, hypotension, agitation, respiratory distress)

      (2) Chest radiograph, with increased volume in one hemithorax, deep sulcus sign (downward displacement of hemidiaphragm), increased radiolucency

      (3) High-risk clinical setting

         (a) Large tidal volumes (> 12 ml/kg)

         (b) PEEP > 15 cm H_2O

         (c) High peak airway pressures (> 50–60 cm H_2O)

         (d) ARDS

         (e) Pneumonia

   b. Acute pleural fluid collections

   c. Diaphragmatic elevation resulting from abdominal process

   d. Valsalva maneuver

E. Hypoxemia. Causes include:

1. Ventilator-related problems

2. Progression of underlying disease

   a. ARDS

   b. Cardiogenic pulmonary edema

   c. Pneumonia, sepsis

   d. Acute exacerbation of asthma or COPD

3. New medical problem

   a. Pneumothorax

   b. Atelectasis or lobar collapse

   c. Aspiration

   d. Sepsis, pneumonia

   e. Pulmonary embolism

   f. Fluid overload

g. Bronchospasm

h. Shock

4. Medications (e.g., bronchodilators, vasodilators, β-blockers)

5. Effects of outside intervention

    a. Endotracheal suctioning

    b. Change in body position

    c. Bronchoscopy

    d. Thoracentesis

    e. Dialysis

F. Sinusitis

  1. Most common in nasotracheal intubation

  2. Diagnosis: aspiration of infected material from the infected sinus

G. Laryngeal injury

  1. Signs: ulceration, granulomas, vocal cord paresis, or laryngeal edema

  2. Resolution: usually within a few weeks of extubation

H. Bleeding (bright-red blood) from endotracheal tube

  1. Etiology

    a. Iatrogenic: suction catheter–related trauma

    b. Pneumonia

    c. Pulmonary secretions (pink frothy sputum with cardiogenic etiology)

    d. PE

    e. Pulmonary artery catheters: associated with pulmonary artery dissection and rupture

    f. Erosion secondary to endotracheal tube cuff: tracheonominate artery fistula

    g. Underlying disease: neoplasms, vasculitis, DIC

  2. Management

    a. Perform physical examination.

    b. Obtain a chest radiograph.

    c. Consult a cardiothoracic surgeon for hemorrhage.

Direct pressure and overinflation of a cuff may serve to tamponade tracheonominate fistulae in emergency situations.

---

    d. Perform bronchoscopy.

    e. Administer antibiotics.

I. Ventilator-associated pneumonia (VAP). This form of pneumonia occurs in 20% to 40% of patients who are ventilated for more than 48 hours.

  1. For diagnosis of VAP, a new radiographic infiltrate must be evident. In addition, one of the following conditions must be present:

    a. Histopathologic evidence of pneumonia

    b. Positive blood or pleural fluid cultures matching tracheal aspirates

    c. Positive quantitative BAL fluid culture

2. Predisposing factors include immunosuppression, renal failure, hepatic insufficiency, and major CNS disease.

Routine empiric antibiotics should be avoided in VAP.

XV. **Weaning from the Ventilator**
    A. **Indications for extubation** (Table 19–6)
    B. **Conditions necessary for weaning**

Evaluate patients on mechanical ventilators daily.

---

1. Resolution or improvement in cause of respiratory failure
2. Cessation of sedative drugs and neuromuscular blocking agents
3. Normal state of consciousness and muscular function
4. Absence of sepsis, anemia, or hyperthermia
5. Cardiovascular stability
6. Correction of electrolyte and metabolic disorders
7. Adequate gas exchange
    a. $Pao_2 > 60$ mm Hg and $Sao_2 > 90\%$, with $Fio_2 \leq 40\%$ and PEEP ≤ 5 mm H_2O
    b. $Pao_2:PAo_2$ ratio ≥ 0.35
    c. $Pao_2/Fio_2 \geq 200$
    d. Alveolar-arterial gradient < 350 mm Hg
8. Adequate respiratory system capacity
    a. Respiratory rate < 35 breaths/min
    b. Spontaneous tidal volume > 5 ml/kg

Table 19-6. Indications for Extubation*

- Patient is alert and oriented and is able to clear and protect the airway
- Respiratory rate < 30 breaths/min
- $Pao_2 > 60–70$ mm Hg on $Fio_2 < 40\%$
- $Paco_2 < 50$ mm Hg
- Negative inspiratory force < -20 cm H_2O
- Tidal volume $> 5–8$ ml/kg
- Vital capacity > 10 ml/kg
- pH > 7.25 (unless chronic COPD)
- Correction of infection, sepsis, malnutrition, electrolyte abnormalities, respiratory muscle weakness, CHF, pulmonary embolus is complete
- Tidal volume/respiratory rate ratio > 10

CHF = congestive heart failure; COPD = chronic obstructive pulmonary disease.

*These are only relative reasons for extubation. Each patient must be evaluated, taking into consideration individual pathophysiology.

      c. Rapid shallow breathing index: respiratory rate/tidal volume < 100

      d. Vital capacity > 10 ml/kg

      e. Minute ventilation < 10–15 L/min

      f. Maximal inspiratory pressure ≤ -20 cm H_2O

    9. Adequate cuff leak, indicating no laryngeal edema

    10. Intact gag reflex

C. Causes of weaning failure

    1. Inadequate respiratory center output

      a. Residual sedation

      b. CNS damage

      c. Metabolic acidosis

    2. Increased respiratory workload

      a. Increased minute ventilation [e.g., hyperventilation (anxiety, pain), increased metabolic rate (feeding, sepsis), increased dead space]

      b. Low thoracic or lung compliance

      c. Intrinsic PEEP

      d. Lower airway obstruction

      e. Copious secretions

      f. Endotracheal tube size (too small)

      g. COPD

    3. Respiratory pump failure

      a. Thoracic wall abnormality or disease (e.g., flail chest, rib fracture)

      b. Peripheral neurologic disorder

      c. Muscular dysfunction (e.g., malnutrition, pulmonary hyperinflation, electrolyte or metabolic disorder, prolonged neuromuscular blockade)

    4. LV failure or coronary artery disease

XVI. Weaning Methods

    A. T-piece weaning

Patients must be under constant supervision during the T-piece weaning process.

---

    1. Short-term (< 7 days) ventilation without COPD

      a. Obtain baseline vital signs, ABG, and saturation.

      b. Discontinue sedation, put patients in the sitting position, and provide bronchodilators and suctioning.

      c. Attach the endotracheal tube to the T-piece.

      d. After 5 minutes, resume mechanical ventilation and draw ABG.

      e. If the 5-minute ABG is acceptable, try intervals of 15 and 30 minutes.

      f. If the 30-minute ABG is acceptable, attempt an interval of 2 hours. If the ABG is acceptable, consider extubation.

      g. Some physicians allow patients to be on T-piece weaning as long as they can and extubate at 24 hours.

    2. **Long-term ventilation or COPD**
        a. Continue the method described previously (see XVI A 1) by following the period of 30 minutes with intervals of 1, 2, 4, 8, and 16 hours.
        b. Return to the shorter interval if the patient deteriorates.
        c. Consider extubation once 24 hours is reached.
        d. This wean can be progressive over several days, with the patient resting at night.

B. IMV weaning
    1. Short-term (< 7 days) ventilation and no COPD
        a. Obtain baseline vital signs and ABG.
        b. Decrease IMV rate at 30-minute intervals by 1–3 breaths/min at each step.
        c. If each step is well tolerated and ABGs are adequate, consider extubation when IMV is zero, CPAP is < 10 cm H_2O, and PEEP is $\leq$ 5 cm H_2O.
        d. Some physicians favor a minimum IMV rate of 4 breaths/min for safety; however, there is no adjustment in minute ventilation.
    2. Long-term ventilation or COPD
        a. Monitor vital signs, saturation, end-tidal carbon dioxide, and ABGs.
        b. Begin IMV at a frequency of 8 breaths/min.
            (1) If the patient tolerates the change poorly, increase the rate until the ABG stabilizes.
            (2) If the patient tolerates 8 breaths/min after 1 hour, decrease the rate to 6 breaths/min. Monitor at 30 minutes and 1 hour.
            (3) If the patient remains stable, the IMV may be repeatedly decreased in the same manner.
        c. If the patient tolerates a CPAP of 10 cm H_2O without deterioration, place on a T-piece and monitor for 4 hours before considering extubation.
        d. If the patient deteriorates, increase the IMV to the previously stable rate.

C. Pressure-support weaning
    1. Place the patient on CPAP.
    2. Increase pressure support until the patient is comfortable.
    3. Keep the respiratory rate < 30 breaths/min and the minute ventilation < 15 L/min. Set the pressure support so that the respiratory rate is approximately 25 breaths/min, the tidal volume is 5–8 ml/kg, and the patient is comfortable.
    4. Gradually decrease pressure support as tolerated (2–4 cm H_2O at a time). Make 1–2 changes per day.
    5. Weaning is complete when the pressure support is $\leq$ 5 cm H_2O and the patient is comfortable.

> **Pressure-support ventilation, which may also be used to assist in IMV weaning, helps overcome the resistance of the endotracheal tube and provides additional pressure to distend the alveoli.**

D. **Problems with weaning**
   1. **Rapid breathing.** This condition must be distinguished from anxiety due to respiratory fatigue or cardiopulmonary insufficiency.
      a. Anxiety is associated with hyperventilation where the tidal volume is increased.
      b. Muscle fatigue and cardiopulmonary disease cause rapid shallow breathing and a decrease in tidal volume.
   2. **Abdominal paradox.** Abnormal movement of the weak diaphragm into the chest under negative intrathoracic pressure creates a decreased intraabdominal pressure and an inward displacement of the abdomen with inspiration. This is a sign of labored breathing.

PNEUMONIA

See Chapter 12.

PULMONARY EMBOLISM (PE)

(See Chapter 10, DEEP VENOUS THROMBOSIS)
   I. **Pathogenesis**
      A. **Venous clot formation** secondary to hypercoagulability, venous stasis, or endothelial injury
      B. **Clot dislodgment and embolization** into the pulmonary circulation
      C. **Release of vasoactive substances** (i.e., serotonin) from activated platelets into the pulmonary circulation
         1. Increased pulmonary vascular resistance, which can lead to increased right ventricular afterload, dilation, and ultimately ischemia
         2. Bronchoconstriction
   II. **Epidemiology**
      A. **Incidence:** about 1 in 1000 per year
      B. **Mortality** (1-year): 15%
   III. **Risk Factors** (Table 19–7)
   IV. **Diagnosis** (Figure 19–3)
      A. **Clinical features** (Table 19–8)

> **If a pulmonary embolus is massive, it may cause hypotension, syncope, and/or circulatory collapse.**

B. **ECG**
   1. Sinus tachycardia

Table 19-7.   Risk Factors for Pulmonary Embolism

Associated medical disease
Congestive heart failure
Myocardial infarction
Inflammatory bowel disease
Hypertension
Malignancy
Heavy cigarette smoking
Age > 60
Pregnancy
Oral contraceptive use

Thrombophilia
Deficiency of protein C, protein S, or antithrombin III
Activated protein C resistance
Antiphospholipid antibodies
Hyperhomocysteinemia

Surgery
Malignant disease–related surgery
Hip surgery
Knee surgery

---

    2. T-wave inversion in anterior precordial leads
  C. Chest radiograph
    1. Usually normal
    2. Hampton's hump: a peripheral wedge-shaped density, abutting the pleural surface
    3. Westermark's sign: region of apparent oligemia
  D. ABG: hypoxemia or hypocarbia (nonspecific)
  E. D-dimer assay [enzyme-linked immunosorbent assay (ELISA)]
    1. High sensitivity. D-dimer levels are elevated in over 90% of patients with PE.
    2. High negative predictive value. A normal D-dimer excludes 90% of PEs.
    3. Low specificity. Recent surgery, infection, or malignancy all falsely elevate D-dimer levels.
  F. Lung scans (nuclear imaging). Normal or high likelihood results are extremely helpful, but low or intermediate likelihood scans rarely aid in decision-making (Table 19–9).
    1. Perfusion scanning. Labeled albumin microaggregates are injected into a peripheral vein and trapped in the pulmonary capillaries, reflecting pulmonary blood flow.
    2. Ventilation scanning. Inhaled radioactive aerosols are distributed to peripheral alveoli.

Mismatched defects (normal ventilation, abnormal perfusion) are most likely to be caused by PE.

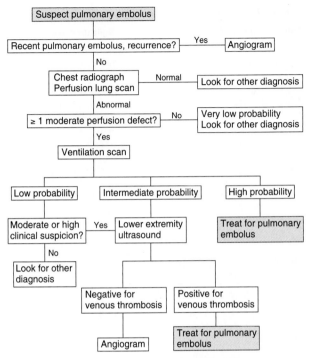

Figure 19-3. Algorithm for the diagnosis of suspected pulmonary embolism (PE).

G. **Lower extremity venous ultrasonography**
1. In patients with documented deep venous thrombosis (DVT), 50% have pulmonary emboli. Nevertheless, DVT ultrasound is noninvasive and easy to perform. The treatment of DVT and PE is usually identical.
2. Conversely, in patients with documented PE, only 30% have abnormal lower extremity ultrasonography.

H. **Spiral chest CT.** This procedure is useful for proximal (i.e., major) pulmonary emboli.
1. It misses small, distal pulmonary emboli that may herald larger, proximal emboli.
2. It may be useful in the exclusion of other diagnoses.

> **If the clinical suspicion for PE is high,
> a chest CT should not be pursued.**

I. **Transthoracic echocardiography (TTE)**

Table 19-8. Clinical Features of Pulmonary Embolism

Symptoms (frequency)	Signs (frequency)
Dyspnea (80%)	Tachypnea (88%)
Apprehension (60%)	Tachycardia (63%)
Pleurisy (60%)	Increased P_2 (60%)
Cough (50%)	Rales (51%)
Hemoptysis (27%)	S_3 or S_4 (47%)
Syncope (22%)	Pleural rub (17%)
Chest pain	Fever
Right-sided heart failure	Wheeze
Hypotension	Jugular venous distention
Arrhythmias	Decreased breath sounds
	Cyanosis
	Splinting
	Mental status change
	Shock

Table 19-9. Probability of Pulmonary Embolism (PE) Using Clinical Suspicion and Ventilation–Perfusion (V-Q) Scans

Clinical Suspicion	Liklihood (V-Q scan)	Probability of PE (%)
High	High	96
Moderate	High	80
Low	High	50
Low	Low	5

1. **Lack of sensitivity.** TTE is abnormal in 40% of patients with PE.
2. **High specificity.** Right ventricular hypokinesis (of the free wall) with normal apical wall motion is diagnostic of PE.
3. **Use.** TTE can be used to **exclude other diagnoses** [e.g., acute myocardial infarction (MI), valvular dysfunction].
J. **Pulmonary angiography.** The gold standard for the diagnosis of PE, this procedure is virtually 100% sensitive and specific.

V. **Grading System** (Table 19–10)
VI. **Treatment**
   A. **Heparin** (IV, unfractionated). Give a bolus of 5000 U (or 80 U/kg) and follow it with a continuous infusion of 1000 U/hr (or 18 U/kg/hr).
      1. **Goal:** maintenance of an activated PTT (aPTT) of 60–80 seconds. Check the aPTT about 6 hours after initiation of therapy and at least daily thereafter. The infusion rate should be adjusted to achieve this goal.

Table 19-10.   Grading System for a Pulmonary Embolism

Grade	PA Distribution (%)	Pao₂ (mm Hg)	Paco₂ (mm Hg)	Response
Minor	20–30	< 80	< 35	Tachycardia
Major	30–50	< 65	< 30	pPA > 20 mm Hg
Massive	> 50	< 50	< 30	pPA > 25 mm Hg
Chronic	> 50	< 70	30–40	pPA > 40 mm Hg

PA = pulmonary artery; pPA = pressure in the pulmonary artery.

2. **Duration of therapy:** discontinuation once oral (or subcutaneous) therapeutic anticoagulation has been achieved
B. **Warfarin.** This agent can be started within 24 hours of initiating heparin therapy.
   1. **Goal:** INR of 2.0–3.0
   2. **Duration of therapy:** 3–6 months
      a. 3 months: patients with an identifiable and reversible risk factor
      b. 6 months: patients without an identifiable or reversible risk factor
C. **Low–molecular-weight heparins**
   1. Randomized, prospective trials have demonstrated that low–molecular-weight heparin is as efficacious as unfractionated heparin in the treatment of DVT and more efficacious in prevention of recurrence.
   2. Low–molecular-weight heparins do not require laboratory monitoring.
D. **Thrombolysis** [tissue plasminogen activator (tPA) or urokinase]
   1. This procedure is **strongly indicated** for patients with a PE and hemodynamic instability secondary to cardiogenic shock.
   2. This procedure is **relatively indicated** for patients with a hemodynamically stable PE and severe cardiac or pulmonary disease.
E. **Pulmonary embolectomy**
   1. Pulmonary embolectomy is **indicated** for patients with PE and hemodynamic instability for whom thrombolysis is either contraindicated or has failed. Unfortunately, most patients who would benefit from embolectomy die before reaching the operating room.
   2. The embolus may be surgically excised via median sternotomy (open) or fragmented with a transvenous catheter.
   3. Pulmonary embolectomy has proved beneficial in patients with pulmonary hypertension secondary to chronic, large-vessel emboli.

20

Radiology in the ICU

I. **Interpretation of Radiographs in the ICU**
A. Know the patient (i.e., know what you are looking for).
B. Understand the limitations of the study ordered. Discuss the appropriateness of a study with a radiologist if you are not sure.
C. Develop a systematic approach (i.e., look at all structures in a deliberate order).
D. Examine all of the information on the films provided, including patient identification, image quality, and technical limitations (e.g., over- or underexposure, processing artifacts).
E. Pay attention to edges, boundaries, superimposition or summation of shadows, and patient position.
F. Do not stop if you see an obvious finding; complete your systematic process of observation.
G. Know your own limitations. Seek help when needed, especially in clinically suspicious situations.

II. **Chest Radiographs in the ICU**
A. **Systematic evaluation.** When evaluating chest films, check the following:
1. Film **quality** and **technique**
2. **Film type** [upright, supine, decubitus, posteroanterior (PA) or anteroposterior (AP), inspiration or expiration, straight or rotated]
3. **Patient positioning** (judge from the centering of the medial ends of the clavicles over the spine)
4. **Lung fields** [lung markings (just vessels in a normal patient), overall aeration, vascularity, infiltrates, masses, interstitial markings, left versus right symmetry (i.e., midline shift)]
5. **Hila** (masses, adenopathy, dilation of pulmonary vessels, retraction, displacement, calcifications)
6. **Heart** (size, position, chamber prominence, calcifications)

7. **Aorta** (narrow mediastinum, distinct aortic knob)
8. **Mediastinum** (masses, shift, widening, pneumomediastinum, calcifications)
9. **Tracheobronchial tree** (tracheal air shadow, position, patency, masses, extrinsic or intrinsic compression)
10. **Hemidiaphragms** and structures below the hemidiaphragms (gastric air bubble, bowel gas)
11. **Pleura** (effusions, pneumonia, thickening, masses, calcifications)
12. **Bony framework** (includes all visible ribs and areas of the spine, clavicles, scapulae, and humeri)
    a. The technique for a chest radiograph is designed to study the lungs, not the bones, and a conscious effort is made to remove the bones from the lung fields.
    b. Flipping the film on its side or upside down makes the skeletal structures stand out more.
    c. Look for masses, rib expansion or destruction, fractures, rib notching, and calcifications.
13. **Soft tissues** (e.g., breast tissue)
    a. These tissues are a common source of artifacts and superimposed shadows.
    b. Asymmetry or absence of these tissues may be a clue to other findings.
    c. Look for masses and calcifications.
14. The **film as a whole**

B. **Evaluation of masses and densities**
   1. **Localization** is best accomplished by viewing the abnormality in more than one view.
      a. In the ICU patient, it is almost impossible to get a regular lateral view.
      b. If necessary, oblique or "shoot-through" lateral views may be attempted.
   2. The following information can be used to localize the site of an abnormality.
      a. **Silhouette sign**
         (1) When there is a density (e.g., mass, fluid, collapse, consolidation) adjacent to another structure, it obliterates the margins of that structure (e.g., hemidiaphragms, heart borders).
         (2) Thus, anterior consolidation (i.e., consolidation of the right middle lobe and left lingula) obliterates the right and left margins of the heart, respectively.
         (3) An effusion adjacent to the diaphragm will hide the diaphragm.
      b. **Ov erlay sign**
         (1) Masses that over- or underlay structures allow the structures to be visualized through them (i.e., the counterpart of the silhouette sign).
         (2) Thus, the hilar structures are visualized through a mass that may be anterior or posterior to the

hilum rather than involving the hilum itself (i.e., hilum overlay sign).

3. **Pleural versus parenchymal masses**
   a. Usually, a pleural mass has obtuse margins with the chest wall, and a parenchymal mass has acute margins.
   b. A pleural mass generally has a different size, shape, and configuration on a lateral film versus a PA film.
4. **Adjacent structures** may show changes (e.g., chest wall or rib destruction, tracheal deviation).
5. **Alveolar versus interstitial disease** (Figure 20-1)

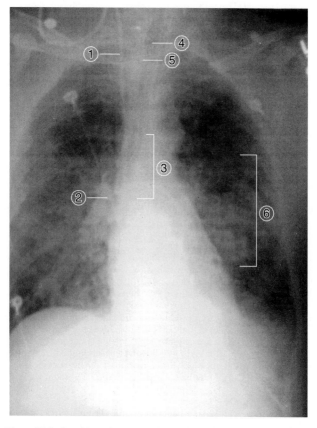

Figure 20-1. Portable supine anteroposterior chest radiograph. *1* = Swan-Ganz catheter; *2* = tip of Swan-Ganz catheter; *3* = nasogastric tube; *4* = endotracheal tube; *5* = external portion of the nasogastric tube; *6* = pulmonary edema.

   a. Air bronchograms showing air in the bronchial structures with surrounding densities in the alveoli are hallmarks of alveolar disease.
   b. Lacy, linear, or granular patterns point toward interstitial disease.
   c. This differentiation is not always possible; it depends on the severity of disease. These processes can mimic each other and are often concomitant (i.e., pulmonary edema is often both interstitial and alveolar).
C. Placement of lines and tubes (Figure 20-2)
   1. Endotracheal tube

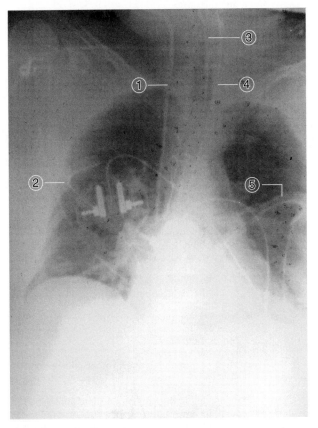

Figure 20-2. Evaluation of lines and tubes on a portable anteroposterior chest radiograph. *1* = Swan-Ganz catheter; *2* = chest tube; *3* = endotracheal tube; *4* = nasogastric tube; *5* = chest tube.

    a. The ideal position for an endotracheal tube in an adult, with the head in neutral position, is the middle of the trachea, approximately 5 cm from the carina.

    b. Flexion and extension of the neck may cause the tube to move approximately 2 cm downward and upward, respectively.

    c. Rotation of the head may cause the tube to move approximately 1 cm downward or upward.

2. Tracheostomy tube

    a. The tip of the tube should be at approximately the level of the third thoracic vertebra (i.e., one half to two thirds the distance between the tracheal stoma and the carina).

    b. The lumen of the tracheostomy tube should occupy two thirds of the tracheal diameter. The cuff should fit, not distend, the trachea.

    c. A posttracheostomy chest radiograph should be obtained to check position and to check for pneumomediastinum and pneumothorax. Subsequent films should be obtained only to resolve specific clinical queries.

3. Thoracostomy tube

    a. The ideal position depends on the reason for the tube and the sight of pathology. For example, closed thoracostomy tubes are placed for hydrothorax, pneumothorax, pyothorax, and hemothorax and should be positioned accordingly.

    b. A chest radiograph should be obtained after placement and manipulation but is not required routinely. If the tube fails to work satisfactorily after reposition and manipulation of the tube, another view (e.g., oblique, "crosstable" lateral, or "shoot-through" lateral) should be considered.

4. Central venous lines and peripherally inserted central lines

    a. The ideal position for these central catheters is between the right atrium and the jugular–subclavian vein confluence with the brachiocephalic vein.

    b. Postplacement chest radiographs are essential. Subsequent films should be obtained only to resolve specific questions.

5. Pulmonary artery catheters

    a. The ideal position for the tip of the pulmonary artery catheter is 5–6 cm distal to the bifurcation of the main pulmonary artery.

    b. On deflation, the catheter tip should not be left beyond the level of the proximal interlobar pulmonary artery to reduce the risk of complication (e.g., infarction, pulmonary artery rupture).

6. Intra-aortic balloon pumps. The extent of the balloon should be between the origins of the great vessels of the head, neck, and upper extremities and the vessels to the abdominal organs (i.e., in the descending aorta between the arch and the diaphragm).

7. **Transvenous pacers and defibrillators.** There are many possible combinations of leads and patches. Each type requires specific information to check appropriate radiographic positioning.

8. **Nasogastric tubes.** The most distal side hole should be within the stomach (i.e., below the diaphragm).

D. **Common radiographic evaluations in the ICU**

1. **Barotrauma** (Figure 20-3) is a significant complication in patients on mechanical ventilation. It is common in patients with ARDS and those on positive end-expiratory pressure ventilation. Common radiographic findings after chest trauma or barotrauma include pulmonary interstitial emphysema (PIE), pneumothorax, pneumomediastinum, pneumopericardium, and pneumoperitoneum.

a. **PIE** is caused by rupture of alveoli adjacent to the interlobular septa into the interstitium. The air dissects along the vascular sheaths to the hilum, leading to pneumomediastinum. PIE is a precursor to pneumothorax. Radiographic findings include:

(1) Increased mottled radiolucency

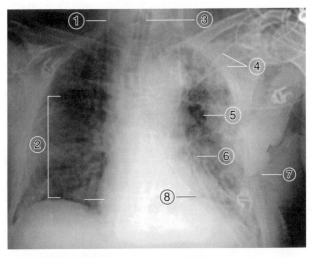

Figure 20-3. Portable supine anteroposterior chest radiograph. *1* = internal jugular central venous line; *2* = ARDS; *3* = nasogastric tube; *4* = ECG/ monitor leads; *5* = pulmonary interstitial emphysema; *6* = chest tube; *7* = staples; *8* = ECG lead.

(2) Nonbranching, disorganized, streaky lucencies radiating from the hila to the periphery

(3) Subpleural air cysts

b. Pneumothorax is obvious when it is large and in the usual location (i.e., apical). However, it may be in an unusual location (e.g., anteromedial, posteromedial, apicolateral, subpulmonic), especially if the patient is very sick and the films are AP and supine with limited technique.

(1) The size of a pneumothorax can be deceptive and is best compared with prior images to look for increase or resolution.

(2) When evaluating for a pneumothorax, look for supportive signs, including:

(a) Pneumomediastinum

(b) Pneumopericardium

(c) Subcutaneous emphysema

(d) Rib fractures

(e) Hydropneumothorax (i.e., air–fluid levels in the pleura)

(3) **Subpulmonic pneumothorax** may present with the deep sulcus sign [i.e., the costophrenic angle on the involved side is lucent (darker) and very deep].

(4) Always assess for signs of **tension pneumothorax,** which may have grave consequences. When pressure in pleural space exceeds atmospheric pressure, "tension" in adjacent structures results. Radiographic signs include:

(a) Shift of the mediastinum

(b) Flattening of the heart border

(c) Flattening of the superior and inferior vena cava

(d) Inversion of the diaphragm

c. In cases of barotrauma, pneumomediastinum, pneumopericardium, and pneumoperitoneum may also be seen radiographically.

2. The etiology of **ARDS** (see Figure 20-3) is considered to be injury to the alveolar epithelium, leading to passage of proteinaceous fluid into the alveolar space at normal hydrostatic pressures. Radiographic diagnosis is often complicated by concomitant pneumonia, pulmonary edema, and barotrauma. Radiographic findings include:

a. Nonuniform, patchy areas of consolidation that are usually bilateral

b. Air bronchograms

c. Small bilateral or unilateral pleural effusions

E. Portable chest radiographs

1. The portable ("bedside") chest radiograph continues to be the most commonly used radiologic study despite the increasing use of portable ultrasound and regular CT scans. Portable chest radiographs are always obtained in an AP manner.

2. Portable chest radiographs are used for evaluation of:
    a. Clinically unstable patients with cardiorespiratory symptoms
    b. Postoperative cardiac or thoracic surgery patients
    c. Trauma and its sequelae
    d. Patients with monitoring or life-support devices
    e. Patients with a clinical condition that does not permit safe transport to the radiology department

3. Portable chest radiographs do have limitations.
    a. The digital technique commonly uses an edge-enhancing algorithm, making the blood vessels slightly more obvious, which gives the appearance of slight pulmonary vascular congestion as compared to regularly obtained radiographs.
    b. Usually only a single supine view can be obtained; therefore, more vigilance is required for location of findings.
    c. The patient is often rotated and not well centered.
    d. Portable units often do not provide enough power, leading to underexposed films.
    e. Most patients are not able to hold their breath.
    f. There are more external artifacts to read through.
    g. On an AP radiograph, the heart appears larger than it does on a standard PA radiograph. Although this may limit evaluation of heart size, it provides useful comparative information in patients followed with serial films.

III. **Abdominal Radiographs in the ICU.** When evaluating abdominal radiographs in the ICU, check the following in a **systematic** manner (Figure 20-4):

A. Film **quality** and **technique**

B. Film **type** (e.g., supine, decubitus, upright, lateral)

C. **Gas patterns** (i.e., displacement and distention)
    1. The stomach and colon normally contain gas, and gas in the small bowel in the absence of dilation also may be normal.
    2. To differentiate between **ileus and obstruction,** obtain upright and decubitus views in addition to a supine view.
        a. In **paralytic ileus,** diffuse distention of the small and large bowel by gas and fluid is seen with air–fluid levels in upright and decubitus films. Involvement of the small versus large bowel may be asymmetrical. Ileus may be limited to a portion of the GI tract (i.e., colonic ileus) or it may be focal (i.e., sentinel loop).
        b. In cases of **mechanical obstruction,** the obstruction may be at any level of the small or large bowel.
            (1) Proximal to the obstruction, the bowel will be distended with air–fluid levels classically in a stepladder fashion. Occasionally, the bowel prox-

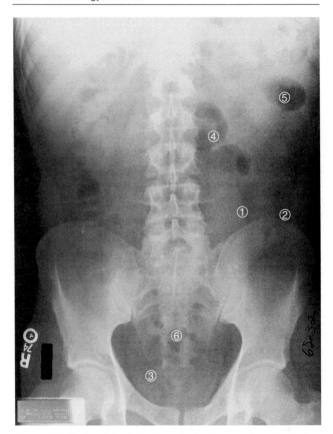

Figure 20-4. Supine abdominal radiograph. *1* = iliopsoas stripe; *2* = flank stripe; *3* = urinary bladder silhouette (full urinary bladder); *4* = air in small bowel; *5* = air in colon (hepatic flexure); *6* = air in colon (rectosigmoid).

imal to the obstruction will be completely filled with fluid.

(2) Distal to the obstruction, the bowel will be decompressed. However, the picture can be complicated by partial or intermittent obstruction, which will allow gas and fluid to escape distal to the obstruction.

(3) An enema or rectal examination just before the radiographs are taken may result in air–fluid levels in the colon.

3. A **sentinel loop** is a focal area of paralysis and dilation sec-

ondary to a localized process (e.g., pancreatitis, cholecystitis, closed-loop obstruction, abscess, appendicitis).

D. Liver, spleen, and **kidneys** (position, size)

E. Pelvis (urinary bladder, rectal air, pelvic fat)

F. Fat and muscle planes (psoas margins, flank stripes)
   1. Normally, the flank stripes are radiolucent.
   2. The psoas margins and flank stripes may be obliterated by an adjacent mass or fluid collection (e.g., appendiceal abscess, retroperitoneal hematoma).

G. Bones: lower ribs, spine, pelvis, and **femoral heads** (fractures, lytic and sclerotic lesions, congenital anomalies)

H. Extraabdominal soft tissues (i.e., subcutaneous, gluteal, and inguinal soft tissues)

I. Lung bases and **diaphragm**

J. Air in abnormal locations
   1. Free air may be seen under the hemidiaphragms on an upright film or over the free edge of the liver on the right-side-up decubitus film. However, because both of these views may not be possible in the ICU patient, more reliance has to be put on the supine view.

Free air may be innocuous if the patient is on peritoneal dialysis or has had recent surgery.

---

   2. Any abnormal air collection in the right upper quadrant requires a more focused or coned-down view of this area. If there is any doubt, a CT scan should be obtained.
   3. Additional abnormal findings include biliary air, portal venous air, air within the bowel wall (pneumotosis), and air that is outside of the bowel but contained (e.g., in an abscess).

K. Fluid in abnormal locations (i.e., ascites)
   1. Small amounts of fluid may accumulate in dependent areas. This can be normal, especially in females.
   2. The amount of ascites required to give the "ground-glass" appearance should be clinically evident. However, the "ground-glass" appearance also may be seen in healthy patients resulting from various factors (e.g., obesity, underpenetration or underexposure of film).
   3. Ascites in the pelvis layers posteriorly on a supine film and appears as a mass superior to the bladder.
      a. In the pelvis, 200–300 ml of fluid may be detectable.
      b. As the volume increases beyond 500 ml, the fluid tracks superolaterally, giving the "dog-eared" appearance.
      c. The colon is displaced anteromedially from the gutters, the margins of the spleen and liver are lost, and bowel loops may float to the center of the abdomen.

L. Abnormal calcifications
   1. Significant findings include biliary, urinary, renal, pancreatic, appendiceal, arterial, and aneurysmal calcifications.

2. Insignificant findings include costal cartilage, phleboliths, atherosclerosis, granulomas in the liver and spleen, mesenteric nodes, uterine fibroids, and injection granulomas.

IV. Computed Tomography in the ICU

A. CT is currently the imaging modality of choice after routine radiographs for evaluating complex fractures and many intrathoracic, intraabdominal, and intracranial diseases.

B. Optimal use of the CT scanner requires knowledge of anatomy and pathophysiology and familiarity with CT techniques.

C. Indications for the use of CT include:

1. Evaluation of abnormalities seen on radiographs
2. Evaluation of patients with clinically suspected occult pathology
3. Staging of malignancies
4. Evaluation of suspected intracranial bleed, infarct, and mass effect
5. CT-guided biopsies and drainage procedures
6. Evaluation of suspected vascular abnormalities (e.g., aneurysms, dissections, leaks, ruptures)
7. Evaluation of trauma and its sequelae
8. Evaluation of septic patients and patients with fever of unknown origin
9. Postsurgical follow up and evaluation

D. There are no absolute contraindications to CT. As with all procedures, the relative benefits and risks of the procedure should be evaluated and appropriate precautions should be taken to minimize patient risk.

V. Ultrasonography in the ICU

A. Ultrasonography is perhaps the most versatile and underutilized tool in imaging of the ICU patient. Its primary advantage is easy bedside availability of multiaxial cross-sectional imaging.

B. Indications for the use of ultrasonography include:

1. Evaluation of suspected vascular abnormalities (e.g., thrombosis, dissections, stenosis, leaks, pseudoaneurysms, fistulas)
2. Evaluation of transplanted organs
3. Evaluation of organ-specific pathology, especially in the abdomen
4. Ultrasound-guided biopsies and drainage procedures

VI. Interventional Radiology.
Interventional radiologic procedures are increasingly being performed on ICU patients. These procedures include:

A. Venous access and central line placement (e.g., peripherally inserted central catheter, transhepatic and translumbar inferior vena cava central lines)

B. Swan-Ganz catheter placement

C. Percutaneous needle aspiration and drainage (e.g., abscess, cholecystostomy)

D. Percutaneous arterial embolization for bleeding
E. Transjugular intrahepatic portosystemic shunting
F. Inferior vena cava filter placement
G. Thrombolysis
H. Visualization studies (e.g., percutaneous cholangiogram, venogram)
I. Arteriography

Renal Disorders

ACUTE RENAL FAILURE

I. Definitions

A. Acute renal failure (ARF) is a functional disorder in which there is an acute loss of renal function over a period of hours to weeks. Commonly used clinical definitions include:

1. An increase in serum creatinine (SCr) of ≥ 0.5 mg/dl over baseline if the baseline level is ≤ 2.0 mg/dl
2. An increase in SCr of ≥ 1.0 mg/dl over baseline if the baseline level is > 2.0 mg/dl
3. A 50% decrease in the calculated creatinine clearance (Ccr)

B. Oliguria is arbitrarily defined as a urine output of < 400 ml/24 hr.

C. Anuria occurs when urine output is < 50 ml/24 hr. Acute anuria suggests a postrenal etiology.

II. Etiology

A. Hospital- versus community-acquired ARF

1. ARF is hospital acquired if the patient had normal SCr on admission. Iatrogenic causes of hospital-acquired ARF include:

   a. Nephrotoxic drugs
   b. Invasive procedures or operations
   c. Radiocontrast dye
   d. Inadequate fluid management
   e. Malfunctioning Foley catheter

2. ARF is community acquired if the patient had established renal failure on admission.

B. Posttransplant ARF

1. The effects of volume depletion are amplified by the vasoconstrictive effect of cyclosporine and tacrolimus (FK-506).

2. Obstruction of the transplant ureter should always be considered as a cause of ARF, as a result of either techni-

cal problems or extrinsic compression (e.g., lymphocele, urinoma).

3. Thrombosis of the main renal artery and vein can result in ARF.

4. Acute rejection should always be considered as a cause of ARF.

C. **Pathophysiologic approach to etiology**

1. **Prerenal azotemia** is precipitated by decreased renal perfusion (i.e., impaired renal plasma flow) [Table 21-1].

2. **Intrinsic renal failure** is a loss of renal function caused by

Table 21-1. Causes of Prerenal Azotemia

Volume depletion or redistribution
Active blood loss
Decreased intake or inadequate fluid replacement
Excessive diuresis or renal salt wasting
Gastrointestinal losses (vomiting, diarrhea)
Hypovolemia
Skin losses (burns, extensive exudative rashes)
Third spacing (peritonitis, pancreatitis, intestinal obstruction, extensive tissue trauma, massive ascites)

Hypoalbuminemia
Malnutrition
Chronic liver disease, cirrhosis
Nephrotic syndrome

Inappropriate peripheral vasodilatation
Chronic liver disease
Hepatorenal syndrome
Sepsis syndrome
Interleukin-2 therapy

Impaired renal perfusion from:
Vascular etiology
Renovascular disease (renal artery stenosis)
Renal vein thrombosis
Aortic disease or dissection involving the renal arteries
Abnormal autoregulation or vasoconstriction
Excessive blood pressure reduction with any drug
Nonsteroidal anti-inflammatory drugs
Angiotensin-converting enzyme inhibitors
Cyclosporine
Tacrolimus (FK-506)
Epinephrine, norepinephrine, phenylephrine, high-dose dopamine
Cardiac dysfunction

disease of intrarenal structures (e.g., microvasculature, glomeruli, tubules, interstitium) [Table 21-2].

3. **Postrenal failure** is due to obstruction of urinary flow at any point along the urinary tree. Possible causes include:
   a. Obstruction of the collecting system by stones, blood clots, sloughed papillae, cancer, or crystals
   b. Extrinsic compression due to inadvertent operative ligation, masses, or retroperitoneal fibrosis
   c. Bladder outlet obstruction due to prostatic hypertrophy, cancer of the prostate or cervix, or an obstructed urinary catheter
   d. Congenital or acquired malformations (e.g., neurogenic bladder)

Table 21-2. Causes of Intrinsic Renal Failure

Vascular disease
  Malignant hypertension
  Vasculitis
  Hemolytic uremic syndrome
  Thrombotic thrombocytopenic purpura
  Eclampsia and preeclampsia
  Atheroembolic renal disease
Glomerular disease
  Systemic lupus erythematosus
  Goodpasture's syndrome
  Cryoglobulinemia
  Vasculitides (Wegener's granulomatosis, polyarteritis nodosa, Henoch-Schönlein purpura)
  Postinfectious glomerulonephritis
Tubular disease
  Interstitial nephritis
    Drug-induced (β-lactam antibiotics, sulfa drugs, nonsteroidal anti-inflammatory drugs, cimetidine, allopurinol, phenytoin)
    Infiltrative (leukemias, lymphomas, sarcoidosis)
    Infectious (staphylococcal bacteremia, pyelonephritis, leptospirosis)
  Acute tubular necrosis
    Renal ischemia
    Nephrotoxic drugs (aminoglycosides, amphotericin B, iodinated contrast dye)
    Nephrotoxic pigments (myoglobinuria, hemoglobinuria)
  Cast nephropathy (myeloma), light-chain nephropathy
  Hypercalcemia, nephrocalcinosis
  Crystal nephropathies (urate, oxalate, sulfadiazine, acyclovir, indinavir, methotrexate)

III. **History**

    A. Determine the presence or absence of symptoms associated with the following disorders:

        1. Volume depletion (vomiting, diarrhea, excessive urine output, thirst, exposure to excessively hot temperatures, orthostatic dizziness, weight loss)

        2. Urinary obstruction (hesitancy, frequency, urgency, nocturia, decreased stream force, history of stones or renal colic)

        3. Heart failure (edema, dyspnea, orthopnea, paroxysmal nocturnal dyspnea)

        4. Uremia (decreased level of energy, anorexia, nausea and vomiting, abdominal pain, metallic taste, abnormal sleep patterns, difficulty with mental activities, pruritus, leg cramping, restless legs)

    B. Take a detailed medication history, including prescription and over-the-counter medications.

    C. Obtain the patient's past medical and surgical history.

IV. **Physical Examination**

    A. Evaluate volume status.

        1. Volume depletion is indicated by low blood pressure, increased pulse rate, absent jugular pulses in the supine position, poor skin turgor, and decreased axillary and mucous membrane moisture.

        2. Volume overload is indicated by elevated jugular venous pressure, S_3, crackles, ascites, and edema.

    B. Examine the abdomen for bladder distention, masses, or ascites.

    C. Perform a rectal examination to evaluate the prostate.

    D. Review charts of weights, intakes, and outputs.

> **Daily weights are the most accurate measure of fluid balance.**

    E. Evaluate urine output and the trend over time. Flush the Foley catheter to clear clots or mucus that may alter urine output.

V. **Diagnostic Tests**

    A. **Laboratory tests**

        1. Obtain relevant blood work, including BUN/creatinine, electrolytes, calcium, phosphate, glucose, liver enzymes, uric acid, and creatine phosphokinase (to rule out rhabdomyolysis). Some factors increase serum BUN and SCr without affecting glomerular filtration rate (GFR) [Table 21-3].

        2. Obtain an ABG and CBC with differential.

        3. Obtain a urinalysis (Table 21-4) to evaluate concentrating ability, presence or absence of proteinuria, and signs of an "active" sediment (i.e., WBCs, RBCs, casts).

        4. For suspicion of glomerulonephritis, obtain specific serologic tests, including:

Table 21-3. Factors that Increase BUN and Creatinine Without Reducing Renal Function

Increased BUN
  Increased urea production or GI absorption caused by:
    Hypercatabolic states
    Increased protein intake or parenteral nutrition
    Upper GI bleeding
    Corticosteroids
    Outdated tetracycline
  Increased urinary tract absorption caused by:
    Volume depletion*
    Heart failure*
    Obstructive uropathy*

Increased creatinine
  Increased release from muscle caused by:
    Rhabdomyolysis
  Decreased tubular secretion caused by:
    Cimetidine
    Trimethoprim
  Altered laboratory assay caused by interference with:
    Ketones
    Cephalosporins (especially cefoxitin)

---

*These factors only increase BUN and creatinine without reducing renal function when mild and adaptive mechanisms maintain the glomerular filtration rate.

      a. Antinuclear antibodies
      b. Complements
      c. Antineutrophil cytoplasm antibodies
      d. Antiglomerular basement membrane antibodies
      e. Hepatitis B and C serologies
      f. Cryoglobulins
      g. Serum and urine protein electrophoresis
      h. Antistreptolysin O titers
  B. Urinary indices (Table 21-5)
    1. Urinary indices are evaluated in the presence of oliguric ARF; extrapolation to nonoliguric ARF may not result in similar test accuracy.
    2. The fractional excretion of sodium (FE_{Na}) is the most useful urinary index. To obtain an accurate FE_{Na}, urine should be obtained before the administration of diuretics or mannitol and before volume resuscitation.
    3. Urinary sodium (U_{Na}) excretion is decreased in states of decreased renal perfusion, suggesting prerenal azotemia, although this can be deceiving when baseline renal perfusion is impaired (e.g., severe liver disease). In these cases,

Table 21-4. Urinalysis Findings in Acute Renal Failure

	Disease State	**Findings**
Dipstick	Prerenal azotemia	High specific gravity (> 1.020) Absent proteinuria
	Intrinsic renal disease	Specific gravity approximately 1.010 (isosthenuria)
	Rhabdomyolysis	Positive hemoglobin
Sediment	Prerenal azotemia	Bland sediment or hyaline casts
	Obstruction	Frequent RBCs, WBCs, and crystals
	Glomerulonephritis	Dysmorphic RBCs, RBC casts, WBCs
	Acute tubular necrosis	Epithelial cells; coarse, granular ("muddy-brown") casts
	Interstitial nephritis	RBCs, WBCs, WBC casts, eosinophils
	Atheroembolic disease	Eosinophils
	Rhabdomyolysis	No RBCs, heme-positive on urine dipstick due to myoglobin

low U_{Na} (< 10 mEq/L) and low FE_{Na} ($< 1\%$) can be seen even in the presence of acute tubular necrosis (ATN).

4. High U_{Na} (> 40 mEq/L) and high FE_{Na} ($> 3\%$) are suggestive of intrinsic ARF (typically ATN). Likewise, prerenal azotemia results in a preserved ability to concentrate urine (i.e., high osmolality) and reabsorb urea [i.e., low fractional excretion of urea (FE_{urea})]. These tubular functions are lost in intrinsic ARF.

5. In patients who received diuretics in the preceding 24–48 hours, the use of FE_{urea} is helpful because diuretics do not directly affect the result.

C. Imaging techniques

1. Renal ultrasound is used to evaluate renal size and parenchymal echotexture and to identify signs of obstruction. Small kidney size, cortical thinning, and increased parenchymal echogenicity suggest a longer duration of renal disease.

2. Doppler interrogation of the renal vessels is used to assess vascular supply.

3. CT scan and MRI are used to evaluate the possibility of a mass.

4. Renal radionuclide scans are useful for evaluating renal perfusion.

5. In selected cases, renal angiography and uroradiologic procedures are better tests for anatomic detail and therapeutic interventions.

Table 21-5. Laboratory Values for the Different Classes of Renal Failure

	Prerenal	Renal (ATN)
BUN	↑	↑
Serum creatinine	Normal	↑
BUN/serum creatinine	> 20:1	< 20:1
Urine specific gravity	> 1.020	~ 1.010
Urine$_{Na}$ (mEq/L)	< 20	> 40‡
Urine$_{Osm}$ (mOsm/kg)	> 500	< 350*
Urine/serum urea (normal = 50)	> 8	< 3
Urine/serum creatinine	> 40	< 20
Urine/serum$_{Osm}$	> 1.2	< 1.2
RFI	< 1	> 1
FE$_{Na}$	< 1†	> 1*
FE$_{Urea}$	0.2–0.3	0.4–0.7

ATN = acute tubular necrosis; BUN = blood urea nitrogen; FE$_{Na}$ = fractional excretion of sodium; FE$_{Urea}$ = fractional excretion of urea; RFI = renal failure index; urine$_{Na}$ = urinary sodium; urine$_{Osm}$ = urine osmolality.
*FE$_{Na}$ is < 1 and the urine$_{Osm}$ is > 500 in glomerulonephritis unless it is associated with tubulointerstitial abnormalities.
†A FE$_{Na}$ < 1 is often nondiagnostic in the elderly and in patients receiving diuretics or who have preexisting renal disease.
‡A urine$_{Na}$ > 40 mEq/L can occur in prerenal conditions in patients with prior renal dysfunction or with ongoing diuretic therapy.

   D. Renal biopsy is useful when the cause of ARF is not clear (e.g., suspected glomerular disease or allograft rejection).
   1. Histologic and immunofluorescence analyses are used to rule out posttransplant rejection, glomerulonephritis, and ATN.
   2. Risk of complications with ultrasound-guided biopsy is < 1%.
VI. Management
   A. General management of established ARF
   1. In all cases of ARF, **identify and correct the inciting factors.**
   2. There is no specific therapy for patients with established ARF; therefore, **supportive therapy** is the key.
      a. Medical therapy
         (1) Avoid nephrotoxins [e.g., radiocontrast agents, aminoglycosides, nonsteroidal anti-inflammatory drugs (NSAIDs), angiotensin-converting enzyme inhibitors, general anesthetics].
         (2) Adjust doses of all medications that are renally excreted.
      b. Dialysis
         (1) **Indications for dialysis**

   (a) Symptomatic uremia (encephalopathy, hemorrhage, pericarditis)
   (b) Volume overload without response to diuretics
   (c) Severe hyperkalemia
   (d) Refractory acidosis
(2) Dialysis modalities (Table 21-6)
(3) General considerations in dialysis
   (a) Hemodynamically unstable patients typically require a continuous technique [continuous venovenous hemodialysis (CVVHD) or automated peritoneal dialysis (APD)].
   (b) Patients in the ICU often have enormous obligatory fluid inputs (e.g., vasopressor drips, parenteral nutrition, sedation drips, antibiotic infusions) that limit the ability of intermittent hemodialysis (IHD) to control volume. In such cases, a continuous modality is helpful and may be the only viable option.
   (c) Hypercatabolic patients often need a continuous technique to match their nitrogen balance and avoid uremia. CVVHD is the only technique that allows adequate solute control in such patients. Solute removal is two- to fivefold higher in CVVHD as compared to standard IHD prescriptions.
 c. Nutritional support

Table 21-6. Dialysis Modalities in Acute Renal Failure

Modality	Advantages	Disadvantages
IHD	Easily performed, good solute control	Central venous access, hemodynamic instability, anticoagulation*
CVVHD	Excellent solute control, precise volume management, hemodynamic stability, possible role in cytokine removal	Central venous access, requires prolonged anticoagulation*, labor intensive, expensive
APD	Technically simple, hemodynamic stability, good solute and volume control, no anticoagulation	Requires intact peritoneum, less precise than CVVHD

APD = automated peritoneal dialysis; CVVHD = continuous venovenous hemodialysis; IHD = intermittent hemodialysis.
*Many patients can be dialyzed with minimal or no anticoagulation.

(1) ARF is a hypercatabolic state, which is further amplified by concomitant organ failure.
  (a) Protein catabolic rates average 1.4–1.8 g protein/kg/day.
  (b) Start aggressive nutritional support by providing 35–50 kcal/kg/day to avoid catabolism.

(2) Protein restriction is not indicated in ARF. It is used only in long-term management of chronic renal insufficiency.

(3) Adjust electrolyte components of enteral and parenteral nutrition and fluids.

(4) Phosphate often needs to be restricted. If the patient is hyperphosphatemic (i.e., phosphate > 5 mg/dl), administer oral phosphate binder with each meal or around-the-clock if the patient is on continuous enteral feeding. Options include:
  (a) Calcium carbonate, 500–1500 mg
  (b) Calcium acetate, 667–2001 mg
  (c) Aluminum hydroxide, 600–1800 mg
  (d) Sucralfate, 1–2 g

B. Management of acute complications of ARF

  1. Volume overload

  a. Patients who are oliguric or anuric and not hypovolemic should receive a diuretic and/or dopamine. It is best to convert oliguric renal failure to nonoliguric renal failure because volume overload is prevented in a patient who is euvolemic and responds to diuretics (i.e., becomes nonoliguric).

  (1) Furosemide (1–3 mg/kg IV q 6–8 hr) is most often used in the treatment of volume overload.
    (a) High doses of furosemide are often needed in the treatment of volume overload associated with ARF.
    (b) In patients requiring > 500 mg/day, an IV drip (0.5–1.0 mg/kg/hr) is preferred.

  (2) Bumetanide (0.025–0.075 mg/kg IV q 6 hr) is a useful alternative to furosemide.

  (3) A thiazide diuretic often adds to the diuretic actions of a loop diuretic. Thiazide diuretics include:
    (a) Metolazone, 2.5–10.0 mg PO bid (administer 30 minutes before furosemide)
    (b) Chlorothiazide, 500–1000 mg IV bid

  (4) "Renal dose" dopamine (< 3 µg/kg/min IV drip) provides a slight increase in cardiac index. It also has a natriuretic effect that increases urine volume. These combined effects result in diuresis, which may be useful in the management of normovolemic ARF.

  b. However, neither diuretics nor dopamine alters the

course of ARF. Diuretics should be used only to make the distinction between oliguric and nonoliguric renal failure and to attempt to avoid dialysis in oliguric patients.

    c. Patients who do not respond to diuretics require dialysis to manage volume overload.

2. Hyperkalemia (see p 196)

    a. Check the ECG for signs of cardiotoxicity (i.e., peaked T waves; depressed P waves; prolonged PR, QT, and QRS intervals).

    b. Definitive therapy includes:

        (1) Insulin, 5–10 U IV, and 50 cc of 50% glucose IV

        (2) Sodium polystyrene sulfonate, 15–30 g PO/PR

        (3) Calcium gluconate, 1 ampule (1000 mg/10 ml) IV

        (4) Furosemide, 20–60 g IV

        (5) Hemodialysis or, less preferably, peritoneal dialysis [for patients with severe hyperkalemia (serum potassium > 7.5 mEq/L)]

        (6) High-dose albuterol nebulizer, 20 mg (used as an additional strategy, especially for severely hyperkalemic patients)

3. Acid–base disorders (see p 189)

    a. The most common acid–base disorder in ARF is uremic metabolic acidosis.

    b. Daily alkali requirements are approximately 1 mEq bicarbonate/kg/day.

        (1) Supplementation as sodium bicarbonate (650 mg PO = 8 mEq) or sodium citrate (1 ml PO = 1 mEq) may be required after the initial base deficit is replaced.

        (2) Bicarbonate or acetate should be added to the total parenteral nutrition prescription in patients who are NPO.

4. Anemia secondary to decreased erythropoietin

    a. Attempt exogenous administration of erythropoietin (50–100 U/kg/dose SQ 2–3 times per week) if the hematocrit is < 30% or the patient requires frequent blood transfusions.

    b. Allow at least 2 weeks for results.

5. Platelet dysfunction. Administer deamino-8-D-arginine vasopressin (dDAVP), 0.3 mg/kg IV over 30–60 minutes, before invasive procedures or for a bleeding episode.

C. Specific management based on classes of renal insufficiency

    1. Prerenal azotemia

        a. Volume depletion

            (1) In prerenal azotemia without associated ischemic renal insult, replace volume with normal saline. Rapid response occurs and SCr rapidly returns to baseline.

                (a) Young patients with intact cardiovascular

function can tolerate large amounts of saline without risk of pulmonary edema.

    (b) Patients with more tenuous cardiopulmonary status benefit from a fluid challenge [i.e., judicious administration of small amounts of saline (100–500 ml) over 15–30 minutes]. Follow the response of blood pressure, pulse, and central venous pressure.

  (2) In many patients, especially patients who are oliguric, a Swan-Ganz catheter is useful.

 b. Volume overload

  (1) Renal function often improves after diuresis.

  (2) Other maneuvers to improve cardiac function (e.g., vasodilators, inotropes, intra-aortic balloon pump) may also improve renal function.

 c. Anuria

  (1) Administer a fluid challenge with crystalloid.

  (2) A pulmonary artery catheter may be required to assess volume status if fluid challenge fails to increase urine output.

  (3) Administer colloids (e.g., albumin, hetastarch, dextran) cautiously because there is a risk of sudden pulmonary edema.

 d. Hepatorenal syndrome

  (1) Hepatorenal syndrome is ruled out when volume replacement is followed by improved urine output and renal function.

  (2) True hepatorenal syndrome only responds to liver transplantation.

2. Postrenal obstruction

 a. Remove the obstructing lesion or percutaneously drain the collecting system as soon as possible.

 b. The reversibility of renal dysfunction is directly related to the duration of the obstruction. Substantial recovery usually occurs if an acute obstruction is relieved within the first week.

3. Intrinsic renal disease

 a. ATN

  (1) ATN is the most common form of intrinsic renal disease.

  (2) In most cases of ATN, no treatment is available.

  (3) Most patients with ATN can be managed **without dialysis.**

    (a) Maintain detailed records of intake (IV, PO, nasogastric) and output (urine, vomiting, nasogastric suctioning, drains, stools and ostomies, open wounds).

    (b) Weigh the patient daily.

    (c) Continuously look for signs of volume overload, volume depletion, and uremic symptoms.

        (d) Consider a pulmonary artery catheter to accurately assess and monitor volume status and optimize cardiac function.

        (e) Treat hypertension with vasodilators to prevent direct reduction in renal blood flow.

        (f) Monitor potassium, phosphate, creatinine, and bicarbonate levels.

  b. Glomerulonephritides and vasculitides

    (1) Many glomerulonephritides and vasculitides can be treated with steroids and cytotoxic agents or plasmapheresis.

    (2) Consult the nephrology service.

  c. Severe acute interstitial nephritis

    (1) Oral prednisone may shorten recovery time.

    (2) Administer prednisone, 1 mg/kg/day PO for 4–6 weeks, followed by a slow taper.

  d. Rhabdomyolysis

    (1) Administer crystalloid (normal saline or lactated Ringer's solution) to keep urine output > 100 cc/hr.

    (2) Alkalinize the urine (i.e., pH > 6.5) with infusions of sodium bicarbonate to increase the solubilization of urine myoglobin.

    (3) Forced diuresis with mannitol (12.5 g IV over 1 hour) or furosemide (40–200 mg IV q 6 hr) may be needed if there is no response to IV fluid.

  e. Crystal deposition processes. Solubilization often can be optimized by altering the urine pH (e.g., alkalinization of urine for uric acid and sulfadiazine; acidification for indinavir).

  f. Acute renal allograft rejection. Therapy with pulse corticosteroids and antilymphocyte antibodies (e.g., antithymocyte gammaglobulin or anti-CD3 monoclonal antibodies) is very effective.

VII. Complications of Acute Renal Failure

  A. Cardiovascular complications include:

    1. Congestive heart failure

    2. Pulmonary edema

    3. Hypertension with occasional hypotension

  B. Infectious complications (30%–70% of patients) are related to the urinary and respiratory tracts and result from indwelling catheters and impaired immune defenses.

  C. Neurologic complications include:

    1. Confusion

    2. Asterixis

    3. Somnolence

    4. Seizures

  D. GI complications include:

    1. Anorexia

    2. Nausea and vomiting

    3. Ileus

> **4.** Bleeding
> **5.** Anemia
> **6.** Gastritis

VIII. Prognosis of Acute Renal Failure

A. Patients with more than five failed organ systems have negligible survival despite maximal supportive therapy. Respiratory failure is a particularly strong predictor of mortality.

B. Causes of death are usually related to the underlying systemic problems (e.g., sepsis, cardiovascular disease, liver disease, GI bleeding).

C. Renal survival varies according to the nature of the injury.

  1. Toxic or ischemic ATN has a good prognosis if the patient survives the underlying illness.

  2. Acute urinary obstruction usually responds well to relief of the obstruction.

  3. Other intrinsic renal processes vary in their course and response to therapy.

D. Mortality has improved in recent years due to better critical care support. However, ARF in the ICU setting requires increased dialysis and has a higher mortality rate (i.e., 25%–40%).

CHRONIC RENAL FAILURE

I. Definition. Chronic renal failure (CRF) is the progressive loss of nephron mass and function, resulting in decreased GFR and characterized by an elevated BUN/creatinine.

II. Management

A. General management of CRF

  1. Nutrition

   a. Do not restrict protein in hospitalized patients with CRF. Although protein restriction may have a beneficial effect in slowing the progression of CRF, acutely ill patients are hypercatabolic and require high protein intake to avoid negative nitrogen balance.

   b. Restrict potassium and phosphates.

  2. Dialysis

   a. If a patient is admitted with CRF, maintain the patient on his or her outpatient dialysis schedule unless additional or different therapy is needed based on the patient's new disease process.

   b. Perform careful inspection of dialysis sites for signs of infection. Obtain blood cultures and peritoneal fluid analysis (cell count and culture) when infection is suspected.

   c. Use prophylactic antibiotics for hemodialysis patients before a potentially bacteremic procedure. The same AHA guidelines used for prevention of bacterial endocarditis can be applied.

B. Management of acute complications in CRF

1. **Volume overload**
   a. Control volume overload with loop diuretics.
   b. Patients on chronic dialysis require volume control with ultrafiltration through hemodialysis or peritoneal dialysis.
2. **Hypertension**
   a. Hypertension should be tightly managed in CRF. Remember the role of volume overload in the hypertension of CRF, especially in patients with end-stage renal disease (ESRD).
   b. The best approach to the management of high blood pressure is to achieve euvolemia and optimize the use of long-acting drugs.
   c. If a short-acting drug is required, administer clonidine (0.1 mg PO q 30 min up to 0.3 mg total) or labetalol (20 mg IV q 15 min in escalating doses up to 300 mg total).
3. **Hypotension**
   a. Dialysis patients may become volume depleted and should be aggressively repleted. **Use caution to avoid overshooting.** Hemodynamic monitoring is often helpful in volume repletion.
   b. Pericarditis with hemodynamically significant pericardial effusion should always be considered as a cause of hypotension given an incidence of 5%–10% in patients with ESRD.
   c. Clotting of an arteriovenous graft or fistula is a common complication of prolonged hypotensive episodes.
4. **Impaired diluting ability and free-water excretion**
   a. CRF patients with impaired diluting ability and free-water excretion are predisposed to hyponatremia.
   b. Free-water restriction may be required.
5. **Bone disease**
   a. Continue calcitriol therapy while the patient is hospitalized.
   b. Calcitriol therapy is especially important in parathyroidectomy patients.
6. **Anemia**
   a. Manage anemia with erythropoietin and iron supplementation.
   b. Limit unnecessary blood draws for laboratory tests.
7. **Platelet dysfunction** is related to CRF and can be managed with dDAVP, 0.3 mg/kg IV over 30–60 minutes.

DRUG DOSING IN RENAL DISEASE

I. **Abnormal Drug Metabolism in Renal Failure**
   A. Absorption may be altered by concomitantly used drugs or autonomic neuropathy with resultant abnormal gastric and bowel motility.

B. Some hepatic first-pass metabolic steps may be impaired in uremia.

C. The volume of distribution of hydrophilic drugs increases if edema or ascites is present and decreases in patients with decreased muscle mass, which is common in renal disease.

D. Decreased protein binding may occur as a result of hypoalbuminemia or intrinsic defects in protein binding. The result is an increased concentration of free drug.

E. Glomerular filtration and tubular secretion are decreased with progressive renal dysfunction.

II. Dosing Guidelines for Commonly Used Drugs (Tables 21–7, 21–8, 21–9, and 21–10)

III. Adjustments in Drug Dosing in Renal Failure

A. Loading doses are usually the same, with rare exceptions (e.g., digoxin). Patients with volume overload and increased extracellular space may require larger loading doses of hydrophilic drugs.

B. Maintenance doses may be adjusted by two methods.

1. Increasing the dose interval while maintaining the same dose is cost effective and most commonly used.

2. Maintaining the dose interval while the individual dose is decreased produces less fluctuations between peak and trough drug levels and is best suited for drugs with a narrow therapeutic index.

C. In the presence of **decreased glomerular filtration and tubular secretion,** adjust drug dosing to the degree of renal insufficiency as estimated by the GFR.

1. The Cockroft-Gault formula is a practical method for estimating Ccr, which is a surrogate marker of GFR. It requires stable SCr. The formula for men is calculated as:

$$Ccr = \frac{(140 - age) \times ideal\ body\ weight\ (kg)}{72 \times SCr\ (mg/dl)}$$

The formula for women is calculated as:

$$Ccr = \frac{(140 - age) \times ideal\ body\ weight\ (kg) \times 0.85}{72 \times SCr\ (mg/dl)}$$

2. Ccr and GFR can be more accurately assessed via a timed urine collection:

$$Ccr = \frac{Urine\ creatinine \times timed\ urine\ volume\ (ml/min)}{Plasma\ creatinine}$$

3. Patients with ARF may have a very low GFR (i.e., < 10 ml/min) despite low SCr levels. Early in the course of ARF, the SCr increases on a daily basis, reflecting renal shutdown. In this situation, Ccr should be calculated by a 2- or 24-hour urine collection and not by the Cockroft-Gault formula.

D. Drug removal by dialysis. Patients on continuous hemofiltration or hemodialysis often have increased drug removal. Tables are available for such adjustments. When this infor-

Table 21-7. Drug Dosing in Renal Failure—Antimicrobials

Drug	Method	GFR 10–50 ml/min	GFR < 10 ml/min*	Dose Suppl
Aminoglycosides				
Amikacin	D + I	30%–70%, q 12–18 hr	20%–30%, q 24–48 hr	Yes
Gentamicin	D + I	30%–70%, q 12 hr	20%–30%, q 24–48 hr	Yes
Tobramycin	D + I	30%–70%, q 12 hr	20%–30%, q 24–48 hr	Yes
Cephalosporins				
Cefaclor	D	50%–100%	50%	Yes
Cefazolin	I	q 12 hr	q 24–48 hr	Yes
Cefoperazone	D	100%	100%	Yes
Cefotaxime	I	q 8–12 hr	q 24 hr	Yes
Cefotetan	D	50%	25%	Yes
Cefoxitin	I	q 8–12 hr	q 24–48 hr	Yes
Ceftazidime	I	q 24–48 hr	q 48 hr	Yes
Ceftizoxime	I	q 12–24 hr	q 24 hr	Yes
Ceftriaxone	D	100%	100%	Yes
Cefuroxime axetil	D	100%	100%	Yes
Cefuroxime sodium	I	q 8–12 hr	q 24 hr	Yes
Cephalexin	I	q 12 hr	q 12 hr	Yes
Penicillins				
Amoxicillin	I	q 8–12 hr	q 24 hr	Yes
Ampicillin	I	q 6–12 hr	q 12–24 hr	Yes
Mezlocillin	I	q 6–8 hr	q 8 hr	No
Penicillin G	D	75%	25%–50%	Yes
Piperacillin	I	q 6–8 hr	q 8 hr	Yes
Ticarcillin	D + I	1–2 g, q 8 hr	1–2 g, q 12 hr	Yes
Other				
Acyclovir	D + I	5 mg/kg, q 12–24 hr	2.5 mg/kg, q 24 hr	Yes
Amphotericin B	I	q 24 hr	q 24–36 hr	No
Azithromycin	D	100%	100%	No
Aztreonam	D	50%–75%	25%	Yes
Chloramphenicol	D	100%	100%	No
Clarithromycin	D	75%	50%–75%	Yes
Clindamycin	D	100%	100%	No
Doxycycline	D	100%	100%	No
Erythromycin	D	100%	50%–75%	No
Fluconazole	D	100%	100%	Yes
Ganciclovir	I	q 24–48 hr	q 48–96 hr	Yes
Imipenem	D	50%	25%	Yes

continued

		GFR 10–50	**GFR < 10**	**Dose**
Drug	**Method**	**ml/min**	**ml/min***	**Suppl**
Metronidazole	D	100%	100%	Yes
Sulfamethoxazole	I	q 18 hr	q 24 hr	Yes
Trimethoprim	I	q 18 hr	q 24 hr	Yes
Vancomycin	D + I	500 mg,	500 mg,	
		q 24–48 hr	q 48–96 hr	Yes

Table 21-7. Drug Dosing in Renal Failure—Antimicrobials

Dose suppl = requirement for dose supplementation after hemodialysis; GFR = glomerular filtration rate; D = decrease dose; I = increase interval.
*Patients on dialysis should be considered to have a GFR < 10 ml/min.

mation is not available for a particular drug, use dosing guidelines for GFR between 10 and 50 ml/min.

PERIOPERATIVE RENAL CARE

I. **Risk Factors for Perioperative Renal Failure.** Patients with underlying renal disease are at an increased risk of perioperative renal failure due to the multiple insults that may occur in the perioperative period.
   A. **High-risk procedures for renal damage**
      1. Open-heart operations with aortic cross-clamping and extracorporeal circulation (e.g., coronary bypass)
      2. Thoracic aortic procedures
      3. Abdominal aortic procedures
   B. **Additional perioperative risks**
      1. Hormonal and metabolic stress of the perioperative period can result from increased catecholamines, corticosteroids, aldosterone, and antidiuretic hormone, all of which lead to sodium and water retention and decreased renal blood flow.
      2. Myocardial depression from anesthetic agents or intraoperative ischemia may result in decreased renal perfusion.
      3. Perioperative hypotension can be caused by general anesthetics, epidural blocks, and bleeding.
      4. Nephrotoxic agents (e.g., IV contrast, nephrotoxic antibiotics) are a leading cause of ATN.
      5. Sepsis is a potential complication in patients on dialysis given their somewhat immunocompromised status.
II. **Preoperative Renal Care.** Preoperative efforts should concentrate on optimizing hemodynamic status.
   A. Achieve euvolemia.
      1. Use adequate amounts of IV fluid or diuretics to achieve euvolemia.

Table 21-8. Drug Dosing in Renal Failure—Cardiovascular Drugs

Drug	Method	GFR 10–50 ml/min	GFR < 10 ml/min*	Dose Suppl
Antihypertensives				
Amlodipine	D	100%	100%	No
Atenolol	D + I	50%, q 48 hr	30%–50%, q 96 hr	Yes
Captopril	D + I	75%, q 12–18 hr	50%, q 24 hr	Yes
Clonidine	D	100%	100%	No
Diltiazem	D	100%	100%	No
Doxazosin	D	100%	100%	No
Enalapril	D	75%–100%	50%	Yes
Hydralazine	I	q 8 hr	q 8–16 hr	No
Lisinopril	D	50%–75%	25%–50%	Yes
Methyldopa	I	q 8–12 hr	q 12–24 hr	Yes
Metoprolol	D	100%	100%	Yes
Minoxidil	D	100%	100%	No
Nifedipine	D	100%	100%	No
Nimodipine	D	100%	100%	No
Nitroprusside	D	100%	100%	No
Prazosin	D	100%	100%	No
Propranolol	D	100%	100%	No
Verapamil	D	100%	100%	No
Antiarrhythmics				
Amiodarone	D	100%	100%	No
Bretylium	D	25%–50%	25%	No
Esmolol	D	100%	100%	No
Lidocaine	D	100%	100%	No
Procainamide	I	q 6–12 hr	q 8–24 hr	Yes
Quinidine	D	100%	75%	Yes
Sotalol	D	30%	15%–30%	Yes
Inotropes				
Digoxin	D + I	25%–75%, q 36 hr	10%–25%, q 48 hr	No
Dobutamine	D	100%	100%	No
Milrinone	D	100%	50%–75%	Unknown
Other				
Isosorbide	D	100%	100%	No
Nitroglycerin	D	100%	100%	No

Dose suppl = requirement for dose supplementation after hemodialysis; GFR = glomerular filtration rate; D = decrease dose; I = increase interval.
*Patients on dialysis should be considered to have a GFR < 10 ml/min.

Table 21-9. Drug Dosing in Renal Failure—CNS Drugs

Drug	Method	GFR 10–50 ml/min	GFR < 10 ml/min*	Dose Suppl
Anticonvulsants				
Carbamazepine	D	100%	100%	No
Phenobarbital	I	q 8–12 hr	q 12–16 hr	Yes
Phenytoin	D	100%	100%	No
Valproic acid	D	100%	100%	No
Sedatives				
Alprazolam	D	100%	100%	No
Diazepam	D	100%	100%	No
Haloperidol	D	100%	100%	No
Lorazepam	D	100%	100%	No
Midazolam	D	100%	50%	No
Propofol	D	100%	100%	Unknown
Analgesics				
Fentanyl	D	75%	50%	Unknown
Ibuprofen	D	100%	100%	No
Ketorolac	D	50%	50%	No
Meperidine	D	75%	Avoid	Avoid
Methadone	D	100%	50%–75%	No
Morphine	D	75%	50%	No
Neuromuscular				
Atracurium	D	100%	100%	Unknown
Pancuronium	D	50%	Avoid	Unknown
Succinylcholine	D	100%	100%	Unknown
Vecuronium	D	100%	100%	Unknown

Dose suppl = requirement for dose supplementation after hemodialysis; GFR = glomerular filtration rate; D = decrease dose; I = increase interval.
*Patients on dialysis should be considered to have a GFR < 10 ml/min.

2. Provide full hemodynamic monitoring during high-risk procedures to anuric patients with ESRD because these patients often have coexisting heart disease.
B. Continue antihypertensives to the time of surgery to control blood pressure.
C. Monitor and adjust electrolyte and acid–base disorders.
D. Correct anemia.
   1. Continue or increase erythropoietin in the perioperative period.
   2. Blood transfusions may still be required.
E. Avoid unnecessary anticoagulation.
   1. Patients on hemodialysis routinely receive systemic heparin anticoagulation during dialysis.

Table 21-10. Drug Dosing in Renal Failure—Miscellaneous Drugs

Drug	Method	GFR 10–50 ml/min	GFR < 10 ml/min*	Dose Suppl
Allopurinol	D	50%	25%	Yes
Azathioprine	D	75%	50%	Yes
Cimetidine	D	50%	25%	No
Cyclophosphamide	D	100%	75%	Yes
Cyclosporine	D	100%	100%	No
Famotidine	D	25%	10%	No
Methylprednisone	D	100%	100%	Yes
Prednisone	D	100%	100%	No
Ranitidine	D	50%	25%	Yes
Sucralfate	D	100%	100%	No
Theophylline	D	100%	100%	Yes

Dose suppl = requirement for dose supplementation after hemodialysis; GFR = glomerular filtration rate; D = decrease dose.
*Patients on dialysis should be considered to have a GFR < 10 ml/min.

  2. Make arrangements with the nephrology service to avoid heparin use if the patient is to undergo an elective procedure shortly after a hemodialysis session.
 F. Adjust drug doses to the degree of renal function.
 G. Avoid specific drugs in patients at risk for renal failure.
  1. Pancuronium and alcuronium are renally excreted and may have a prolonged effect in patients with renal insufficiency.
  2. Succinylcholine causes potassium release from muscles.
  3. Meperidine and propoxyphene have metabolites that may accumulate in patients with renal insufficiency and may be neurotoxic.
  4. NSAIDs decrease preglomerular blood flow.
  5. Aminoglycosides may cause ATN.

22

Thermoregulation

Disorders

HYPERTHERMIA

I. Postoperative Fever [i.e., temperature $> 101.5°F$ ($> 38.5°C$)]

> **The five Ws pertaining to the differential diagnosis of fever in the postoperative period are:**
>
> **Wind**—atelectasis, pneumonia (postoperative days 1–2)
> **Water**—UTI (postoperative days 3–5)
> **Wound**—infection (postoperative days 6–7)
> **Walking**—deep venous thrombosis, pulmonary embolus (postoperative days 7–10)
> **Wonder drugs**—drug fevers

A. **Etiology**
1. **Acute onset of fever**
   a. Pneumonia
   b. Atelectasis
      (1) Atelectasis is a decrease in the functional residual capacity of air in the lungs at end expiration.
      (2) The functional residual capacity decreases 40%–70% after upper abdominal surgery.
   c. Aspiration pneumonitis
   d. Wound infection
   e. Medications (especially antibiotics)
   f. Catheter-related infection
   g. Preexisting infection (i.e., unrelated to procedure)
2. **Persistent fever**
   a. Intraabdominal or thoracic abscess
   b. Pleural effusions (consider sampling; can be infected if sampled)

    c. Ascites (consider sampling; can be infected if sampled)

    d. Sinusitis [especially in patients with long-standing nasotracheal (40%–50% incidence) or nasogastric intubation]

    e. Acalculous cholecystitis

    f. Meningitis (especially in neurotrauma patients)

    g. Deep venous thrombosis and pulmonary embolus

    h. Pancreatitis

    i. Bowel infarction

    j. Endocarditis

    k. Malignant hyperthermia (see II)

    l. *Clostridium difficile* colitis

    m. Necrotizing fasciitis

B. Diagnostic tests

  1. Testing for unknown etiology

    a. Culture blood two times from separate sites.

    b. Obtain urine culture and analysis.

    c. Obtain sputum sample for culture.

    d. Obtain WBC count.

    e. Obtain a chest radiograph.

    f. Send special serum studies (e.g., viral cultures, tuberculosis cultures), depending on the situation (e.g., transplants).

    g. Perform a full fever work-up with a more conservative temperature threshold in patients who are immunosuppressed or on steroids (e.g., transplant and cancer patients).

  2. Testing for specific etiology

    a. Acalculous cholecystitis can be diagnosed by abdominal examination, ultrasound, radionuclide scans, and CT scan.

    b. Diagnosis of bowel infarction often requires laparotomy.

    c. To diagnose endocarditis, listen for a new murmur and obtain an echocardiogram.

    d. To diagnose *C. difficile* colitis, evaluate the stool for the *C. difficile* toxin or perform a colonoscopy if clinically indicated.

    e. Necrotizing fasciitis can be diagnosed with fascial biopsies and culture. Obtain a Gram's stain immediately. MRI is most sensitive for evaluation of soft tissues for infection and gas.

    f. Intraabdominal and thoracic abscesses require CT scan and percutaneous drainage for diagnosis. Send the aspirated fluid for culture.

    g. Diagnosis of sinusitis may require CT scan for evaluation or otolaryngologic consult for drainage and culture, or both.

C. Management

1. Treat the **source** of the fever.
   a. To minimize **atelectasis,** which may lead to pneumonia, order incentive spirometry, chest physiotherapy, and ambulation.
   b. **Wound infection**
      (1) Take down all dressings and evaluate for infection. It may be necessary to remove one or two stitches or staples to further evaluate or culture.
      (2) If infected, open the entire length of the incision and pack, with dressing changes two or three times a day. Use normal saline, half-strength Dakin's solution, or povidone-iodine solution.
      (3) If infection occurs within 24 hours of surgery, consider streptococcal or clostridial wound infection. Treatment involves incision and drainage.
   c. **Catheter-related infection**
      (1) Fever requires central line change.
         (a) If the site appears clean, change the line over a wire.
         (b) If the site is not clean, place a new line in a new location.
         (c) Each hospital has specific guidelines for management of central lines.
      (2) Send the blood from central lines for culture in the work-up of a fever. Send the tip or intradermal portion of the central line for culture if the line is changed.
      (3) Arterial lines are generally not cultured but should be removed if the site is not clean.
      (4) Remove or replace Foley catheters if leukocyte esterase or WBCs are found on urinalysis or if a UTI is diagnosed.
2. Start **broad-spectrum antibiotics** before receiving culture results.
   a. Before culture results are received, antibiotics may be determined empirically and adjusted based on a Gram's stain.
   b. After culture results are determined, narrow the choice of antibiotics to target the specific organism.
3. Order additional diagnostic tests if necessary (e.g., CT scan, ultrasound, spinal tap, chest radiograph, bronchoalveolar lavage, serial blood cultures).

II. Malignant Hyperthermia
A. Incidence
1. Malignant hyperthermia occurs in 1:15,000 pediatric and 1:50,000–100,000 adult anesthetic procedures.
2. Malignant hyperthermia is seen more often in males than in females.
3. The mortality rate is 65% if left untreated and 7%–10% if treated with dantrolene sodium.

B. Pathogenesis

1. There is a rise in end-tidal carbon dioxide, resulting in central venous desaturation (i.e., decreased mixed venous saturation).
2. Metabolic and respiratory acidosis occur.
3. There may be failure to relax after administration of succinylcholine, followed by tachycardia and tachypnea. If this progression goes unrecognized, cyanosis will develop, even with high FIO_2 and adequate ventilation.
4. Rhabdomyolysis then develops.
5. Temperature rises. This occurs in 30% of patients and is usually a late feature of the disease.
6. Arrhythmias and hypertension result.

C. **Etiology**
1. Malignant hyperthermia is a rare disorder caused by increased intracellular calcium secondary to increased release of calcium or decreased uptake of calcium from the sarcoplasmic reticulum.
2. Malignant hyperthermia can be triggered by **potent inhalational agents and depolarizing muscle relaxants** (e.g., halothane, isoflurane, trichloroethylene, diethyl ether, enflurane, methoxyflurane, chloroform, ketamine, succinylcholine).
3. In 50% of cases, malignant hyperthermia occurs with an uneventful anesthetic procedure resulting from the **duration of anesthesia, type of premedication,** and the **state of the sympathetic nervous system** (e.g., stress or exercise state).

D. **Signs and symptoms**

> **Malignant hyperthermia may be delayed in appearance after a procedure, and it may recur once under control.**

1. Tachycardia (96%)
2. Tachypnea
3. Muscle rigidity (84%)
4. Labile blood pressure (e.g., hypertension) [86%]
5. Cyanosis (71%)
6. Fever (31%)
7. Acidosis
8. Electrolyte changes [e.g., hyperkalemia, hyperphosphatemia, elevated creatine phosphokinase (CPK), myoglobinuria]

E. **Management**
1. The treatment of choice for malignant hyperthermia is **dantrolene sodium.**
   a. For acute cases, give 2.5 mg/kg IV bolus. Repeat q 15 min to a maximum of 10 mg/kg.
   b. For maintenance doses, give 1–2 mg/kg PO qid for 3 days.
   c. Dantrolene sodium works at the level of the sar-

coplasmic reticulum by inhibiting the calcium-induced release of calcium.

2. Treat metabolic and respiratory acidosis with **bicarbonate.**
3. **Hyperventilate** with 100% oxygen.
4. Monitor **urine myoglobin, CPK, ABG, electrolytes,** and **glucose.**

F. **Complications.** Late complications of malignant hyperthermia include seizures, disseminated intravascular coagulation, acute renal failure, and pulmonary and cerebral edema.

III. Heat Stroke

A. **Pathophysiology**

1. Heat stroke is a syndrome of acute thermoregulatory failure in warm environments. The primary injury is due to direct cellular toxicity at temperatures $> 107.6°F$ ($> 42°C$).
2. Muscle degeneration and necrosis are common, especially with an exertional etiology. This may lead to significant muscle enzyme elevation and rhabdomyolysis.
3. Cardiac output is usually high due to increased demands and low systemic vascular resistance secondary to vasodilation and dehydration.
4. Direct thermal toxicity to the brain and spinal cord may result in cerebral edema and local hemorrhage. This may lead to stupor and coma and may be preceded by ataxia, dysmetria, and dysarthria.
5. Acute renal failure occurs in 5% of heat stroke patients, mostly from severe dehydration. Dehydration, pigment load, hypoperfusion, and urate nephropathy are thought to contribute to acute tubular necrosis.
6. Hepatic necrosis and cholestasis peak 2–3 days after injury and lead to death in 5%–10% of patients.
7. The effects of the heat may result in platelet aggregation, deactivation of platelet and coagulation factors, and a decrease in coagulation factor synthesis.
8. Hyperthermia produces frequent imbalances in potassium, sodium, calcium, and phosphate levels.

B. **Etiology**

1. **Increased heat production** can lead to heat stroke and can result from:
   a. Exercise
   b. Fever
   c. Thyrotoxicosis
   d. Drugs (e.g., amphetamines, hallucinogens)
2. **Impaired heat loss** can also lead to heat stroke and can result from:
   a. Loss of voluntary control when ambient temperatures are high (increased risk in schizophrenic, comatose, senile, and mentally deficient patients)
   b. Dehydration and impaired cardiovascular performance
   c. Hypokalemia (results in decreased muscle blood

flow, impaired cardiovascular performance, and decreased sweat gland function)

   d. Skin disorders that impair sweat gland function
   e. Inability to sweat effectively (e.g., the elderly)

C. Diagnosis

1. **History and physical examination** will usually be suggestive of heat stroke.

   a. Heat stroke should be suspected in any individual exercising in hot weather or falling in a high-risk group (e.g., age > 65 years, patients with schizophrenia or Parkinson's disease, alcoholics, paraplegics, quadriplegics).
   b. Coma or profound stupor is almost always present.

2. **Diagnostic criteria** include:

   a. Core temperature > 104°F (> 40°C) [may be absent if there is significant time between onset and medical care]
   b. Anhidrosis (may be absent if there is significant time between onset and medical care)
   c. Severely depressed mental state or coma
   d. Elevated serum creatine kinase level
   e. Compatible history

D. Management (i.e., cooling and decreasing thermogenesis)

1. **Methods of cooling**

   a. Evaporative cooling involves continuously wetting the skin and fanning the patient with two electric fans.
   b. Direct external cooling by immersion in cold water or with ice packs is acceptable. However, the skin must be constantly massaged to overcome skin vasoconstriction and to allow circulation to carry heat from the core.
   c. When evaporative and direct external cooling methods fail, peritoneal lavage with iced saline cooled to 68°F–48.2°F (20°C–9°C), gastric lavage, or hemodialysis may be necessary.

2. **Care at the scene** (i.e., before transport to the hospital)

   a. Move victim to a cool or shaded area immediately.
   b. Remove clothes and constantly wet the patient's skin.

3. **ICU care**

   a. Obtain IV access with a large-bore catheter.
   b. Place patient in a cool room.
   c. Use a pulmonary artery catheter for invasive monitoring.
   d. Follow ABG and correct for temperature.
   e. Follow urine output closely. The patient must be volume resuscitated. Given the risk of rhabdomyolysis, use mannitol as needed to maintain brisk urine flow (i.e., > 100 cc/hr).
   f. Continuously monitor the patient's temperature. Stop cooling procedures as the temperature approaches 102.2°F (39°C).

4. **Treatment of complications**

a. **Hypotension** is common in heat stroke.
    (1) Initially, treat hypotension with crystalloid. If necessary, use isoproterenol. Avoid dopaminergic and alpha agents because they tend to produce peripheral vasoconstriction.
    (2) Monitor the patient with a pulmonary artery catheter and arterial catheter to help assess and treat the associated cardiac dysfunction, dehydration, and low peripheral vascular resistance.
b. **Seizures** are common in heat stroke and usually respond to diazepam.
c. Moderate-to-severe **liver failure** is common in heat stroke.
d. **Disseminated intravascular coagulation** requires supportive care and fresh frozen plasma.

E. Prognosis
    1. Morbidity and mortality are directly related to the time spent at elevated temperatures and the peak temperature.
        a. When managed appropriately, mortality ranges from 5%–18% depending on premorbid conditions.
        b. A delay in treatment of only 2 hours may result in 70% mortality.
    2. Neurologic function usually returns rapidly as the patient becomes euthermic. However, some patients may be left with some cerebellar disorder.

IV. **Neuroleptic Malignant Syndrome**
A. Pathophysiology
    1. Muscular rigidity, akinesia, mutism, and tremor are due to hypothalamic dopaminergic imbalance.
    2. Motor abnormalities are typical of the parkinsonian-type extrapyramidal reactions.
    3. Hyperthermia results from an increase in endogenous heat production, impaired heat dissipation, loss of voluntary temperature regulation, and possibly an elevation of the hypothalamic setpoint.
    4. Rhabdomyolysis may occur secondary to hyperthermia and muscle rigidity. Although the CPK level is typically elevated to 1000–5000 IU, it may rise to 10,000 IU.
    5. Acute renal failure occurs in 9%–30% of patients and is due to myoglobin-induced acute tubular necrosis.

B. Etiology
    1. Neuroleptic malignant syndrome may appear in patients receiving agents believed to decrease dopaminergic hypothalamic tone or after withdrawal of dopaminergic agents.
    2. **Drugs** associated with the onset of neuroleptic malignant syndrome include:
        a. Butyrophenones: haloperidol, bromperidol
        b. Thioxanthenes: thiothixene
        c. Phenothiazines: chlorpromazine, levomepromazine, trifluoperazine, fluphenazine
        d. Debenzoxazepines: loxapine

     e. Dihydroindolones: molindone
     f. Tricyclic dibenzodiazepines: clozapine
     g. Dopamine-depleting agents: tetrabenazine, alpha-methyltyrosine, domperidone, metoclopramide
     h. Levodopa, carbidopa, amantadine (withdrawal)

C. Signs and symptoms
    1. The onset of symptoms usually occurs within 1 week of initiation of a neuroleptic drug or within 2 weeks of a dosage increase of a previously prescribed neuroleptic drug.
    2. Symptoms include:
      a. Dysphagia or dysarthria
      b. Muscular rigidity, tremors, muteness, and hypophonia
      c. Hyperthermia (peak temperatures are reached within 48 hours of onset of symptoms)
      d. Mental status changes
      e. Tachycardia, diaphoresis, changes in blood pressure, tachypnea (often secondary to hyperthermia)

D. Laboratory results
    1. Elevations in CPK, lactate dehydrogenase, and WBC counts will parallel body temperature.
    2. CPK levels will peak between 2–3 days and 1 week after diagnosis.

E. Management
    1. Discontinue the neuroleptic agent.
    2. Decrease thermogenesis by reducing muscle contraction.
      a. First-line therapy: dantrolene, 1.0–2.5 mg/kg IV q 6 hr until a dose of 100–300 mg/day PO can be given
      b. Paralysis (may be required to reduce the metabolic rate and muscle contraction): curare, pancuronium
    3. Reduce extrapyramidal side effects.
      a. Amantadine, 100–200 mg PO bid
      b. Bromocriptine, 2.5 mg PO tid
      c. Carbidopa with levodopa, 10–100 mg PO tid
    4. Provide external cooling.
    5. Continue treatment and close observation for 1 week or longer, depending on the rate of excretion of the neuroleptic drug.

COLD INJURY

  I. Local Tissue Cold Injury. The severity of injury depends on the temperature, duration of exposure, environmental conditions, protective clothing, and the patient's general state of health.
    A. Types of injury
      1. Frostnip is the mildest form of local cold injury.
        a. Frostnip is characterized by initial pain, pallor, and numbness.
        b. Frostnip is reversible with warming and does not result in tissue loss unless there are repeated incidences.

2. Frostbite is caused by the freezing of tissue with intracellular ice-crystal formation and microvascular occlusion, which result in tissue hypoxia. Some injury may be a result of rewarming (e.g., reperfusion injury).

    a. The degree of frostbite burn depends on the depth of involvement.

        (1) First-degree burns are characterized by hyperemia and edema without skin necrosis.

        (2) Second-degree burns are characterized by the formation of large, clear vesicles in addition to edema and hyperemia with partial-thickness skin necrosis.

        (3) Third-degree burns are characterized by hemorrhagic vesicle formation and full-thickness necrosis that includes subcutaneous tissues.

        (4) Fourth-degree burns are characterized by bone gangrene and full-thickness skin necrosis that includes muscle.

    b. The depth of burn cannot be accurately assessed until full demarcation has occurred.

3. Nonfreezing injury (e.g., trench foot, immersion foot) is caused by microvascular endothelial damage, stasis, and vascular occlusion. This injury results from extended or repetitive exposure to wet conditions and temperatures just above freezing.

B. Management

    1. General management of local tissue cold injury

        a. Immediate treatment is required to decrease the duration of tissue freezing.

        b. Remove wet clothes, apply blankets, and administer warm fluids PO.

        c. Place injured area in a circulating water bath at 104°F–120°F (40°C–48.8°C) until pink in color and reperfusion occurs (20–30 minutes).

        d. Treat the pain adequately with IV or IM analgesia.

        e. Place the patient on a cardiac monitor.

        f. Administer tetanus prophylaxis.

        g. When treating local cold injury, **do not rewarm if there is a chance of refreezing and do not use dry heat or rubbing.**

    2. Local wound care of frostbite

        a. Preserve damaged tissue by preventing infection, keeping vesicles intact, and elevating the area.

        b. Administer antibiotics if there are signs of infection.

        c. Do not allow the patient to walk until edema resolves.

        d. Advise the patient to avoid nicotine and vasoconstrictive agents.

II. Hypothermia

    A. Classification

        1. Hypothermia is a core body temperature < 95°F (< 35°C).

2. In the absence of traumatic injury, hypothermia may be classified as follows:
   a. Mild: core temperature 89.6°F–95°F (32°C–35°C)
   b. Moderate: core temperature 86°F–89.6°F (30°C–32°C)
   c. Severe: core temperature < 86°F (< 30°C)
3. In trauma patients, hypothermia may be classified as follows:
   a. Mild-to-moderate: core temperature 98.6°F–89.6°F (36°C–32°C)
   b. Severe: core temperature < 89.6°F (< 32°C)
B. **Physiologic profile** in hypothermia
   1. **Cardiac function**
      a. Cardiac output falls proportional to core temperature.
      b. Cardiac irritability begins at 91.4°F (33°C).
      c. Atrial fibrillation occurs at temperatures between 93.2°F and 77°F (34°C and 25°C).
      d. Ventricular fibrillation is more common at temperatures < 82.4°F (< 28°C), and asystole occurs at temperatures < 77°F (< 25°C).
      e. ECG results in a patient with mild hypothermia may show bradycardia with prolongation of the PR, QRS, and QT intervals.
         (1) At temperatures < 86°F (< 30°C), first-degree heart block is not unusual.
         (2) At a temperature of 68°F (20°C), third-degree heart block may be seen.
      f. Hypotension is common at temperatures < 77°F (< 25°C) as systemic vascular resistance decreases.
   2. **Hematologic function.** Hypothermia affects WBCs, RBCs, and platelets.
   3. **Endocrine function.** Hypothermia directly suppresses the release of insulin from the pancreas and increases resistance to insulin action in the periphery.
C. **Etiology**
   1. Advanced age
   2. Exposure to cold (Wetness, wind, and exhaustion contribute to increased loss of body heat.)
   3. Drugs (Alcohol, phenothiazines, barbiturates, and paralytic agents frequently produce hypothermia by depressing sensory afferents, the hypothalamus, and effector responses.)
   4. Endocrine dysfunction (e.g., diabetic ketoacidosis, hyperosmolar coma, hypoglycemia)
   5. CNS disorders (e.g., stroke, primary and metastatic tumors, sarcoidosis, luetic gliosis)
   6. Spinal cord transection (Hypothermia results from an inability to shiver and a loss of body muscle mass.)
   7. Trauma [hypothermia secondary to multiple insults (e.g., shock, massive transfusion)]

    8. Iatrogenic causes (e.g., infusion of blood or fluids at temperatures below body temperature, ultrafiltration at high flow rates, anesthesia and surgery performed in a cool operating room)

D. Signs and symptoms

  1. Decreased core temperature

    a. Measure core temperature using bladder, rectal, tympanic, esophageal, or great-vessel techniques.

    b. It may be helpful to monitor two different temperatures for comparison.

  2. Depressed level of consciousness

    a. Stuporous or confused: core temperature 95°F–89.6°F (35°C–32°C)

    b. Verbally responsive but incoherent: core temperature 89.6°F–80.6°F (32°C–27°C)

    c. Comatose but able to respond to noxious stimuli: core temperature < 80.6°F (< 27°C)

  3. Patient cold to touch and cyanotic

  4. Variable and possibly severely depressed heart rate, respiratory rate, and blood pressure

E. Management

> **A hypothermic patient cannot be pronounced dead until rewarmed to 98.6°F (37°C).**

  1. Follow the **algorithm for suspected hypothermia** (Figure 22-1).

  2. Obtain **central venous access.**

  3. Obtain ABG and maintain **oxygen saturation > 90%.**

  4. Rewarm the patient at < 35.6°F (< 2°C) per hour.

    a. Mild exposure requires passive external rewarming with blankets, clothing, and warm IV fluids.

    b. Moderate exposure requires active external rewarming with hot blankets, electric heating pads, circulating warmed air adjacent to the skin, and immersion in a warm bath.

    c. Severe exposure requires active core rewarming with peritoneal or pleural lavage; gastric lavage; cardiopulmonary bypass; hemodialysis; and humidified, warmed oxygen.

  5. Provide **pharmacologic support.**

    a. Cardiac drugs and defibrillation are not effective in the presence of acidosis, hypoxia, and hypothermia.

    b. Bretylium is the only antiarrhythmic drug that is effective in the setting of hypothermia.

    c. Dopamine is the only inotrope that is effective in the setting of hypothermia.

  6. Electrical defibrillation should be attempted; however, it is unlikely to succeed until the core temperature is > 86°F (> 30°C). Atrial arrhythmias and heart block generally resolve spontaneously on rewarming.

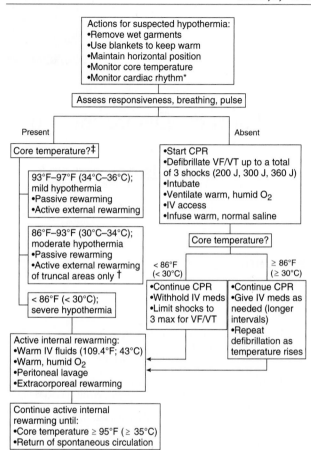

Figure 22-1. Management algorithm for suspected hypothermia. *VF* = ventricular fibrillation; *VT* = ventricular tachycardia.

The following text is contained within the figure:

Actions for suspected hypothermia:
- Remove wet garments
- Use blankets to keep warm
- Maintain horizontal position
- Monitor core temperature
- Monitor cardiac rhythm*

Assess responsiveness, breathing, pulse

Present

Core temperature?‡

93°F–97°F (34°C–36°C); mild hypothermia
- Passive rewarming
- Active external rewarming

86°F–93°F (30°C–34°C); moderate hypothermia
- Passive rewarming
- Active external rewarming of truncal areas only †

< 86°F (< 30°C); severe hypothermia

Active internal rewarming:
- Warm IV fluids (109.4°F; 43°C)
- Warm, humid O_2
- Peritoneal lavage
- Extracorporeal rewarming

Continue active internal rewarming until:
- Core temperature ≥ 95°F (≥ 35°C)
- Return of spontaneous circulation

Absent

- Start CPR
- Defibrillate VF/VT up to a total of 3 shocks (200 J, 300 J, 360 J)
- Intubate
- Ventilate warm, humid O_2
- IV access
- Infuse warm, normal saline

Core temperature?

< 86°F (< 30°C)
- Continue CPR
- Withhold IV meds
- Limit shocks to 3 max for VF/VT

≥ 86°F (≥ 30°C)
- Continue CPR
- Give IV meds as needed (longer intervals)
- Repeat defibrillation as temperature rises

* Monitoring cardiac rhythm may require needle electrodes through the skin.
† Methods of active external rewarming include electric or charcoal warming device, hot water bottles, heating pads, radiant heat source, and warming beds.
‡ The core temperature must be measured by esophageal probe.

23

Thoracic Disorders and

Thoracic Management

HEMOTHORAX

I. Etiology
   A. Penetrating trauma
   B. Blunt trauma
   C. Complication of central lines
   D. Postoperative complications

II. Clinical Presentation
   A. Blood loss into the hemithorax may lead to hypotension and hypoxia.
   B. The neck veins may be flat from severe hypovolemia or they may be distended because of the mechanical effects of the hemothorax.
   C. Physical examination reveals unilateral dullness to percussion and absence of breath sounds.

III. Management
   A. Restore volume deficits with crystalloid and type-specific blood. Continue rapid restoration of volume deficits as the chest cavity is evacuated.
   B. Insert a large thoracostomy tube (i.e., 36–40 Fr) in the fifth intercostal space along the midaxillary line, directed posteriorly. If possible, use a drainage system with a blood autotransfusion unit.
   C. Thoracotomy is required if the initial chest tube output is > 1 liter (i.e., > 20 ml/kg) or if blood loss continues at a rate of > 200 ml/hr for 2 consecutive hours.

In the management of hemothorax, the volume of blood evacuated from the chest initially is not as important as the rate of continuing blood loss.

IV. Complications. Hemothorax may develop into an empyema or fibrothorax if not properly drained. In this case, thoracotomy or thoracoscopy and decortication are required.

PNEUMOTHORAX

I. **Etiology**
   A. Rupture of blebs
   B. Positive-pressure ventilation
   C. COPD
   D. Infection (e.g., *Pneumocystis carinii* pneumonia)
   E. Lung cancer
   F. Connective tissue disease
   G. Trauma (blunt or penetrating)
   H. Endometriosis (catamenial pneumothorax)
II. **Clinical Presentation**
   A. **Tension pneumothorax** may manifest with:
      1. Tracheal deviation
      2. Distended neck veins
      3. Respiratory distress
      4. Hemodynamic instability
      5. Pulseless electrical activity
      6. Cyanosis
   B. Without tension, a **large pneumothorax** usually presents with:
      1. Shortness of breath
      2. Tachypnea
      3. Decreased oxygen saturation
      4. Chest pain
   C. Smaller pneumothoraces may not cause symptoms.
   D. Physical examination reveals decreased breath sounds over the affected lung field and hyperresonance.
III. **Diagnostic Tests**
   A. A chest radiograph will confirm the diagnosis.
   B. A CT scan of the chest may reveal a pneumothorax not visible on chest radiograph (i.e., **occult pneumothorax**). CT scan may also reveal underlying pathology.
IV. **Management**
   A. **Nonoperative management**
      1. **Tension pneumothorax**
         a. Insert a needle into the second intercostal space in the midclavicular line of the affected hemithorax to provide rapid release of pressure.
         b. Definitive treatment requires insertion of a chest tube into the fifth intercostal space anterior to the midaxillary line, directed anteriorly.
      2. **Open pneumothorax** ("sucking chest wound")
         a. Close the defect with a sterile, occlusive dressing taped securely on three sides to create a flutter-valve effect.

    b. Place a chest tube through a separate incision (i.e., away from the open wound).

  3. Large (75% of hemithorax) or symptomatic pneumothorax. Place a thoracostomy tube into the fifth intercostal space anterior to the midaxillary line.

  4. Small (10%–15% of hemithorax) or asymptomatic pneumothorax

    a. If the pneumothorax does not increase in size over a 24- to 48-hour period, discharge the patient. Follow up with serial chest radiographs as an outpatient until the pneumothorax completely resolves.

    b. If the pneumothorax increases in size over a 24- to 48-hour period, place a chest tube.

B. Operative management

  1. Indications for operative treatment include:

    a. Recurrence of pneumothorax (i.e., second episode; approximately 20% recur after treatment with a thoracostomy tube)

    b. Persistent air leak or failure of lung to reexpand for a prolonged period (i.e., > 1 week)

    c. Occupational etiology (e.g., airline pilot)

    d. Associated lung pathology (e.g., tumor, bullous lung disease)

  2. Operative treatments include:

    a. Sclerotherapy with doxycycline, talc, or bleomycin

    b. Stapling of blebs with parietal pleural abrasion

    c. Mechanical pleural abrasion

POSTTHORACOTOMY PATIENTS

I. Physiologic Considerations

  A. Thoracotomy decreases:

    1. Tidal volume

    2. Residual volume

    3. Total lung capacity

    4. Functional reserve capacity

    5. Lung compliance

  B. Chest splinting secondary to pain, retained secretions, fluid overload, and atelectasis also contribute to impaired respiratory function.

  C. Preoperative pulmonary function tests, ABG, and ventilation-perfusion (V/Q) scanning may be useful in predicting residual ventilatory function after pulmonary resection.

II. Function of Thoracostomy Tubes. Thoracostomy tubes are used to:

  A. Remove blood and air from the pleural space

  B. Drain infected spaces

  C. Prevent mediastinal shifts after pneumonectomy

  D. Enable full expansion of the lung while air leaks seal

  E. Allow immediate recognition of bleeding

III. Maintenance of Thoracostomy Tubes

A. General maintenance. Evaluate thoracostomy tubes daily for the presence of air leaks, tube patency, and amount of drainage. If drainage from the tube is < 100 ml over a 24-hour period, the tube may be removed as long as there is full lung expansion and no evidence of an air leak.

B. Maintenance after a pneumonectomy

1. Tubes placed after a pneumonectomy are clamped in the operating room and released to remove fluid or air if a mediastinal shift is apparent on a chest radiograph.

2. The tube may be removed after 48 hours if there is no evidence of an air leak or mediastinal shift.

IV. Management of Postthoracotomy Patients

A. Immediate postoperative period

1. If possible, extubate patients in the operating or recovery room. Benefits of early extubation include:

   a. Elimination of the effects of positive-pressure ventilation on the pulmonary parenchyma, especially at vulnerable sites (e.g., staple lines, bronchial stumps)

   b. Minimized need for sedation

2. Continue ventilatory support for patients with:

   a. Inability to maintain appropriate gas exchange secondary to oversedation

   b. Limited ventilatory reserve

   c. Acute pulmonary compromise (e.g., pneumonia, pulmonary edema)

   d. Extensive chest wall resections

   e. Extensive decortication

B. Prevention of complications

1. **Hypoxemia** is usually related to V/Q mismatch secondary to decreased functional residual capacity, atelectasis, and poor inspiratory effort.

   a. Maintenance of oxygenation and ventilation is required to prevent V/Q mismatch.

   b. Additional considerations include suctioning of retained secretions, aspiration precautions, and prevention of fluid overload.

2. **Atelectasis** decreases pulmonary compliance and increases the work of breathing. Remember the following when attempting to prevent atelectasis.

   a. Incentive spirometry and continuous positive airway pressure masks sustain expansion of the lungs.

   b. Adequate pain control prevents the need for splinting.

   c. Early mobilization improves functional residual capacity.

   d. Fluid management guided by a Swan-Ganz catheter may prevent fluid overload.

   e. Coughing mobilizes secretions.

   f. Endotracheal suctioning or bronchoscopy may be important for lung reexpansion.

      g. Chest physiotherapy and postural drainage may be helpful.

      h. Mucolytic agents can be used to decrease sputum viscosity.

      i. Adequate chest tube function diminishes pleural fluid and air, which improves lung expansion.

  C. Pain control. Modes of pain control include:

      1. Epidural analgesia

      2. Patient-controlled analgesia (IV or epidural)

      3. Intercostal nerve block

      4. Intrapleural analgesia (controversial benefit)

V. Complications Associated with Thoracotomy

  A. Arrhythmia

  B. Atelectasis

  C. Persistent air leak

  D. Bronchopleural and esophagopleural fistulas

  E. Empyema

  F. Pulmonary edema

  G. Lobar torsion

  H. Pulmonary and tumor embolisms

  I. Cardiac herniation

  J. Wound infections

  K. Pneumothorax (must be considered if a patient develops respiratory distress, even with thoracostomy tubes in place)

24

Toxicology

POISONINGS: OVERDOSE AND INGESTIONS

I. **Diagnosis and General Approach**
   A. **Medical history**
      1. Gather **SATS** information:
         a. **S**ubstance
         b. **A**mount ingested and route of ingestion
         c. **T**ime ingested and time last seen
         d. **S**ymptoms
      2. Gather **AMPLE** information:
         a. **A**ge
         b. **M**edications
         c. **P**ast medical history (previous substance abuse)
         d. **L**ast meal
         e. **E**vents leading to present condition(s)
      3. **Maintain a high index of suspicion for poisoning,** which should be suspected in patients who present with the following conditions:
         a. Multiple organ dysfunction
         b. Change in baseline mental status
         c. Head injury or trauma
         d. Chest pain or arrhythmias (young patient)
         e. Unexplained metabolic acidosis

   > **Poisoning should be suspected in patients who are rescued from the scene of a fire or accident at a chemical plant.**

   B. **Emergency management**
      1. **Airway.** Secure the airway while keeping the cervical spine immobilized.
      2. **Breathing**
         a. Establish that breathing is present and adequate.
         b. Evaluate the respiratory pattern.
         c. Intubate patients with any respiratory irregularities or depressed level of consciousness.

523

3. Circulation
   a. Assess pulse rate and quality and skin perfusion.
   b. Establish IV access and place the patient on continuous ECG monitoring.
   c. If hemodynamics are altered, initiate advanced cardiac life support (ACLS) protocols.
4. Blood analysis
   a. CBC, prothrombin time/partial thromboplastin time (PT/PTT), electrolytes, liver function tests, amylase/lipase, BUN/creatinine, albumin, glucose
   b. Drug levels (illicit and prescribed) [acetaminophen, acetylsalicylic acid, benzodiazepines, opioids, cannabis, barbiturates, theophylline, digoxin]
   c. ABG
   d. Immediate fingerstick for blood sugar
5. Treatment
   a. Give the following to all patients: naloxone 2 mg IV/IM, thiamine 100 mg IV. Give to all comatose patients: one ampule of 50% dextrose (avoid in patients with diabetic ketoacidosis).
   b. Consider GI decontamination (**Table 24-1**).
   c. Consider dialysis (**Table 24-2**).
   d. Give specific antidotes (**Table 24-3**).
II. Specific Drugs and Poisons
A. Acetaminophen

Table 24-1.   Toxins Not Absorbed By Charcoal
Acids
Alkalis
Bromide
Cyanide
DDT
Ethanol
Ethylene glycol
Ferrous sulfate
Iodide
Ipecac
Lithium
Iodide
Methanol
N-methylcarbamate
Potassium
Tobramycin
Tolbutamide
DDT = dichlorodiphenyltrichloroethane.

Table 24-2. Agents Not Eliminated by Dialysis
Aluminum
Benzodiazepines
Carbon tetrachloride
Chlorodiazepoxide
Chloroproamide
Cocaine
Cyanide
Cyclophosphamide
Digoxin
Hallucinogens
Iron
Isoniazid
Magnesium
Mercury
Methaqualone
Methotrexate
Narcotics
Organophosphates
PCP
Phenothiazines
Procainamide
Quinidine
Secobarbital
Tricyclic antidepressants

1. **Toxicology**
   a. **Metabolism.** Acetaminophen is metabolized by liver, where it is converted to inactive compounds that can be excreted by the kidneys. Although a minor metabolite, N-acetyl-benzoquinoneimine, is toxic, it combines with glutathione in the liver to produce a nontoxic conjugate.

> **Acetaminophen is absorbed within 2 hours. The ingestion of the drug with food, which slows gastric emptying, increases the time necessary for absorption.**

   b. **Overdose.** Hepatocellular supplies of glutathione become exhausted, resulting in acute hepatic necrosis. In addition, acute renal failure can occur as a primary or secondary insult.
   c. **Toxicity.** In adults, toxicity is likely to result from ingestion of a single dose larger than 10 g (or 140 mg/kg). A single 25-g dose is lethal.

Table 24-3. Antidotes to Specific Toxic Syndromes

Type	Antidote	Initial Dose*
Acetaminophen	N-acetylcysteine (NAC) [Mucomyst]	140 mg PO, then 70 mg/kg PO q 4 hr × 17 doses
Arsenic	BAL	4 mg/kg IM
Atropine	Physostigmine	0.5–2.0 mg over 10 min
β-Blockers	Glucagon	5–10 mg over 1 min
	Atropine	0.01 mg/kg
	Isoproterenol	2–10 μg/min, titrate to a heart rate < 60 beats/min
Botulism	Trivalent antitoxin	1–2 vials
Calcium channel blockers	Calcium chloride (10%)	1 g (10 ml) over 5 min
	Glucagon	0.1–0.3 mg/kg over 1 min as needed
	α- or β-agonists	
Carbamates	Atropine	0.4–2.0 mg
Carbon monoxide	100% oxygen	
Cyanide	Amyl nitrate	Inhale 30 sec over each min
	Sodium nitrite (3%)	0.33 ml/kg over 5 min (max 10 ml)
	Sodium thiosulfate (25%)	1.65 ml/kg over 10 min (max 50 ml)
Cyclic antidepressants	Sodium bicarbonate	0.5–2.0 mEq/kg
Digitalis	Digoxin-specific antibodies	Dose in vials = 0.009 × (serum digoxin level) × weight in kg
Ethylene glycol	Ethanol (100%)	10 ml/kg over 1 hr, then 1 ml/kg/hr to level of 100 mg/dl
Heparin	Protamine sulfate	100 mg/100 U heparin given
Insulin/oral hypoglycemics	$D_{50}W$	50–100 ml
	Glucagon	0.5–1.0 mg
Iron	Deferoxamine	15 mg/kg/hr as infusion
Lead	BAL EDTA/DMSA	Depends on clinical presentation
Magnesium	Calcium gluconate (10%)	1 g (10 ml) over 5 min
Mercury	BAL or penicillamine	4 mg/kg IM; 20–40 mg/kg/day PO

continued

Table 24-3. Antidotes to Specific Toxic Syndromes

Type	Antidote	Initial Dose*
Methanol	Ethanol (10%)	10 ml/kg over 1 hr, then 1 ml/kg/hr to a level of 100 mg/dl
Methemoglobinemia	Methylene blue	2 mg/kg
Opiates	Naloxone	0.8–2.0 mg
Organophosphates	Atropine	2 mg
	Pralidoxime	1 g over 30 min
Phenothiazines	Diphenhydramine	25–50 mg IV/IM
	Benztropine mesylate (dystonic reactions only)	1–2 mg IV/IM
Quinidine	Sodium bicarbonate	0.5–2.0 mEq/kg
Warfarin (Coumadin)	Vitamin K	10 mg over 10–30 min
	Fresh frozen plasma	As necessary
Wernicke's encephalopathy	Thiamine	100 mg

*Administered IV unless otherwise indicated.
BAL = bronchoalveolar lavage; EDTA/DMSA = ethylenediamine-tetra-acetic acid/dimercaptosuccinic acid.

Acetaminophen toxicity may be increased with fasting or as a result of chronic ingestion of barbiturates and antituberculosis medications.

---

2. Clinical presentation
   a. Symptoms and signs
      (1) Nonspecific symptoms (e.g., nausea, vomiting, anorexia, diaphoresis) with early resolution (first 12–24 hours)
      (2) Liver toxicity (onset in 1–4 days)
      (3) Right upper quadrant pain and tenderness
      (4) Myocarditis
      (5) Pancreatitis
   b. **Laboratory results:** elevated transaminases and bilirubin, prolonged coagulation times
   c. **Lethal overdose:** fulminant hepatic failure with bleeding, hypoglycemia, renal failure, hepatic encephalopathy, cerebral edema, multiple organ system failure, and death
3. **Management**

   a. Treat uncomplicated overdoses with GI decontamination and *N*-acetylcysteine (NAC), which supplies
   sulfhydryl groups to glutathione.
     (1) Give NAC enterally as a loading dose of 140 mg/kg,
       then 70 mg/kg q 4 hr for 18 doses. Dilute with fruit
       juice down to a 5% solution (stock solutions:
       10%–20%) and serve on ice. If hepatic failure de-
       velops, continue NAC indefinitely.
     (2) The risk of hepatic failure and death increases
       with delay in administration of NAC.
   b. Administer activated charcoal if within 4 hours of ingestion.
   c. Alternate NAC and charcoal. If these materials are
   coadministered, charcoal will absorb 30% of the NAC.
   d. Measure serum acetaminophen levels 4 hours after
   ingestion **(Figure 24-1)**.

**If acetaminophen ingestion has occurred within 4
hours, measurement of serum concentration does not
help assess risk, because absorption is not complete.**

---

  4. Prognosis
   a. Patients with poor prognosis must be referred for
   liver transplantation as soon as possible, before fulminant hepatic failure and associated complications
   occur.
   b. Mortality rates increase from day 2 to 4. Indicators of
   mortality include:
     (1) Acidemia (pH < 7.30)
     (2) Renal insufficiency
     (3) Grade 3 or grade 4 hepatic encephalopathy
     (4) Elevated PT
B. Salicylates
  1. Toxicology
   a. Metabolism. The liver metabolizes and eliminates a
   single dose in 3 hours. With repeated or toxic doses,
   however, hepatic enzymes are saturated, and serum
   half-life may be as long as 24 hours.
   b. Toxicity. At toxic levels, salicylates interfere with glucose metabolism by uncoupling oxidative phosphory-
   lation. The resulting acidemia is a measure of the degree of salicylate poisoning.

**In salicylate poisoning, the classic initial
disturbance is respiratory alkalosis.**

---

     (1) Mild-to-moderate toxicity. Stimulation of the
   medullary respiratory center is manifested by an
   increase in depth and rate of respiration. This results in **respiratory alkalosis** and a **compensatory
   bicarbonate diuresis.**

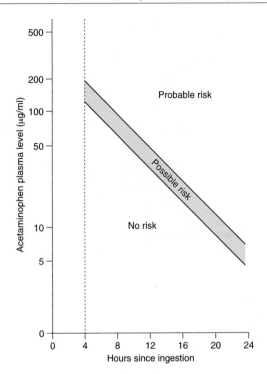

Figure 24-1. Acetaminophen overdose nomogram used to evaluate the need for treatment with N-acetylcysteine, based on time since ingestion and level on presentation. Treatment should be considered when levels fall above the area of "no risk." Determinations prior to 4 hours may not represent peak levels. (Reprinted with permission from Rumack BH: Acetaminophen overdose: 662 cases with evaluation of oral acetylcysteine treatment. *Arch Intern Med* 141[3 Spec No]:380–385, 1981.)

       (2) Severe toxicity. Primary metabolic acidosis with production of ketoacids and lactate develops. The increased acidemia allows more toxin to enter the cells.
  2. Clinical presentation

> **Chronic salicylate ingestion is often accidental and may affect patients with altered mental status.**

    a. Acute ingestion
      (1) Toxicity levels
        (a) Toxic dose: 150 mg/kg

        (b) Lethal dose: 500 mg/kg
- **(2) GI signs (appearing first):** GI bleeding from gastric mucosal irritation, possible gastric perforation
- **(3) CNS signs and symptoms:** tinnitus, hearing impairment, diaphoresis, irritability, hyperventilation

   b. Chronic ingestion. This is more deadly because of the chronically elevated tissue levels, which may have caused baseline cellular dysfunction. **Signs and symptoms** include:

- **(1)** Hyperventilation, anxiety, agitation, and hallucinations, which mimic psychiatric disorders
- **(2)** Abdominal pain and vomiting
- **(3)** Metabolic acidosis and ketonuria, which may be confused with diabetic ketoacidosis
- **(4)** Clinical course that may mimic sepsis, with fever, leukocytosis, pulmonary infiltrates, encephalopathy, coagulopathy, and hypotension

3. Diagnosis
   a. Determine the serum salicylate level (**Figure 24-2**).

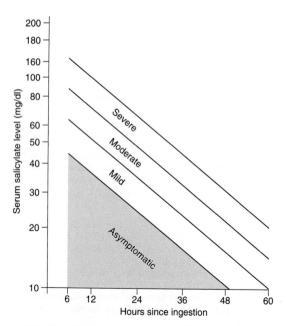

Figure 24-2. Salicylate overdose nomogram used to estimate the severity of salicylate overdose, based on time since ingestion and level on presentation. (Reprinted with permission from Done AK: *Pediatrics* 26:800, 1960.)

b. Interpret salicylate levels cautiously. The therapeutic level is 10–20 mg/dl; a level above 25 mg/dl may be tolerated in an acute ingestion but may have severe manifestations in a chronic overdose.

The serum salicylate values must be interpreted cautiously in conjunction with clinical status and serum pH. A falling salicylate level in the presence of acidemia is a sign of diffusion of salicylate into cells rather than clearance from the body.

---

4. **Management**
   a. Use supportive measures such as resuscitation with volume and administration of sodium bicarbonate.
   b. Promote salicylate clearance and prevent further absorption.
      (1) Administer activated charcoal, 1 g/kg, for acute ingestion. Add sorbitol to the first dose to reduce further absorption. Repeat frequently.
      (2) Perform gastric lavage in between charcoal administrations if within 4 hours of ingestion.
   c. Treat moderate-to-severe toxicity in acute or chronic ingestion.
      (1) First stabilize airway, ventilation, and vital signs.
      (2) Correct temperature dysregulation.
      (3) Provide aggressive fluid resuscitation. Marked diuresis occurs as a result of the respiratory alkalosis and ketosis.
      (4) Maintain the serum pH between 7.45 and 7.5. Administer sodium bicarbonate, 1–2 mmol/kg IV hourly, as needed to control pH.
      (5) Replace potassium aggressively.
      (6) Maintain adequate serum glucose with frequent monitoring.
   d. Perform charcoal hemoperfusion or dialysis.
C. **Tricyclic antidepressants (TCAs)**
   1. **Toxicology**
      a. Metabolism. TCAs are readily absorbed from the GI tract by body tissues. The half-life of these agents, which usually bind to plasma proteins, is 3 hours to 3 days.
      b. Toxicity. Ingestion of > 10 mg/kg leads to toxicity.
   2. **Clinical presentation**
      a. Anticholinergic effects (occur in mild overdoses or in the acute phases of severe ingestion)
         (1) Mydriasis, blurred vision, dry mouth, hyperpyrexia
         (2) Sinus tachycardia
         (3) Ileus, urinary retention
         (4) Agitation, psychosis
      b. Other severe signs
         (1) Hypotension, arrhythmias

       (2) Coma, seizures

       (3) Noncardiogenic pulmonary edema, aspiration

       (4) Syndrome of inappropriate secretion of antidiuretic hormone (SIADH)

       (5) Neuroleptic malignant syndrome

  3. Management

    a. Closely monitor for cardiac arrhythmias and cardiovascular collapse.

      (1) Monitor heart block and bradyarrhythmias, which do not routinely respond to atropine. Use temporary pacing in high-degree block.

      (2) Use isoproterenol to maintain cardiac rhythm while providing temporary pacing.

      (3) Treat hypotension initially with fluid and sodium bicarbonate. If there is no response, start vasopressors.

    b. Provide GI decontamination with activated charcoal and a cathartic or gastric lavage.

    c. Administer sodium bicarbonate, which may antagonize the quinidine-like effect of the TCAs on myocardial conduction and help resolve arrhythmias. Maintain pH at 7.5 (avoid acidosis).

    d. Treat anticholinergic effects. Physostigmine, which has been advocated, may transiently improve these symptoms but may potentially precipitate seizures, bradycardia, asystole, and vomiting.

D. Antipsychotic drug toxicity

  1. Clinical presentation

    a. Acute dystonia: spasms of the muscles of the tongue, face, neck, and back

    b. Akathisia: motor restlessness

    c. Parkinsonism: bradykinesia, rigidity, mask facies, tremor, shuffling gait

    d. Neuroleptic malignant syndrome: fever, rigidity, unstable blood pressure

    e. Perioral tremor (rare, late finding)

    f. Tardive dyskinesia: oral-facial dyskinesia (rare, late finding)

    g. Other effects: anticholinergic toxicity, priapism, agranulocytosis, photosensitivity, lower seizure threshold

  2. Management

    a. Treatment is largely **supportive.**

      (1) Stabilize the airway.

      (2) Administer activated charcoal.

      (3) Provide fluid hydration.

    b. Treatment for **acute dystonic reactions** includes the following:

      (1) Discontinue the antipsychotic drug.

      (2) Administer diphenhydramine, 25–50 mg IV/IM, or benztropine mesylate, 1–2 g IV/IM.

E. Benzodiazepines

1. **Toxicology and clinical presentation**
   a. **Metabolism.** Benzodiazepines are rapidly absorbed from the GI tract with primarily hepatic metabolism. Although the half-life may range from hours to days, it is usually short with acute overdoses.
   b. **Signs and symptoms.** Manifestations of overdose are usually mild.
      (1) Dizziness, weakness, disorientation, somnolence
      (2) Possible cerebellar dysfunction with ataxia, dysarthria, and diplopia
   c. **Synergistic effects.** Benzodiazepines, which are often part of a multidrug overdose with ethanol, narcotics, or TCAs, promote the depressant effects of these drugs, leading to **respiratory failure.**

2. **Management**
   a. Assess for use of other drugs, and admit to the ICU if the toxicity is part of a multidrug overdose.
   b. Rule out hypoxemia and hypoglycemia.
   c. Provide GI decontamination with activated charcoal. Give the first dose with a cathartic.
   d. Consider administration of flumazenil, a benzodiazepine antagonist. This may be diagnostic and therapeutic (not first-line therapy).
      (1) Reliable reversal of the benzodiazepine effect on CNS depression
      (2) Dose: 0.3–0.5 mg IV q 30 sec up to a total dose of 3 mg
      (3) Possible risk of resedation, because the half-life is 1 hour
      (4) Side effects including nausea, vomiting, and pain at the injection site
      (5) Possible removal of protective effect of benzodiazepine
         (a) Initiation of withdrawal in chronic user
         (b) Occurrence of seizures in patients with epilepsy who have taken other seizure-causing drugs
         (c) Ventricular tachycardia in patients who have ingested chloral hydrate or a TCA

F. β-Blockers

1. **Toxicology**
   a. Stimulation of β_1-receptors in the heart, kidney, and eye causes increased inotropy and chronotropy, increased renin secretion, and increased production of aqueous humor.
   b. Stimulation of β_2-receptors in the vascular, uterine, intestinal, and bronchial smooth muscle results in smooth muscle relaxation. β_2-Receptors in the liver and pancreas affect lipogenesis, gluconeogenesis, and insulin release.

2. **Clinical presentation** (often dependent on medical history and drug ingested)
   a. **Cardiac signs**
      (1) Bradycardia, delay in myocardial conduction, decreased contractility (most drugs)
      (2) First-degree block, interventricular conduction delays, bundle branch block, atrioventricular (AV) dissociation
      (3) Hypotension due to decreased contractility
      (4) CHF and pulmonary edema in patients with underlying cardiac disease
   b. **CNS signs:** lethargy, stupor, coma, seizures
3. **Specific management**
   a. Perform gastric emptying, using activated charcoal.
   b. Administer glucagon, 5 mg bolus IV, then 1–5 mg/hr by continuous infusion, for reversal of bradycardia and myocardial depression. Prepare it in dextrose; do not use the diluent (phenol) that comes with the drug.
   c. Provide cardiac pacing for resistant bradycardia.
   d. Provide cardiovascular support with intra-aortic balloon pump.

G. Calcium channel blockers

1. **Toxicology**
   a. Clinical effects are apparent in 30–60 minutes.
   b. Overdoses of 5–10 times the therapeutic dose are toxic.

2. **Clinical presentation**
   a. Cardiac manifestations
      (1) Hypotension resulting from peripheral vasodilation and myocardial depression (verapamil, nifedipine)
      (2) Arrhythmia, including bradycardia, second- and third-degree heart block, sinus arrest, asystole
   b. Pulmonary edema
   c. Lethargy and confusion; coma from cerebral hypoperfusion
   d. Nausea and vomiting; hyperglycemia

3. **Management**
   a. Perform gastric lavage or catharsis.
   b. Use activated charcoal; repeat doses in case of sustained-release preparations of calcium channel blockers.
   c. Perform whole bowel lavage with polyethylene glycol.
   d. Treat hypotension with volume infusion and IV calcium. The amount of calcium required depends on ingestion.
      (1) Start with 0.2 ml/kg of 10% calcium chloride IV over 5 minutes.
      (2) Repeat every 15–20 minutes to a total of 4 doses. Check serum level after first 30 minutes and then every 2 hours.

     e. Administer glucagon, 3.5–5 mg IV, followed by an infusion of 1–5 mg/hr.

     f. Treat refractory hypotension with pressor agents.

     g. Use isoproterenol to increase heart rate or cardiac pacing. Atropine is often ineffective for bradycardia.

H. Digitalis

  1. Toxicology. Digitalis acts by decreasing activity of the Na^+-K^+–ATPase pump, secondarily increasing intracellular calcium. Patients with the following conditions are particularly subject to digitalis toxicity.

     a. Renal insufficiency. A lower dose of digitalis is effective in this condition, because the volume of distribution is lower.

     b. Electrolyte abnormalities include hypomagnesemia (causes arrhythmias) and hypercalcemia (causes ventricular arrhythmias).

     c. Thyroid abnormalities. Digoxin clearance is abnormal in patients who are hypothyroid, and the volume of distribution is increased in those who are hyperthyroid.

  2. Clinical presentation

     a. Possible hypoxemia and hypercapnia, which may predispose to arrhythmias, in patients with severe respiratory disease

     b. Increased risk of arrhythmias from β_2-agonists

     c. Cardiac signs

        (1) AV junctional block and increased ventricular automaticity

        (2) Prolonged AV nodal refractory period, paroxysmal atrial tachycardia, sinus arrest, premature ventricular contractions, ventricular tachycardia, or ventricular failure

     d. Headaches, visual disturbances, confusion, fatigue, anorexia

  3. Management

     a. Give atropine for sinus arrest, bradycardia, and AV block.

     b. Provide temporary cardiac pacing.

     c. Administer digoxin-specific Fab fragments.

        (1) The large volume of distribution of these high-affinity polyclonal antibodies effectively removes digoxin from the myocardium and other binding sites.

        (2) Digoxin-specific Fab fragments are indicated in severely intoxicated patients with serious arrhythmias.

        (3) Give 800 mg IV over 30 minutes for massive overdose and severe toxicity. Consider using a bolus if cardiac arrest is imminent. Serum levels are unreliable for days after administration.

I. Theophylline

1. **Clinical presentation**
    a. Therapeutic range = 10–20 mg/L
    b. **Acute intoxication**
        (1) Adrenergic and CNS hyperstimulation, with irritability, agitation, confusion, and uncontrollable seizures

---

Seizures due to theophylline toxicity may lead to coma, hypoventilatory respiratory failure, rhabdomyolysis, and compartment syndrome.

---

   (2) Hypotension
   (3) Dyspnea, respiratory alkalosis
   (4) Leukocytosis
   (5) Hypokalemia, hypophosphatemia, hypomagnesemia, hyperglycemia
   (6) Cardiac arrhythmias such as sinus tachycardia, atrial fibrillation, paroxysmal supraventricular tachycardia, and multifocal premature ventricular contractions
    c. **Chronic intoxication**
        (1) Potentially lethal manifestations occur at lower serum levels than in acute intoxication.
        (2) Nausea, vomiting, and tachycardia may not be present.
        (3) Hypotension, electrolyte abnormalities, or rhabdomyolysis are unlikely.
2. **Management**
    a. **Systemic support**
        (1) Administer β-blockers (propranolol or esmolol) for cardiac toxicity.
        (2) Give lidocaine for ventricular tachycardia.
        (3) Treat hypotension with volume infusion first.
        (4) Treat seizures, which are usually prolonged, recurrent, and resistant to therapy.
            (a) Give loading dose of phenobarbital.
            (b) Give benzodiazepines to terminate seizures.
        (5) Replace potassium conservatively. Rebound hyperkalemia may develop once theophylline toxicity is resolved.
    b. **GI decontamination**
        (1) Provide prompt gastric lavage if within 2 hours of ingestion or longer with sustained-release preparations
        (2) Administer activated charcoal, 20–40 g q 2 hr, several times to reduce systemic symptoms of the absorbed drug until the theophylline level is < 25 mg/L. This shortens the half-life of the drug by 50%.
        (3) Give cathartics.

      (4) Administer antiemetics to permit GI decontamination.

   c. In instances of **severe poisoning,** with rising levels of theophylline and GI decompression, use extracorporeal decontamination.

      (1) Use hemoperfusion (procedure of choice) or hemodialysis.

      (2) Attempt before severe life-threatening events occur.

        (a) Start at serum levels of 60–100 mg/L in acute poisoning or 30–60 mg/L in chronic poisoning.

        (b) Continue until theophylline level is < 25 mg/L.

J. Alcohols. Low-molecular-weight aliphatic alcohols include methanol, ethylene glycol, and isopropanol. (See SUBSTANCE ABUSE AND WITHDRAWAL, p 540, for discussion of ethanol intoxication.)

  1. General overview of alcohols

   a. Toxicity. These agents are weak toxins on their own, which cause gastric irritation, inebriation, and CNS depression.

      (1) They are metabolized by the hepatic enzyme alcohol dehydrogenase to metabolites of varying toxicities.

      (2) Alcohol dehydrogenase has a higher affinity for ethanol. Thus, an ethanol level > 100 mg/dl virtually "turns off" metabolism of these other alcohols, forcing methanol and ethylene glycol to be metabolized by nonhepatic routes.

   b. Presence of an osmolar gap. Differential diagnosis includes alcohol ingestion, ketotic states, hyperlipidemia, and hyperproteinemia.

   c. Management. Diagnosis and treatment should be prompt. Treatment of inebriation is supportive.

  2. Methanol

   a. Toxicology

      (1) Metabolism. Alcohol dehydrogenase metabolizes methanol to formaldehyde, which is further metabolized by aldehyde dehydrogenase to formic acid. Metabolism of formic acid (with folate as a cofactor) leads to carbon dioxide.

      (2) Toxicity. Small quantities (30 ml or 0.4 ml/kg) may result in significant morbidity and mortality because of metabolites.

        (a) Absorption through the skin or lungs may lead to toxicity.

        (b) High anion gap acidosis occurs. As acidemia develops, formic acid concentrates in the eyes and CNS.

b. Clinical presentation

(1) Early symptoms (< 12 hours after ingestion): nausea, vomiting, abdominal pain, headache, vertigo

(2) Serious manifestations (12–24 hours after ingestion): stupor, coma, respiratory arrest

(3) Ocular damage: edema and inflammation

    (a) Patient complaints: snowstorms or flashes before the eyes

    (b) Diminished visual acuity

    (c) Visual field defects

    (d) Fixed or dilated pupils

(4) CNS damage (occurs at higher levels): cerebral dysfunction (e.g., stupor, coma, seizures), which may be irreversible

c. Diagnosis

(1) Confirmation by methanol level

(2) High suspicion (metabolic acidosis)

d. Management

(1) Correct acidosis. Consider using sodium bicarbonate.

(2) Administer ethanol to slow the breakdown of methanol. An ethanol level of 13–30 mg/dl fully saturates alcohol dehydrogenase, effectively "turning off" production of metabolites.

    (a) Use the recommended dose: 10% solution 0.6–0.8 g/kg IV bolus over 30–60 minutes, followed by a maintenance dose of 0.08–0.15 g/kg/hr. [The enteral preparation (20%–40%) may be used.]

    (b) Continue before and after dialysis, and try to maintain an ethanol level of 100–200 mg/dl.

(3) Accelerate removal with hemodialysis. Indications include:

    (a) Serum methanol level > 50 mg/dl

    (b) Ingestion of potentially lethal amount

    (c) Presence of significant or refractory metabolic acidosis

    (d) Evidence of neurologic or ocular dysfunction

(4) Continue dialysis until acidosis resolves and the serum methanol level is < 25 mg/dl. The level may rebound from equilibration with intracellular stores. Dialysis removes ethanol, which must be replaced. Add ethanol, 100–200 mg/dl, to the dialysate or increase the maintenance rate by 0.25–0.35 mg/kg/hr.

3. Ethylene glycol

a. Toxicology. This component of antifreeze, solvents, paints, and lacquer has a sweet and pleasant taste that encourages ingestion.

(1) **Metabolism.** Ethylene glycol is rapidly absorbed in the GI tract, reaching peak levels in 2 hours.

      (2) **Toxicity.** Ingestion of 1.0–1.5 ml/kg can be fatal to an adult. Like methanol, ethylene glycol may produce severe delayed toxicity.

  b. Clinical presentation

    (1) Within 12 hours: acute inebriation

    (2) Within 12–18 hours

      (a) Metabolic acidosis

      (b) CNS dysfunction: hallucinations, encephalopathy, seizures, coma

      (c) Ocular motility is affected, with papilledema and diminished visual acuity

      (d) Cardiopulmonary: hypertension, tachycardia, arrhythmias, myocardial dysfunction, shock

      (e) ARDS

    (3) Within 24–72 hours

      (a) Renal failure (calcium oxalate crystals and RBCs on urinalysis)

      (b) Precipitation of calcium oxalate in tissues (possible)

    (4) Within 6–18 days: cranial nerve palsies

  c. Diagnosis

> **Ethylene glycol poisoning must be diagnosed early to avoid irreparable damage.**

    (1) Obtain a serum ethylene glycol level.

    (2) Use the following list of features to make a clinical diagnosis if an ethylene glycol level cannot be obtained.

      (a) Inebriation

      (b) Elevated ethanol level

      (c) Elevated serum osmolar gap

      (d) High anion gap acidosis

      (e) Hypocalcemia

      (f) Calcium oxalate crystals in urine

      (g) Fluorescence from Wood's lamp evaluation of skin, urine, or gastric contents (from sodium fluorescein)

  d. Management

    (1) Provide GI decontamination within the first 2 hours.

    (2) Correct acidosis with sodium bicarbonate.

    (3) Administer ethanol to halt production of toxic metabolites.

    (4) Perform dialysis; 12 hours of continuous dialysis may be necessary to remove toxins. Indications include an ethylene glycol level > 20–50 mg/dl, significant acidosis, renal failure, or cardiovascular deterioration.

    (5) Provide supplemental pyridoxine and thiamine,

which are cofactors in the metabolism of some toxic metabolites.

    (a) Pyridoxine, 50 mg IM q 4 hr for 2 days

    (b) Thiamine, 100 mg IM q 4 hr for 2 days

4. Isopropanol

  a. Toxicology

    (1) Metabolism. Alcohol dehydrogenase metabolizes most isopropanol to acetone, which is excreted slowly via the kidneys (urine), lungs (breath), and liver (bile).

      (a) GI absorption occurs rapidly (within 30 minutes).

      (b) The half-life of isopropanol is 8–26 hours.

    (2) Toxicity. Found in rubbing alcohol, skin lotions, and window cleaners, isopropanol is a potent CNS depressant.

      (a) Ingestion of 2–4 ml/kg or 200 ml of 70% solution is potentially lethal.

      (b) Toxicity may arise from extensive dermal contact or via inhalation.

  b. Clinical presentation

    (1) CNS depression (prolonged): headache, dizziness, blurred vision, weakness, ataxia, nystagmus, dysarthria, areflexia or hyperreflexia, confusion, cognitive deficits

    (2) GI effects: nausea, vomiting, abdominal pain

    (3) Cardiovascular effects: hypotension from hypovolemia (fluid loss), vasodilation, or myocardial depression

> **Acidosis is not characteristic of isopropanol poisoning, except in cases of concomitant lactic acidosis secondary to hypovolemia.**

    (4) High serum creatinine levels (falsely elevated because of high levels of acetone)

  c. Management

    (1) Provide supportive care.

    (2) Perform GI lavage if within first few hours.

    (3) Perform hemodialysis in severe ingestion associated with coma, refractory hypotension, or isopropanol levels > 400 mg/dl.

SUBSTANCE ABUSE AND WITHDRAWAL

I. Ethanol

  A. Toxicology

    1. Metabolism. Ethanol is chiefly degraded in the liver. Most individuals can metabolize about 150 mg/kg/hr (15–20 mg/dl per hour in nonalcoholics; 40 mg/dl in alcoholics).

2. Acute toxicity

a. Clinical manifestations

(1) **CNS:** decreased inhibition, slow reaction time, visual disturbances, incoordination, slurred speech, lethargy, stupor, coma

(2) **Cardiovascular:** vasodilation, arrhythmias, myocardial depression

(3) **Respiratory:** hypoventilation, aspiration

(4) **Metabolic:** hypoglycemia, hypophosphatemia, hypomagnesemia, acidosis

(5) **GI:** gastritis, peptic ulcers, pancreatitis, hepatitis, GI bleeding

(6) **Bone marrow suppression**

b. Toxicity levels

(1) Most persons exhibit gross intoxication at levels > 150 mg/dl.

(2) Obtundation occurs at levels > 300 mg/d, and death may result from respiratory and cardiovascular collapse at levels > 400–500 mg/dl.

c. Acid–base disorders

(1) Respiratory acidosis and hypoventilation due to depression of respiratory centers occur in intoxicated patients.

(2) Nausea and vomiting may cause hypokalemia and metabolic alkalosis.

(3) Alcoholic ketoacidosis may develop in chronic alcoholics.

3. Chronic ingestion

a. Chronic use depresses central α- and β-adrenergic receptors. The CNS increases neuronal activity to compensate. When alcohol consumption stops, this enhanced neuronal activity leads to the hyperadrenergic state that causes the symptoms characteristic of withdrawal.

b. Centrally acting α_2-agonists such as clonidine have been shown to ameliorate the adrenergically mediated signs and symptoms of alcohol withdrawal.

c. Treatment with high doses of benzodiazepines has been used but often has only a moderate effect. Some patients can tolerate very large ingestions without assistance.

B. Treatment of acute intoxication

1. Provide supportive therapy.

2. Draw stat blood chemistries (including ethanol level), ABG, and fingerstick blood glucose

3. Administer thiamine, 50–100 mg IM; $D_{50}W$, 1 ampule IV; and naloxone, 2 mg IV, to patients with altered mental status.

a. If the patient responds, then start IV with $D_{10}W$ continuous infusion. Evaluate blood glucose levels with fingerstick measurements.

  b. If the patient is obtunded or comatose, then *intubate*.
  4. Correct hypothermia and electrolyte imbalances.
C. Withdrawal: symptoms, prophylaxis, and treatment
  1. Minor withdrawal
   a. Symptoms. These conditions appear within a few hours after reduction or cessation of alcoholic consumption and resolve in 48 hours.
     (1) Tremulousness, irritability
     (2) Anorexia
     (3) Nausea
   b. Withdrawal prophylaxis. Use one of the following:
     (1) Lorazepam, 0.5–2.0 mg PO/IV q 6 hr
     (2) Diazepam, 5–20 mg PO q 6 hr
     (3) Chlordiazepoxide, 25–100 mg PO q 6 hr
   c. Treatment of alcohol withdrawal. Use one of the following:
     (1) Lorazepam, 2 mg q 6 hr for 4 doses, then 1 mg q 6 hr for 8 doses
     (2) Diazepam, 10 mg q 6 hr for 4 doses, then 5 mg q 6 hr for 8 doses
     (3) Chlordiazepoxide, 50 mg q 6 hr for 4 doses, then 25 mg q 6 hr for 8 doses
   d. Additional replacements for patients with intoxication
     (1) Multivitamins, 1 PO qd
     (2) Folate, 1 mg PO qd
     (3) Thiamine, 100 mg IM qd for 3 days, then 100 mg PO qd
  2. Alcohol withdrawal seizures. These self-limited seizures, which tend to be tonic-clonic (grand mal), occur between 6 and 48 hours after the last ethanol use.
  3. Delirium tremens (DTs)
   a. Onset: usually 2–5 days after the last use
   b. Symptoms
     (1) Tremor
     (2) Confusion, disorientation
     (3) Delusions, hallucinations
     (4) Tachycardia, hypertension
     (5) Hyperreflexia
     (6) Cardiovascular collapse. During the DTs, the CI increases by 36%, and oxygen delivery and consumption are both 25% higher.
     (7) Seizures. The more times a patient has experienced detoxification or DTs, the higher the risk of tonic-clonic (grand mal) seizures.

> **An underlying cerebral insult such as trauma is possible in an alcoholic patient. This may need to be investigated if mental status remains altered. A subacute subdural hematoma may go unnoticed.**

   c. Treatment

        (1) ICU monitoring

        (2) IV fluids

        (3) Cooling blanket if patients are hyperthermic

        (4) Benzodiazepines

II. Cocaine

A. General aspects

1. Means of administration

    a. Intranasal snorting involves placing 30–60 mg in each nostril. The euphoria lasts 1–5 hours after the last administration.

    b. Smoking free-base cocaine may occur either through a pipe or in a cigarette rolled with tobacco. The vaporized cocaine is absorbed by the pulmonary vascular bed, and the euphoria lasts 20–30 minutes.

    c. IV administration involves injection of 16–32 mg alone or in combination with heroin ("speedball").

2. Actions. Major neurochemical actions of cocaine include the following:

    a. CNS stimulation with release of dopamine

    b. Inhibition of neuronal catechol uptake with resultant sympathetic stimulation

    c. Release or blockade of serotonin uptake

    d. Inhibition of sodium current in neuronal tissue, resulting in a local anesthetic effect

B. Toxicity

1. Cocaine hydrochloride numbs the tongue, lips, nose, and other mucosal surfaces. Most mucosal surfaces absorb cocaine.

2. In large doses, cocaine may cause a generalized impairment of neuronal impulse transmission, leading to coma, respiratory depression, and respiratory arrest.

3. At low doses, cocaine leads to stimulation with euphoria.

4. Excessive CNS stimulation may occur. CNS manifestations include tremulousness, agitation, sleeplessness, paranoia, and frank psychosis. Aggressive behavior is common with overdose.

5. Cocaine lowers the seizure threshold. Seizures are usually short and self-limited; sustained or repeated seizures suggest hyperthermia, intracranial hemorrhage, metabolic abnormality, or massive intake of cocaine ("body packers").

6. Intracranial effects include stroke, transient ischemic attacks, subarachnoid hemorrhage, cerebral infarction, or cerebral atrophy with chronic use.

7. Cocaine inhibits neuronal uptake of norepinephrine, leading to intense vasoconstriction and even end-organ ischemia.

8. Cocaine may induce myocardial infarction (MI). Attacks are manifested by chest pain, often within 30 minutes of use of IV cocaine, 90 minutes of smoking cocaine, or 120 minutes of intranasal cocaine. Acute MI results from thrombus formation.

> ### Chronic cocaine use may cause CHF, cardiomyopathy, or silent ischemia.

   a. The ischemia is due to α-adrenergic coronary vasoconstriction, which is worsened by β-adrenergic
   blockers.
   b. The mainstay of treatment is oxygen. Aspirin and nitroglycerin provide pain relief. If pain persists, patients may be candidates for thrombolytic therapy.
   c. Phentolamine is the drug of choice to decrease
   cocaine-induced myocardial ischemia. Start with 5
   mg IM/IV and titrate to effect.
   9. Cocaine is highly arrhythmogenic in large quantities.
   10. **Severe hypertension may occur,** leading to subarachnoid hemorrhage, stroke, intracerebral bleed, or MI.
   11. **Hypoventilation and respiratory depression may lead to
   respiratory arrest.**

> ### Septic pulmonary emboli and pulmonary vascular obstruction may result from foreign body granulomas or angiothrombosis secondary to IV abuse.

   12. Cocaine snorting and crack inhalation may lead to pneumomediastinum or pneumothorax.
   13. Hyperpyrexia from muscle hyperactivity and rhabdomyolysis is common
 C. **Treatment of acute intoxication**
   1. Stabilize and closely monitor airway and cardiac
   rhythm.
   2. Administer benzodiazepines for agitation, psychosis,
   and seizures associated with cocaine overdose.
   a. Diazepam: 5–20 mg IV
   b. Lorazepam: 2–4 mg IV
   c. Midazolam: 5–10 mg IV
   3. Induce paralysis, if necessary, for patients with persistent muscle hyperactivity or severe hyperthermia.
   a. Pancuronium, 0.1 mg/kg IV
   b. Vecuronium, 0.1 mg/kg IV (better suited for patients
   with tachyarrhythmias or unstable cardiac status)
   4. If seizures have caused the hyperactivity or hyperthermia or there is a possibility of seizures, use continuous
   EEG monitoring.
   5. Treat cocaine-intoxicated patients with elevated blood
   pressure with nitroprusside, labetalol, or phentolamine.
 D. **Withdrawal.** Clinical manifestations include the following:
   1. Depression, irritability
   2. Sleep and appetite dysfunction
   3. Intense desire for cocaine
   4. Necessity of cocaine for sensation of well-being
III. Opioids

A. **Toxicity**
   1. **Administration.** IV (mainlining), IM, SC, and intradermal (skin popping) routes are used.

Illicit opioids for IV injection are rarely pure. Mixed with microcrystalline cellulose, talc, or cellulose, they may produce angiothrombosis or foreign body granulomas or induce endocarditis and septic emboli.

---

   2. **Clinical presentation.** Toxic manifestations are mediated by μ receptors in the CNS. The typical presentation of intoxication involves coma, miotic pupils, and shallow respirations.
      a. Other CNS effects such as seizures or apathy
      b. Bronchospasm, urticaria, and pruritus as a result of opioid-induced release of histamine from mast cells
      c. Respiratory complications such as aspiration, pulmonary edema, pulmonary hypertension, ARDS
      d. Preload reduction, decreased cardiac output, and hypotension as the result of venous capacitance dilation
      e. Constipation and urinary retention
B. **Treatment of acute intoxication**
   1. Stabilize the airway (essential). Maintain adequate oxygenation and ventilation.
   2. Administer naloxone to antagonize the effects of opioids. This drug has a short half-life (20–30 minutes) and may need to be readministered at regular intervals until opioids have been completely metabolized.
      a. Dosage
         (1) Patients without respiratory depression: 0.4–0.8 mg IV
         (2) Patients with signs of ventilatory depression: 2 mg IV
      b. It may be necessary to repeat these doses every 4 minutes to total dose of 20 mg. If no effect is evident after 20 mg, other etiologies of respiratory depression must be sought.
C. **Withdrawal: symptoms and treatment**
   1. **Clinical presentation**
      a. **Early (4–10 hours):** yawning, lacrimation, rhinorrhea, sneezing, sweating
      b. **Intermediate (12–18 hours):** restless sleep, piloerection, restlessness, irritability, anorexia, flushing, tachycardia, tremor, hyperthermia
      c. **Late (> 24 hours):** fever, nausea, vomiting, abdominal pain, diarrhea, difficulty sleeping, muscle spasm, joint pain, involuntary ejaculation, suicidal thoughts
   2. **Treatment**
      a. **Buprenorphine**
         (1) This semisynthetic partial opioid agonist (mixed agonist antagonist) has high affinity but low ac-

tivity at the μ-opioid receptor. Toxicity is low because μ-antagonistic effects limit the opioid effects of sedation, respiratory depression, and hypotension.

(2) When taken chronically, buprenorphine produces less physical dependence than pure agonists (methadone), but addiction is possible.

    (a) Remember that 2–4 mg of buprenorphine is equivalent to 20–30 mg of methadone.

    (b) The features of buprenorphine withdrawal are prolonged (8–10 days) but much less intense compared to those associated with methadone.

b. Clonidine, 15–20 μg/kg, can suppress the signs and symptoms of opiate withdrawal within 24 hours. This agent shortens acute withdrawal reactions by 3–4 days.

Transplantation

ALLOGRAFT REJECTION

I. **Definitions**
   A. **Types of allograft rejection**
      1. Humoral (antibody–mediated)
      2. Cellular (T lymphocyte–mediated)
   B. **Classification of allograft rejection**
      1. Hyperacute rejection
      2. Accelerated acute rejection
      3. Acute rejection
      4. Chronic rejection

II. **Hyperacute rejection.** Grafts that involve cardiac and renal tissue are particularly susceptible.
   A. **Onset:** < 48 hours (often within minutes of reperfusion of the transplant). Classically, it appears immediately after unclamping vessels with intraoperative vascular thrombosis.
   B. **Pathophysiology**
      1. Preformed cytotoxic antibodies are deposited onto the vascular endothelium.
         a. Anti-HLA: most common cause in the rare instances of hyperacute rejection of liver transplants
         b. Antivascular endothelium
         c. Isohemagglutinins against ABO blood group antigens
      2. Aggregation of antibodies results in complement activation with platelet and fibrin aggregation and thrombosis of the graft.
   C. **Graft function:** none
   D. **Diagnosis:** ultrasound of graft vessels to rule out thrombosis

III. **Accelerated Acute Rejection**
   A. **Onset:** 7–10 days
   B. **Mechanisms:** cellular and humoral
      1. Possibly due to anti-HLA antibodies
      2. T lymphocyte–mediated, likely the result of prior sensitization
   C. **Graft function:** failure

> **With accelerated acute allograft rejection,
> the rate of graft loss is 60% or more.**

IV. **Acute Rejection**
  A. **Onset:** most commonly 7 days–3 months after transplantation, with possible occurrence at any time after loss of effective immunosuppression
  B. **Mechanisms:** cellular and humoral
  C. **Clinical presentation**
    1. **Surveillance laboratory testing** usually detects the condition before symptoms begin to develop.
    2. **Signs and symptoms** are rarely seen unless immunosuppression is poorly monitored.
        a. Graft pain, swelling, or warmth
        b. Fever
        c. Malaise and fatigue
        d. Signs of reduced graft function by organ
            (1) Renal: edema, weight gain, hypertension
            (2) Hepatic: hepatosplenomegaly, ascites, oligobilia, elevated transaminases
            (3) Cardiac: arrhythmia, hypotension, dyspnea
            (4) Pancreatic: elevated serum trypsinogen, decreased urinary amylase (if bladder drainage), hyperglycemia (late effect; infiltration of islets can be less severe than rest of pancreas)
  D. **Diagnostic tests**
    1. **Ultrasound**
    2. **Biopsy**
        a. **Heart transplant.** Grades of rejection and associated biopsy findings are:
            (1) **Mild:** mild perivascular lymphocytic infiltrate with edema
            (2) **Moderate:** increased infiltrate extending into the interstitium
            (3) **Severe:** diffuse infiltrate with neutrophils, hemorrhage, and necrosis
        b. **Liver transplant.** Mild inflammation with focal damage to < 50% of the bile ducts is nondiagnostic. Grades of rejection and associated biopsy findings are:
            (1) **Mild:** portal infiltrate, endothelialitis, < 50% of bile ducts damaged
            (2) **Moderate:** portal infiltrate, endothelialitis, > 50% of bile ducts damaged
            (3) **Severe:** arteritis, centrilobular ischemia, and/or paucity of bile ducts
        c. **Pancreatic transplant** (mononuclear infiltrate, endovasculitis, glandular invasion, blunted epithelium, vascular occlusion, necrosis)
        d. **Lung transplant.** Grades of rejection and associated biopsy findings are:

      (1) Minimal: slight perivascular lymphocytic infiltrate

      (2) Mild: perivascular and subendothelial infiltrate

      (3) Moderate: dense perivascular infiltrate with extension into the alveolar septa and air spaces

      (4) Severe: diffuse mononuclear infiltrate surrounding blood vessels and extending into the interstitium and alveolar air spaces

    e. Kidney transplant (lymphocytic infiltrate, interstitial edema, tubulitis, vasculitis, more frequent involvement of cortex than medulla, glomerular thrombosis, cortical infarcts, hemorrhage)

E. Management. Treatment options include:

    1. Corticosteroids

    2. Monoclonal anti–T cell antibody (OKT3)

    3. Antithymocyte globulin (ATG)

V. Chronic Rejection

A. Onset: months to years after transplantation

B. Etiology: controversial

C. Clinical presentation

    1. Liver rejection: hyperbilirubinemia

    2. Pancreas rejection: decreased urinary amylase, hyperglycemia

    3. Lung rejection: hypoxemia, decreased pulmonary function tests

    4. Kidney rejection: hypertension, proteinuria, elevated creatinine

D. Diagnostic test. Biopsy of a typical lesion shows concentric vessel narrowing and ischemic end-organ disease. However, biopsy findings vary based on the organ involved. Specific organs and associated biopsy findings are:

    1. Heart: myofibrointimal proliferation, medial scarring, accelerated graft atherosclerosis

    2. Liver: fibro-obliterative endarteritis, portal fibrosis, "vanishing bile duct" syndrome

    3. Pancreas: fibrointimal proliferative endarteritis, vascular occlusion, infarction, fibrosis, loss of islets

    4. Lungs: "bronchiolitis obliterans" obstruction of bronchioles with submucosal scarring, fibrointimal thickening of vessels

    5. Kidney: intimal hyperplasia, arterial occlusion, ischemic damage, atrophy, fibrosis, thickened basement membrane, glomerular scarring

CADAVERIC DONOR SELECTION AND SUPPORT. See also BRAIN DEATH in Chapter 14.

I. Selection of Cadaveric Donors (Table 25-1)

II. Guidelines for Donor Support

A. End points to maintenance therapy

    1. Systolic blood pressure: 100–120 mm Hg

Table 25-1. Indications and Contraindications for Selection of a Cadaveric Donor

Organ	Indications	Contraindications	
		Absolute	Relative
Kidney	Age < 65 years (older only with normal biopsy) Normal renal function	Sepsis Lentivirus infection Tuberculosis HIV or AIDS Hepatitis A, B, and C Herpes simplex virus Fungal disease Malignancy (except primary intracranial neoplasm or basal cell carcinoma)	History of pyelonephritis Chronic systemic disease Hypertension
Liver	Age < 65 years (older only with normal biopsy) Normal hepatic function	Diabetes mellitus Chronic liver disease Sepsis Lentivirus infection Tuberculosis HIV or AIDS Hepatitis A, B, and C Herpes simplex virus Fungal disease Malignancy (except primary	Chronic systemic disease Hypertension

		intracranial neoplasm or basal cell carcinoma)
Heart	Age < 60 years (older only with normal biopsy) Normal cardiac function	Cardiac disease Pulmonary disease Cardiac arrest Sepsis Lentivirus infection Tuberculosis Fungal disease Malignancy (except primary intracranial neoplasm or basal cell carcinoma)	Chronic systemic disease Hypertension
Pancreas	Age < 55 years (older only with normal biopsy) Normal pancreatic function Normoglycemia	Pancreatic disease (past or present) Diabetes mellitus Chronic liver disease (cirrhosis) Hepatitis A, B, C Herpes simplex virus Collagen-vascular disease Sepsis Lentivirus infection Tuberculosis HIV or AIDS	History of pancreatic disease Previous duodenal or pancreatic surgery Serum amylase > 100 U/L Age > 55 years Chronic systemic disease Hypertension

continued

Table 25-1. Indications and Contraindications for Selection of a Cadaveric Donor

Organ	Indications	Contraindications	
		Absolute	**Relative**
Pancreas *(continued)*		Fungal disease	
		Malignancy (except primary intracranial neoplasm or basal cell carcinoma)	
		Direct blunt or penetrating trauma to the pancreas	
		Acute or chronic pancreatitis at the time of donation	

    2. Central venous pressure: 8–10 mm Hg

    3. Core temperature: $\geq 95°F$ ($\geq 35°C$)

    4. PaO_2: 80–100 mm Hg

    5. SaO_2: $\geq 95\%$

    6. Urine output: 100–300 ml/hr

    7. pH: 7.37–7.45

    8. Hemoglobin: 10–12 g/dl

    9. Hematocrit: 30%–35%

B. Restore normal circulatory volume. Use Ringer's lactate, blood, or colloid as necessary.

C. Maintain brisk diuresis.

    1. Keep urine output $\geq 1–2$ ml/kg/hr.

    2. Support with increased fluids or blood as necessary.

    3. Give maintenance fluid as necessary.

        a. If urine output is 1–2 ml/kg/hr, administer D_5W 1/2 normal saline with 70 mEq KCl/L at 2 ml/kg/hr.

        b. If urine output is > 2 ml/kg/hr, match IV intake with urine output (i.e., cc for cc).

    4. Use diuretics (e.g., mannitol, furosemide) as appropriate.

D. Monitor electrolytes and correct as needed.

    1. If hypernatremia develops, change IV fluid to D_5W mixed with 1/4 normal saline.

    2. If the hourly IV rate is ≥ 500 cc/hr, decrease the dextrose to 1%.

E. Support blood pressure. Provide adequate hydration and administer dopamine for hemodynamic instability. Try to keep dopamine as low as possible.

F. Maintain core temperature $\geq 95°F$ ($\geq 35°C$).

G. Diagnose and treat diabetes insipidus.

    1. Suspect diabetes insipidus under the following circumstances:

        a. Urine volume > 500 ml/hr (i.e., 7 ml/kg/hr)

        b. Serum sodium > 150 mEq/L

        c. Serum osmolality > 310 mOsm/L

        d. Low urinary sodium

    2. Give deamino-8-D-arginine vasopressin; desmopressin acetate (dDAVP) [Pitressin], 1–2 µg IV over 30 minutes; repeat q 2–12 hr if necessary to keep urine output at 100–300 ml/hr.

    3. See SODIUM AND OSMOLALITY DISTURBANCES in Chapter 8

H. Treat hyperglycemia (i.e., serum glucose > 180 mg/dl) with an insulin drip.

I. Treat cardiac arrest with vigorous resuscitation and advanced cardiac life support. If this is successful, reassess suitability for organ donation.

HEART TRANSPLANTATION

I. Indications

    A. Congenital heart disease and cardiomyopathy

B. Acquired cardiomyopathy
1. Ischemic heart disease (most common indication)
2. Dilated cardiomyopathy, including idiopathic, viral, alcoholic, hypertensive, postpartum, familial, and doxorubicin-related disease
3. Valvular cardiomyopathy
4. Restrictive cardiomyopathy, including idiopathic disease, endocardial fibrosis, postradiation or chemotherapy-induced disease, and sarcoidosis

II. Candidates for Heart Transplantation
A. Severe heart failure despite maximal medical therapy
B. Unacceptable quality of life due to disabling symptoms of congestive heart failure (CHF)
C. Unacceptable risk of cardiac death within the next year, despite limited symptoms of CHF
D. No other reasonable surgical option (e.g., coronary artery bypass graft, valve replacement)

III. Contraindications
A. Absolute contraindications
1. Active infection
2. Recent or active malignancy
3. End-stage extracardiac disease
4. Severe psychosocial dysfunction
5. Diabetes mellitus with end-organ damage
6. Recent pulmonary infarct
7. Severe peripheral vascular disease
8. Amyloidosis
9. Active peptic ulcer or diverticular disease
10. Chronic bronchitis

B. Relative contraindications
1. Age > 65 years
2. Transpulmonary gradient > 15 mm Hg
3. Renal insufficiency
4. Hepatic dysfunction

IV. Management
A. Preoperative evaluation
1. Cardiac evaluation, including right and left heart catheterization
2. Pulmonary function tests, chest radiography
3. Laboratory tests: CBC, platelets, coagulation profile, chemistry, thyroid, renal and liver function, histocompatibility, blood typing
4. Skin testing
5. Consults (psychiatry, social work, financial counseling)

B. Pretransplant care
1. Maximal heart failure management, including angiotensin-converting enzyme inhibitors, diuretics, anticoagulation, antiarrhythmic agents, and β-blockers
2. Status and listing with United Network of Organ Sharing (UNOS)

    3. Determination of need for mechanical assist device as a bridge to transplant

C. Donor criteria

    1. The **size** of the heart of the donor should match that of the recipient. This is the most important part of the selection process.

    2. The **blood type** of the donor should match that of the recipient.

    3. Donor hearts should have **normal cardiac function** and be free from any abnormalities, with good cardiac output on minimal inotropic support. In an effort to increase the donor pool, some centers have used hearts with less-than-perfect function in brain-dead donors. These hearts may have wall motion abnormalities, coronary disease, or increased needs for inotropic support.

D. Immunosuppression. Treatment varies according to the institution. Most centers use a regimen with three or four drugs, depending on treatment indications (e.g., induction, maintenance, rejection).

    1. Cyclosporine A (CSA) or FK-506 for induction and maintenance

    2. Azathioprine or mycophenolate mofetil (MMF) for induction and maintenance

    3. Prednisone for induction and maintenance

    4. OKT3 in select patients with renal failure for induction and for treatment of hemodynamically compromised rejection

E. Postoperative issues

    1. Right-sided failure is the most common early complication.

        a. The right ventricle tolerates ischemia poorly.

        b. Pulmonary artery pressures and right ventricular afterload are higher in the recipient than in the donor. The right heart may take time to adjust to this new work load.

    2. Control of heart rate may prove difficult in the newly transplanted heart. Isoproterenol is started postoperatively and continued for 2–3 days. Isoproterenol is the chronotrope of choice, because it has excellent inotropic and chronotropic activity and decreases pulmonary vascular resistance.

    3. Postoperative complications include:

        a. Bleeding

        b. Cardiac tamponade

        c. Renal failure

        d. Respiratory failure

    4. Endomyocardial biopsies are used for surveillance for rejection. Initially, pulse steroids are given for 3 days. If the steroids are unsuccessful, the patient is given antithymocyte gamma-globulin (ATGAM) or OKT3.

IMMUNOSUPPRESSIVE THERAPY

I. **Cyclosporin A (CSA)**
   A. **Pharmacology**
      1. **Drug type.** CSA is a cyclic undecapeptide of fungal origin that is lipid soluble.
      2. **Mechanism of action**
         a. Binds to intracellular cyclophilin to form the cyclophilin–CSA complex, which inhibits calcineurin, an intracellular second messenger that regulates T-cell activation
         b. Blocks transcription of interleukin-1 (IL-1), IL-2, IL-2 receptors, IL-3, IL-4, and interferon
         c. Blocks IL-2–stimulated autocrine T-cell proliferation
      3. **Metabolism.** CSA is degraded by the liver and excreted in the bile.
   B. **Indications**

Initiation of immunosuppression can be delayed for induction therapy or for oliguria after renal transplantation.

---

   1. Preoperative use in living, related kidney transplantation
   2. After kidney, heart, lung, pancreas, and liver transplantation
   C. **Preparations and dosage**
      1. **Oral microemulsion** (Neoral)
         a. Improved bioavailability; available as a liquid and soft gel capsule
         b. Dosage

The therapeutic window for CSA is narrow. If levels are erratic, a pharmacokinetic profile should be performed.

---

   (1) **Early postoperative therapy**
      (a) Dosage: 8–10 mg/kg/day bid
      (b) Objective: whole blood trough level of 200–250 ng/ml (350–450 ng/ml for hepatic transplantation)
   (2) **Maintenance therapy**
      (a) Dosage: 4–5 mg/kg bid
      (b) Objective: whole blood trough level of 150–200 ng/ml
      2. **Oral tablets or capsules** (Sandimmune)
         a. More irregular GI absorption, with bioavailability of 5%–89%
         b. Dosage: 10 mg/kg qd
      3. **IV preparation** (Sandimmune IV)
         a. 1 mg IV = 3–5 mg PO
         b. Dosage
            (1) Adult: 2 mg/kg/day as a continuous drip

        (2) Pediatric: if weight is < 20 kg, 3 mg/kg/day as a continuous drip

        (3) Objective: steady-state level of 250–275 ng/ml

D. Toxicity

  1. Side effects

    a. Nephrotoxicity

    b. Hypertension

    c. Hyperkalemia

    d. Hyperuricemia, gout

    e. Gingival hypertrophy

    f. Hirsutism

    g. Neurologic abnormalities

    h. Hyperglycemia

    i. Hepatotoxicity

  2. Drug–drug interactions. These are a major management problem.

    a. CSA levels are decreased by carbamazepine, nafcillin, phenobarbital, phenytoin, rifampin, and valproic acid.

    b. CSA levels are increased by diltiazem, erythromycin, ketoconazole, and verapamil.

  3. Treatment of toxicity

    a. Taper CSA to a minimum of 2.5 mg/kg bid.

    b. Consider triple therapy (CSA, corticosteroid, and MMF or azathioprine].

      (1) Acute rejection: reduce to 4–5 mg/kg/day

      (2) Nephrotoxicity: reduce to 50 mg/day (minimum of 2.5–3 mg/kg/day)

II. FK-506 (tacrolimus)

A. Pharmacology

  1. Drug type. FK-506 is a macrolide antibiotic of fungal origin.

  2. Mechanism of action. The action of FK-506 is similar to that of CSA, but FK-506 is 10 to 100 times as potent.

    a. Binds to intracellular FK-binding protein, forming a complex that inhibits calcineurin

    b. Blocks T-cell activation, IL-2 receptor expression, and cytokine production

  3. Metabolism. FK-506 undergoes hepatic metabolism via the cytochrome P_{450} system.

B. Indications

  1. Refractory rejection

  2. Induction immunosuppression with corticosteroids

  3. Primary maintenance immunosuppression (some centers)

C. Dosage

  1. 0.15 mg/kg/day PO qd or bid

  2. 0.075 mg/kg IV q 12 hr

D. Toxicity

  1. Nephrotoxicity (should not be used with CSA)

  2. Headaches, tremors, light sensitivity, insomnia, mood changes

III. Rapamycin (RPM). RPM is also a macrolide antibiotic of fungal origin. Similar in structure to FK-506, it has a different method of action (i.e., it does not bind to calcineurin).

IV. Corticosteroids (e.g., prednisone, methylprednisolone)
  A. Pharmacology
    1. Mechanism of action
      a. Binds to cytoplasmic steroid receptors, which translocate to the nucleus to regulate transcription
      b. Decreases synthesis of IL-1, IL-6, and other cytokines
      c. Inhibits thymocyte activation and mixed lymphocyte reaction
    2. Metabolism
      a. Prednisone is converted to prednisolone by the liver, which then degrades it.
      b. A large majority of prednisone (80%) and all of prednisolone (100%) are enterally absorbed.
    3. Drug–drug interactions. The half-life of corticosteroids is decreased by phenytoin, phenobarbital, and rifampin.
  B. Indications
    1. Intraoperative and postoperative immunosuppression induction
    2. Maintenance of immunosuppression
    3. Acute allograft rejection

Corticosteroids can be instituted following a delay to allow bronchial anastomosis healing after pulmonary transplantation.

  C. Dosage
    1. Initial therapy
      a. Give methylprednisolone, 7 mg/kg IV (maximum of 500 mg intraoperatively).
      b. Give prednisone, 1–2 mg/kg/day (maximum of 120 mg qid).
      c. Taper gradually to a maintenance dose of 0.1–0.2 mg/kg/day.
    2. Maintenance immunosuppression: prednisone, 0.1–0.2 mg/kg/day bid, qd, or qod
    3. Rejection
      a. Adult: methylprednisolone, 5–15 mg/kg/day IV for 3–5 days
      b. Pediatric: methylprednisolone, 7 mg/kg/day for 3–5 days
      c. Adults and children: prednisone, 2 mg/kg/day PO for 3–5 days; taper over 2–4 weeks
  D. Toxicity
    1. Cushingoid features
    2. Hypertension
    3. Weight gain
    4. Hyperglycemia
    5. Cataracts

      6. Poor wound healing

      7. Thin skin

      8. GI effects: pancreatitis, peptic ulcer disease, GI bleeding

V. Mycophenolate Mofetil (MMF) [Cellcept]

  A. Pharmacology

    1. Drug type. MMF is an antimetabolite.

    2. Mechanism of action. MMF inhibits purine metabolism. It is more lymphocyte selective than azathioprine.

  B. Indication. MMF is used as part of triple therapy with CSA and corticosteroids.

  C. Dosage

    1. Adult: 1.0–1.5 g PO bid

    2. Pediatric: 600 mg/m^2 PO bid

VI. Azathioprine (Imuran)

  A. Pharmacology

    1. Drug type. Azathioprine is a thiopurine that is metabolized by the liver to active forms.

    2. Mechanism of action. This agent inhibits purine synthesis by interfering with (i.e., diminishing) DNA and RNA metabolism, lymphocyte proliferation, and cytokine production.

  B. Indications

    1. Used in combination with CSA and corticosteroids to decrease nephrotoxicity (triple therapy)

    2. Used preoperatively with donor-specific transfusion

    3. Maintenance immunosuppression (dual therapy with corticosteroids) [less frequent]

  C. Preparations [IV and PO (45% absorbed)] **and dosage**

    1. Give 5 mg/kg qd up to a maximum of 350 mg.

    2. Taper to 1–3 mg/kg/day (more if WBC count remains > 5000 cells/mm^3).

    3. If used as part of triple therapy, the dose is 2 mg/kg/day.

    4. Reduce dosage 25%–50% with concomitant allopurinol administration.

  D. Toxicity

    1. Symptoms

      a. Fever

      b. Hypotension

      c. Bronchospasm

      d. Mental status changes

      e. Hepatotoxicity, hepatitis, cholestasis, pancreatitis

      f. Leukopenia, thrombocytopenia, megaloblastic anemia

      g. Dermatitis, alopecia

      h. Neoplasms

    2. Options for treatment of toxicity

      a. Adjust dosage to keep WBC count > 3000 cells/mm^3.

      b. Substitute cyclophosphamide (rarely used), but halve the dose.

      c. Discontinue azathioprine.

VII. Cyclophosphamide (Cytoxan) [rarely used]

    A. Pharmacology. The mechanism of action involves the alkylation of DNA.

    B. Indication. Cyclophosphamide may be used in cases of azathioprine intolerance.

    C. Dosage. Give 0.5–1.5 mg/kg/day, adjusted to maintain the WBC count > 3000 cells/mm^3.

    D. Toxicity
        1. Leukopenia, thrombocytopenia
        2. Hemorrhagic cystitis
        3. Nausea, vomiting

VIII. Antithymocyte Globulin (ATG)

    A. Pharmacology
        1. Drug type. ATG is a polyclonal antiserum from animals such as horses, goats, or rabbits that is active against human thymocytes.
        2. Mechanism of action. ATG depletes circulating T lymphocytes and thymus-dependent areas of the lymph node and spleen.

    B. Indications
        1. Postoperative induction of immunosuppression
        2. Postoperative oliguria
        3. Treatment of rejection

    C. Dosage and administration
        1. Dosage. Give 10–30 mg/kg/day IV over 6 hours for 5–7 days.
        2. Administration
            a. Administer a test dose. Before therapy, perform intradermal forearm skin testing with 0.1 ml 1:1000 ATG in one arm and saline in the opposite arm.
            b. Administer ATG through central line only.
            c. Premedicate with diphenhydramine and acetaminophen.
            d. Monitor for anaphylaxis (1% of patients).
            e. Adjust corticosteroids to 0.4 mg/kg/day (maximum of 30 mg/day).
            f. Reduce CSA by 50% until 2 days before giving the last ATG dose.
            g. Withhold azathioprine until 4 days before giving the last ATG dose.

    D. Toxicity
        1. Side effects
            a. Anaphylaxis, bronchospasm
            b. Fever, chills
            c. Nausea, vomiting, diarrhea
            d. Hypotension
            e. Mental status changes
            f. Leukopenia, thrombocytopenia
            g. Development of intolerance to horse, goat, or rabbit products
            h. Rash, pruritus, urticaria
            i. Phlebitis, tissue necrosis

    2. **Treatment of toxicity**

       a. If the WBC count < 3000 cells/mm^3, then reduce ATG dose by 50%.

       b. If the WBC count < 2000 cells/mm^3, then hold the dose of ATG.

       c. If the platelet count $< 80,000$ cells/mm^3, then reduce ATG by 50%.

       d. If the platelet count $< 50,000$ cells/mm^3, then hold the dose of ATG.

IX. Antilymphocyte Globulin (ALG)

  A. Drug type. ALG is a polyclonal antiserum from animals such as horses, goats, or rabbits that is active against human thymocytes.

  B. Indication, dosage, and toxicity. These are similar to those of ATG (see VIII).

X. Monoclonal Anti–T cell Antibody (OKT3).

Other monoclonal antibodies undergoing clinical evaluation are anti-CD4, anti-CD5, anti-IL-2 receptor, anti-α-β TCR, anti-CD2, anti-CD45, and B7KD28.

  A. Pharmacology

    1. Drug type. OKT3 is a monoclonal antibody.

    2. Mechanism of action. OKT3 binds to T cells, which results in T-cell destruction by the reticuloendothelial system.

       a. Binds to T-cell CD3 proteins and modulates the T-cell receptor–CD3 complex

       b. Blocks class I and class II antigen recognition

       c. Inhibits generation and function of effector T cells

  B. Indications

    1. Induction of immunosuppression (intra- or postoperative)

    2. Postoperative oliguria

    3. Treatment of rejection

  C. Dosage and administration

    1. Dosage

       a. 2.5–10 mg IV qd for 30 minutes for 10–14 days

       b. If weight < 30 kg: 2.5 mg IV qd for 10–14 days

    2. Administration

OKT3 may be given by peripheral IV.

---

       a. Premedicate with acetaminophen, diphenhydramine, corticosteroids, or indomethacin.

       b. Monitor for anaphylaxis (1% of cases).

       c. Reduce CSA by 50% until 48 hours before completion of OKT3.

       d. Withhold MMF or azathioprine until 4 days before completion of OKT3.

  D. Toxicity

    1. Fever, chills, headache

    2. Nausea, vomiting, diarrhea

3. Dyspnea, wheezing, pulmonary edema
4. Tachycardia, hypotension
5. Aseptic meningitis, seizure, coma
6. Allergy to mouse products

KIDNEY TRANSPLANTATION

I. Preoperative Issues

> **Kidney transplantation is usually an elective procedure unless the patient is losing access to dialysis.**

A. Candidates
1. Patients have end-stage renal disease on maintenance dialysis or declining renal function nearing dialysis.
2. Patients may range in age from newborn to 70 years.

B. Indications
1. **Adults**
   a. Diabetes mellitus (31%)
   b. Chronic glomerulonephritis (28%)
   c. Polycystic disease (12%)
   d. Nephrosclerosis (hypertension) [9%]
   e. Pyelonephritis, systemic lupus erythematosus, IgA nephropathy, and interstitial nephritis (8%)
   f. Miscellaneous (12%)
2. **Children**
   a. Congenital renal disease (50%)
   b. Acquired renal disease (50%)

C. Recipient evaluation
1. ABO blood typing
2. Negative lymphocytotoxicity cross-matching
3. HLA matching

D. Donor-related issues
1. **Living, related donors**
   a. Account for 20% of kidney transplants
   b. Types of histocompatibility matches
      (1) **Perfect match.** Both HLA haplotypes match (i.e., offspring receive one haplotype from each parent); therefore, a sibling–sibling transplant has a 25% chance of a perfect match. One-year graft survival is 95%.
      (2) **Half match.** One of two HLA haplotypes matches; therefore, siblings have a 50% chance of a half match. A parent–child transplant is always a half match. One-year graft survival is 90%.
      (3) **Zero match.** Neither haplotype matches; therefore, siblings have a 25% chance of a zero match. One-year graft survival is 92%.
2. **Cadaveric donors**
   a. Account for 80% of kidney transplants

       b. Matching of anywhere from zero to six of HLA antigens

       c. One-year graft survival

          (1) Six-antigen match: 90%

          (2) All other matches: 85%

          (3) Retransplants (second cadaveric graft): 70%

  3. Living, unrelated donors

     a. Account for < 1% of kidney transplants

     b. Similar to cadaveric donors in terms of degree of matching

E. Survival issues

  1. All types of transplants from living donors fare better than those from cadaveric donors.

  2. Retransplantation adversely affects graft survival.

II. Operative Concerns

A. Indications for nephrectomy of native kidney

  1. Chronic persistent pyelonephritis

  2. Severe cyst complications from polycystic kidneys

  3. Persistent upper tract stones

  4. Vesicoureteral reflux

  5. Severe unmanageable high renin–induced hypertension

B. Placement of graft and anastomoses

  1. Graft placed heterotopically in the retroperitoneal iliac fossa

  2. Renal vessel anastomoses

     a. Adults: iliac artery and vein

     b. Children: aorta and inferior vena cava

  3. Ureter implanted into bladder

III. Postoperative Issues

A. Graft function

  1. Immediate function (70%–90% of cases)

     a. Rapid drop in creatinine

     b. Brisk diuresis

  2. No immediate function (10%–30% of cases)

     a. This condition is usually temporary, with return of function in 7–14 days.

     b. Acute tubular necrosis (ATN) must be differentiated from early rejection.

       (1) ATN is rare in living, related kidney recipients, while in cadaveric kidneys, the incidence is approximately 35%.

       (2) ATN may occur immediately after revascularization or within a few hours of revascularization in grafts that initially diuresed.

       (3) Both ischemic and immunologic factors can increase the incidence of ATN.

          (a) Ischemic factors include long ischemia time, donor hypertension, advanced age of donor, and the use of vasopressors.

          (b) Immunologic factors include retransplants and poor HLA matching.

(4) Patients with posttransplant ATN have a higher incidence of acute rejection.

(5) Many patients who develop ATN require short-term hemodialysis. In 95% of cases, renal allograft function returns.

B. Immunosuppression. Treatment involves:

1. CSA

2. Corticosteroids (e.g., prednisone, methylprednisolone)

C. Complications

1. **Rejection**

a. **Acute rejection**

(1) Affects 50% of recipients

(2) May be treated with pulse steroids or antilymphocyte antibody

(3) Reversible in 80% of cases

b. **Chronic rejection**

(1) May be predicted by prior episode of acute rejection (strongest predictor)

(2) Results in graft failure

2. **Technical complications**

a. **Hemorrhage**

(1) **Etiology.** Hemorrhage is usually a result of unligated vessels in the hilum of the renal allograft.

(2) **Complications.** Hemorrhage may cause a hematoma, which results in renal venous thrombosis or deep venous thrombosis.

b. **Renal artery thrombosis**

(1) **Etiology.** Renal artery thrombosis can be caused by unidentified intimal flaps, arterial damage, size discrepancy between the donor and recipient, and presence of multiple renal arteries.

(2) **Diagnosis**

(a) If urine output suddenly ceases, gently irrigate the Foley catheter to rule out plugging by a clot.

(b) If the CVP is low and the patient does not respond to fluid, order Doppler studies to assess arterial blood flow.

(c) If blood flow is reduced but not absent, an arteriogram may be necessary.

c. **Aneurysms or stenoses**

(1) **Diagnosis.** A suspected aneurysm or stenosis can be confirmed with an arteriogram.

(2) **Treatment.** Aneurysms require surgery while stenosis may be percutaneously dilated or surgically repaired.

d. **Venous thrombosis**

(1) **Etiology.** Venous thrombosis can be caused by anastomotic kinking, intimal injury during harvest, pressure on the vein from a lymphocele, a uri-

noma, a teratoma, or an extension of ileofemoral thrombosis.

(2) **Characteristics.** Venous thrombosis usually occurs within the first few days after transplant and is characterized by sudden onset of pain and graft swelling.

(3) **Diagnosis.** Venous thrombosis can be diagnosed by ultrasound and Doppler studies.

(4) **Treatment**

   (a) If the thrombosis is incomplete, perform an embolectomy or administer thrombolytic agents.

   (b) If the thrombosis is complete, consider surgical embolectomy or administration of thrombolytic agents. However, nephrectomy is usually required.

e. Hematuria

(1) **Complications.** Bleeding from the distal ureter or cystotomy suture lines usually lasts 12–24 hours. More extensive bleeding may lead to clot formation and obstruction of the urinary tract.

(2) **Treatment**

   (a) Initial treatment involves continuous bladder irrigation.

   (b) If clot formation continues or the clot does not dissolve, cystoscopy is needed.

f. Urinary leakage

(1) **Diagnosis**

   (a) Physical examination will reveal graft swelling and tenderness; fever; wound drainage; and edema of the scrotum, labia, or thigh.

   (b) The serum BUN/creatinine may rise if there is peritoneal absorption.

(2) **Treatment.** Options for treatment include percutaneous nephrostomy or surgical repair with stenting.

g. Lymphocele

(1) **Complications.** A lymphocele may cause deep venous thrombosis or impaired graft function.

(2) **Treatment.** Preferred treatment options include laparoscopic or open surgical drainage into the peritoneal cavity.

LIVER TRANSPLANTATION

I. Preoperative Issues

A. Candidates

1. Patients have end-stage liver disease manifested by the following conditions:

   a. Encephalopathy
   b. Refractory ascites with increasing associated complications
   c. Esophageal varices associated with recurrent hemorrhage or hepatic decompensation
   2. Death within 1–2 years is likely without transplantation.
   3. Most candidates are between 6 months and 70 years of age.
B. Indications. Approximately 90% of patients who undergo liver transplants have chronic hepatic disease, and 10% have fulminant hepatic failure.
   1. Adults (chronic diseases)
      a. Postnecrotic cirrhosis, including cirrhosis secondary to hepatitis B (HBV) or C (HCV), alcoholic cirrhosis, and cryptogenic cirrhosis (55%)
      b. Primary biliary cirrhosis (15%)
      c. Primary sclerosing cholangitis (15%)
      d. Other rare causes of cirrhosis (15%)
   2. Children (> 50% of cases are secondary to biliary atresia)
C. Controversial indications
   1. Alcoholic cirrhosis. Preoperative screening is required to evaluate a patient's ability to maintain sobriety posttransplant.
   2. Fulminant hepatic failure. Psychiatric screening is necessary in patients who have attempted suicide. Fulminant hepatic failure is also associated with development of cerebral edema and subsequent herniation and death.
   3. Chronic HBV. There is a risk of recurrent HBV in the transplanted liver.
   4. Primary liver tumors. The risk of recurrence of disease is high. Transplantation is limited to those patients with no more than three lesions, with the largest being < 5 cm in size.
D. Recipient evaluation. Only ABO compatibility is necessary.

Negative lymphocytotoxicity cross-matching is not required for liver transplantation. In addition, HLA matching is not necessary.

E. Donor-related issues
   1. An **ABO blood group match** improves survival.
   2. The **size** of the donor liver should match that of the recipient. This issue is particularly critical in children.
      a. An adult cadaveric liver can be split.
      b. A living donor (adult) can donate the left lateral segment of the liver.
II. Operative Procedure
   A. Removal of liver
      1. The structures in the porta hepatis are dissected.
      2. The inferior vena cava is dissected below, behind, and above the liver.

    3. The retroperitoneal and diaphragmatic attachments are dissected.

    4. The liver is removed (the patient is temporarily anhepatic).

B. Transplantation of graft

    1. External venovenous bypass involves cannulation of the inferior vena cava and portal vein to decompress the lower extremities and splanchnic circulation. This blood is then delivered into the subclavian vein via an automated pump.

    2. Anastomoses are made in the suprahepatic vena cava, infrahepatic vena cava, and portal vein.

    3. Venous anastomoses are unclamped.

        a. The liver is oxygenated.

        b. Caval flow is established.

Reperfusion of a cold ischemic donor liver may induce severe hypotension and hypothermia, which usually resolve within 5–10 minutes of the reperfusion.

---

    4. The hepatic artery is anastomosed.

    5. The biliary tract is reconstructed. Options include:

        a. End-to-end (duct-to-duct) anastomosis (choledochocholedochostomy)

        b. Roux-en-Y choledochojejunostomy

III. Postoperative Issues

  A. Graft function

    1. Signs of graft function include:

        a. Bile production

        b. Uptake of potassium by hepatocytes

        c. Ability to correct coagulopathy

        d. Metabolism of anesthetics (i.e., Can the patient be awakened?) and return of normal mental status

        e. Resolution of hypoglycemia and hyperbilirubinemia and clearance of serum lactate

---

In liver transplantation, graft nonfunction requires urgent retransplantation.

---

    2. Signs of graft nonfunction include:

        a. No bile production

        b. Persistent coagulopathy

        c. Inability to awaken from anesthesia

  B. Immunosuppression. Treatment involves:

    1. CSA or FK-506

    2. Corticosteroids

    3. Azathioprine

  C. General postoperative care

    1. Determine the need for **mechanical ventilation,** which is usually necessary for 24–48 hours posttransplant.

    2. Perform **continuous hemodynamic monitoring.** The preoperative hemodynamic profile will persist into the postoperative period until hepatic function improves.

   a. Myocardial dysfunction seen early after reperfusion may persist, with decreased compliance and contractility. Optimize preload and afterload using inotropic agents such as dopamine and dobutamine.

   b. Hypertension is common in the early postoperative period and is usually responsive to calcium channel blockers.

3. Assess for bleeding.

   a. Initially, check hemoglobin and hematocrit levels every 4–6 hours.

   b. Assess coagulation parameters [i.e., platelet count, prothrombin time (PT), partial thromboplastin time (PTT)] every 6 hours.

   c. If bleeding is confirmed, administer fresh frozen plasma, cryoprecipitate, platelets, and blood as needed until graft function begins.

4. Check fluid and electrolytes.

   a. Most liver recipients have an increased extravascular volume and a decreased intravascular volume.

   b. Follow potassium levels.

      (1) Potassium levels may be elevated due to poor renal function, reperfusion effect, or CSA.

      (2) Potassium levels may be reduced due to needed diuretic therapy.

   c. Keep magnesium levels > 2 mg/dl and phosphate levels 2–5 mg/dl to prevent seizures.

   d. Treat hyper- and hypoglycemia.

      (1) Hyperglycemia may result from steroid use and should be treated with insulin.

      (2) Hypoglycemia is often an indication of poor hepatic function and should be treated immediately with glucose.

5. Maintain GI bleeding prophylaxis.

   a. Histamine (H_2) blockers are preferred.

   b. Sucralfate may bind CSA and therefore should be avoided.

6. Provide adequate nutrition. The GI tract can be used 3–5 days after the transplant. If the patient has prolonged ileus, total parenteral nutrition (TPN) should be instituted early.

7. Maintain infection prophylaxis with:

   a. Perioperative antibiotics with third-generation cephalosporin

   b. Trimethoprim and sulfamethoxazole (when patient is able to take pills PO) [protect against *Pneumocystis* species, *Nocardia* species, *Legionella* species, and *Listeria* species]

   c. Nystatin (protects against fungal infections)

   d. Ganciclovir (protects against viral infections)

D. Complications
 1. Primary nonfunction
   a. The **incidence** is approximately 5% with an associated mortality rate of 80%, unless retransplanted.
   b. The **etiology** is unknown; however, several risk factors have been associated with nonfunction. These include:
    (1) Advanced age
    (2) Increased fat content of donor's liver
    (3) Long donor hospital stay before procurement
    (4) Cold ischemia > 18 hours
    (5) Reduced-size grafts (split-liver transplants)
   c. Signs of nonfunction include:
    (1) No return of consciousness
    (2) Increased renal dysfunction
    (3) Hemodynamic instability
    (4) Rising PT
    (5) Persistent hypoglycemia
   d. Early **diagnosis** is valuable to identify a need for retransplant.
    (1) Before deciding to retransplant, it is necessary to rule out hepatic artery thrombosis (HAT), accelerated acute rejection, and severe infection.
    (2) The following combined factors are 100% predictive of nonfunction:
      (a) Aspartate aminotransferase levels > 5000 IU/L
      (b) Factor VIII levels < 60%
      (c) PT > 20 seconds at 4–6 hours postreperfusion
      (d) Bile production < 50 ml/24 hr
   e. Treatment includes:
    (1) Retransplant (the only viable option)
    (2) Prostaglandin E_1 (vasodilates the splanchnic circulation with enhanced blood flow to the new liver)
      (a) Administer an initial dose of 0.005 µg/kg/min.
      (b) Increase as tolerated by systolic blood pressure to a maximum dose of 0.03 µg/kg/min.
 2. Rejection
   a. Acute rejection
    (1) The **incidence** of acute rejection is 50%.
    (2) Signs of acute rejection include:
      (a) Elevated bilirubin or transaminase levels (associated with symptoms of fever and malaise)
      (b) Decreased bile production
      (c) Pale, watery bile
    (3) Diagnosis requires liver biopsy.
    (4) With **treatment,** acute rejection is almost always

reversible. Treatment is based on the severity of episodes.

  (a) Mild-to-moderate episodes are treated with high-dose corticosteroids.
  (b) Severe episodes are treated with ATG or OKT3.

b. Chronic rejection

  (1) **Pathophysiology.** Chronic rejection involves immunologic attack on bile ducts and associated small arteries.
  (2) The primary **clinical manifestation** is "vanishing bile duct" syndrome.
  (3) **Treatment** involves retransplantation.

3. Surgery-related complications. These problems often relate to any of the five anastomoses.

a. Postoperative hemorrhage

  (1) **Incidence.** Postoperative bleeding is common and is usually multifactorial.
  (2) **Etiology.** Hemorrhage is caused by a large raw surface created during recipient hepatectomy.
  (3) **Complications.** Coagulopathy often exists due to deficits in coagulation, fibrinolysis, and platelet function.

b. HAT

  (1) **Incidence.** HAT occurs in 5% of adults and 10% of children.
  (2) **Signs and symptoms.** Patients may be asymptomatic or they may present with:
    (a) Severe liver failure due to extensive necrosis
    (b) Marked elevation of serum transaminases, septic shock, hepatic encephalopathy (if HAT occurs in early postoperative period)
    (c) Biliary leak or stricture (Because the donor bile duct receives its blood supply from the hepatic artery, once the artery becomes ischemic, the common bile duct may leak or stricture.)
  (3) **Diagnosis** is made by Doppler ultrasound.
  (4) **Treatment** requires:
    (a) Prompt reexploration with thrombectomy and revision (70% graft salvage rate if diagnosis is made quickly)
    (b) Retransplantation if necrosis is extensive

c. Portal vein thrombosis

  (1) **Incidence.** Portal vein thrombosis occurs in < 2% of recipients.
  (2) **Etiology.** Related conditions include "purse stringing" of the anastomosis and excessive length of the portal vein with kinking.
  (3) **Symptoms** may include severe liver dysfunction with generation of ascites and variceal bleeding

from increased portal pressures. If thrombosis occurs late, there may be no symptoms because function is preserved by collateral flow.

(4) **Diagnosis** requires Doppler ultrasound.

(5) **Treatment** based on early diagnosis requires thrombectomy and revision of the anastomosis, which may be successful.

d. **Bile leaks** (within 30 days posttransplant)

(1) **Locations.** Leaks usually occur from the T-tube site or from the biliary anastomosis, which has a tenuous blood supply.

(2) **Symptoms** include fever, abdominal pain, and peritoneal irritation.

(3) **Diagnosis.** Ultrasound may demonstrate fluid collection, but cholangiography is the test of choice. Pathways include via the T-tube, by endoscopic retrograde cholangiopancreatography, or percutaneously transhepatic cholangiography. Bile in the drains suggests a leak; however, absence of bile in the drains is not conclusive for ruling out a leak.

(4) **Treatment** involves either biliary stenting or operative drainage of fluid collections and revision of the biliary anastomosis.

e. **Biliary obstruction** (late in postoperative period)

(1) **Etiology.** Obstruction is usually secondary to stricture. Strictures at the anastomosis are related to ischemia while other strictures are related to HAT, prolonged cold ischemia, and ABO-incompatible donors.

(2) **Symptoms.** Patients present with cholangitis and cholestasis.

(3) **Diagnosis** requires cholangiography.

(4) **Treatment** involves balloon dilation or stenting initially. If these fail, surgical revision is indicated.

4. **HBV recurrence**

E. **Overall prognosis**

1. Children fare slightly better than adults; in children, the 5-year graft survival rate is 74%, whereas in adults, it is 63%.

2. Patients who are less ill at time of transplantation do better.

3. Poorer outcomes are associated with cancer, fulminant hepatic failure, and chronic HBV.

PANCREAS TRANSPLANTATION

I. **Preoperative Issues**

A. **Candidates and specific indications**

1. Patients who have insulin-dependent diabetes (type I) and fall into the following three groups:

      a. Patients with end-stage renal disease, who are candidates for simultaneous pancreas–kidney transplants (SPKs)

      b. Patients with renal failure, who are candidates for renal transplantation followed by pancreas [pancreas after kidney (PAK)] transplant

      c. Patients without renal complications but with other severe diabetic complications, who are candidates for pancreas transplantation alone (PTA)

   2. Patient age: usually 25–45 years

B. Contraindications

   1. Age > 55 years

   2. Severe peripheral vascular disease

   3. Severe coronary artery disease

   4. Obesity

   5. Type II diabetes

C. Recipient evaluation

   1. ABO compatibility

   2. Negative lymphocytotoxicity cross-match

   3. HLA matching

D. Donor-related issues

   1. Use insulin as needed to keep serum glucose levels at 100–150 mg/dl.

   2. Pancreas donors also donate iliac artery bifurcation for arterial reconstruction.

   3. The spleen is removed from the graft.

II. Operative Procedure. Pancreatic transplantation involves the following steps:

A. The splenic artery and the superior mesenteric artery of the donor pancreas are joined by a Y graft (bifurcation of donor common iliac artery).

B. The pancreas is placed into the right iliac fossa.

C. The portal vein is anastomosed to the iliac vein.

D. The common iliac artery graft is anastomosed to the right common iliac artery.

E. The pancreatic duct is anastomosed to the bladder via the duodenal conduit (or more rarely, the small bowel). Exocrine secretions pass into the urine.

F. In SPK transplants, the kidney is placed in the left iliac fossa.

III. Postoperative Issues

A. Initial postoperative care

   1. During the first postoperative day, check serum glucose levels every 1–2 hours and CBC every 6 hours. Thereafter, check serum glucose levels every 2–4 hours and CBC, electrolytes, and serum amylase daily.

   2. In SPK transplants, urine output is replaced on a ml-per-ml basis for the first 48 hours and then tapered to a maintenance dosage.

   3. In the early postoperative period, keep blood glucose levels < 150 mg/dl. Many patients will have elevated graft function, which may require dextrose infusions. However, some patients may require an insulin drip.

4. Keep patients on broad-spectrum antibiotics and antifungal agents until duodenal cultures are negative.

5. Patients with bladder drainage require specific treatment.
   a. For patients with bladder drainage of the pancreas, keep the Foley catheter in place for 10–14 days.
   b. Because bicarbonate is lost in the urine in bladder-drained patients, it should be replaced with oral supplements.
   c. In patients with bladder drainage, urine amylase levels should be monitored by a timed 8-hour collection.

B. Graft function

1. **Endocrine.** Successful transplantation restores plasma glucose to normal. Elevated serum glucose often indicates substantial loss of graft function.

2. **Exocrine.** If the pancreas is connected to the bladder, exocrine function can be evaluated by measurement of urinary amylase.

C. Immunosuppression

1. Induction immunosuppression that often includes antilymphocyte serum
2. CSA
3. Corticosteroids

D. Complications

1. **Rejection.** An episode of acute rejection occurs in up to 60% of SPK transplants.
   a. **Signs** that indicate rejection and should provoke consideration of a biopsy include:
      (1) A 25% decline in urine amylase levels from baseline on two consecutive hourly measurements
      (2) Further rise in serum amylase levels
      (3) Further rise in glucose levels
   b. **Treatment**
      (1) Begin with IV boluses of methylprednisolone, 250–500 mg/day. If the methylprednisolone is not effective within 48 hours, begin antilymphocyte antibody therapy.
      (2) Administer ganciclovir with OKT3 and ATGAM until discharge. After discharge, replace ganciclovir with acyclovir and administer with OKT3 and ATGAM for a total of 6 weeks. The total doses of OKT3 and ATGAM are > 1 dose during the first 4 months posttransplant.
      (3) If necessary, corticosteroids are used as adjuncts.

2. **Other problems**
   a. **Graft pancreatitis** may be due to ischemic or preservation injury, cytomegalovirus infection, or urine reflux. Treatment involves fasting, IV fluids, and other standard therapies.

      b. Pancreatic leaks and fistulae

      c. Graft thrombosis usually occurs during the first few days posttransplant and is associated with hyperglycemia and a fall in urine amylase levels.

      d. Bleeding

      e. Bladder complications may be secondary to exposure to pancreatic enzymes or drainage from a duodenal remnant.

      f. Dehydration

E. Survival

    1. Rejection is the most common cause of graft loss. Rejection of the pancreas graft is difficult to monitor, except in SPK transplants, where kidney may serve as marker of pancreas graft rejection.

    2. One-year graft survival is approximately 90%.

SMALL BOWEL TRANSPLANTATION

I. Preoperative Issues

  A. Candidates. Characteristics include:

    1. Irreversible intestinal failure

    2. Permanent dependence on TPN

    3. Some associated TPN-induced liver failure, which requires combined small bowel and liver transplantation

  B. Indications

    1. Adults

      a. Crohn's disease

      b. Trauma

      c. Vascular accidents

      d. Volvulus

    2. Children

      a. Congenital atresias

      b. Volvulus

      c. Necrotizing enterocolitis

      d. Gastroschisis

II. Operative Procedure

  A. The portal or systemic veins serve as routes of venous outflow.

  B. Options include:

    1. No anastomoses and two stomas

    2. Two anastomoses and no stomas

    3. One anastomosis and one stoma (preferred method, because it allows proximal bowel continuity and distal stoma for biopsy access)

III. Postoperative Issues

  A. Immunosuppression. FK-506 is usually used.

  B. Complications

    1. Rejection. Graft-versus-host disease is more prevalent because the bowel is rich in lymphoid tissue.

      a. Intestinal manifestations include sloughing, shortening, and blunting of villi.

        b. Skin rash, diarrhea, altered liver function tests, and anemia may also occur.
  2. Sepsis
  3. Stoma complications (e.g., retraction, ischemia)
  4. Vascular thrombosis or hemorrhage
  5. Lymphatic drainage problems: usually short-term
C. Survival. One-year survival is 70% (experience is still limited).

26

Trauma

GENERAL ASSESSMENT AND MANAGEMENT

I. Goals of Trauma Management
  A. Establish a secure airway.
  B. Establish cardiovascular stability.
  C. Control hemorrhage.
  D. Keep the patient warm.
  E. Maintain adequate immobilization until the spine is evaluated.
  F. Correct coagulopathy.

**Time is a crucial factor for management
of the complicated trauma patient.**

II. Primary Survey and Resuscitation
  A. Airway maintenance
    1. Assessment
      a. Ascertain patency of the airway and assess for airway obstruction (e.g., foreign body, facial and mandibular fractures).
      b. A patient who is able to speak has an adequate airway.
    2. Management
      a. Establish a patent airway using a chin-lift or jaw-thrust maneuver.
      b. Establish a definitive airway by intubation or surgical cricothyroidotomy (see Chapter 32).
      c. Maintain the cervical spine in a neutral position.

**Assume all trauma patients have a
cervical spine injury until proved otherwise.**

  B. Breathing (i.e., ventilation and oxygenation)
    1. Assessment
      a. Determine the rate and depth of respirations.

    b. Auscultate the chest bilaterally and assess movement of the chest (i.e., symmetry).

    c. Inspect and palpate the neck for tracheal deviation and wounds.

    d. Palpate the chest for crepitus and chest wall deformity.

2. Management

    a. Administer oxygen by facemask.

    b. Ventilate the patient with a bag-valve-mask unit or a facemask device, if needed.

    c. Attach the patient to a pulse oximeter.

    d. Treat pneumothorax, if present.

       (1) Seal an open pneumothorax with an occlusive dressing taped on three sides.

       (2) Decompress a tension pneumothorax with a 14-gauge angiocatheter in the second intercostal space in the midclavicular line on the affected side. A thoracostomy tube may be placed subsequently.

    e. Intubate patients with compromised oxygenation or ventilation.

C. Circulation (with hemorrhage control)

  1. Assessment

    a. Identify any sources of external, exsanguinating hemorrhage.

    b. Evaluate the pulse (i.e., quality, regularity, rate, pulsus paradoxus) and blood pressure (BP).

       (1) A palpable radial pulse corresponds to a BP of at least 80–90 mm Hg.

       (2) A palpable femoral pulse corresponds to a BP of at least 70 mm Hg.

       (3) A palpable carotid pulse corresponds to a BP of at least 60 mm Hg.

    c. Evaluate the skin color (e.g., pallor, mottling).

    d. Perform an ECG and check manual BP.

  2. Management

    a. Apply **direct pressure to any external bleeding site or expanding hematoma.**

    b. Close scalp lacerations quickly because they can be the source of significant hemorrhage.

    c. Insert two large-caliber (i.e., 14- to 16-gauge) IV catheters.

    d. Obtain blood for CBC, chemistry analysis, type and cross-match, prothrombin time (PT), partial thromboplastin time (PTT), and ABG.

    e. Initiate vigorous IV fluid therapy with warmed Ringer's lactate solution. Use high-flow fluid warmers when possible to avoid hypothermia.

       (1) If the patient does not respond to 2 liters of Ringer's lactate solution, proceed with blood transfusions.

(2) Use type O negative uncross-matched blood until type-specific blood is available.

Do not treat hypovolemic shock with vasopressors.

---

    f. Insert a urinary catheter unless contraindicated by signs of urethral injury (e.g., blood at urethral meatus, blood in scrotum, high-riding prostate).

    g. Insert a nasogastric (NG) tube (orogastric if patient is intubated) unless contraindicated (e.g., fracture to the base of the skull, facial fracture).

    h. Initiate continuous ECG monitoring because dysrhythmias are common in trauma patients.
        (1) Tachycardia, atrial fibrillation, premature ventricular contractions, and ST segment changes may represent cardiac contusion or injury.
        (2) Pulseless electrical activity may indicate cardiac tamponade, tension pneumothorax, or profound hypovolemia.
        (3) Bradycardia, aberrant conduction, and premature beats may indicate hypoxia or hypoperfusion.

    i. See assessment of the pulseless trauma patient (Figure 26-1).

D. Disability (with brief neurologic examination)
    1. Assessment
        a. Determine level of consciousness using the Glasgow coma scale (GCS) [see Table 14-2].
        b. Assess the size, equality, and reactivity of the pupils.
        c. Assess the patient's ability to move and sense extremities.
    2. Management. Ensure in-line stabilization of the cervical spine.

E. Exposure and environment
    1. Assessment. It is necessary to completely undress the patient to fully assess for all injuries.
    2. Management. Prevent hypothermia with blankets, warm fluid, and a warm trauma room.

III. Secondary Survey
    A. History should include information about (**AMPLE**):
        1. Allergies
        2. Medications
        3. Past medical history
        4. Last meal
        5. Events related to injury
            a. For blunt trauma, determine the cause of injury [e.g., seat belt, air bag, steering wheel (steering wheel deformation), collision, intrusion into passenger compartment, ejection from vehicle].
            b. For burns, determine the cause of the burn, the environment in which it occurred, and any substances consumed by the flames.

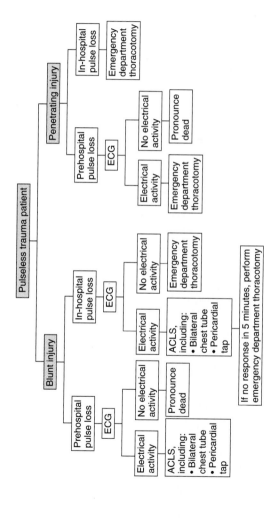

Figure 26-1. Assessment of the pulseless trauma patient. *ACLS* = advanced cardiac life support.

    c. For exposure injuries, determine what the patient was exposed to (e.g., toxins, chemicals, radiation).

B. Physical examination

  1. Head and maxillofacial injury

    a. Reevaluate level of consciousness using the GCS.

    b. Check the pupils and evaluate the eyes for visual acuity, hemorrhage, and contact lenses.

    c. Check the ears (especially the tympanic membranes) and nose for blood and CSF.

  2. Cervical spine and neck injury

    a. Look for signs of blunt or penetrating injury and tracheal deviation.

    b. Palpate down to the T1 spinous process to evaluate for tenderness, deformity, bony crepitus, and subcutaneous emphysema.

    c. Do not remove helmet until the cervical spine is cleared (i.e., fully assessed with no evidence of injury), unless an emergent airway is needed. The cervical spine can be cleared clinically if the following criteria are met:

      (1) Patient is alert and oriented with no history of alcohol or drug use

      (2) No major distracting injury (e.g., femur fracture, multiple broken ribs, pelvic fracture)

      (3) No pain on palpation of the cervical spine

      (4) No pain on extension, flexion, or rotation of the neck

      (5) Intact neurologic function

    d. Auscultate the carotid arteries for bruits.

  3. Thoracic and lumbar injury

    a. Logroll the patient to both sides to fully visualize the back and axillas.

    b. Palpate and inspect the thoracic and lumbar spine for tenderness, contusions, lacerations, and deformities.

  4. Chest injury

    a. Inspect and palpate the anterior, lateral, and posterior chest wall for signs of injury and bilateral respiratory excursions.

    b. Auscultate the chest for bilateral breath sounds and heart sounds.

  5. Abdominal injury

    a. Inspect the abdomen for signs of injury and internal bleeding.

    b. Assess the abdomen for tenderness, rebound, and guarding.

  6. Perineal, rectal, and vaginal injury

    a. Evaluate for contusions, hematomas, and lacerations.

    b. Check for urethral or rectal blood.

    c. Check anal sphincter tone and prostate position.

    d. Fully visualize the anus, scrotum, and labia for evidence of injury.

7. Musculoskeletal injury
   a. Inspect the extremities for signs of injury.
   b. Palpate the extremities and joints for tenderness and range of motion.
   c. Palpate all peripheral pulses.
8. Neurologic injury
   a. Reevaluate the pupils.
   b. Reevaluate level of consciousness using the GCS (see Table 14-2).
   c. Evaluate for evidence of paralysis or paresis.
C. Radiographic evaluation
   1. All trauma patients should receive a cervical spine series as well as films of the chest and pelvis, unless these areas can be cleared clinically.
   2. The location of the injury can also be used to determine the appropriate radiographic studies.
      a. Cervical spine injury. Obtain lateral, anteroposterior (AP), and odontoid (open-mouth) views of the cervical spine.
         (1) A lateral view will reveal the base of the occiput and the spinous processes of C1–T1.
         (2) An AP view will reveal the body and lateral masses of C2–T1.
         (3) An odontoid (open-mouth) view will reveal the lateral masses of C1 and the entire odontoid process.
      b. Thoracic and lumbar injury
         (1) AP and lateral views of the thoracic and lumbar spine are required if the circumstances of the injury involve a fall from a height, ejection from a motor vehicle, or direct trauma or if there is tenderness along the thoracic or lumber spine.
         (2) If a cervical spine fracture is found, the thoracic and lumbar spine should be evaluated given a high incidence of associated fractures.
      c. Chest injury. A chest radiograph will assess for pneumothorax, contusion, hemothorax, and aortic injury.
         (1) If aortic injury is suspected by chest radiograph or clinical suspicion, a CT scan of the chest may be used to evaluate the aorta and mediastinum.
         (2) However, aortography remains the gold standard for diagnosis of aortic injury.
      d. Abdominal injury
         (1) A CT scan of the abdomen and pelvis may be obtained in stable patients with the appropriate mechanism of injury for abdominal and pelvic trauma.
         (2) A **f**ocused **a**bdominal **s**onogram for **t**rauma (FAST) will allow for rapid evaluation of the abdominal compartment for free fluid and of the pericardium for tamponade.

     e. Head injury. Head injuries that involve neurologic deficits (e.g., loss of consciousness) or a patient > 80 years of age require a CT scan of the head.

ABDOMINAL COMPARTMENT SYNDROME

I. Definitions
  A. The **abdominal cavity** may be considered a single compartment with a wall that has limited compliance.
  B. Abdominal compartment syndrome is a condition in which sustained increased intraabdominal pressure (IAP) adversely affects the function of the GI tract and associated extraperitoneal organs.
  C. Intraabdominal hypertension (IAH) is a condition of sustained increased IAP. It is a common cause of abdominal compartment syndrome.

II. Pathophysiology (Table 26-1)
  A. Respiratory
    1. Ventilated patients require increased airway pressures to deliver a set volume.
    2. Impairments in respiratory mechanics are seen starting at an IAP of 20 mm Hg.
    3. Increased IAP leads to reduced total lung capacity, functional residual capacity, and residual volume. These conditions then lead to ventilation-perfusion (V/Q) abnormalities and hypoventilation, producing hypoxia and hypercarbia.
    4. Upward-pushing hemidiaphragms also cause a decrease in total lung capacity and predispose patients to pneumonia.
  B. Renal effects of IAH include:
    1. Reduced absolute and proportional renal arterial flow
    2. Increased renovascular resistance with changes in intrarenal blood flow
    3. Reduced glomerular filtration rate
    4. Increased tubular absorption and sodium retention
  C. Intraabdominal (i.e., abdominal wall) effects of IAH include:
    1. Reduction in abdominal wall blood flow
    2. Development of local ischemia and edema
    3. Loss of wall compliance
    4. Abdominal wall muscle and fascial ischemia (may contribute to wound complications)
  D. Intracranial effects of IAH. Acute changes of IAP > 15 mm Hg have been known to result in:
    1. Elevated intracranial pressure (ICP)
    2. Reduced cerebral perfusion pressures

III. Etiology
  A. Acute
    1. Peritoneal tissue edema secondary to peritonitis or severe abdominal trauma
    2. Fluid overload due to hemorrhagic or septic shock

Table 26-1. Physiologic Changes with Elevated Intraabdominal Pressure (IAP)

Patient Status	Cardiovascular Changes	Renal Changes	Splanchnic Changes
Stable (IAP 10–15 mm Hg)	Preload increases, contractility and afterload remain unchanged, CO increases	Urine output remains unchanged or is slightly reduced (reversible)	Low-grade intestinal ischemia, hepatic ischemia
Mildly unstable (IAP 16–20 mm Hg)	Preload decreases, contractility remains unchanged, afterload increases, CO decreases	Oliguria, azotemia	Increased intestinal ischemia, increased hepatic ischemia
Circulatory collapse (IAP $\geq$ 30 mm Hg)	Preload markedly decreases, contractility decreases, afterload markedly increases, CO is marginal	Anuria, worsening azotemia with renal failure	Bowel infarction, hepatic insufficiency, bacterial translocation possible

3. Retroperitoneal hematoma from trauma or aortic rupture
4. Peritoneal injury due to elective or emergency abdominal surgery
5. Reperfusion injury after bowel ischemia
6. Retroperitoneal and mesenteric inflammation from acute pancreatitis
7. Ileus and bowel obstruction
8. Abdominal packing for control of hemorrhage
9. Closure of the abdomen under undue tension

B. Chronic
1. Large intraabdominal tumor or mass
2. Congestive heart failure
3. Continuous ambulatory peritoneal dialysis
4. Tense ascites
5. Pregnancy

IV. Diagnosis

A. Diagnostic findings that indicate abdominal compartment syndrome include:
1. IAP > 20–25 mm Hg
2. Peak airway pressures > 45 cm H_2O
3. Urine output < 0.5 ml/kg/hr
4. Elevated central venous pressure (CVP)

B. Measurement of IAP can be performed by direct intraabdominal catheters, gastric tonometry, or a transvesicle technique. The **transvesicle technique** is quick, reliable, and easy to perform.

1. Place the patient in the supine position, which is best for measuring IAP.
2. Drain the bladder with a Foley catheter.
3. Introduce 50–100 ml of saline into the bladder via the Foley catheter.
4. Cross-clamp the drainage tubing and insert a 16-gauge needle, connected to a manometer, through the aspiration port.
5. The recorded pressure is the IAP.

V. Management

A. Nonoperative management

1. If the patient is intubated, switch to pressure-control ventilation.
2. Provide hemodynamic support.
3. Consider pharmacologic paralysis.
4. If the abdomen is full of ascites, perform paracentesis.

B. Operative abdominal decompression

1. **Indications.** Abdominal decompression is the treatment of choice for **severe IAH** due to peritoneal or visceral edema and large tumors. The determination of whether IAH is severe is based on the clinical picture.

   a. **Grades I and II (mild)**
      (1) Sustained IAP: 10–20 mm Hg (Physiologic effects are usually well compensated and thus clinically insignificant.)
      (2) Urinary bladder pressure: < 25 mm Hg
      (3) Suggested treatment: maintenance of adequate intravascular volume or hypervolemic resuscitation (may be adequate to preserve organ function)

   b. **Grade III (moderate)**
      (1) Sustained IAP: 21–35 mm Hg
      (2) Urinary bladder pressure: 26–35 mm Hg
      (3) Suggested treatment: decompression

   c. **Grade IV (severe)**
      (1) Sustained IAP: > 35 mm Hg
      (2) Urinary bladder pressure: > 35 mm Hg
      (3) Suggested treatment: exploration

2. **Technique of decompression**
   a. To prevent hemodynamic decompensation during decompression, restore intravascular volume, maximize oxygen delivery, and correct hypothermia and coagulation defects.
   b. Open the abdomen in the operating room under optimal conditions, if stability permits.
   c. To prevent any possibility of reperfusion injury, volume load with crystalloid solution along with mannitol and bicarbonate may be beneficial.
   d. After decompression, leave the abdominal compart-

ment (i.e., the fascia) open. Use a temporary, tension-free closure technique to cover the viscera.

3. **Reclosure of the abdomen**
   a. Reclosure should only be entertained when the patient is well resuscitated and when the probability of achieving complete fascial closure is highest.
   b. Reclosure of the abdomen is usually possible 3–4 days after the primary insult and decompression, when the following have occurred:
      (1) Brisk diuresis
      (2) Negative fluid balance
      (3) Diminished abdominal girth
      (4) Decreased peripheral edema

4. **Prognosis**
   a. After decompression, cardiac, respiratory, and renal function are immediately improved.
   b. There is an overall survival rate of 59% in all patients with abdominal compartment syndrome.

ABDOMINAL TRAUMA

I. **Penetrating Abdominal Trauma**
   A. **Gunshot wounds**
      1. All abdominal gunshot wounds that penetrate the peritoneum require exploratory celiotomy.
      2. Tangential wounds to the anterior abdominal wall that do not penetrate the peritoneum may be assessed by peritoneal lavage or laparoscopy.
      3. Local wound exploration is an additional way of determining the depth of injury; however, local damage caused by the blast effect may be missed.
   B. **Stab wounds**
      1. Mandatory, immediate laparotomy is required for patients with stab wounds under the following conditions:
         a. Hemodynamic instability
         b. Peritoneal signs
         c. Evisceration
      2. See Figure 26-2 for management of an anterior abdominal stab wound in a stable patient.
      3. Stab wounds to the flanks and back need to be evaluated by a CT scan of the abdomen and pelvis with triple contrast (i.e., oral, IV, and rectal) [if the patient is stable].
   C. **Penetrating wounds to the colon**
      1. **Nondestructive** colon wounds can undergo primary repair if there is no evidence of peritonitis.
      2. **Destructive** colon wounds
         a. Patients can undergo resection and primary anastomosis if they are hemodynamically stable, have no underlying disease, have minimal associated injuries, and do not have peritonitis.

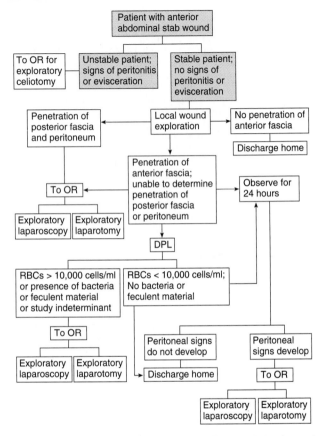

Figure 26-2. Algorithm for management of an anterior abdominal stab wound.

        b. Resection and colostomy should be performed on all patients with shock, peritonitis, or significant comorbidities.

    3. Colostomies for trauma may be closed as early as 2 weeks if contrast enema shows distal colon healing. The patient must be otherwise healthy.

  II. Blunt Abdominal Trauma

    A. Blunt abdominal trauma in an unstable patient (Figure 26-3)

    B. Blunt abdominal trauma in a stable patient (Figure 26-4)

  III. Grading System for Organ Injuries

    A. Liver (Table 26-2)

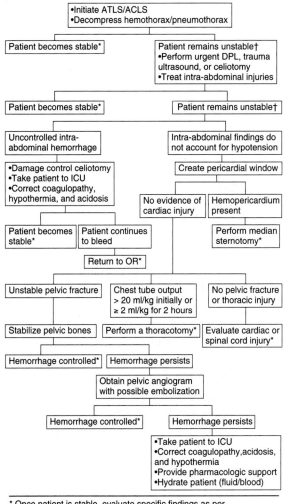

* Once patient is stable, evaluate specific findings as per standard trauma protocols.

† Never send an unstable patient to the CT scanner.

Figure 26-3. Management of a hemodynamically unstable patient with blunt abdominal trauma. *ACLS* = advanced cardiac life support; *ATLS* = advanced trauma life support; *DPL* = diagnostic peritoneal lavage. (Adapted with permission from Holcroft JW: *Bull Am Coll Surg* 13:34, 1997.)

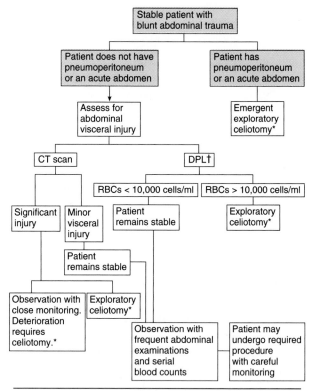

* In some patients, laparoscopy may be used to visually inspect the abdomen for injury; however, it is less sensitive than celiotomy for occult perforations.

† Remember that DPL cannot evaluate retroperitoneal injuries.

Figure 26-4. Management of a hemodynamically stable patient with blunt abdominal trauma. *DPL* = diagnostic peritoneal lavage.

- **B. Pancreas** (Table 26-3)
- **C. Spleen** (Table 26-4)
- **D. Kidney** (Table 26-5)

BURN MANAGEMENT

I. Acute Resuscitation and Management
A. Initial actions
1. Evaluate and manage airway, breathing, and circulation.

Table 26-2.	Liver Injury Scale
Grade	**Injury Description**
I	
Hematoma	Subcapsular, nonexpanding hematoma ($<$ 10% surface area)
Laceration	Capsular tear, nonbleeding, with $<$ 1-cm deep parenchymal disruption
II	
Hematoma	Subcapsular, nonexpanding hematoma (10%–50% surface area); intraparenchymal, nonexpanding hematoma ($<$ 2 cm in diameter)
Laceration	Parenchymal depth $<$ 3 cm, length $<$ 10 cm
III	
Hematoma	Subcapsular hematoma ($>$ 50% surface area or expanding); ruptured subcapsular hematoma with active bleeding; intraparenchymal hematoma ($>$ 2 cm in diameter)
Laceration	Parenchymal depth $>$ 3 cm
IV	
Hematoma	Ruptured central hematoma
Laceration	Parenchymal destruction involving 25%–75% of hepatic lobe
V	
Laceration	Parenchymal destruction involving $>$ 75% of hepatic lobe
Vascular	Juxtahepatic venous injuries (retrohepatic caval/major hepatic veins)
VI	
Vascular	Hepatic avulsion

  a. Assess the adequacy and stability of the airway.
  b. Apply high-flow, 100% oxygen.
  c. Intubate at any time for air hunger or suspected airway burns.

If in doubt, always intubate.

---

  d. Establish IV access.
 2. If there is concern for inhalation injury (see III), perform immediate direct laryngoscopy and bronchoscopy.
B. Physical examination
 1. Examine the face, nares, and mouth for smoke and thermal burns.
 2. Remove all clothing and examine the patient for associated injuries per the trauma assessment protocol (see GENERAL ASSESSMENT AND MANAGEMENT: III B).
C. Diagnostic tests

Type	Definition	Treatment
I	Contusion and laceration without duct injury	External drainage, infrequent distal pancreatectomy
II	Distal transection and/or parenchymal injury with duct injury	Distal pancreatectomy
III	Proximal transection or parenchymal injury with probable duct injury	Distal pancreatectomy or Roux-en-Y pancreaticojejunostomy
IV	Combined pancreatic and duodenal injury with ampulla and blood supply intact	Repair/exclude duodenum, repair pancreas as per I, II, and III
	Massive injury (i.e., ampulla destroyed, devascularization)	Pancreaticoduodenectomy

Table 26-3. Pancreatic Injury Scale

1. ABG with carboxyhemoglobin level
2. CBC and platelet count
3. PT and PTT
4. Electrolytes, magnesium, calcium, phosphate
5. BUN/creatinine
6. Albumin and total protein
7. Urinalysis
8. Urine myoglobin
9. Type and cross-match

D. **Management**
   1. Determine the **degree and extent of thermal surface injury** (Table 26-6), and calculate the percentage of first-, second-, and third-degree burns (Figure 26-5).
   2. Determine the need for admission.
      a. Indications for **surgical ICU or burn center admission** include:
         (1) Second-degree burn covering > 25% of body surface area (BSA) in adults or 20% BSA in children
         (2) Third-degree burn covering > 10% BSA in adults and children
         (3) Burns of the face, hands, feet, eyes, ears, or perineum
         (4) Inhalation injury
         (5) Electrical injury
         (6) Burn associated with other major trauma
         (7) Presence of comorbid medical conditions (e.g., diabetes, cardiac disease, pulmonary insufficiency, immunosuppression)
      b. Indications for **standard hospital admission** include:

Table 26-4. Splenic Injury Scale

Grade	Injury Description
I	
Hematoma	Subcapsular, nonexpanding hematoma ($<$ 10% surface area)
Laceration	Capsular tear, nonbleeding, with $<$ 1-cm deep parenchymal disruption
II	
Hematoma	Subcapsular, nonexpanding hematoma (10%–50% surface area); intraparenchymal, nonexpanding hematoma ($<$ 2 cm in diameter)
Laceration	Capsular tear with active bleeding, parenchymal depth 1–3 cm, no involvement of trabecular vessels
III	
Hematoma	Subcapsular hematoma ($>$ 50% surface area or expanding); ruptured subcapsular hematoma with active bleeding; intraparenchymal hematoma ($>$ 2 cm or expanding)
Laceration	Parenchymal depth $>$ 3 cm or involvement of trabecular vessels
IV	
Hematoma	Ruptured intraparenchymal hematoma with active bleeding
Laceration	Involvement of segmental or hilar vessel producing major devascularization ($>$ 25% of spleen)
V	
Laceration	Completely shattered spleen
Vascular	Hilar vascular injury that devascularizes the spleen

Table 26-5. Renal Injury Classification

Grade	Injury Description
I	Contusion or subcapsular hematoma without laceration
II	Nonexpanding perirenal hematoma or cortical laceration $<$1 cm deep without urinary extravasation
III	Laceration $>$1 cm deep into cortex without urinary extravasation
IV	Laceration into corticomedullary junction and into collecting system, or main renal artery or vein injury (two fragments)
V	Shattered kidney or renal pedicle injury (three fragments)

  (1) Second-degree burn covering 15%–25% BSA in adults or 10%–20% BSA in children
  (2) Third-degree burn covering 5%–10% BSA in adults and children

Table 26-6. Types of Burns

Type of Burn	Tissue Involvement	Physical Presentation	Prognosis
First-degree	Minimal tissue damage; only involves the epidermis	Erythematous skin, mild edema	Usually heals without scarring
Second-degree*	Involves all of the epithelium and much of the dermis (partial thickness)	Redness, blisters	Superficial: minimal scarring unless infected; takes 10–14 days Deep: heals with scars in 25–35 days
Third-degree*	Full thickness	Dry, tough, leathery, charred surface; blisters are uncommon; areas are anesthetic due to loss of pain receptors; no capillary refill	Scarring will occur

*If there is doubt as to whether the burn is a second-degree or a third-degree burn, assume it is a third-degree burn.

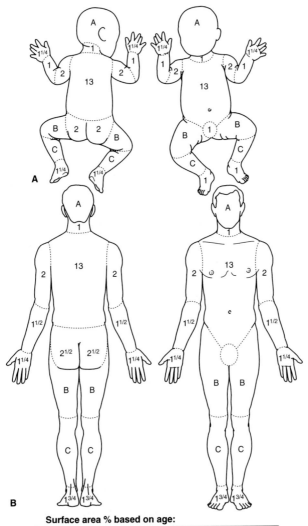

Surface area % based on age:

	0	1 yr	5 yr	10 yr	15 yr	Adult
A	9.5%	8.5%	6.5%	5.5%	4.5%	3.5%
B	2.75%	3.25%	4.0%	4.25%	4.5%	4.75%
C	2.5%	2.5%	2.75%	3.0%	3.25%	3.5%

Figure 26-5. Guidelines for calculating percentage of body surface area burned in (*A*) children and (*B*) adults.

3. Administer **IV narcotics and sedatives** for pain management (especially for débridement and dressing changes).
4. Administer a **tetanus booster.**
5. Administer **stress ulcer prophylaxis** (e.g., H_2 blockers, sucralfate). GI bleeding in burn patients is due to erosive gastritis (Curling's ulcer).
6. Place a **Foley catheter** and **NG tube.**
7. **Determine fluid resuscitation** using the **Parkland formula.** This formula only provides general guidelines; therefore, the absolute resuscitation should be modified according to the clinical scenario. This formula is based on the percentage of second- and third-degree burns.
   a. **First 24 hours postburn** (not postadmission)
      (1) Adults require lactated Ringer's solution at 2–4 ml/kg/% burn.
      (2) Children require lactated Ringer's solution at 3–4 ml/kg/% burn plus maintenance, which is calculated as follows:
         (a) First 10 kg = 4 ml/kg/hr
         (b) Second 10 kg = 2 ml/kg/hr
         (c) Each additional kg = 1 ml/kg/hr
      (3) In all patients, of the total volume of lactated Ringer's solution administered, infuse 50% in the first 8 hours postburn and the other 50% in the remaining 16 hours.
      (4) Avoid dextrose, except in the very young burn patient (< 2 years). Start within 12–18 hours.
   b. **Second 24 hours postburn**
      (1) Adjust maintenance fluid for urine output, base deficit, and mixed venous gases.
         (a) Adults require D_5W maintenance plus colloid (5% albumin in normal saline) at 0.5 ml/kg/% burn.
         (b) Children require D5/0.5% normal saline plus colloid (5% albumin in normal saline) at 0.5 ml/kg/% burn.
      (2) Rule out the possibility of osmotic diuresis.
      (3) Decrease the initial resuscitation infusion rate as tolerated by 25% every 3 hours.
8. **Monitor fluid resuscitation hourly.** Urine output is the most available index for evaluating fluid resuscitation and can be measured by inserting a Foley catheter.
   a. Adequate urine output is defined as a minimum of 1–2 ml/kg/hr in adults and 2–3 ml/kg/hr in children weighing < 30 kg.
   b. Low urine output is usually prerenal. If present, administer IV fluid in boluses.
   c. High urine output indicates overhydration and is defined as > 75 ml/hr in adults and > 3 ml/kg/hr in children. Rule out glucosuria before adjustment of fluids.

9. Determine the need for **invasive pulmonary artery monitoring.** Indications include:
   a. Poor response to fluid resuscitation
   b. Extremes of age
   c. Underlying cardiac disease
10. **Weigh the patient** on admission and daily. Weight should increase 10%–20% in the first 2 days because of edema, and then it should decrease slowly.
11. Provide **thermal burn wound care.**
    a. Examine the wound daily for infection, indicated by:
       (1) Conversion of a second-degree burn (i.e., partial-thickness necrosis) to a third-degree burn (i.e., full-thickness necrosis)
       (2) Focal dark-brown or black discoloration of the wound
       (3) Degeneration of the wound with neoeschar formation
       (4) Unexpected rapid eschar formation
       (5) Hemorrhagic discoloration of subeschar fat
       (6) Erythematous or violaceous edematous wound margin
       (7) Metastatic septic lesions in unburned tissues (ecthyma gangrenosum)
       (8) Green discoloration of subcutaneous fat (indicates *Pseudomonas* infection)
    b. Perform gentle daily débridement.
    c. Apply topical antimicrobials.
       (1) Silver sulfadiazine (1%) has poor eschar penetration and is painless.
       (2) Silver nitrate (0.5%) is used for patients who are allergic to sulfur. It has no eschar penetration and is painless.
       (3) Mafenide acetate (11.1%) has excellent eschar penetration and is painful in areas of partial-thickness burns.
    d. Burn wound excision may be necessary. Administer systemic antibiotics before the procedure and apply biologic dressing.
12. Consider **escharotomy** in all burns that are circumferential (i.e., burns on the forearm, upper arm, thigh, calf, abdomen, and chest) [Figure 26-6].
    a. Indications for escharotomy include an absent, decreased, or diminishing arterial pulse.
    b. Do not use anesthesia because the procedure is done through third-degree burns.
    c. Carry the incision down through the superficial subcutaneous fat, along the entire length of the full-thickness injury, and across involved joints.

II. **Nutrition in the Severely Burned Patient**
   A. **Nutrition in the adult burn patient**
      1. **Caloric needs**

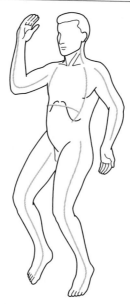

Figure 26-6. Preferred sites for escharotomies.

a. Standard formulas are inadequate to predict caloric needs because of the unique needs of burn patients based on:
   (1) Different environmental temperatures and humidity
   (2) Different types of inhalation injuries
   (3) Dressing changes
   (4) Skin grafting
   (5) Different levels of pain and anxiety
   (6) Use of sedatives
   (7) Varying activity levels
b. Use the Harris-Benedict equation (see p 384) to determine basal energy expenditure. Then, to determine caloric needs, multiply the basal energy expenditure by the following amounts based on total body surface area (TBSA) burned:
   (1) < 20% TBSA = 1.2–1.4
   (2) 20%–25% TBSA = 1.6
   (3) 25%–30% TBSA = 1.7
   (4) 30%–35% TBSA = 1.8
   (5) 35%–40% TBSA = 1.9
   (6) 40%–45% TBSA = 2.0
   (7) > 45% TBSA = 2.1

2. **Caloric distribution** goals are approximately 20% protein, 50% carbohydrates, and 30% fat.
   a. **Protein**
      (1) Give 1.5–3.0 g/kg ideal body weight (IBW)/day.
      (2) Protein requirements increase for gluconeogenesis, healing of wounds, and replacement of nitrogen losses.
      (3) Administration of intact protein results in better weight maintenance and survival than administration of free amino acids.
   b. **Carbohydrates**
      (1) Optimal delivery is 5 mg glucose/kg IBW/min.
      (2) Glucose promotes sparing of lean body mass.
      (3) Excess carbohydrates result in excess carbon dioxide production and hyperglycemia.
   c. **Fat**
      (1) The minimal amount of linoleic acid needed to prevent essential fatty acid deficiency is 4% of the total calories consumed.
      (2) Large amounts of fat, especially omega-6 fatty acids, can have an immunosuppressive effect by stimulating the release of prostaglandins.
      (3) Omega-3 fatty acids, which are mainly found in fish oil and marine products, may have a beneficial effect on immunocompetence.
   d. **Vitamins** (similar regimen as that used for pediatric patients)

B. **Nutrition in the pediatric burn patient**
   1. The following characteristics, unique to pediatric patients, need to be considered:
      a. Limited fat and lean body mass
      b. High basal metabolic requirements
      c. Increased BSA in proportion to weight
      d. Extra needs for growth and development
   2. **Caloric needs** are determined using the **Davies method:**

   Caloric needs = 60 kcal/kg/day + 35 kcal/% TBSA burned/day

   3. **Caloric distribution**
      a. **Protein**
         (1) For children < 1 year of age, use 3–4 g protein/kg IBW.
         (2) For children 1–3 years of age, use 3 g protein/kg IBW.
         (3) For children > 3 years of age, use 1.5–2.5 g/kg IBW.
         (4) When preburn weight is not known, use the 50 percentile weight for age as IBW.
         (5) To calculate insensible nitrogen losses in pediatric patients:
            (a) Birth–4 years: urine urea nitrogen + 2
            (b) 4–10 years: urine urea nitrogen + 3

(c) Older than 10 years: urine urea nitrogen + 4

b. **Carbohydrates**

(1) Carbohydrates should provide 40%–50% of total calories consumed.

(2) For infants, initiate a parenteral infusion of D_5W at a rate of 5 mg/kg/min and advance over 2 days to 15 mg/kg/min.

(3) For older infants and children, restrict D_5W to a maximum of 5–7 mg/kg/min.

c. **Fat**

(1) Fat intake of 2%–3% of total calories consumed is needed to prevent fatty acid deficiency.

(2) Give IV lipids at a maximum of 4 mg/kg IBW/day.

d. **Vitamins**

(1) Give one multivitamin daily.

(2) Use age to determine the dose of:

(a) Ascorbic acid

(i) Younger than 3 years: 250 mg bid

(ii) Older than 3 years: 500 mg bid

(b) Vitamin A

(i) Younger than 3 years: 5000 IU qd

(ii) Older than 3 years: 10,000 IU qd

(c) Zinc sulfate

(i) Younger than 3 years: 100 mg qd

(ii) Older than 3 years: 220 mg qd

4. **Feeding guidelines**

a. Feed the gut whenever possible. Enteral feeds theoretically protect the gut mucosa and prevent bacterial translocation. One option for enteral feeding is 10–20 cc via an NG tube or long feeding tube.

b. Limit total parenteral nutrition to those patients without a functioning gut.

c. Use commercial infant formulas when aggressive nutritional support is needed in children < 1 year of age.

(1) Infant formula with 20 calories/ounce can be increased with glucose polymers (e.g., Polycose, Moducal) or lipid emulsion (e.g., Microlipid) to 24–30 calories/ounce.

(2) For children 9 months–6 years of age, use isotonic products with higher calorie and protein densities.

III. **Inhalation Injury**

A. **Types of inhalation injuries**

1. Inhalation of **super-heated steam or air** leads to direct thermal injury to the upper airway.

2. Inhalation of **chemicals** leads to toxic damage to lung parenchyma.

a. Particles ≥ 10 μ are trapped in the nasopharynx.

b. Particles ≤ 2 μ are deposited throughout the airway.

     c. Particles $< 0.06\ \mu$ are deposited in the alveoli.
  3. Inhalation of **carbon monoxide** leads to carbon monoxide poisoning.
     a. Carbon monoxide binds to hemoglobin 230 times stronger than oxygen and then binds to cytochrome oxidase.
     b. The use of cellular oxygen is prevented and tissue hypoxia intensifies.

B. Clinical presentation
  1. Signs of **carbon monoxide poisoning** include:
     a. Blurred vision or diplopia
     b. Nausea
     c. Headaches
     d. Dizziness
     e. Coma
  2. Signs of **thermal inhalation injury** include:
     a. Singed nose hairs
     b. Carbonaceous sputum
     c. Facial burns
     d. History of burn within a confined space
     e. Carbon deposits in the oropharynx

C. Diagnostic tests
  1. Bronchoscopy allows direct visualization of large airways.
  2. A xenon-133 lung scan is a ventilation scan that noninvasively assesses the presence of an inhalation injury.

D. Management
  1. For **carbon monoxide poisoning,** place the patient on 100% oxygen, which reduces the half-life of carbon monoxide from 4.5 hours to 50 minutes. Hyperbaric treatment usually is not helpful due to the time factor.
  2. **Inhalation injury** patients with respiratory failure do better on high-frequency ventilation, which helps to keep small airways open.

IV. Electrical Injury
  A. Assessment. The severity and extent of tissue damage is determined by the resistance of the skin and deep tissues and the intensity, pathway, frequency, and duration of the current.
    1. Skin with high resistance results in high thermal damage but less penetration.
    2. Skin with low resistance (i.e., high skin/water ratio, as seen in children) results in minimal thermal damage and serious internal organ damage.
  B. Management. Treat in the same manner as thermal burns (see I D 1–12).

EXTREMITY VASCULAR TRAUMA

I. Classification of Extremity Vascular Trauma
  A. Penetrating trauma accounts for the majority of extremity vascular injuries in urban settings.

1. Low-velocity gunshot wounds and stab wounds are the most prevalent causes of penetrating trauma and are associated with lower rates of primary amputation than high-velocity gunshot wounds and shotgun blasts.
2. Penetrating vascular injury occurs as a result of direct trauma to the vessel or blast injury.

B. Blunt trauma accounts for the majority of extremity vascular injuries in rural settings.
   1. Mechanisms of blunt injury include:
      a. Compression
      b. Shear or distraction (especially when associated with displaced fractures)
      c. Direct trauma from bony fragments
   2. A high index of suspicion is needed to diagnose vascular injuries in patients with displaced long-bone fractures and posterior dislocation of the knee.

II. Diagnostic Work-up

A. History and physical examination are the most important elements when assessing a potential extremity vascular injury.
   1. A **history** is taken to assess the:
      a. Direction and type of trauma
      b. Amount and location of blood loss
      c. Degree of sensory and motor loss
      d. Degree of circulatory impairment or shock
   2. The **physical examination** is used to assess the hard and soft signs of vascular injury and the degree of associated tissue loss. Document the baseline vascular examination for later comparison.
      a. Hard signs, which mandate exploration, include:
         (1) Active arterial bleeding
         (2) Distal ischemia or pulse deficit
         (3) Thrill or bruit over the area of injury
         (4) Expanding or pulsatile hematoma
      b. Soft signs, which mandate further investigation, include:
         (1) Proximity of injury to a major vessel
         (2) Adjacent nerve injury
         (3) Stable hematoma
         (4) Diminished but palpable pulses
         (5) Unexplained shock
      c. Although the presence of hard and soft signs suggests vascular injury, absence of these signs does not rule out vascular injury.

B. Noninvasive diagnostic studies
   1. **Doppler studies** and the **ankle-brachial index (ABI)** can be used as adjunctive measures of vascular injury to add to the accuracy of the physical findings.
      a. An ABI < 0.90 in the affected limb versus the unaffected limb is suggestive of significant vascular injury and warrants angiography or exploration.
      b. An ABI > 0.90 does not rule out vascular injury be-

cause small intimal flaps or pseudoaneurysms may be missed. These patients may be followed carefully.
2. **Duplex ultrasound** may prove beneficial in the diagnosis of vascular injury; however, lack of available personnel may limit its usefulness in trauma cases.

C. **Invasive diagnostic studies—angiography**
1. Angiography is the **gold standard for detection of arterial injuries.**
2. **Indications** include:
   a. Physical examination suspicious for abnormal ABI
   b. Known vascular injury
   c. Evaluation of anatomy before operative procedure
   d. Proximity of insult to a major vascular structure (relative indication)
3. **Contraindications** (i.e., situations in which angiography may delay operative intervention) include:
   a. Unequivocal physical examination
   b. Evidence of ischemia
4. Angiography should be limited to those patients in whom it would eliminate the need for operative intervention or facilitate the operative procedure.

III. Management

A. Initial management of any trauma patient should follow the **standard trauma assessment** protocol (see GENERAL ASSESSMENT AND MANAGEMENT).

B. **Nonoperative management** has limited indications, which include:
1. Asymptomatic injury
2. Minimal injury based on angiogram
3. Injury limited to vessels that would cause minimal morbidity and no mortality if injury were to progress
4. Close follow-up needed

C. **Operative management** includes primary amputation, vascular repair, and adjunctive procedures.
1. **Primary amputation** should be considered only after formal operative exploration of the extremity and consultation with orthopaedic, plastic, and reconstructive surgical teams. Rarely is vascular injury the deciding factor.
2. **Vascular repair** involves débridement of all devitalized soft tissue and bone, including transmurally injured vessel walls.
3. **Adjunctive procedures**
   a. **Prophylactic fasciotomy** is indicated for:
      (1) Prolonged hypotension
      (2) Ischemia of ≥ 4 hours' duration
      (3) Combined arterial and venous injuries
      (4) Severe distal trauma or limb swelling
   b. **Soft tissue coverage** involves covering the vessels with adequate muscle or skin flaps at the conclusion of the procedure.

D. **Postoperative management**

1. Continue resuscitation after the patient returns to the ICU. Focus on correction of coagulopathy and reversal of shock.
2. Treat any complications that develop.
   a. Closely monitor the patient for development of myoglobinuria and acute lung injury. If necessary, institute supportive measures.
   b. Bleeding and thrombosis are both indications for operative reexploration. A high index of suspicion must be maintained.
   c. Diagnosis of a compartment syndrome requires a high index of suspicion and close observation, especially if a primary fasciotomy was not performed.

HEAD TRAUMA

I. **Brain Injury Classification**
   A. **Primary** injury is an initial mechanical, traumatic, or vascular insult that may be partial or complete.
   B. **Secondary** injury is a global sequela arising from the initial injury and includes:
      1. Hypotension (systolic BP < 90 mm Hg)
      2. Hypoxia (PO_2 < 60 mm Hg, apnea, cyanosis)
      3. Hyperthermia
      4. Hyperglycemia or hypoglycemia
      5. Intracranial hypertension
      6. Edema
      7. Vasospasm
      8. Seizures
II. **Physical Examination**
   A. Initially, focus on airway, breathing, and circulation (see GENERAL ASSESSMENT AND MANAGEMENT: II A–C).
   B. Obtain the initial **neurologic examination** before intubation, sedation, or paralysis, if possible. During the examination, evaluate:
      1. Level of consciousness using the GCS (see Table 14-2)
      2. Baseline neurologic function
      3. Patient's ability to follow commands
      4. Pupil size and reaction to light
      5. Cranial nerve and brainstem function (e.g., facial asymmetry, dysconjugate gaze, pinpoint pupils)
      6. Sensory deficits (see Figure 14-1)
   C. Evaluate extremity tone, movement, and strength.
   D. Look for facial and scalp lacerations, which indicate possible skull fracture.
   E. Evaluate for periorbital and mastoid ecchymosis.
   F. Look for CSF drainage from the nose or ears.
III. **Diagnostic Test: CT Scan**
   A. Obtain a CT scan of the head after the patient has been stabilized. However, it is important to **obtain the CT scan as quickly as possible.**

B. When evaluating the CT scan, consider the following questions:

1. Are basal cisterns present or absent?
2. Is there a chronic or acute hematoma (epidural or subdural) [Figures 26-7 and 26-8]?
3. Is there a subarachnoid hemorrhage and where is it located (e.g., cisterns, ventricles, sulci)?
4. Is there evidence of diffuse axonal injury (i.e., small punctate hemorrhages in the gray–white matter junction predominantly seen in the corpus callosum, brainstem, or cortices)?
5. Is there a coup–contrecoup parenchymal hematoma or contusion?
6. Are there linear or depressed skull fractures, particularly underlying an open laceration or traversing the middle meningeal artery groove of the temporal and parietal bones?
7. Is there evidence of pneumocephalus?

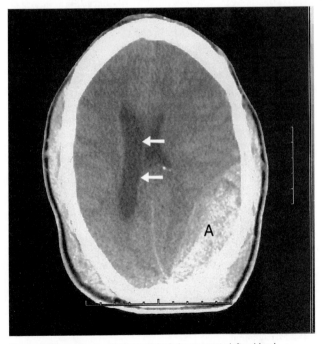

Figure 26-7. A CT scan of the head depicting an acute left epidural hematoma (*A*) following head trauma. Notice the lenticular shape of the hematoma with characteristic hyperintense signal. Notice midline shift (*arrows*) exerted by the epidural hematoma.

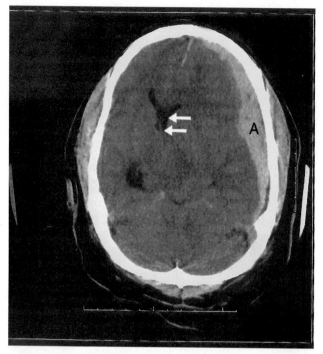

Figure 26-8. A CT scan of the head revealing a 1-cm left acute subdural hematoma (*A*). Notice that in contrast to chronic subdural hematomas, the acute subdural hematoma is hyperintense in relation to the brain. Also notice mass effect on the ventricular system with some degree of midline shift (*arrows*).

8. Are there skull-base fractures, particularly involving the foramen lacerum (indicate carotid artery involvement)?
9. Is there fluid in the sphenoid or ethmoid sinuses (indicates CSF leak)?
10. What is the size of the ventricular system and is there a mass effect?
11. How much midline shift is present, if any?
12. What is the effacement pattern of gyri and sulci?

IV. **Management**
   A. **Goals of management**
      1. Avoid hypotension and hypoxia.
      2. Keep the patient euvolemic, but ensure full resuscitation.
   B. **Evaluation of patient for approach to treatment**

1. Evaluate the risk-to-benefit ratio before deciding on an operative approach.
2. Reevaluate the neurologic examination frequently by correlating neurologic findings with location and mass effect of the lesion. Intubate the patient if the neurologic examination reveals a GCS score of < 8.

It is important to maintain a secure airway during assessment of a head injury.

---

3. After the neurologic examination, the second priority in decision making is the CT scan.
   a. If the CT scan shows diffuse cerebral injury, use a 1-g IV bolus of **phenytoin,** then continue with 100 mg IV tid.
   b. If the CT scan shows a large lesion causing mass effect, perform emergent **craniotomy.**
4. Indications for immediate neurosurgery consultation include:
   a. Trauma and depressed level of consciousness
   b. Head pathology on CT scan
      (1) Intracranial hemorrhage [epidural, subdural, intraparenchymal (Figure 26-9), subarachnoid]
      (2) Skull fracture
      (3) Pneumocephalus
C. **Nonoperative management of closed head injury**
   1. If **stable,** transfer the patient to the ICU for sedation, ventilation, and monitoring.
   2. **Gunshot wounds** to the head do not require emergent surgery, unless a significant mass lesion requires emergent evacuation.
      a. It is best to stabilize the patient and follow the neurologic examination because the operative outcome is not favorable.
      b. A craniotomy for the débridement of extracranial particles at entry and exit sites can be performed on a semiurgent or elective basis.
   3. Patients with **epidural, chronic subdural, or intracranial hematomas** who are awake, alert, and following commands are monitored nonoperatively with daily CT scans until the lesion is stable.
   4. **Hemodynamically unstable** patients or those with **multiple trauma** require an ICP monitor or ventriculostomy.
D. An **ICP monitor** (see Chapter 35), with or without a ventricular drain, is placed intraoperatively if the patient is taken to the operating room emergently or it may be placed in the ICU. A ventricular drain is preferable because it allows therapeutic drainage of CSF.
   1. Additional factors favoring the placement of an ICP monitor with or without a ventricular drain include:
      a. Low GCS score (i.e., 3–8) on admission

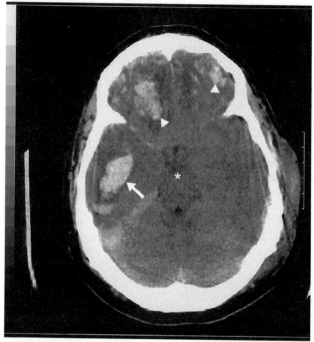

Figure 26-9. CT scan of an intraparenchymal bleed showing multiple contusions involving the right temporal lobe (*arrow*) and bilateral frontal contusions (*arrowheads*). Notice effacement of basal cisterns (*asterisk*) secondary to diffuse cerebral edema.

      b. Evidence of diffuse cerebral injury (e.g., hematoma, contusion, edema, loss of basal cisterns) on CT scan without reliable neurologic examination

      c. Inability to perform reliable neurologic examination because of prolonged sedation or paralysis (patient must be able to follow commands)

      d. Two of the following with a normal CT scan:
          (1) Age > 40 years
          (2) Unilateral or bilateral motor posturing
          (3) Systolic BP < 90 mm Hg

2. When attempting to control ICP (Figure 26-10), keep the following in mind:

      a. Corroborate changes with the neurologic examination, if possible.

      b. The goal is to maintain adequate cerebral perfusion pressure (CPP), which equals mean arterial pressure

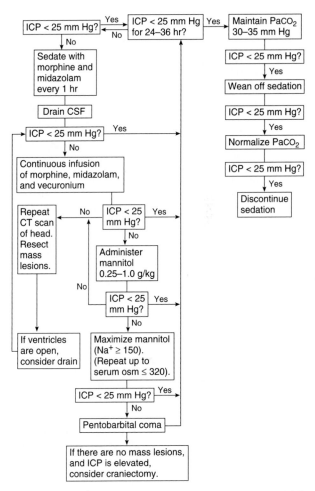

Figure 26-10. Algorithm for management of intracerebral pressure (ICP).

(MAP) minus the ICP. CPP in the range of 50–70 mm Hg has a favorable outcome.

c. Dopamine may be used at a maximum rate of 12 μg/kg/min to elevate the MAP if it is not contraindicated.

d. ICP treatments should be initiated at an upper

threshold of 20–25 mm Hg. Drain CSF to keep ICP < 20–25 mm Hg.

   e. For treatment of symptoms of transtentorial hernia-tion or progressive deterioration, use an intermittent bolus of mannitol, 0.25–1 g/kg IV (avoid hypo-volemia). This can be repeated as long as serum os-molarity is < 310 mOsm.

   f. Hyperventilation is not indicated for long periods of time because it will compromise perfusion. It can be used intermittently for the control of ICP (aim for PCO_2 of 30–35 mm Hg). Indications for hyperventila-tion include acute deterioration of neurologic status or an increase in ICP refractory to other measures.

E. **Operative management of closed head injury**

   1. In patients who are **hemodynamically unstable** or who have **multiple trauma,** if the ICP rises despite nonopera-tive management, surgical evacuation of a focal lesion causing a mass effect may be beneficial.

   2. One third of patients with severe head injuries require surgical evacuation of mass lesions.

   3. **Lesions in basal cisterns** (i.e., medial temporal lobes and posterior frontal lobes) require surgery more promptly. Lesions can obstruct CSF outflow, causing hydrocephalus and brainstem compression.

   4. **Acute subdural hematomas** (see Figure 26-8) with mass effect, midline shift, and resultant focal neurologic find-ings in a semicomatose patient should be emergently evacuated. Prompt evacuation results in a favorable out-come.

   5. **Chronic subdural hematomas** (Figure 26-11) create an osmotic gradient and increase in size with a subsequent mass effect. They are often evacuated on a semielective basis, and can be done electively if the patient is neuro-logically stable.

   6. **Open, depressed skull fractures** require emergent surgery if the fracture involves full-skull thickness. The goals of surgery include skull repair, assessment of dura for lacerations, and cleansing of the area to prevent ab-scess formation.

   7. Elevated ICP with no mass lesions is usually managed with an ICP monitor. However, extreme efforts include uni-lateral or bilateral craniectomy and duraplasty.

F. **Antiseizure prophylaxis** is recommended in the early (i.e., 1–7 days) and not the late posttraumatic period. It has not been shown to improve outcome.

NECK TRAUMA

I. **Zones of the Neck** (Figure 26-12)

   A. **Zone 1** extends from the level of the cricoid cartilage down

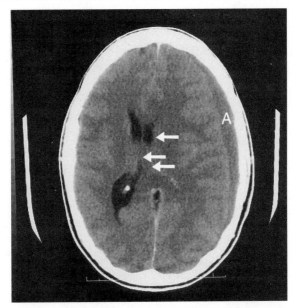

Figure 26-11. CT scan of the head showing a left chronic subdural hematoma (*A*). Notice extra-axial collection (1–2 cm) pushing the brain to the right. Also notice midline shift (*arrows*) and effacement of the left ventricular bodies.

to the level of the clavicle and sternal notch. Zone I contains the:

1. Proximal carotid artery
2. Subclavian vessels
3. Major vessels in the lungs, chest, upper mediastinum, esophagus, trachea, and thoracic duct

B. **Zone 2** extends from the cricoid cartilage to the angle of the mandible.

C. **Zone 3** extends from the angle of the mandible to the base of the skull.

II. **History.** The history should include:

A. Mechanism of injury

B. Chain of events after injury and progression of symptoms

C. Difficulty breathing, swallowing, or talking

D. Location and character of pain

E. Patient's neurologic history

III. **Physical Examination**

> **In cases of neck trauma, physical examination is generally inaccurate for signs of injury.**

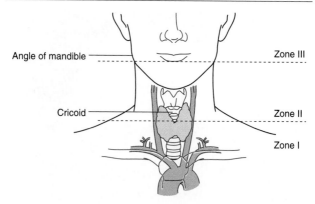

Figure 26-12. Zones of the neck.

A. Evaluate ventilatory exchange.
B. Evaluate for subcutaneous emphysema, hemoptysis, difficulty with phonation, and stridor.
C. Determine the presence of laryngeal trauma, indicated by tenderness, voice change, and shortness of breath.
D. Evaluate for vascular injury by examining all pulses and looking for expanding hematomas. Many vascular injuries may be asymptomatic and clinically occult.
E. Determine if the platysma muscle has been penetrated.
F. Perform a neurologic examination.

IV. **Diagnostic Tests**
   A. Obtain a cervical spine series to evaluate for fractures, retained foreign bodies, subcutaneous emphysema, and bullet marks.
   B. Obtain a chest radiograph to rule out thoracic and parenchymal injury and mediastinal air.

**Massive bleeding may be hidden
in the mediastinum and chest.**

   C. Arteriography is recommended for injuries in zones 1 and 3. Zone 2 arteriography is controversial (i.e., some believe in nonoperative management, whereas others explore all wounds in which the platysma muscle has been penetrated).
      1. Indications for arteriography include blunt injury to the carotid region with signs of hematoma, Horner's syndrome, transient ischemic attacks, nonlucid intervals, and limb paresis in an awake patient.
      2. Arteriography helps to define vascular anatomy (i.e., collaterals) for definitive treatment.
      3. All arteriograms should include both carotid and both vertebral arteries.

D. Perform direct laryngoscopy to evaluate for possible tracheal injury.

E. Perform direct esophagoscopy and barium swallow to evaluate for esophageal injury.

V. Management

A. Initial management. Complete a primary and secondary trauma survey (see GENERAL ASSESSMENT AND MANAGEMENT: II and III).

B. General management

1. Suspected or proved laryngeal injury necessitates tracheostomy if mechanical ventilation is required.

2. Never probe or explore a wound because a clot could dislodge and result in uncontrollable bleeding.

3. Do not place an NG tube until bleeding is controlled because of the risk of retching, which could lead to loss of a hemostatic clot.

4. **Indications for immediate surgery** include:

   a. Expanding hematoma

   b. Active, uncontrolled bleeding

   c. Hemodynamically unstable patient

SPINAL TRAUMA

I. Anatomy of the Spine

A. Spinal column

1. The spinal column consists of 7 cervical, 12 thoracic, and 5 lumbar vertebrae.

2. The vertebral bodies are separated by intervertebral discs and are held together anteriorly and posteriorly by the anterior and posterior longitudinal ligaments.

3. Posterolaterally, two pedicles form the pillars on which the roof of the vertebral canal (i.e., the lamina) rests.

4. The facet joints, interspinous ligaments, and paraspinal muscles work for spinal stability.

B. Spinal cord

1. The spinal cord originates at the caudal end of the medulla oblongata at the foramen magnum and ends at the level of the first lumbar vertebrae as the conus medullaris. The cauda equina continues to the end of the spinal column.

2. The spinal cord is made up of the corticospinal tract, spinothalamic tract, and posterior columns.

   a. The corticospinal tract lies in the posterolateral aspect of the cord and controls motor power on the same side of the body. It is tested by voluntary muscle contraction and involuntary response to painful stimuli.

   b. The spinothalamic tract is located in the anterolateral aspect of the cord. It transmits pain and temperature sensation from the opposite side of the body. It is tested by pinprick and light touch.

      c. The posterior columns carry position sense (i.e., proprioception), vibration sense, and some light touch from the same side of the body. They are tested with vibration and position.

II. Classification of Spinal Injuries

A. An injury is **complete** if there is no demonstrable sensory or motor function below a certain spinal level.

B. An injury is **incomplete** if any motor or sensory function remains. An injury does not classify as incomplete based on preserved sacral reflexes (e.g., bulbocavernosus reflex, anal wink).

C. **Sacral sparing** may be demonstrated by preservation of some sensory function.

D. Spinal injuries are also described based on the **neurologic level,** which includes sensory and motor levels.

    1. The **sensory level** is determined by the most caudal segment of the spinal cord with normal sensory function on both sides of the body.

    2. The **motor level** is determined by the most caudal segment of the spinal cord with motor function of at least three-fifth grade on both sides of the body.

III. Types of Spinal Injuries

A. Atlanto-occipital dislocation

    1. Dislocation results from severe traumatic flexion and distraction.

    2. Most patients die of brainstem destruction.

B. Atlas fracture (C1)

    1. A **Jefferson fracture** is a stable burst fracture that results from impaction of the ring of C1 against the occipital condyles.

    2. Forty percent of atlas fractures are associated with fracture of C2.

C. Axis fracture (C2)

    1. Odontoid fractures are a common result of falls, blows to the head, and motor vehicle crashes.

        a. Type 1 involves the tip of the odontoid.

        b. Type 2 occurs through the base of the dens.

        c. Type 3 occurs at the base of the dens and extends into the body of the axis.

    2. Hangman's fracture is a fracture of the pedicle of C2 from severe overextension and consequent dislocation of C2 on C3.

D. Fracture and subluxation of C3–C7

    1. C5 is the most common site of vertebral fracture.

    2. C5 on C6 is the most common level of subluxation.

E. Thoracic spine fractures

    1. Anterior wedge compression injuries are caused by axial loading with flexion.

    2. Burst injuries are caused by vertical-axial compression.

    3. Chance fractures may be associated with retroperitoneal injuries. Distraction applied in flexion (e.g., seat belt) results in a splitting injury, which begins posteriorly and moves anteriorly through the vertebral body or disc.

4. Fracture and dislocations are relatively uncommon from T1–T10.

F. Fractures of the thoracolumbar junction (T11–L1)

1. Fractures are caused by the immobility of the thoracic vertebrae compared to the lumbar vertebrae.

2. Injuries of the thoracolumbar junction are usually unstable.

3. The nerve roots forming the cauda equina begin at this level; therefore, an injury at the thoracolumbar junction may result in bladder and bowel dysfunction.

G. Lumbar spine fractures should be evaluated with AP and lateral radiographs.

IV. Spinal Cord Syndromes (Table 26-7)

V. Physical Examination

A. Start with evaluation of airway, breathing, circulation, and disability.

1. **Airway:** ensure the airway is clear and open. Consider intubation if the airway is compromised.

2. **Breathing:** evaluate the adequacy of oxygenation and ventilation.

3. **Circulation:** if patient is hypotensive, differentiate between hypovolemic and neurogenic shock.

   a. Hypovolemic shock is indicated by decreased BP, increased heart rate, and cool extremities.

   b. Neurogenic shock results from impairment of the descending sympathetic pathways and is indicated by decreased BP and heart rate and warm extremities. There is a loss of vasomotor tone and loss of sympathetic innervation to the heart, which results in bradycardia or an inability to become tachycardic when required.

4. **Disability:** determine level of consciousness using the GCS (see Table 14-2), assess pupils, and recognize paralysis and paresis.

B. Assess the spine.

1. Palpate the entire spine carefully to assess for deformity; swelling; crepitus; increased pain with palpation; and evidence of contusions, lacerations, and wounds.

2. Evaluate the patient for pain, paralysis, and paresthesia. Determine the presence or absence, the location, and the neurologic level of any pain or dysfunction.

3. Test sensation to pinprick in all dermatomes and determine the most caudal dermatome that feels the prick (see Figure 14-1).

4. Evaluate motor function to determine the lowest neurologic level with adequate motor function.

   a. The deltoid (C5) raises the elbow to the level of the shoulder.

   b. The bicep (C6) flexes the forearm.

Table 26-7 Comparison of Spinal Cord Syndromes

Syndrome	Cause	Characteristics
Central cord syndrome	Vascular compromise caused by hyper-extension injury (e.g., fall with facial impact) in a patient with preexisting cervical canal stenosis	Disproportionately greater loss of motor power in the upper extremities than in the lower extremities
Anterior cord syndrome	Infarction of the cord in the distribution of the anterior spinal artery	Paraplegia and dissociated sensory loss with loss of pain and temperature sensation
Brown-Séquard's syndrome	Hemisection of spinal cord	Ipsilateral motor loss (corticospinal tract) and loss of position sense (posterior columns) associated with contralateral dissociated sensory loss one to two levels below the injury (spinothalamic tract)

    c. The tricep (C7) extends the forearm.
    d. C8 flexes the wrist and fingers.
    e. T1 abducts the small finger.
    f. The iliopsoas (L2) flexes the hip.
    g. The quadricep (L3) extends the knee.
    h. The tibialis anterior (L4) dorsiflexes the ankle.
    i. The extensor hallucis longus (L5) extends the big toe.
    j. The gastrocnemius (S1) plantar flexes the ankle.

  5. Evaluate the strength of each muscle and score on a scale of 0–5.
    a. Total paralysis = 0
    b. Palpable or visual contraction = 1
    c. Full range of motion with gravity eliminated = 2
    d. Full range of motion against gravity = 3
    e. Full range of motion, but less than full strength = 4
    f. Normal strength = 5

  6. Test the deep tendon reflexes.
  7. Document and repeat the neurologic examination at serial intervals.

VI. Diagnostic Tests

  A. Plain films of the spine must be obtained immediately.
  B. A CT scan of the spine should be done to assess bony injury.
  C. An MRI of the spine should be done to examine for hematoma within the spinal canal, direct cord or root injury, ischemia, or ligamentous injury.

VII. Management

  A. Perform **primary and secondary trauma assessments** (see GENERAL ASSESSMENT AND MANAGEMENT: II and III).
  B. Perform a detailed **neurologic examination.**
  C. Maintain spinal stability with a **cervical-spine collar** and **logrolling.**
  D. Consult a **neurosurgeon** and **orthopaedic surgeon.**
  E. If spinal cord injury is likely on examination, begin **methylprednisolone** protocol with a bolus of 30 mg/kg. This can be done in the field or in the emergency department; the earlier the better.
    1. If the initial bolus is **within 3 hours of injury,** give methylprednisolone, 5.4 mg/kg/hr for **23 hours.** Start the continuous infusion 1 hour after the initial bolus or as soon as possible thereafter.
    2. If the initial bolus is **within 3–8 hours after injury,** give methylprednisolone, 5.4 mg/kg/hr for **47 hours.** Start the continuous infusion 1 hour after the initial bolus or as soon as possible thereafter.
  F. Treat **neurogenic shock,** if present.
    1. Guide fluid therapy by CVP or pulmonary artery catheter; however, volume replacement usually is not successful in restoring BP.
    2. Administer inotropes, if necessary, to improve cardiac output.

      3. Administer vasopressors and atropine for bradycardia.
  G. Continually reassess the neurologic examination.

THORACIC TRAUMA

  I. Initial Assessment and Management of Thoracic Trauma
    A. Diagnostic work-up
      1. Follow the standard trauma assessment protocol (see GENERAL ASSESSMENT AND MANAGEMENT: II and III).
        a. The primary survey should identify immediately life-threatening injuries, including:
          (1) Airway obstruction
          (2) Tension pneumothorax
          (3) Open pneumothorax
          (4) Massive hemothorax
          (5) "Flail chest"
          (6) Cardiac tamponade
        b. The secondary survey should identify potentially life-threatening injuries, including:
          (1) Pulmonary contusion
          (2) Myocardial contusion
          (3) Aortic disruption
          (4) Diaphragmatic hernia
          (5) Tracheobronchial disruption
          (6) Esophageal disruption
      2. Inspect and palpate the chest wall for evidence of lacerations, penetrating wounds, sucking chest wounds, abrasions, contusions, and tenderness overlying injured areas.
      3. Auscultate the chest to identify any asymmetry, which may indicate underlying hemothorax or pneumothorax.
      4. Obtain a chest radiograph in the trauma room, which may indicate hemothorax, pneumothorax, pulmonary contusion, mediastinal widening, rib fractures, diaphragm rupture, or missile location.
    B. Initial management
      1. Establish a **secure airway.** Depending on the nature of the injuries, choose one of the following methods:
        a. Natural airway
        b. Orotracheal intubation
        c. Nasotracheal intubation
        d. Surgical cricothyroidotomy
      2. Needle decompression, tube thoracostomy, or emergent thoracotomy may be necessary to **improve oxygenation and ventilation.**
        a. Needle decompression
          (1) In patients with a suspected tension pneumothorax, immediately perform needle decompression with a 14- to 16-gauge IV catheter.
          (2) Place the catheter in the second or third intercostal space in the midclavicular line on the side of the suspected tension pneumothorax.

        (3) After needle decompression, perform tube thoracostomy.

   b. Tube thoracostomy

        (1) Indications for tube thoracostomy include:

           (a) Hemothorax

           (b) Pneumothorax

           (c) Hemopneumothorax

        (2) Place thoracostomy tubes in the midaxillary line at the fourth or fifth intercostal space. Use a minimum of a 36-Fr tube to ensure optimal drainage of clotting blood.

        (3) For patients without hemothorax, tension pneumothorax, or hemopneumothorax who have penetrating chest wounds and are about to undergo positive-pressure ventilation for exploratory laparotomy, place the thoracostomy tube on the side of the chest injury.

   c. Emergent thoracotomy

        (1) Emergent thoracotomy (see Chapter 47) is indicated for penetrating trauma to the chest or abdomen with witnessed and documented loss of pulse and BP but with myocardial electrical activity.

        (2) The prognosis is related to the type of injury and length of time without vital signs.

C. Postoperative management of thoracic trauma patients

  1. Excellent pulmonary toilet is critical in patients with significant thoracic trauma and should be given top priority.

  2. Missed injuries after significant thoracic trauma may be life threatening. Maintain a high index of suspicion for missed injuries when caring for thoracic trauma patients.

  3. Encourage early ambulation, which may reduce many pulmonary complications.

II. Blunt Thoracic Trauma

A. Blunt trauma to the chest wall

  1. Rib fractures

   a. Rib fractures are the most common blunt chest wall injuries.

   b. Treatment consists of adequate pain relief. This prevents muscle splinting and subsequent hypoventilation.

        (1) Place an epidural catheter for analgesia when multiple rib fractures are present.

        (2) Use mechanical ventilation in patients with sufficient lung injury to lead to respiratory failure.

  2. "Flail chest"

   a. "Flail chest" results when multiple consecutive ribs in two separate locations are fractured (or dislocated both anteriorly and posteriorly), allowing paradoxical chest wall motion. The degree of pulmonary compromise depends on the underlying parenchymal injury and the size of the flail segment.

   b. Place an epidural catheter for analgesia.

  c. Intubation and mechanical ventilation may be required for respiratory failure.

B. Blunt cardiac trauma

 1. Signs and symptoms are usually not reliable indicators and include:

  a. External chest trauma (e.g., fractures, imprint of steering wheel)

  b. Chest pain (similar to anginal symptoms but not relieved by nitroglycerin)

 2. Diagnosis

  a. Blunt cardiac injury should be suspected in patients with an appropriate mechanism of injury or in patients who manifest an inappropriately or abnormally poor cardiovascular response to injury.

  b. An **ECG** should be obtained on admission for all patients with a suspected blunt cardiac injury. It is the most significant independent predictor of a complication of myocardial contusion.

   (1) If the ECG is normal, no further work-up is needed.

   (2) If the ECG is abnormal (e.g., arrhythmias, ST changes, ischemia, heart block), the patient should be admitted for monitoring for 24–48 hours.

  c. If the patient is unstable, a **transthoracic or transesophageal echocardiogram** should be performed in addition to the ECG.

C. Blunt vascular trauma

 1. Classification

  a. Aortic transection occurs in over 8000 patients per year in the United States. It usually occurs at the descending aorta just beyond the takeoff of the left subclavian artery.

  b. Undiagnosed **aortic rupture** results in an in-hospital mortality rate of 50% in the first 48 hours; therefore, prompt diagnosis is crucial and a high index of suspicion is mandatory when evaluating patients with significant blunt chest trauma and deceleration injuries.

 2. Etiology. Causes of blunt vascular trauma include:

  a. Motor vehicle accident with or without ejection, air bag deployment, and side impact

  b. Fall from a height

  c. Crushing injury

 3. Diagnostic tests

  a. Angiography is the gold standard for diagnosis of blunt vascular trauma.

  b. Chest radiograph findings that warrant further investigation by aortography include:

   (1) Mediastinal widening > 8 cm on an AP chest radiograph

   (2) Apical cap

(3) Fracture of the first or second ribs or scapula, or multiple rib fractures on the left side
(4) Massive left hemothorax
(5) Depression of the left mainstem bronchus
(6) Fracture or dislocation of the thoracic spine
(7) Loss of the aortic knob
(8) Deviation of the trachea or NG tube to the right

> **High clinical suspicion is the key to diagnosis of blunt vascular trauma.**

4. **Management**
   a. Angiographic evidence of aortic rupture should prompt immediate repair. In this case, aggressively control BP (i.e., keep systolic BP < 140 mm Hg) with nitroprusside and β-blockers until repair is completed.
   b. Postoperative complications include paraplegia, acute renal failure, hemorrhage, and death.

D. Cardiac tamponade
   1. **Signs and symptoms**
      a. Venous pressure elevation (elevated jugular venous distention)
      b. Decreased arterial pressure (hypotension)
      c. Muffled heart sounds
      d. Electromechanical dissociation
      e. Decreased voltage on ECG
      f. Pulsus paradoxus
   2. **Differential diagnosis**
      a. Tension pneumothorax
      b. Massive pulmonary embolus
      c. Hypovolemic shock
   3. **Management**
      a. Administer fluid to increase venous return.
      b. Perform a pericardiocentesis (see Chapter 42) or create a pericardial window.
      c. Perform an exploratory left thoracotomy or sternotomy if the pericardiocentesis is positive (i.e., there is aspiration of nonclotting blood).

E. Blunt pulmonary trauma
   1. **Pulmonary contusion**
      a. **Pathophysiology**
         (1) Pathologic changes include capillary damage resulting in interstitial and intra-alveolar edema.
         (2) A progressive decrease in compliance and an increasing physiologic response results.
         (3) Hypoxia gets worse over 24–72 hours as a result of increasing physiologic shunting and a progressively greater oxygen-diffusion barrier.
         (4) Pulmonary vascular resistance usually increases, and pulmonary blood flow tends to decrease.

(5) Poor outcomes are seen in the following situations:

    (a) Pulmonary contusion on admission radiograph

    (b) Three or more rib fractures

    (c) Chest tube required

    (d) PaO_2/FIO_2 ratio on admission < 250

b. Etiology

(1) Pulmonary contusions result from penetrating, explosive, compressive, and decelerating trauma to the chest.

(2) The force delivered to the chest wall results in a decrease in the size of the chest cavity and compression of the lung.

(3) Physical effects generated by the force include the spalling effect, inertial effect, and implosion effect.

    (a) The spalling effect occurs when the compressive wave generated from the impact meets the liquid–air interface at the alveolus.

    (b) The inertial effect appears to result from different rates of acceleration of the pulmonary tissues, causing stripping of the low-density alveoli from the high-density bronchi.

    (c) The implosion effect is generated by the rebound effect of overexpansion of lung tissue following its compression after injury.

c. Diagnostic tests. Chest radiograph is the standard diagnostic method; however, CT scan is an extremely sensitive method.

(1) In the majority of patients, chest radiograph changes appear during the first 4–6 hours after injury. In the remaining patients, changes develop in the next 24 hours. Chest radiograph changes frequently progress during the first 24–48 hours after injury.

(2) Common pulmonary changes include patchy infiltrates and consolidation of the lung at the site of injury.

(3) Repeat chest radiographs and ABGs should be performed at 6- to 12-hour intervals.

(4) Chest radiographs often underestimate the severity of lung contusions and usually lag at least 24 hours behind ABGs.

d. Management

(1) The primary goals in the management of a pulmonary contusion are to maintain adequate ventilation and prevent pneumonia.

(2) Chest physiotherapy, nasotracheal suctioning, intercostal nerve blocks, and epidural analgesia are used as needed.

(3) If mechanical ventilation is needed, the use of in-

termittent mandatory ventilation and positive end-expiratory pressure usually provides better V/Q matching.

(4) Fluid therapy should be titrated to keep an hourly urine output of 0.5 cc/kg. Blood loss should be replaced with packed red blood cells.

(5) In severely injured patients, continuous monitoring of pulmonary artery wedge pressure and cardiac performance should be considered.

2. Tracheobronchial injury

a. **Incidence.** Tracheobronchial injuries are rare.

b. **Location.** Tracheobronchial injuries usually occur at the carina or within 2 cm of the carina. Tracheal injury may also occur in the neck.

c. **Signs and symptoms** of tracheobronchial injury include:

(1) Massive air leak after thoracostomy

(2) Pneumomediastinum

(3) Subcutaneous emphysema

(4) Large pneumothorax

(5) Round, undeformed endotracheal cuff on chest radiograph

(6) Inability to reexpand lung

d. **Diagnosis** is by tracheobronchoscopy.

e. **Management**

(1) Most tracheobronchial injuries require operative repair. Cardiopulmonary bypass may be necessary if the patient cannot be ventilated by single-lung ventilation.

(2) Avoid high airway pressures postoperatively so that repair will not be jeopardized.

III. Penetrating Thoracic Trauma

A. **Penetrating trauma to the chest wall.** Most penetrating chest wall injuries are relatively innocuous, except for shotgun blasts and injuries to the intercostal and internal mammary arteries.

1. Shotgun blasts may require extensive chest wall reconstruction and prolonged mechanical ventilation.

2. Injuries to intercostal and internal mammary arteries may cause significant hemothorax. Urgent thoracotomy is indicated for the treatment of hemothorax in the following situations:

a. Initial placement of thoracostomy tube results in 1000–1500 cc of blood

b. Drainage > 200–300 cc/hr for the first 4 hours after placement of a thoracostomy tube

B. **Penetrating cardiac trauma**

1. The right ventricle is most often injured in cases of penetrating anterior thoracic trauma.

2. Common **complications** of penetrating cardiac wounds are bleeding and pericardial tamponade.

3. **Management**

    a. All patients with penetrating cardiac wounds should undergo transesophageal echocardiography intraoperatively or in the immediate postoperative period to rule out internal cardiac injuries.

    b. For patients who undergo emergent thoracotomy, open the pericardium and digitally control the cardiac defect. Wounds may be suture repaired or stapled to allow for stabilization and transport to the operating room.

    c. Posterior wounds may require institution of cardiopulmonary bypass for repair.

    d. Avoid high filling pressures and inotropic agents postoperatively, if possible, because they may compromise myocardial repair.

C. Penetrating trauma to the great vessels

    1. Great vessel injuries result from trauma to the base of the neck or to the chest.

    2. Management ranges from simple bypass grafting to hypothermic arrest and cardiopulmonary bypass. Stable patients should undergo arteriography to identify injuries and plan definitive operative repair.

D. Penetrating pulmonary trauma

    1. Manifestations of penetrating pulmonary trauma include:

        a. Pneumothorax

        b. Hemothorax

        c. Pulmonary contusion or hematoma

        d. Systemic air emboli

        e. ARDS

    2. Most pulmonary injuries can be managed by tube thoracostomy and mechanical ventilation.

    3. Injuries that cause massive hemothorax, continuing hemorrhage, persistent air leak, or pulmonary necrosis require thoracotomy and possibly simple repair, stapled wedge resection, formal lobectomy, or pneumonectomy.

    4. Aim postoperative ventilatory management at keeping airway pressures < 40 mm Hg. Limit coughing, straining, and Valsalva maneuver with sedation or paralytic agents to prevent subsequent bronchoalveolar–pulmonary venous fistula and systemic air emboli.

E. Penetrating esophageal trauma

    1. Symptoms of esophageal injury include:

        a. Chest pain

        b. Dysphagia

    2. Diagnosis

        a. Perform Gastrografin esophagography in all patients with suspected esophageal injury.

        b. Some physicians believe that esophagogastroduodenoscopy (EGD) should also be performed in all patients with suspected esophageal injury. For those surgeons who do not perform EGD in all patients, indications for EGD include:

   (1) Assessment of a suspicious lesion seen on esophagography
   (2) Follow-up for a technically imperfect esophagography
   (3) Patients with a high likelihood of esophageal injury

3. **Management**
   a. Operative intervention should rapidly follow diagnosis and may consist of:
      (1) Primary repair with drainage if the injury is < 6 hours old
      (2) Diversion (e.g., cervical esophagostomy) and mediastinal drainage for complex injuries or those > 6 hours old
   b. After repair, keep patients strictly NPO. Maintain nutrition through total parenteral nutrition or a surgically placed jejunal feeding tube. Have patients undergo a Gastrografin swallow 5–7 days after repair to look for a leak.

27

Vascular Disease

AORTIC ANEURYSMS

I. **Anatomy of the Aorta** (Figure 27-1)
II. **Risk Factors for Aortic Aneurysm Formation and Growth**
A. **Size of the aneurysm**
   1. As aortic aneurysms enlarge, the growth rate, rate of aortic dissection, and rate of aortic rupture increase.
   2. Size is perhaps the single most important factor in the decision to intervene surgically on a nonemergent basis.
B. **Hypertension**
   1. Hypertension is known to be independently predictive of aortic rupture.
   2. Because hypertension correlates with a large aortic diameter, it is considered a risk factor for aortic rupture based on Laplace's law (tension = pressure × radius).
C. **Smoking and COPD**
   1. Both smoking and COPD promote aneurysm formation and increased aneurysm growth rates.
   2. The mechanism for this effect is related to increased proteolytic (i.e., collagenase and elastase) activity.
D. **Syphilis**
   1. Before antibiotics, syphilis accounted for 75% of aortic aneurysms.
   2. Since the discovery of appropriate antibiotics, aortic aneurysms secondary to syphilis are rare.
E. **Normal aging**
   1. The aorta becomes increasingly less distensible with age, leading to gradual weakening and subsequent dilation.
   2. Elastin, smooth muscle cells, collagen, and ground substance all change with advancing age.
      a. Elastic fibers fragment.
      b. Smooth muscle cells diminish.
      c. Collagen becomes more prominent.
      d. Ground substance increases.

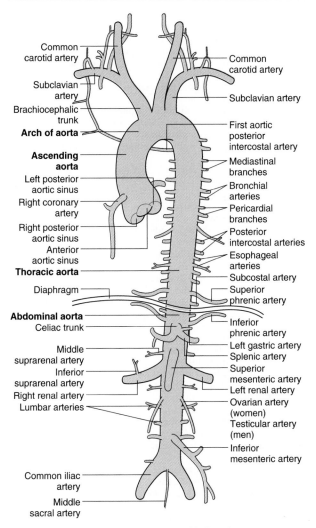

Figure 27-1. The aorta and its branches.

F. Atherosclerosis

1. Atherosclerosis was previously considered a cause of aneurysms of the descending aorta.

2. However, rather than a cause, atherosclerosis may be a concomitant process.

III. Complications of Aortic Aneurysms
A. Complications of untreated aneurysms
1. Rupture (risks include an aneurysm > 5 cm in diameter, elevated blood pressure, presence of COPD, use of steroids, and the presence of a clot in the wall of the aorta)
2. Distal embolization
3. Sudden, complete thrombosis
4. Infection
5. Chronic consumption coagulopathy
6. Development of an arteriovenous fistula

B. Postoperative complications
1. **Early postoperative complications** (i.e., up to 30 days after surgery)
   a. Cardiac events (e.g., ischemia, MI, arrhythmia, CHF)
   b. Pulmonary insufficiency
   c. Renal failure (correlates with preoperative creatinine clearance)
   d. Bleeding
   e. Distal thromboembolism
   f. Wound infection
   g. Ischemic colitis, stroke, and paraplegia
   h. Paralytic ileus
   i. False aneurysms (may occur at the suture line and present as abdominal masses)
   j. Changes in potency and retrograde ejaculation
2. **Late postoperative complications** (i.e., 3–5 years after surgery)
   a. Graft infection (< 1% of cases)
   b. Aortoenteric fistula
   c. Graft occlusion
   d. Anastomotic aneurysms

IV. Aneurysms of the Ascending Aorta
A. Etiology reflects degenerative connective tissue disease of the aortic media and includes:
1. Inherited metabolic derangements (e.g., Marfan's syndrome, Ehlers-Danlos syndrome)
2. Acquired defects (e.g., cystic medial necrosis) in the aortic media
3. Annuloaortic ectasia
4. Idiopathic conditions
5. Chronic type A dissections
6. Infection
7. Mycotic conditions
8. Syphilis
9. Trauma
10. Poststenotic dilation secondary to aortic stenosis

B. Clinical presentation
1. Patients are often asymptomatic at the time of diagnosis.
2. Congestive heart failure (CHF) secondary to aortic insufficiency is commonly the first clinical manifestation.

C. Physical examination

1. Examination of a patient with an aneurysm of the ascending aorta will reveal aortic insufficiency with the associated **diastolic murmur** and a **widened pulse pressure.**
2. Rupture is indicated by pain consistent with rupture and unexplained by other causes, compression of adjacent organs, and significant aortic insufficiency.

D. Diagnostic tests

1. Dilation of the ascending aorta on radiograph indicates an aneurysm.
2. The diagnosis can be confirmed with a CT scan, MRI, or angiogram.
3. Cardiac catheterization is recommended before operative repair to assess for aortic valvular insufficiency, aortic root disease, and associated coronary artery displacement.

E. Management

1. **Indications for surgery** include:
   a. Rupture and symptomatic states (require emergent surgery because of progressive nature of aortic insufficiency)
   b. Enlargement ≥ 1 cm/yr
   c. Aneurysm approaching or already at absolute aortic diameter in the ascending aorta (i.e., 5.0 cm in patients with Marfan's syndrome and 5.5 cm in patients without a documented collagen-vascular disease)
2. The **surgical procedure** depends on the nature of the disease.
   a. In cases of isolated disease of the ascending aorta, a graft is placed between the aorta just above the coronary ostia and innominate artery.
   b. If aortic insufficiency is present, an aortic valve replacement is performed in addition to placement of a graft.
   c. If the aortic annulus is dilated, it is replaced to prevent a recurrent aneurysm. In this case, the ostia of the coronary arteries are reimplanted.

V. Aneurysms of the Aortic Arch

A. Pathology. Aneurysms of the aortic arch may be isolated or associated with aneurysms in other locations in the aorta.

B. Etiology

1. Aortic dissection (e.g., chronic type A dissection)
2. Atherosclerosis
3. Idiopathic conditions
4. Infection
5. Mycotic conditions
6. Syphilis
7. Trauma

C. Clinical presentation. Patients are often asymptomatic at the time of diagnosis.

D. Diagnostic tests

1. Dilation of the aortic arch on radiograph indicates an aneurysm.

    2. The diagnosis can be confirmed with a CT scan, MRI, or angiogram.

  E. Management

    1. Indications for surgery are the same as those for aneurysms of the ascending aorta (see IV E 1).

    2. The **operative technique** is complex and involves both myocardial and cerebral protection employing cardiopulmonary bypass with deep hypothermia and circulatory arrest.

VI. Aneurysms of the Descending Thoracic Aorta (TAAs)

  A. Pathology

    1. TAAs usually originate in the proximal part of the thoracic aorta, just distal to the left subclavian artery.

    2. TAAs may extend a variable distance.

    3. In general, TAAs are fusiform rather than saccular.

  B. Etiology

    1. Atherosclerosis

    2. Infection

    3. Chronic dissection of the aortic wall

    4. Cystic medial necrosis

    5. Aortitis

    6. Traumatic transection

  C. Clinical presentation

    1. Patients are often asymptomatic at the time of diagnosis.

    2. Symptoms may result from enlargement of the aneurysm.

      a. Dyspnea may result from the aneurysm compressing the left mainstem bronchus.

      b. Vocal cord paralysis and associated hoarseness may result from the aneurysm compressing the left recurrent laryngeal nerve where it encircles the ligamentum arteriosum.

    3. Hemoptysis may be secondary to erosion into a bronchus or pulmonary parenchyma.

  D. Diagnostic tests

    1. Dilation of the thoracic aorta on a radiograph indicates an aneurysm.

    2. The diagnosis can be confirmed with a CT scan, MRI, or angiogram.

  E. Management

    1. Indications for surgery (see IV E 1)

    2. Surgical procedures

      a. Graft replacement is performed during a standard left posterolateral thoracotomy.

      b. Options for bypass protect against spinal cord ischemia and include a partial left atrial-femoral bypass or a femoral artery–femoral vein bypass.

      c. The "clamp-and-sew" technique is also used by some surgeons.

      d. Risks associated with aortic replacement with cross-clamping include paraplegia and renal failure.

      e. Somatosensory evoked potential monitoring may be

used to evaluate spinal cord function while the aorta is occluded.

VII. **Aneurysms of the Descending Abdominal Aorta (AAAs)**

A. **Pathophysiology–structural basis for aneurysm formation**

1. Elastin degradation of the aortic wall manifests first in the intimal and medial layers, causing degeneration of these layers. However, elastin disruption and depletion are complete at the stage of relatively small aneurysms. Ultimately, the forces that lead to medial elastin degradation also cause degradation of the elastic lamellae within the inner third of the adventitia.

2. Therefore, aneurysmal disease is primarily a disease of the adventitial layer of the aortic wall. This explains why patients who undergo an endarterectomy do not generally develop aneurysmal vessels.

B. **Pathology—size and rate of expansion of AAAs**

1. **Large AAAs** (i.e., > 5 cm in diameter) expand more rapidly than small aneurysms. The risk of rupture is 25%–41% within 5 years.

2. Of all **small AAAs** (i.e., < 4 cm in diameter), 15%–20% do not expand substantially, and 80% increase progressively, including those that increase by > 0.5 cm/yr. The risk of rupture is approximately 2% within 5 years.

C. **Signs and symptoms**

1. Many AAAs are asymptomatic at the time of diagnosis.

2. Patients may experience pain, which can range from vague discomfort to severe pain. The nature and location of the pain can aid in the diagnosis.

   a. Severe pain in the back or flank suggests a rupture or leak.

   b. Pain that radiates to the groin or pelvis suggests a contained rupture.

3. The **classic triad** of symptoms indicating rupture includes **hypotension, abdominal pain,** and a **pulsatile abdominal mass.** This triad is only present in 50% of patients with an AAA.

D. **Physical examination**

1. Palpate for a pulsatile abdominal mass.

2. Examine all pulses (i.e., carotid, femoral, popliteal, dorsalis pedis, and posterior tibial). Evaluation of pulses helps to determine possible iliac involvement and provides a baseline for postoperative changes.

E. **Diagnostic tests**

1. **Significant findings** on diagnostic tests include:

   a. Suprarenal extension of the aneurysm

   b. Demonstration of stenotic lesions in the renal arteries, superior mesenteric artery (SMA), or celiac trunk

   c. Presence of a thrombus in the aorta

   d. Patency of the inferior mesenteric artery

2. **Abdominal ultrasound**

   a. Sensitivity approaches 100%.

     b. Size is reproducible within 0.6 cm.

     c. Abdominal ultrasound is technician-dependent and does not use contrast or radiation.

     d. Abdominal ultrasound cannot evaluate the longitudinal extent of the aneurysm or the visceral vessels, but it is appropriate for sequential follow-up.

  3. CT scan

     a. CT is highly sensitive.

     b. CT scans provide information about intraluminal and mural thrombi, the size and shape of the aneurysm, and the anatomic relationships of the visceral and renal vessels.

     c. Contrast and radiation are required.

     d. CT scans are appropriate for sequential follow-up or preoperative evaluation.

  4. MRI

     a. MRI is a noninvasive test that does not have any practical advantages over ultrasound or CT.

     b. MRI scans provide accurate measurements and views of relevant vascular anatomy.

     c. Clarity approaches that of aortography.

  5. Aortography

     a. Aortography is used for better definition of the aorta and visceral vessels before repair.

     b. Use of aortography preoperatively is helpful in the following conditions:

       (1) Suspected renovascular hypertension

       (2) Suspected chronic mesenteric ischemia

       (3) Signs or symptoms of lower extremity peripheral vascular disease

       (4) Juxtarenal or suprarenal aneurysm

F. Management

  1. Nonoperative management

     a. If operative management is contraindicated, perform repeat ultrasound examinations every 6 months for aneurysms 4–5 cm in diameter and every 3 months for aneurysms > 5 cm in diameter. The patient may also be followed by CT scans. The rule is to make all judgments between similar examinations.

     b. There is some evidence that the administration of a β-blocker (e.g., propranolol) significantly diminishes the expansion rate of aneurysms > 5 cm in diameter.

  2. Operative management

     a. Indications for surgery

       (1) Ruptured AAA

         (a) The presence of hypotension and abdominal pain with a known AAA or pulsatile abdominal mass is suggestive of rupture and mandates surgery.

   (b) Overall mortality is 90%, and approximately 50% of patients who reach the hospital survive.
   (2) Asymptomatic aneurysm > 5 cm in diameter
   (3) Aneurysm 4–5 cm in diameter in a patient at low operative risk (50% of these aneurysms will expand to > 5 cm in diameter)
   (4) Aneurysms twice the diameter of the normal infrarenal aorta
   (5) Rapid expansion of the aneurysm (i.e., > 0.5 cm in 6 months)
   b. Contraindications to elective surgery
   (1) Myocardial infarction (MI) within the last 6 months
   (2) Intractable CHF or angina
   (3) Severe pulmonary insufficiency with dyspnea at rest
   (4) Severe chronic renal insufficiency
   (5) Life expectancy < 2 years

ARTERIAL INSUFFICIENCY OF THE LOWER EXTREMITIES, CHRONIC

I. Epidemiology
   A. Incidence. The incidence of asymptomatic lower extremity arterial disease with a reference ankle-brachial index (ABI) ≤ 0.9 is 10% in patients 55–74 years of age.
   B. Prevalence
   1. In symptomatic patients 55–74 years of age diagnosed by interview or questionnaire, the prevalence is 4.6% for men and women.
   2. In symptomatic patients 55–74 years of age diagnosed by ABI ≤ 0.9, the prevalence is 16% for men and 13% for women. Male predominance diminishes after 70 years of age.
   C. Natural history. When patients with intermittent claudication are followed over 5 years, 50% show either no change in symptoms or improvement, 16% show progression of symptoms, and < 4% require major amputation.

II. Pathophysiology
   A. Complete or partial atherosclerotic arterial obstruction reduces blood flow.
   B. Intimal damage occurs.
   C. Platelet and fibrin thrombi form.
   D. Cholesterol and low-density lipoproteins accumulate in the vessel wall.
   E. Atherosclerotic plaque forms and stenosis occurs.
   F. Hemorrhage into the plaque and mural thrombi further narrow the vessel.

G. Segmental distribution occurs at bifurcations and angulations, causing the disruption of laminar flow.

H. Collateral vessels form around occluded segments.

I. Exercise increases the metabolic demand and metabolic waste production of the muscles, which results in pain.

III. Risk Factors

A. Cigarette smoking (90% of patients with chronic arterial insufficiency are smokers)

1. Smoking 11–20 cigarettes/day increases relative risk 1.75 times.

2. Smoking > 20 cigarettes/day increases relative risk 2.11 times.

B. Diabetes (results in neuropathy and peripheral atherosclerosis)

C. Systolic hypertension (relative risk: women = 4, men = 2)

D. Hyperlipidemia (A fasting cholesterol level > 270 mg/dl is associated with a doubling of the incidence of claudication.)

E. Male gender if < 70 years of age

F. Age > 50 years

IV. Clinical Presentation

A. Claudication

1. Claudication is exercise-induced leg pain caused by insufficient blood flow through the arteries of the lower extremities (Figures 27-2 and 27-3)

a. Pain is only experienced with sufficient exercise.

b. Pain is relieved with rest.

2. The level of pain is in one muscle group below the arterial lesion.

a. Aortoiliac disease results in buttock and thigh claudication.

b. Iliofemoral disease results in thigh and calf claudication.

c. Femoropopliteal disease results in calf claudication.

d. Tibial disease results in critical foot ischemia.

e. Leriche's syndrome encompasses thigh and buttock claudication, impotence, and absent femoral pulses.

3. Claudication worsens with age and causes a debilitating reduction in activity and quality of life.

B. Critical ischemia

1. Pain occurs in the affected muscle group at rest.

2. Nonhealing ulcers and gangrene may be present.

3. Physical examination reveals signs of ischemia, including:

a. Pallor

b. Pulselessness

c. Pain and coolness

d. Ulcers

e. Dependent rubor

f. Clubbing

4. The ABI is < 0.5, ankle pressure is ≤ 50 mm Hg, and toe pressure is ≤ 30 mm Hg.

V. Differential Diagnosis

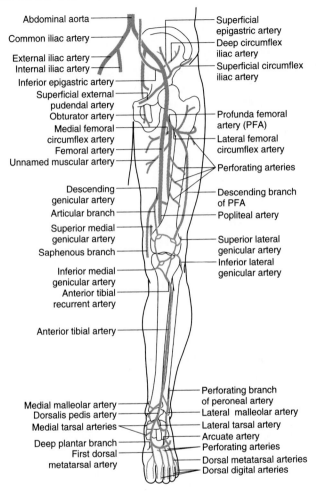

Figure 27-2. Anterior view of lower extremity vascular anatomy.

  A. Nocturnal muscle cramps (not induced by exercise)
  B. Chronic compartment syndrome (occurs after vigorous exercise; slow recovery from pain)
  C. Osteoarthritis (variable severity and onset; slow recovery)
  D. Spinal stenosis (neurogenic claudication)
    1. Radicular leg pain begins with upright posture.
    2. Symptoms (i.e., paresthesia, burning, tingling) are relieved in the recumbent position.

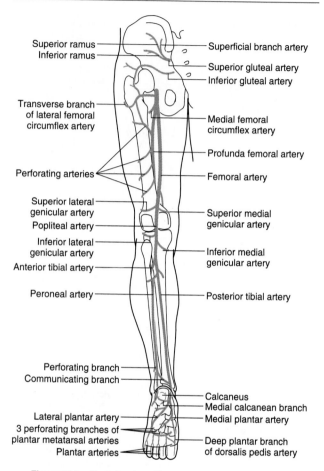

Figure 27-3. Posterior view of lower extremity vascular anatomy.

VI. **Comorbid Conditions**
  A. Coronary artery atherosclerosis
  B. Cerebrovascular disease
  C. Aortic aneurysm
  D. Hyperhomocystinemia
VII. **Diagnostic Tests**
  A. **ABI** (see Chapter 29) is a predictor of arterial insufficiency. If there are no signs of insufficiency at rest, then the ABI should be measured, along with absolute pressures, after the patient has walked on a treadmill with a 12-degree grade for

5 minutes at 2 miles per hour. When measuring ABI, the most important variable is the extent to which ankle pressure falls ($> 20\%$ of the baseline value and requires > 3 minutes for recovery). Following are some reference values to consider when measuring ABI.

1. Normal ankle pressure is 20 mm Hg $>$ brachial pressure (i.e., ABI ≥ 0.9).
2. In claudication, ankle pressure is 30 mm Hg $<$ brachial pressure (i.e., ABI $= 0.5–0.84$).
3. In critical ischemia, the ABI is < 0.5 or there is a pressure drop > 50 mm Hg from the level above.

B. **Doppler segmental pressures** and **pulse volume recordings** help to identify the level of occlusion. An ABI can be calculated from the segmental pressures (Figure 27-4).

C. **Toe systolic pressure index (TSPI)** is a ratio of the pressure recorded from the arm compared to the toe systolic pressure.
  1. A normal TSPI is > 0.6.
  2. If the absolute pressure is ≤ 30 mm Hg, healing is unlikely to occur on the foot without intervention.

D. **Duplex ultrasonography** can be used to assess for areas of arterial stenosis (Table 27-1) or occlusion and for surveillance of bypass grafts. The most reliable method for determining the degree of arterial narrowing is to compare peak systolic velocity changes from one segment of the artery to the next (Table 27-2).

E. **Angiography** is performed preoperatively for definitive identification and characterization of arterial disease. Some patients have other diseases that are overshadowed by the primary symptoms.

VIII. **Management** (Figure 27-5)
  A. **Nonoperative management**
    1. **Reduce the risk factors,** which involves:
      a. Glycemic control in diabetes
      b. Control of hypertension
      c. Smoking cessation
      d. Control of hyperlipidemia (keep low-density lipoprotein cholesterol < 100 mg/dl)
      e. Optimization of body weight
      f. Hormone replacement after menopause
    2. Recommend **progressive exercise therapy** for claudication.
      a. Instruct the patient to exercise from 30 minutes to 1 hour each day to or through the onset of claudication.
      b. After claudication begins, the patient should rest until relief and then resume exercise.
      c. Progressive exercise therapy increases pain-free walking time 134% and peak walking time 96%. The main factor limiting success is lack of patient motivation.
      d. Conditions excluding patients from exercise include

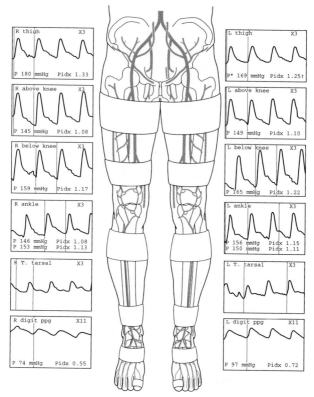

Figure 27-4. Pulse volume recordings of the lower extremity arterial system. The *asterisk* denotes the arterial pressure at each level and the *dagger* denotes the index of the segmental pressure over the brachial pressure (i.e., 169/125 = 1.25).

unstable angina, debilitating COPD or CHF, and severe manifestations of limb ischemia.

3. Prescribe **antiplatelet and rheologic agents.**
   a. Antiplatelet agents include:
      (1) Aspirin, 81–325 mg PO qd (may improve the natural history of patients with intermittent claudication by preventing progression of the arterial disease)
      (2) Ticlopidine, 250 mg PO bid
   b. Consider rheologic agents (e.g., pentoxifylline, 400 mg PO tid) for patients who cannot engage in exer-

Table 27-1. Ultrasonographic Criteria for Arterial Stenosis

Percentage of Stenosis	Ultrasound Finding
None	Triphasic waveform
1%–19% (minimal wall lesion)	Spectral broadening alone
20%–49%	Increase in peak systolic velocity > 30% but < 100% from the preceding segment with preserved reverse flow
50%–99% (critical)	Increase in peak systolic velocity > 100%–150% from one segment to the next segment
100%	No flow

Table 27-2. Peak Systolic Velocity of Various Arteries

Artery	Peak Systolic Velocity
Abdominal aorta	100 ± 20 cm/s
Common external iliac arteries	119 ± 22 cm/s
Proximal superficial femoral artery	91 ± 14 cm/s
Distal superficial femoral artery	94 ± 14 cm/s
Popliteal artery	69 ± 14 cm/s

cise therapy or do not respond to exercise. The actual degree of improvement is unpredictable.

4. Administer a **3-hydroxy-3-methylglutaryl–coenzyme A (HMG-CoA) reductase inhibitor** to lower lipid levels in patients with claudication and elevated serum cholesterol.

5. Provide **foot care** (i.e., prevent and treat injury and infection).

B. Operative management

1. **Indications for surgery**
   a. Activity limited by claudication
   b. Rest pain
   c. Nonhealing ulcer
   d. Gangrene
   e. Vasculogenic impotence

2. **Operative procedures**
   a. **Percutaneous transluminal angioplasty with or without an intra-arterial stent** has a major complication rate of 2%–3%. This procedure is used for:
      (1) Short-segment aortoiliac disease
         (a) Initial success rate: 90%
         (b) 5-year patency rate: 63% in patients with good runoff and 51% in patients with poor runoff

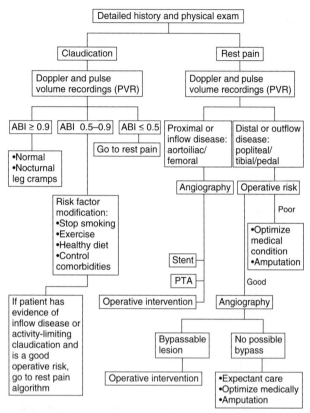

Figure 27-5. Algorithm for the management of peripheral vascular disease. *ABI* = ankle-brachial index; *PTA* = percutaneous transluminal angioplasty.

  (2) Femoropopliteal disease
    (a) Initial success rate: 90%
    (b) 5-year patency rate: 40%–60%
  b. **Surgical bypass grafting** has a morbidity rate of up to 30% and a mortality rate that is usually < 5%. Specific procedures include autologous saphenous vein graft (patency rate is greater than the patency rate for artificial graft or vein transplant) and prosthetic infrainguinal bypass. Bypass grafting is used for:
    (1) Aortobifemoral bypass (5-year patency rate > 90%)
    (2) Femoropopliteal bypass (5-year patency rate 70%–85%)

C. **Postoperative management**
1. Meticulous attention to detail is required to avoid postoperative complications.
2. Consider invasive cardiac monitoring with a pulmonary artery catheter and arterial line in all patients with preexisting cardiac disease.
3. Carefully monitor postoperative renal function.
4. Administer heparin and warfarin sodium for postoperative anticoagulation in patients with small target vessels and poor-quality conduits.
   a. Anticoagulation is a trade-off between postoperative bleeding and potential graft thrombosis.
   b. The level of anticoagulation must be closely monitored and the patient must be routinely examined for signs of bleeding.
5. Administer low-molecular-weight dextran 40 and aspirin to inhibit platelet aggregation and function. Monitor patients for the development of CHF and signs of bleeding with the use of IV dextran 40.
6. Carefully monitor postoperative graft function by following clinical examination, distal pulses, graft Doppler signals, and occlusion pressures. Any changes in the quality of these measurements should prompt consideration of ultrasound, angiography, thrombectomy, or revision of the bypass graft if limb salvage is to be successful.
7. Although postoperative diagnostic imaging may be useful in evaluating graft function, it should not delay operative intervention when indicated. It may also be used to follow graft patency.

IX. **Prognosis for Claudication**
A. Five-year risk of amputation: 4%
B. Five-year risk of worsening claudication or limb-threatening ischemia: 16%
C. Five-year mortality rate: 29% (60% from cardiac complications, 15% from cerebrovascular complications)
D. Ten-year mortality rate: 50%
E. Stabilization of disease or improvement with nonoperative treatment: 75%

ARTERIAL OCCLUSION, ACUTE

I. **Pathophysiology**
A. After obstruction, the vasculature distal to the obstruction begins to spasm. The spasms propagate to a site of adequate collateral flow.
B. After approximately 8 hours, the spasms subside and a clot forms distal to the obstruction, obliterating collateral flow and worsening distal ischemia.
C. Peripheral nerves and muscles withstand acute ischemia for 6–8 hours without permanent damage. Skin withstands acute ischemia for approximately 24 hours.

II. Etiology
A. Embolic etiology
1. **Cardiac embolisms** can result from rheumatic valve disease, atrial fibrillation, and a mural thrombus after MI or a ventricular aneurysm. These embolisms usually occlude larger vessels (i.e., vessels > 5 mm in diameter).
2. **Paradoxical embolisms** are venous in origin and pass through patent atrial or ventricular septal defects.
3. **Intra-arterial embolisms** originate from proximal atherosclerotic or aneurysmal disease and occlude smaller vessels (i.e., vessels < 5 mm in diameter). Blue toe syndrome is an example in which there are palpable pulses with distal digit ischemia due to cholesterol emboli.
4. **Iatrogenic embolisms** can occur after arterial catheterization, angioplasty, and aortic balloon pump placement with dislodgment of atheromatous debris.
B. **Thrombotic etiology.** Spontaneous thrombosis of existing atherosclerotic lesions or aneurysmal disease (e.g., popliteal aneurysms) is less likely to be limb threatening if the patient has preexisting claudication, collateral development, and greater efficiency of oxygen use in the ischemic limb.

III. Signs and Symptoms
A. Pain
B. Paresthesia
C. Paralysis
D. Pallor
E. Pulselessness
F. Poikilothermia

IV. Diagnostic Work-up

**Early diagnosis of acute arterial occlusion
is critical to successful limb salvage.**

A. Careful **history and physical examination** will reveal the level of obstruction, probable cause, and degree of ischemia.
1. History will reveal preexisting cardiac, aortic, or arterio-occlusive disease.
2. Physical examination will reveal limb viability and the level of arterial occlusion, which is determined by color and temperature changes, pulse examination, and Doppler signals.
B. **Diagnostic tests** are important but must not delay prompt therapeutic intervention in the setting of an acutely ischemic limb.
1. Blood work is used to assess hydration, oxygen-carrying capacity, renal function, cardiac function, and muscle loss.
2. Urinalysis is used to assess for myoglobinuria.
3. ECG is used to evaluate cardiac function.
4. An arteriogram is performed only if the diagnosis and therapeutic decision are in question (i.e., absent femoral pulses or acute ischemia overlying chronic arterio-occlu-

sive disease). **Obtaining an arteriogram must not delay intervention in acute ischemia, especially in the presence of sensory motor deficits.**

V. Management

A. Heparinization

1. All patients with limb-threatening acute arterial occlusion should be therapeutically heparinized without delay (see Appendix E, Drug Index, p 757).
2. Heparin prevents clot propagation while natural fibrinolysis occurs.
3. Supratherapeutic doses have been advocated to provide therapeutic levels distal to the arterial obstruction.

B. Embolectomy

1. Acceptable-risk patients who present with ischemia of < 8 hours' duration that is likely embolic in origin should proceed to the operating room for embolectomy.
2. The groin and both legs should be prepped into the field for possible extra-anatomic bypass.
3. A femoral or popliteal approach may be necessary, depending on the level of occlusion.
4. Bypass of atherosclerotic or aneurysmal lesions may be necessary and completion angiography should be obtained.

C. Fasciotomy

1. Four-compartment fasciotomy should be considered in patients after restoration of flow to an acutely ischemic extremity.
2. Fasciotomy is especially indicated if ischemia has persisted for > 6–8 hours.

D. Thrombolytic therapy

1. **Indications for thrombolytic therapy** include:
   a. Acute thrombosis of a previously patent saphenous vein graft or native artery
   b. Acute arterial embolus not accessible to embolectomy
   c. Thrombosis of a popliteal artery aneurysm resulting in severe ischemia, provided that all runoff vessels are also thrombosed
   d. Thromboembolic occlusions in situations in which surgery carries a high potential of mortality
2. **Contraindications to thrombolytic therapy** are listed in Table 5-8 (see p 105).
3. Thrombolytic therapy is not effective in the primary treatment of an advanced acutely ischemic limb because it requires a prolonged period of time to effectively restore blood flow, and tissue loss becomes irreversible after 6–8 hours.
4. Thrombolytic therapy may be effective in patients with subacute ischemia related to thrombosis in whom limb loss is not imminent.
5. Thrombolytic therapy may unmask underlying disease and allow further therapeutic options.

E. **Primary amputation**
1. If tissue loss is imminent or ischemia has been long-standing, primary amputation may be necessary.
2. Critically ill patients or patients with significant preexisting cardiac, pulmonary, or renal disease may not tolerate the systemic effects of restoration of blood flow to an acutely ischemic extremity, and may fare better with primary amputation.

F. **Postoperative management**
1. Observe patients in an ICU setting.
2. Continue heparin anticoagulation or administration of dextran 40.
3. Look for evidence of continued or persistent ischemia and compartment syndrome.
4. Consider inotropic and ventilatory support, alkalinization of the urine, and hemodialysis in the care of patients with myocardial depression, acute respiratory distress, or renal failure that may result from washout of toxic metabolites of anaerobic metabolism after reperfusion.
5. If the source of ischemia is uncertain preoperatively, perform a full work-up (e.g., cardiac and aortic imaging) to rule out hypercoagulable state and determine the underlying cause of acute ischemia.

CEREBROVASCULAR DISEASE

I. **Definitions**
A. **Stroke** (cerebrovascular accident) is a permanent neurologic deficit resulting from disturbed blood flow to the brain.
B. **Transient ischemic attack (TIA)** is a temporary, reversible loss of neurologic function that usually resolves within 24 hours.
C. **Reversible ischemic neurologic deficit** is a temporary, reversible loss of neurologic function lasting > 24 hours.

II. **Anatomy and Pathology**
A. **Cerebral blood supply**
1. The right and left carotid arteries each supply 40%–45% of the blood flow to the brain.
2. The right and left vertebral arteries each supply 5%–10% of the blood flow to the brain.
B. **Atherosclerosis**
1. Atherosclerosis occurs in a segmental distribution.
2. The carotid bifurcation is commonly involved, from the carotid bulb to 1–2 cm into the internal carotid artery.
C. **Collaterals that bypass an occluded carotid artery**
1. External carotid artery → ophthalmic artery → distal internal carotid artery
2. External carotid artery → muscular branches in the neck → distal vertebral artery
3. Anastomoses across the face between the right and left external carotid arteries
4. Vertebral-basilar system

     5. Circle of Willis

III. Incidence of Stroke. In the United States, there are 500,000 strokes per year.

IV. Risk Factors for Stroke

    A. History of TIA and carotid stenosis

       1. First year after TIA and carotid stenosis: 12%–13% risk

       2. Five years after TIA and carotid stenosis: 30%–35% risk

    B. History of previous stroke

       1. First year after stroke: 5%–9% risk

       2. Five years after stroke: 25%–45% risk

    C. Echolucent, heterogeneous plaques of the carotid artery by ultrasound in symptomatic patients

    D. Asymptomatic patients with carotid stenosis > 75%

       1. First year after stenosis: 2%–5% risk

       2. Two to five years after stenosis: 11% risk

Most patients (i.e., 83%) have no warning symptoms before a stroke.

    E. Rapid progression of carotid stenosis between examinations

    F. History of smoking

    G. Male gender

    H. Recent onset of symptoms (i.e., < 30 days)

    I. Anatomic factors (lead to an increased incidence of perioperative stroke)

       1. Contralateral siphon stenosis

       2. Long external carotid artery plaque

       3. Female gender (due to narrower internal carotid arteries)

    J. Comorbid medical conditions

       1. Hypertension (i.e., systolic blood pressure $\geq$ 180 mm Hg and diastolic blood pressure > 90 mm Hg)

       2. Prior MI

       3. CHF

       4. Diabetes mellitus

       5. Hypercholesterolemia, hyperlipidemia

       6. Intermittent claudication

V. Etiology of Stroke

    A. Atheromatous or thrombotic emboli (60%)

    B. Cardiocerebral emboli (15%)

    C. Subarachnoid or intracerebral hemorrhage (15%)

    D. Other (10%)

VI. Signs and Symptoms of Cerebrovascular Disease. The clinical manifestations of cerebrovascular disease depend on the vascular distribution affected.

    A. Left internal carotid artery: aphasia, right facial and body paralysis, left amaurosis fugax

    B. Right internal carotid artery: left facial and body paralysis, right amaurosis fugax

    C. Vertebral artery: incoordination

VII. Differential Diagnosis of a Neurologic Deficit

    A. Seizure

      B. Arrhythmia
      C. Cardiac embolus
      D. Intracranial tumor
      E. Trauma
      F. Thoracic aortic aneurysm
      G. Subclavian steal
      H. Fibromuscular dysplasia
      I. Vagal reflex
      J. Hypoglycemia
      K. Hypoxia
      L. Pulmonary embolus
      M. MI
      N. Aortic stenosis

VIII. Physical Examination
    A. Perform a detailed neurologic examination.
    B. Listen for carotid bruits, a sign of extracranial carotid stenosis, and heart murmurs.
    C. Look for Hollenhorst plaques in the eye fields.
    D. Check the blood pressure in both arms.
    E. Check for pulse regularity.

IX. Diagnostic Tests
    A. Laboratory tests (CBC, platelet count, prothrombin time, activated partial thromboplastin time, electrolytes, BUN/creatinine)
    B. ECG
    C. Duplex ultrasound (combined B-mode and pulsed Doppler)
      1. Ultrasound accurately and noninvasively detects lesions at the carotid bifurcation and along the extracranial internal carotid artery.
      2. Addition of arteriography to ultrasound does not change the operative plan in 98% of patients.
    D. Angiography (gold standard for diagnosis)
      1. Indications for angiography include:
        a. Inadequate ultrasound imaging
        b. Ultrasound suggests more proximal or distal disease
        c. Symptoms do not correlate with ultrasound pathology
      2. Complications associated with angiography include:
        a. Stroke or TIA (1.0%–1.2%)
        b. Death (0.1%)
        c. Contrast-induced acute tubular necrosis (1%)
    E. Magnetic resonance angiography
    F. Cranial CT scan
      1. Abnormal CT scans are seen in 30% of patients with TIA.
      2. Patients with new strokes on CT scan are at higher risk for intraoperative stroke.
    G. Ocular pneumoplethysmography

X. Management
    A. Nonoperative management
      1. Reduce risk factors, which involves:
        a. Control of hypertension

    b. Smoking cessation

    c. Reducing hyperlipidemia

    d. Reducing obesity

    e. Avoiding excessive alcohol consumption

    f. Regular exercise

2. Administer **antiplatelet therapy.**

    a. Enteric-coated aspirin, 325 mg PO qd, reduces the risk of stroke from 10% to 8% in the first year after diagnosis in symptomatic patients.

    b. Administer ticlopidine, 250 mg PO bid, to patients who fail aspirin therapy.

    c. Dipyridamole has not proven beneficial.

3. **Acute carotid occlusion** and **acute carotid dissection** are best treated **medically.** Surgery should be chosen for patients on an individual basis.

B. Operative management

    1. **Indications for surgery** (i.e., carotid endarterectomy)

        a. Symptomatic, good-risk patients are candidates for surgery by a surgeon with mortality and morbidity rates < 5%. Qualities of symptomatic, good-risk patients include:

           (1) TIA or mild stroke in the past 6 months and carotid stenosis > 70%

           (2) TIA, mild or moderate stroke in the past 6 months, and carotid stenosis of 50%–69%

           (3) Progressive stroke and carotid stenosis ≥ 70%

           (4) TIA, ipsilateral stenosis ≥ 70%, and previous or simultaneous coronary artery bypass grafting (CABG)

        b. Asymptomatic, good-risk patients are candidates for surgery by a surgeon with mortality and morbidity rates < 3%. Asymptomatic patients with carotid stenosis ≥ 60% are considered a good risk. In these patients, carotid endarterectomy reduces stroke and death risk from 11% to 5% over 5 years.

        c. Combined carotid artery disease and coronary artery disease may require both CABG and carotid endarterectomy.

           (1) If carotid endarterectomy precedes CABG, there is a greater frequency of MI and death (stroke, 5%; MI, 11%; death, 9%).

           (2) If CABG precedes carotid endarterectomy, there is a greater frequency of stroke (stroke, 10%; MI, 3%; death, 4%).

           (3) Simultaneous procedures (i.e., CABG and carotid endarterectomy) are an option and result in similar frequencies of stroke, MI, and death (stroke, 6%; MI, 5%; death, 6%).

    2. **Operative procedure—carotid endarterectomy**

        a. Use either general or local anesthesia.

           (1) General anesthesia reduces the metabolic rate.

(2) Local anesthesia allows neurologic monitoring.
   b. Use intraoperative heparin.
   c. If indicated, use intraoperative carotid–carotid shunting. Some surgeons shunt all patients, especially under general anesthesia. However, indications for shunting vary by surgeon and can include:
   (1) Symptoms or electroencephalogram changes on clamping
   (2) Internal carotid back pressure < 50 mm Hg
   (3) Contralateral carotid occlusion
   (4) Prior stroke
   d. Avoid emboli during surgery.
   e. The carotid artery is often closed with a patch.
3. **Postoperative management**
   a. Admit patient to an ICU setting for careful monitoring.
   b. Frequently assess the patient's neurologic status. Any changes in the following areas must be reported immediately:
   (1) Speech and phonation
   (2) Strength and movement
   (3) Sensation
   (4) Facial symmetry
   (5) Location of tongue [i.e., tongue should stick out in midline (hypoglossal nerve)]
   c. Inspect the incision for bleeding and hematoma. Check for airway compromise.
   d. Keep systolic blood pressure between 110 and 160 mm Hg.
   (1) If systolic blood pressure is > 160 mm Hg, use nitroprusside to control hypertension.
   (2) If systolic blood pressure is < 110 mm Hg, use phenylephrine, 0.1 mg/kg/min, to desired effect.
   e. Administer antiplatelet therapy, including:
   (1) Aspirin, 325 mg PO daily
   (2) Low-molecular-weight dextran 40 (use in immediate postoperative period)
XI. Prognosis
   A. Morbidity and mortality
   1. Symptomatic and asymptomatic patients: 4.8%–9.0%
   2. Asymptomatic patients: 0%–4.3%
   3. AHA-acceptable levels for operative morbidity for institutions performing carotid endarterectomies are:
   a. Recurrent stenosis: 10%
   b. Stroke: 7%
   c. TIA: 5%
   d. Complications for an asymptomatic patient: 3%
   B. Risk of stroke after carotid endarterectomy
   1. In patients with a history of stroke, there is a 2%–3% risk per year.

2. In patients with a history of TIA, there is a 1%–2% risk per year.
3. In patients with asymptomatic carotid stenosis, there is a 0.7%–2.0% risk per year.

DIABETIC FOOT INFECTION

I. **Incidence.** Foot problems are the reason for 20% of hospitalizations of diabetic patients.

II. **Susceptibility.** Complications of diabetes and severe atherosclerotic disease leave patients susceptible to foot infection.
   A. Peripheral sensory neuropathy may develop in patients with diabetes. These patients may not notice a foreign body or foot lesion because of poor vision or an insensate foot.
   B. An anatomic foot deformity (e.g., Charcot foot) alters the weight-bearing portion of the foot, which increases the likelihood of skin breakdown.
   C. Dry, hyperkeratotic skin is prone to cracking, which can harbor infection.
   D. Tissue ischemia leads to poor wound healing, especially with transcutaneous oximetry values < 20 torr.
   E. Poor neutrophil chemotaxis due to hyperglycemia decreases the ability to combat infection.

III. **Signs and Symptoms.** Patients may present with local or systemic symptoms, including:
   A. Fever
   B. Discoloration
   C. Purulent discharge
   D. Cellulitis
   E. Abscess
   F. Gangrene
   G. Diabetic ketoacidosis or sepsis

IV. **Diagnostic Work-up**

Early diagnosis and treatment of foot infection are imperative to healing.

   A. **Physical examination**
      1. Vigilance is mandatory to rule out deep-space infection.
      2. Pain or even minimal discomfort over the dorsum of the foot may indicate a severe deep-space infection.
   B. Required **blood tests** include CBC, blood chemistries, and blood cultures.
   C. **Plain radiographs** may reveal osteomyelitis and gas, which indicate a deep-space infection.

V. **Management**

Diabetic foot infection should be considered a vascular emergency.

A. **Preoperative and operative management**
1. Stabilize the patient with IV fluids, urine output monitoring, and invasive hemodynamic monitoring as needed. Stabilization may not be possible until definitive drainage is performed.
2. Initiate broad-spectrum, IV antibiotics after blood cultures are drawn.
3. Perform **operative drainage,** which is the cornerstone of treatment.
   a. **Remove all necrotic tissue and drain all pus** during the initial operative procedure to prevent loss of life or limb. Failure of adequate initial débridement may lead to future limb loss.
   b. Digit, transmetatarsal, or leg amputation may be necessary and should be performed as a life-saving measure without hesitation.
   c. Leave wounds open and frequently change the dressing. Formal amputation, closure, or skin grafting can be performed at a later date.
4. Revascularization may be required if pulse volume recordings and transcutaneous oximetry are indicative of poor healing.
   a. Perform revascularization after the extremity has been adequately débrided and the infection has been removed.
   b. **Do not place a fresh arterial graft into an area of acute infection.**

B. **Postoperative management**
1. Frequently change the wound dressing.
2. Perform bedside débridement.
3. Apply antibiotic creams (e.g., Silvadene)
4. Send the patient for hydrotherapy and physical therapy.
5. Consider skin grafting of the wound at a later date.

C. **Preventive care**
1. Meticulous foot care with a team that includes the primary care provider, podiatrist, and vascular surgeon is most beneficial to avoid potentially lethal and morbid complications of diabetic foot infections.
2. Educate the patient to perform surveillance and preventive care.

VI. **Prognosis**
   A. Limb loss occurs in approximately 10%–20% of patients hospitalized for diabetic foot infection.
   B. The outcome of diabetic foot infection depends on immediate recognition, correction of metabolic derangement, and complete surgical excision and drainage.

MESENTERIC ISCHEMIA

I. **Acute Mesenteric Ischemia (AMI)**
   A. In AMI, **intestinal viability is threatened.**

B. Classification of AMI
 1. Arterial AMI
   a. SMA thromboses occur at areas of chronic athero-sclerosis and narrowing, usually at the origin of the SMA. AMI is commonly superimposed on chronic mesenteric ischemia (CMI). Patients have atherosclerotic disease of multiple vascular beds.
   b. SMA emboli are usually cardiac in origin and account for 40%–50% of episodes of AMI. These lesions are usually 3–10 cm past the origin of the SMA (i.e., distal to the middle colic artery).
   c. Nonocclusive mesenteric ischemia (NOMI) results from splanchnic vasoconstriction due to low-flow states (e.g., hypotension, low cardiac output) or medications. NOMI accounts for 20%–30% of episodes of AMI.
 2. Venous AMI—acute mesenteric vein thrombosis
   a. Acute mesenteric vein thrombosis accounts for < 5% of cases of AMI.
   b. It is associated with hypercoagulable states, portal hypertension, retroperitoneal and intraabdominal inflammatory processes, postoperative state, and trauma.

C. Risk factors
 1. Age > 50 years
 2. CHF
 3. Cardiac arrhythmias
 4. Recent MI or hypotension
 5 Previous or synchronous emboli

D. Signs and symptoms
 1. Abdominal pain occurs in 75%–98% of patients with AMI. Pain out of proportion to physical findings, especially in conjunction with rapid and forceful bowel evacuation, is highly suggestive of AMI.
 2. Development of peritonitis suggests developing full-thickness bowel necrosis.

E. Diagnostic tests
 1. Abdominal radiograph is usually normal early in the course of disease (i.e., before infarction). Late findings include "thumbprinting," free air after perforation, and pneumatosis or portal venous gas.
 2. Laparoscopy does not allow mucosal evaluation.
 3. Ultrasound may show portal and mesenteric venous thromboses. However, it is technician-dependent and is difficult if an ileus is present.
 4. Angiography is the gold standard for the diagnosis of occlusive and nonocclusive AMI and is the mainstay of treatment for nonocclusive disease. The false-negative rate may be as high as 50%. Early diagnosis depends on a high index of suspicion.
 5. Findings on **laboratory tests** include leukocytosis, hyper-

amylasemia, abnormal liver function, occult blood in the stool (75% of patients), and elevated lactic acid.

6. **ECG** can rule out MI and atrial fibrillation.

7. **Endoscopy** can be used to evaluate colonic mucosa.

F. **Management** (Figure 27-6)

1. **General management of AMI**

   a. Treat **underlying or predisposing factors** (e.g., hypovolemia, CHF).

   b. Keep patient **NPO.**

   c. Provide **fluid resuscitation.** Use invasive blood pressure monitoring and a Swan-Ganz catheter to guide preoperative, intraoperative, and postoperative fluid resuscitation.

   d. Obtain **plain radiographs** to rule out a perforated viscus and other diagnoses.

   e. Perform selective **angiography.**

   f. Administer **broad-spectrum antibiotics.**

   g. Insert a **Foley catheter** and a **nasogastric tube.**

2. **Management of an SMA embolus**

   a. If an SMA embolus is identified on angiography, place a catheter and begin infusion of **papaverine.** For small emboli, begin **urokinase** infusion. Failure of urokinase success within 4 hours is an indication for surgery.

   b. If an SMA embolus is seen with peritoneal signs, proceed to **laparotomy with resection of gangrenous bowel, embolectomy, and reconstruction of the SMA,** and then make an **assessment of viable bowel** (in that order).

   c. Continue papaverine infusion postoperatively for at least 12–24 hours, then obtain an **angiogram** to evaluate for persistent vasospasm.

   d. If a second-look laparotomy is planned, continue papaverine infusion through the second operation and postoperative angiogram.

3. **Management of SMA thrombosis**

   a. Differentiate thrombosis from embolus. Good collateralization may indicate a chronic state with longstanding occlusion and no acute thrombus.

   b. Start an infusion of **papaverine or urokinase.**

   c. **Revascularize** with reimplantation, thrombectomy and endarterectomy, bypass grafting (with or without stenting), or angioplasty.

4. **Management of NOMI**

   a. Correct shock and sepsis and **discontinue vasopressors.**

   b. Infusion of **papaverine** (30–60 mg/hr) or **glucagon** (2–4 mg/hr) via the SMA catheter is the mainstay of treatment.

   c. **IV heparinization** is necessary to prevent cannula thrombosis.

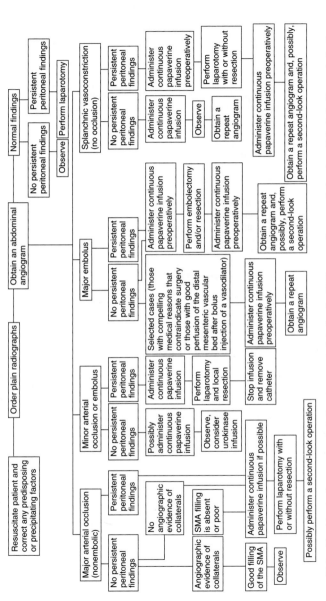

Figure 27-6. Algorithm for the management of acute mesenteric ischemia. *SMA* = superior mesenteric artery. (Adapted with permission from Reinus JF, Brandt LJ, Boley SJ: Algorithm for the management of acute mesenteric ischemia. *Clin North Am* 19:319, 1990.)

    d. Patients with peritoneal signs require laparotomy and resection of obvious gangrenous bowel.

    e. Continue papaverine infusion while reassessing the bowel with a **second-look laparotomy** 24–36 hours later.

II. Chronic Mesenteric Ischemia (CMI)

A. In CMI, intestinal viability is not threatened, but **blood flow is inadequate** to support functional demands.

B. **Signs and symptoms** mimic nonspecific findings of GI malignancy and include:

    1. **Weight loss** (most common finding)

    2. Food aversion

        a. Food aversion is secondary to postprandial abdominal pain.

        b. Patients usually take frequent, small meals or do not eat at all to avoid the pain.

    3. Chronic abdominal discomfort

C. **Diagnostic test—aortic angiography**

    1. The involvement of at least two visceral vessels is necessary for the diagnosis of CMI.

    2. Eighty-five percent of CMI patients have significant stenosis of the SMA and celiac artery on lateral projection.

D. **Management. Elective bypass grafting** is the treatment of choice.

PART III

Procedures

28

Abscess: Incision and

Drainage

I. **Definition.** An abscess is a localized collection of purulent material.

II. **Diagnosis**
   A. **Physical examination** may reveal fever, malaise, evidence of prior trauma, swelling or deformity, erythema, local warmth, induration, fluctuance, tenderness, drainage, a fistula, or a loss of function in the affected area.
   B. **Aspiration** by a 14-gauge "finder needle" may be used to localize purulence.
   C. **Imaging studies** are reserved for cases in which the abscess is deep, there is a possibility of extension of a superficial abscess, or there is concern for osteomyelitis.
   D. **Laboratory studies** include complete blood count and blood culture.

III. **Management**
   A. **Treatment of an abscess is guided by several factors:**
      1. **Location** (determines accessibility and threat to adjacent structures)
      2. **Etiology** (e.g., trauma, hematogenous seeding, microorganisms present)
      3. **Host immune function**
      4. Presence of **cellulitis**
      5. Need for **anesthesia** to incise and drain
   B. **Procedure**
      1. Administer anesthesia.
         a. Anesthesia may not be required for simple abscesses.
         b. In the case of perirectal abscesses or wounds requiring substantial debridement, local infiltration of lidocaine (0.5%–2.0%) with or without epinephrine, sedation, or general anesthesia may be required.

2. Position the patient for free access to the abscess on a bed or table at a sufficient height with bright lighting.
3. Prepare the area using iodine solution.
4. Place sterile drapes.
5. Aspirate with a 14-gauge needle to help localize collection and to improve comfort by reducing pressure.
6. Incise the abscess.
   a. Ensure that the area is anesthetized.
   b. Use a sterile #11 blade.
   c. Avoid injury to local neurovascular structures.
   d. Start the incision small and extend it to eventually span the entire diameter of the abscess.
   e. In the case of perirectal abscesses, make a crusciate- or T-shaped incision to prevent the skin from sealing over.
7. Drain all accessible purulence using external pressure, suction, or irrigation.
8. Swab the wound for Gram stain, culture, and sensitivity.
9. Break loculations crossing the abscess space by repeatedly opening a curved hemostat or by using a finger.
10. Sharply debride any gangrenous, necrotic, or devitalized tissue.
11. Probe the fascial planes to evaluate for fasciitis.
12. Inspect the wound for hemostasis and control brisk bleeding.
13. Irrigate the wound well with copious amounts of warm, sterile saline solution.

If an abscess cannot be adequately drained in a procedure room or if necrotizing fasciitis is detected, proceed to the operating room.

---

14. All but the smallest abscesses require packing.
    a. Pack the full extent of the cavity.
    b. Use sterile tapes, gauze, or sponges.
    c. Use the smallest number of the largest packs to avoid losing packing material within the wound.
    d. Packs should be wet-to-dry dressings with normal saline changed twice a day until the wound heals from the base up.
    e. The first pack can be soaked with iodine solution.
15. Some wounds require drains (e.g., abscesses secondary to animal bites).
    a. Wounds usually require open drainage with a Penrose drain.
    b. Perirectal abscesses with fistula-in-ano can be treated with silk suture "seton" passed through the fistula tract until the fistula can be resected or as the definitive treatment.
16. Cover the wound with dry, sterile dressing.

17. Consider antibiotics in the following cases:
    a. Associated cellulitis
    b. Immune compromise
    c. Sepsis
    d. Ongoing infection from the primary source
18. Consider admission to the hospital based on the patient's condition and ability to care for the wound.

29

Ankle-Brachial Index

I. Indications

A. The ankle-brachial index (ABI) is a useful screening test for **peripheral vascular disease.**

B. An ABI should be performed on any patient suffering **extremity trauma** (e.g., gunshot wound, fracture, crush injury) or when perfusion is questioned.

C. The ABI is used to provide an indication of the **arterial circulation** to the extremities; however, it is insensitive in identifying the progression of other sclerotic disease.

D. Signs of vascular insufficiency (injury) that may indicate the need to check the ABI include:

1. Pain
2. Pulselessness
3. Pallor
4. Paresthesias
5. Paralysis
6. Poikilothymia
7. Pulsatile hemorrhage
8. Thrill or bruit

II. Procedure

A. Allow 5 minutes after any exercise (e.g., walking) to perform the examination. The patient should be in the supine position.

B. Place a Doppler probe over the selected artery at the ankle or foot.

C. Inflate a sphygmomanometer cuff at the calf until the signal becomes inaudible.

D. Release the cuff pressure slowly and record the pressure at which the signal returns.

E. Repeat the procedure at the brachial artery.

F. Calculate the ABI (ABI = ankle occlusion pressure/brachial occlusion pressure).

G. Make comparisons to the contralateral limb.

III. Evaluation

A. Nontraumatic conditions

1. The ABI value can be used to confirm the diagnosis of a suspected condition (Table 29-1).
2. An ankle pressure less than 40 mm Hg indicates severe disease regardless of the ABI.

B. Trauma to an extremity

1. Measure the occlusion pressure of the injured extremity and divide by the occlusion pressure of an uninjured arm (use a leg if both arms are injured).
2. A difference of greater than 20 mm Hg or a ratio of less than 0.9 mm Hg requires an evaluation by angiography, which guides exploration and repair by a vascular surgeon. The following guidelines are for the angiographic evaluation of injured extremities.
   a. Use opaque markers to identify surface injuries.
   b. Position the patient and catheters such that orthogonal views of the entire extremity are available.
   c. Evaluate for early arteriovenous fistula filling and late pseudoaneurysm contrast retention.
   d. Hydrate the patient before and after the procedure to reduce nephrotoxicity.
   e. After the procedure, the patient must lie flat and the distal pulse and groin must be monitored for adequacy of flow and bleeding.

Table 29-1. Significance of the Ankle-Brachial Index (ABI)

Condition	Typical ABI Value
Normal	1.1 mm Hg
Subcritical stenosis of lower extremity blood vessels	1.1 mm Hg*
Significant arterial disease	<0.9 mm Hg
Arterial injury	<0.9 mm Hg
Claudication	0.60 ± 0.15 mm Hg
Revascularization indicated	<0.5 mm Hg
Revascularization inevitable	<0.3 mm Hg
Ischemic ulcer	0.4 ± 0.1 mm Hg
Rest pain	0.25 ± 0.13
Impending gangrene	0.05 ± 0.08 mm Hg

*With subcritical stenosis of lower extremity blood vessels, the ABI will be normal at rest. With exercise, the ABI will drop to below normal, gradually returning to normal at rest. This dip in the ABI corresponds with symptoms of claudication.

30

Bronchoscopy and

Bronchoalveolar Lavage

I. **Lobar Lung Anatomy (Figure 30-1)**
II. **Bronchoscopy**
   A. **Indications**
   1. **Malignancy** (yields diagnosis in 55%–85% of central lesions; variable results with peripheral lesions)
   2. **Interstitial lung disease** (sarcoidosis, lymphangitic spread of cancer, hypersensitivity)
   3. **Immunosuppressed patients** (human immunodeficiency virus positive, post-transplant; high yield for pneumocystis pneumonia)
   4. **Nonresolving pneumonia** [in conjunction with bronchoalveolar lavage (BAL) or biopsy]
   5. **Hemoptysis**
   6. Assist with **intubation**
   B. **Basic technique of flexible bronchoscopy**
   1. **Premedication** regimen includes:
      a. **Antisialogogues** (atropine, glycopyrrolate, or scopolamine) to reduce oral secretions
      b. Sedation with **narcotics** (meperidine with hydroxyzine), **benzodiazepines** (midazolam, lorazepam, or diazepam), or both
   2. **Preoxygenate** the patient with 100% oxygen by face mask or ventilator.
   3. For **nonintubated** patients:
      a. Insert a bite block into the mouth.
      b. Insert the flexible bronchoscope through the bite block and over the tongue. Maintain the tip slightly upward until the epiglottis is encountered.
      c. When the epiglottis is directly visualized, straighten the tip and advance the bronchoscope through the center of the vocal cords.

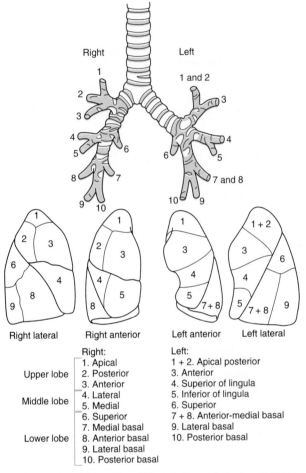

Figure 30-1. Lobar lung anatomy. (Adapted with permission from Sabiston D: *Sabiston Textbook of Surgery,* 15th ed. Philadelphia, WB Saunders, 1997, p 1777.)

d. Advance the scope until the trachea and carina come into view.

e. Advance the tip into the orifices of the left and right mainstem bronchi.

f. To prevent coughing during the procedure, instill topical lidocaine into the upper trachea, the mainstem bronchi, and the lobar bronchi bilaterally.

4. For **intubated** patients:
   a. Insert the flexible bronchoscope directly through the endotracheal tube.
   b. Follow the steps for nonintubated patients.
C. **Complications of flexible bronchoscopy**
   1. **Airway obstruction** resulting in increased work of breathing, hypoxia, hypercarbia, and arrhythmias
   2. **Oversedation** resulting in decreased respiratory drive, hypoxemia, and hypercarbia
   3. **Lidocaine toxicity** resulting in seizures, tachyarrhythmias, bradyarrhythmias, and hypotension
   4. **Mechanical trauma** resulting in dental damage and postprocedure hemoptysis
   5. **Fever and flu-like symptoms** (33% of patients) secondary to cytokine release from alveolar macrophages

III. Bronchoalveolar Lavage (BAL)

A. **Common diseases investigated with BAL**
   1. **Diffuse interstitial lung disease** (sarcoidosis, pulmonary fibrosis, hypersensitivity pneumonitis)
   2. **Environmental or occupational lung diseases** (asbestos, silica, beryllium)
   3. Genetic or acquired **deficiency diseases** [cystic fibrosis, α_1-antitrypsin deficiency, acquired immune deficiency syndrome (AIDS)]
   4. **Alveolar airway disease** (asthma, chronic obstructive pulmonary disease, alveolar proteinosis)
   5. **Malignancy**
   6. **Adult respiratory distress syndrome**
   7. **Pneumonia**
B. **Technique of BAL**
   1. Follow the steps for flexible bronchoscopy (see p 660).
   2. Instill warm saline (in aliquots of 20 ml to 60 ml) through the working channel of the bronchoscope.
   3. Aspirate the instilled fluid after it has dwelled briefly in the lung segment to be studied. An internal control can be used (i.e., the opposite lung).
   4. Send specimens for chemical analysis, cytology examination, bacterial culture, and Gram stain.
C. **Protected BAL** is a variation of conventional BAL in which distally protected catheters are used. This procedure avoids contact between BAL fluid and the suction channel, which may be contaminated with oral-tracheal organisms.

IV. Nonbronchoscopic Bronchoalveolar Lavage (BAL) [Catheter-Directed BAL]

A. **Indications**
   1. Patient with AIDS with a possible presence of **pneumocystis pneumonia**
   2. **Ventilator-associated pneumonia**
      a. Quantitative culture is required to ensure proper specificity.
      b. The cutoff point for bacterial growth varies from 10^3

to 10^5, depending on the dilution of the lung secretions in the BAL fluid.

   c. Typical dilution varies from 10–100 times, so a **count of 10^4 colonies is equivalent to 10^5-10^6 bacteria/ml** of lung secretion, a figure considered indicative of infection.

   d. In the presence of antibiotic treatment, the sensitivity of nonbronchoscopic BAL is reduced.

B. Technique for Ballard (directional) catheter BAL in mechanically ventilated patients

   1. Apply the catheter adapter to the end of the endotracheal (tracheostomy) tube.

   2. Insert the catheter through the endotracheal tube adapter.

   3. Direct the catheter clockwise (i.e., to the right mainstem bronchus).

   4. Instill 20–60 ml of warm saline, allow it to dwell for 1–2 minutes, and then aspirate it.

   5. Direct the catheter counterclockwise (i.e., toward the left mainstem bronchus). Use a new catheter if the procedure is for cultures.

   6. Instill 20–60 ml of warm saline, allow it to dwell for 1–2 minutes, and then aspirate it.

   7. Send each fluid sample separately for quantitative culture.

C. Advantages of nonbronchoscopic BAL (as compared to conventional BAL)

   1. Easy to obtain alveolar specimens

   2. Safe

   3. Rapid

   4. Does not require extensive training

   5. Disposable catheters

   6. Inexpensive

   7. Protected specimen is not contaminated by upper airway flora

D. Disadvantages of nonbronchoscopic BAL (as compared to conventional BAL)

   1. Random sample (no direct visualization)

   2. Semiquantitative study (unknown dilution)

31

Chest Tube Placement

and Removal

I. Chest Tube Placement Techniques

A. **Posterolateral approach** is used for trauma and spontaneous pneumothorax.

1. Choose the appropriate size chest tube.

a. In the case of trauma with a high incidence of hemothorax, a large-caliber chest tube (i.e., greater than 36 Fr) should be used to drain blood and fluid adequately.

b. In the case of a spontaneous pneumothorax, a relatively small chest tube (i.e., 20–34 Fr) may be used. The size varies according to individual choice.

2. Determine the insertion site.

a. The chest tube is usually inserted just below the nipple level (i.e., the fifth intercostal space) anterior to the midaxillary line.

b. The incision is over the sixth rib.

3. Surgically prepare the chest with povidone-iodine and drape in a sterile fashion.

4. Locally anesthetize the skin, rib, and intercostal muscles. Remember that the neurovascular bundles run along the inferior aspect of the ribs.

a. Use 1% lidocaine and make a large skin wheal.

b. Anesthetize the underlying muscle.

5. Make a 2- to 3-cm transverse incision over the rib at the predetermined site and bluntly dissect through the subcutaneous tissues to a point just over the top of the rib. It is important to maintain adequate anesthesia and analgesia.

6. Insert the lidocaine syringe through the incision and enter the chest cavity with the needle while the plunger is

pulled back. When in the pleural space, there will be a rush of air. Slowly withdraw the needle and inject the lidocaine.

7. Prepare the chest tube with a large Kelly clamp placed over the proximal chest tube longitudinally.

8. With another Kelly clamp, puncture through the remaining muscle and the parietal pleura; do not plunge into the chest. Place a gloved finger into the hole to avoid injury to other organs and to clear any adhesions or clots. When in the thorax, it may be necessary to use the clamp to dilate the opening.

9. Advance the chest tube on the Kelly clamp into the hole, in a posterior and superior direction. When the chest tube is in the chest, release the clamp and guide the chest tube to the desired length.

10. Look for fogging of the chest tube or fluid return to assure placement within the thorax.

11. Connect the end of the chest tube to a water seal apparatus and apply negative 20 cm water suction.

12. Suture the chest tube in place with a silk or monofilament suture. Make sure there is a tight seal to the skin.

13. Apply an occlusive dressing and secure the chest tube and the tubing to each other and to the chest.

14. Obtain a chest x-ray to check tube placement and to assess for pneumothorax.

B. **Anterior approach** is most often used for spontaneous pneumothorax. It **should not be used for trauma or fluid drainage.**

1. Obtain a 24-Fr chest tube or smaller.

2. Identify the second intercostal space in the midclavicular line as the insertion site.

3. Surgically prepare the chest with povidone-iodine and drape in a sterile fashion.

4. Locally anesthetize the skin, rib, and intercostal muscles. Remember that the neurovascular bundles run along the inferior aspect of the ribs.

   a. Use 1% lidocaine and make a large skin wheal.

   b. Anesthetize the underlying muscle and carefully enter the pleural space with constant back pressure on the syringe.

   c. When air returns in the syringe, slowly withdraw the needle while instilling local anesthesia.

5. Make a 1-cm transverse incision over the rib at the predetermined site and bluntly dissect through the subcutaneous tissues to a point just over the top of the rib.

6. Follow the steps for posterior approach.

II. Chest Tube Removal

A. Make sure that the chest tube has been placed on water seal for 6 hours or longer before removal.

    B. Make sure the patient has no pneumothorax on upright posteroanterior chest x-ray when on water seal.

    C. While the patient is still on water seal, make sure there is no air leak.

    D. Place the patient in a supine position.

    E. Prepare a few gauze sponges with Xeroform gauze and bacitracin ointment in the center.

    F. Cut multiple strips of wide or elastic tape.

    G. Remove the dressing and cut the stay suture. Make sure not to cut the U-stitch if present.

    H. Place the gauze and Xeroform to the insertion site on top of the chest tube and maintain firm pressure.

    I. Have the patient inhale fully and perform the Valsalva maneuver, at which time the chest tube is removed in one constant, brisk pull.

    J. Without releasing pressure on the gauze (tie the U-stitch if present), apply strips of tape over the full surface of the dressing.

    K. Obtain a repeat chest x-ray to rule out recurrent pneumothorax. Allowing a 2- to 6-hour interval between removal and chest x-ray provides better accuracy.

III. Three-Bottle Suction (Figure 31-1)

    A. Collection bottle ("fluid trap")

        1. A series of clear chambers with graduated markings is used to measure the amount of fluid or blood drained.

        2. Fluid drained from the patient via the chest tube is trapped while gas continues on to the water seal bottle.

    B. Water seal bottle

        1. The tip of the tube that leads to the collection bottle is submerged under water.

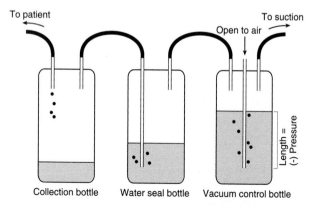

Figure 31-1. Diagram of standard three-bottle suction apparatus.

2. Gas exiting the patient via the collection tube bubbles through the water in the water seal bottle. The gas cannot return to the patient because the liquid blocks passage back to the collection bottle.

3. Air leaks are exhibited by air bubbling through the water in the water seal bottle. Small or slow air leaks are detected by disconnecting the vacuum control bottle from suction, asking the patient to cough, and observing for bubbles during coughing.

C. **Vacuum control bottle**

1. The vacuum control bottle is connected to wall suction or a portable vacuum generator.

2. Outside suction must be increased until bubbles are seen in the vacuum control bottle.

3. Vacuum is transmitted to the patient via the collection and water seal bottles.

4. As vacuum increases, outside air will be drawn down the center tube.

5. If the negative pressure (measured in cm H_2O) exceeds the submerged length of the tube open to air, outside air will bubble into the bottle, thereby limiting the vacuum transmitted to the patient.

6. Adding or removing water adjusts the amount of negative pressure.

IV. **Chest Tube Apparatus** (Figure 31-2)

A. The **water seal pressure scale** determines the negativity in the patient's chest cavity. Oscillation of this compartment demonstrates patency in the system. Oscillations may not be present with suction, when the lung is fully inflated, or the tubing is locked or kinked.

1. If there is no suction attached, the pressure in the chest cavity is read by the fluid level on this scale.

2. If there is suction attached, add the reading from the suction control chamber to the reading of the water seal pressure scale.

B. The **patient air leak meter** indicates the approximate degree of air leak. The greater the number, the greater the leak.

C. The **positive pressure relief valve** opens with increases in positive pressure, preventing pressure accumulation.

D. The **high negativity float valve** preserves the water seal in the presence of high negativity and may be used to reduce negativity.

E. The **filtered high negativity relief valve** vents excessive negativity. Depress the button to reduce negativity, at which time filtered air enters the unit and the water level in the water seal drops.

F. The **self-sealing diaphragm** is used to add or reduce the water level in the water seal.

G. **Suction control pressure scale.** When suction is applied and bubbling occurs, the approximate level of suction imposed

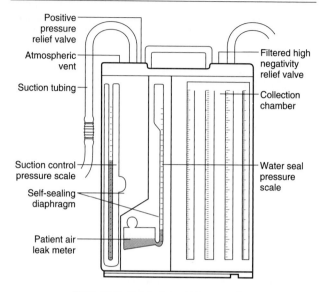

Positive pressure relief valve

Atmospheric vent

Suction tubing

Suction control pressure scale

Self-sealing diaphragm

Patient air leak meter

Filtered high negativity relief valve

Collection chamber

Water seal pressure scale

Figure 31-2. Standard chest tube apparatus.

is determined by the original fluid level. Evaporation may cause a decrease in the fluid level and should be closely monitored. Suction needs to be gentle.

H. The **suction tubing** connects to the suction source. If suction is not required, the tubing should remain unclamped and uncapped to allow air to exit.

32

Cricothyrotomy

> **Cricothyrotomy is contraindicated in children less than 12 years of age. In these cases, transtracheal needle insufflation should be used if unable to intubate.**

I. **Surgical Cricothyrotomy** (Figure 32-1)
   A. Place the patient in the supine position with the neck in a neutral position.
   B. Palpate the thyroid cartilage, the thyroid-cricoid junction, and the sternal notch for orientation.
   C. Surgically prepare the area and anesthetize if needed.
   D. Stabilize the thyroid cartilage with the left hand.
   E. Make a midline **vertical** skin incision (2.5 cm) down to the cricothyroid membrane.
   F. Carefully incise through the membrane **horizontally.**
   G. Insert the scalpel handle or a hemostat into the incision to open the airway.
   H. Insert an appropriate-sized endotracheal tube or a tracheostomy tube, directing the tube distally into the trachea.
   I. Inflate the cuff and ventilate the patient.
   J. Check placement and adequate ventilation by auscultation and chest movement.
   K. Secure the airway to the patient.
   L. Obtain a chest x-ray to ascertain tube position.

II. **Needle Cricothyrotomy**
   A. Place the patient in the supine position with the neck in a neutral position.
   B. Palpate the thyroid cartilage, the thyroid-cricoid junction, and the sternal notch for orientation.
   C. Surgically prepare the area and anesthetize if needed.
   D. Stabilize the thyroid cartilage with the left hand.
   E. Attach a 5-ml syringe to a 12- to 14-gauge IV catheter. Insert the needle over the cricothyroid membrane in the midline and direct the needle inferiorly at a 45° angle.
   F. Advance the catheter slowly with constant back pressure on

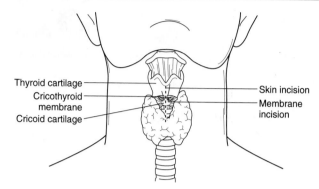

Figure 32-1. Anatomy for cricothyrotomy. A vertical incision is made in the skin and a horizontal incision is made in the cricothyroid membrane.

the plunger. When air is aspirated, do not advance further; the catheter is in the trachea. Slowly advance the catheter only over the needle and down the tracheal lumen.

G. Connect a 3-mm pediatric tube adaptor to the catheter. Then attach a Y connector to the hub as well as to the oxygen source.

H. Maintain oxygen flow at 15 ml/min by the wall gauge.

I. Cover the second Y port intermittently to administer oxygen, which prevents the escape of oxygen out of the second Y port and forces it into the patient.

33

Electrocardiogram

Evaluation

I. **Systematic Evaluation**
   A. Read the name, date, and time of the electrocardiogram (ECG).
   B. Obtain the previous ECG for comparison if possible.
   C. Evaluate **rate.**
   D. Evaluate **rhythm.**
      1. What is the rate of the QRS complex?
      2. What are the characteristics of the QRS complex (e.g., regular or irregular, narrow or wide)?
      3. Are there P waves?
      4. Does a P wave precede every QRS complex?
      5. Is the PR interval constant?
   E. Evaluate the **axis** ($-30°-110°$) [Figure 33-1].
      1. Identify the lead that is isoelectric for the QRS complex (upward deflection is equal to downward reflection). The axis is perpendicular to this line.
      2. The correct perpendicular axis lies in the quadrant determined by the deflections in leads I and aVF.
   F. Evaluate the **intervals.**
      1. **PR interval** (0.12–0.20 seconds)
         a. In first-degree atrioventricular (AV) block, the PR interval is greater than 0.20 seconds.
         b. In second-degree AV block, not every P wave yields a QRS complex.
            (1) Mobitz type I (Wenckebach)—the PR interval progressively lengthens and eventually a QRS complex is dropped.
            (2) Mobitz type 2—the PR interval is constant, but P waves do not always lead to a QRS complex.
         c. In third-degree AV block, the P waves and QRS com-

671

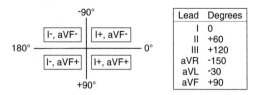

Figure 33-1. Electrocardiogram lead orientation (axes).

plex are no longer related to each other (complete AV dissociation).

2. **QRS complex** (< 0.12 seconds)

   a. A **wide** QRS complex is present in premature ventricular contraction, ventricular tachycardia, aberrant conduction, paced ventricle, and bundle branch block (BBB).

   b. A **narrow** QRS complex is normally present in sinus rhythm and other supraventricular rhythms.

3. **QT interval**

   a. Measure from the start of the QRS complex to the end of the T wave. It is dependent on the heart rate.

   b. The correct formula is:

   $$QTc = QT\ interval/square\ root\ of\ R\text{-}R\ interval$$

   c. A prolonged QT complex is caused by antiarrhythmic drugs, tricyclic antidepressants, hypothermia, electrolyte abnormalities, and idiopathic causes.

4. The different leads represent different areas of the heart. Each of these areas is supplied by specific arteries (Table 33-1)

G. Evaluate **PQRST.**

1. **P wave morphology**

   a. Right atrial enlargement results in peaked P waves more than 2.5 mm in lead II.

   b. Left atrial enlargement results in a biphasic P wave in lead V_1 and a double-peaked P wave in lead II.

   c. Abnormal conductance results in inverted P waves in leads II, III, and aVF.

2. **Q wave morphology.** A hallmark of infarction is a Q wave that is one box wide and one box deep on ECG.

3. **R wave progression**

   a. There should be dominant deflection by lead V_3 or lead V_4.

   b. Early progression reflects posterior or lateral wall infarct or right ventricular or septal hypertrophy.

   c. Late progression reflects infarct or injury of the anterior left ventricle.

4. **ST segments**

Table 33-1. Myocardial Territory and Representative Electrocardiogram Leads

Territory	Lead	Artery
Anterior	V_2 through V_6	Left anterior descending
Inferior	II, III, aVF	Right coronary artery
Lateral	I, aVL, V_5 through V_6	Circumflex artery
Posterior	Tall R wave in V_1 through V_2	Variable arteries

      a. Never evaluate on rhythm strip.
      b. Elevation is a hallmark of myocardial injury.
      c. Depression indicates ischemia.
      d. Nonspecific ST segment changes indicate ischemia until proved otherwise.
   5. T waves
      a. T waves are normally inverted in leads aVR and are upright in leads I, II, and V_3 through V_6.
      b. Flattened T waves may indicate ischemia.
      c. Tall T waves may follow a myocardial infarction.
      d. Peaked T waves are a sign of hyperkalemia.

II. Interpretation
  A. Arrhythmias (Table 33-2)
  B. Ventricular tachycardia versus supraventricular tachycardia with aberrancy
   1. Ventricular tachycardia is indicated by:
      a. QRS complex > 0.14 seconds
      b. Left axis deviation
      c. Constant axis
      d. AV dissociation
      e. Concordancy in leads V_1 through V_6
      f. Fusion and capture beats
   2. Supraventricular tachycardia with aberrancy is indicated by:
      a. QRS complex < 0.14 seconds
      b. Prior premature atrial contractions
      c. Responsive to vagal maneuvers
  C. Hypertrophy
   1. Left ventricle hypertrophy is indicated by:
      a. R wave in lead aVL > 11 mm or the sum of S wave in lead V_1 and R wave in lead V_5 or V_6 > 35 mm
      b. Early transition in anterior (V) leads
      c. Left atrial enlargement
      d. QRS complex > 0.10 seconds
      e. Left axis in absence of left BBB or left anterior fascicular block
   2. Right ventricle hypertrophy is indicated by:
      a. Right axis deviation > 110° in the absence of right BBB, posterior fascicular block, or inferior anterolateral myocardial infarction

Table 33-2. Arrhythmias

Rhythm	Rate (beats/min)	Morphology
Sinus bradycardia	< 60	Slow rate
Junctional bradycardia	40–60	Narrow QRS complex, P waves absent or dissociated
Ventricular escape	30–40	Wide QRS complex, slow ventricular tachycardia, P waves absent or dissociated
Accelerated junctional	60–100	P waves retrograde, narrow QRS complex
Accelerated idioventricular	50–100	Wide QRS complex
Atrial fibrillation	50–200	Narrow QRS complex, irregularly irregular rhythm; no P waves seen
Atrial flutter	50–200	Narrow QRS complex, regular QRS complex; no P waves; often sawtooth
Sinus tachycardia	100–160	P waves upright
Paroxysmal atrial tachycardia	140–220	Regular rhythm, abnormal P waves
Multifocal atrial tachycardia	100–200	Three separate P wave morphologies
Junctional tachycardia	140–220	P wave may be hidden
Ventricular tachycardia	150–250	Wide QRS complex, P waves absent or dissociated
Torsades de pointes	200–250	Ventricular tachycardia with varying amplitude of QRS complex
Ventricular fibrillation	> 250	Chaotic

   b. Late transition in anterior (V) leads
   c. Dominant R wave > 5 mm in lead V_1
   d. R:S ratio > 1 in lead V_1
D. BBB (infranodal)
   1. Left BBB is indicated by:
      a. Wide QRS complex directed leftward and posterior
      b. QRS complex > 0.12 seconds
      c. Broad or notched R waves in leads V_6 through V_6, I, and aVL
      d. No Q or S waves
      e. Left axis $< 30°$
   2. Right BBB is indicated by:
      a. QRS complex directed rightward and anterior
      b. Large R waves in lead V_1 and large S waves in lead V_4
      c. rSR' pattern in leads V_1 through V_3 with ST segment depression and T wave inversion
      d. Wide S wave in leads V_5 through V_6 and I
   3. Left anterior hemiblock is indicated by:
      a. Normal QRS complex duration
      b. Left axis $-30°$ to $-90°$
      c. Small Q waves in leads I and aVL
      d. R waves in leads II, III, and aVF
      e. rS complex in lead II with positive T waves
   4. Left posterior hemiblock is indicated by:
      a. Right axis $> 90°$
      b. Small Q waves in leads II, III, and aVF
      c. Deep S waves in leads I and aVL
      d. R waves in leads II, III, and aVF
E. Disease states
   1. Pericarditis is indicated by:
      a. Concave ST segment elevated diffusely
      b. PR segment diffusely depressed
      c. Evidence of effusion (e.g., low-voltage QRS complex, electrical alterans)
   2. Cor pulmonale is indicated by:
      a. Increased RV voltages
      b. Right axis $> 100°$
      c. R:S ratio in lead $V_6 < 1$
   3. Pulmonary embolus is indicated by:
      a. Sinus tachycardia
      b. Nonspecific ST segment and T wave changes
F. Electrolyte abnormalities
   1. Hyperkalemia. As potassium rises above 6 mEq/L, the following progression may occur:
      a. Tall, peaked T waves
      b. Depressed ST segments
      c. Decreased amplitude R waves
      d. Prolonged PR interval
      e. Absent P waves
      f. Widening of the QRS complex
      g. Torsades de pointes

       h. Asystole
- **2. Hypokalemia** may cause:
  - **a.** Flattened T waves
  - **b.** ST segment depression
  - **c.** U waves
- **3. Hypercalcemia** may cause:
  - **a.** Decreased ST segments
  - **b.** Shortened QT interval
  - **c.** Bradycardia
- **4. Hypocalcemia** is indicated by prolonged QTc.

G. Drug effects
- **1. Digoxin** causes:
  - **a.** Sloped ST segment depression (J point depression)
  - **b.** Atrial tachycardia and accelerated junctional or ventricular tachycardia/ventricular fibrillation
  - **c.** AV block
- **2. β-Blockers** cause sinus bradycardia with AV block.
- **3. Calcium channel blockers** cause sinus arrest with AV block.
- **4. Quinidine/procainamide/disopyramide** cause a prolonged QT interval or torsades de pointes.
- **5. Amiodarone** causes bradycardia, complete heart block, or a prolonged QT interval.

Gastrointestinal Tubes

PLACEMENT OF NASOGASTRIC AND FEEDING TUBES

I. Placement in the Stomach. Although a soft tube with a stylet and a radiopaque stripe is preferred for feeding, a nasogastric tube may be used.

    A. Elevate the head of the bed 45° and flex the neck. Brace the head to prevent extension during placement.

    B. Measure from the ear to the xiphoid (add 25 cm for the duodenum).

    C. Coat the tip generously with lidocaine jelly.

    D. Place the tip in the most widely patent nostril and direct posteriorly, not superiorly.

    E. Have the patient sip water.

    F. Insert the tube smoothly and gently and have the patient swallow it down.

    G. Remove the stylet and confirm the position by auscultating injected air at the epigastrium, aspirating gastric contents, and performing a chest x-ray.

II. Placement in the Duodenum. In addition to the following technique, the tube also may be placed with the assistance of fluoroscopy.

    A. Follow the technique for placement in the stomach.

    B. Place the patient in the right lateral decubitus position for 1–2 hours and then on the left side for 1–2 hours.

    C. Allow time and gut peristalsis to move the tube.

    D. Check the position with serial abdominal x-rays.

PLACEMENT OF SMALL BOWEL TUBES

I. Technique

    A. Using a needle and syringe, inject 5 ml of saline into the balloon at the end of the tube.

   B. With the patient in an upright sitting position, roll up the balloon, apply lubricant, and insert it into a patent naris.
   C. Carefully manipulate the tube so the balloon falls into the nasopharynx. Be careful not to obstruct the airway.
   D. Instruct the patient to swallow the balloon and the tube as it is lowered into the pharynx.
   E. After it has been swallowed, confirm that the patient can speak clearly and breathe easily. Then advance it into the stomach.
   F. Insert the tube to the point where the "D" is at the nose. Place the patient in a right decubitus position for 1–2 hours.
      1. The tube should not be fixed to the nose.
      2. Intermittent suction may be applied.
   G. Obtain an abdominal x-ray to confirm that the tip is in the duodenum. If the tube is coiled in the stomach, it may need to be withdrawn for a short distance.
   H. Place the patient in a supine position for 1–2 hours and then in a left decubitus position for 1–2 hours to help guide the tube through the C-loop of the duodenum.
   I. Confirm the position of the tube by an abdominal x-ray. If the tube is still in the stomach, it can be guided through the pylorus under fluoroscopy or by upper endoscopy.
   J. When the tube is beyond the C-loop of the duodenum, it can be advanced 2–3 cm every 15 minutes.
II. Removal
   A. When the small bowel tube is no longer needed, it should be removed slowly, over a few hours, to prevent intussusception.
   B. Withdraw the tube 3–5 cm every 15 minutes.

PLACEMENT OF A SENGSTAKEN-BLAKEMORE TUBE

   I. Indication—patient exsanguinating from esophageal varices.
   II. Technique (Figure 34-1)

> **Patient should be closely monitored in an ICU during the placement of a Sengstaken-Blakemore tube. Perforation is a risk with the Sengstaken-Blakemore tube and its use should be supervised by someone who is experienced.**

   A. Before starting the procedure, endotracheal intubation is recommended to secure the airway and prevent aspiration.
   B. Place a nasogastric tube to empty the stomach, then remove it.
   C. Test the esophageal and gastric balloons with air for leaks.
   D. Apply a lubricant to the balloons.
   E. Insert the tube into a patent naris with the patient's head flexed.
   F. Advance the tube into the nasopharynx and instruct the patient to swallow the tube.

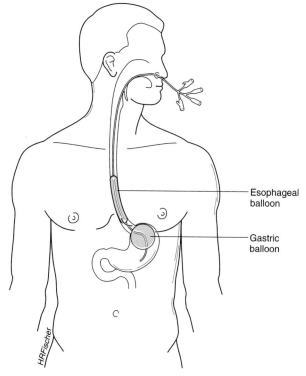

Figure 34-1. Positioning of a Sengstaken-Blakemore tube. (Adapted with permission from Chen H, Sola JE, Lillemoe KD: *Manual of Common Bedside Surgical Procedures*. Baltimore, Williams & Wilkins, 1995, p 144.)

    G. When the tube has been swallowed, make sure the patient can breathe and speak clearly, then advance the tube to approximately 45 cm.

    H. Place the gastric port to low intermittent suction.

        1. Return of blood confirms the placement in the stomach.

        2. If there is no blood return, inject air and auscultate over the epigastric area.

    I. When the placement in the stomach is confirmed, inject 100 ml of air into the gastric balloon, then clamp the balloon port to maintain balloon volume. Stop inflating the balloon if the patient complains of pain.

        1. If pain occurs, the balloon is most likely in the esophagus.

        2. Deflate the balloon and advance it 10 cm and then repeat.

    J. With the gastric balloon inflated, slowly withdraw the tube until the balloon lodges up against the lower esophageal sphincter. Anchor the tube in this position.

K. Obtain a chest x-ray to confirm gastric balloon position.

L. When the position is confirmed, add 150 ml of air to the gastric balloon and reapply the clamp.

M. Irrigate the gastric port with saline and then aspirate.

    1. If no bleeding is encountered, leave the esophageal balloon deflated.

    2. If bleeding persists, continue with the following procedure.

        a. Connect the esophageal balloon port to the pressure monitor and inflate the esophageal balloon to 25–45 mm Hg.

        b. Transiently deflate the esophageal balloon every 4 hours to check for further bleeding by aspirating from the gastric port.

        c. Apply low intermittent suction to both gastric and esophageal ports.

        d. If there is no evidence of bleeding for 24 hours, deflate both balloons.

N. The tube may be removed when bleeding is absent for an additional 24 hours.

35

Intracranial Pressure

Monitoring

I. **Placement of an Intracranial Pressure (ICP) Monitor/Ventricular Catheter** (Figure 35-1)

A. Shave the area over the right frontal parietal bone extending from the hairline to 3–5 cm posterior to the coronal suture and from 2–3 cm lateral to the midline on the left side and 4–5 cm lateral to the midline on the right side.

B. Outline with marker the midpupillary line and the perpendicular intersection between the external auditory meatus line and the lateral canthus. This identifies Kocher's point (3–5 cm lateral to midline and 2–3 cm anterior to coronal suture), which is anterior to the motor strip and lateral to the sagittal sinus (see Figure 35-1).

C. Prepare the area with povidone-iodine.

D. Inject 1% lidocaine with epinephrine over Kocher's point 2 minutes before the incision.

E. Drape the area and allow visualization of the outlined landmarks.

F. Make a 3-cm incision with a #15 blade down to the periosteum. Mobilize the periosteum laterally using a small Kelly clamp to allow contact with the underlying bone.

G. Using a twist drill with a 5.8-mm bit, drill perpendicular to the bone.

Always maintain control when drilling to avoid plunging into the brain or dura.

---

1. When drilling, you will feel the outer cortex, then the diploe (less resistance), then the inner cortex (higher resistance).

2. At this point be very careful until you feel another change

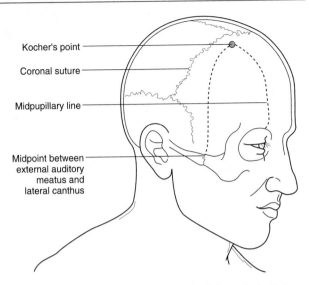

Figure 35-1. Surface landmarks for placement of intracerebral catheters.

in resistance, at which point you have reached the epidural-periosteal interspace.

  H. With a small Kelly clamp, remove all bone particles and hair from the wound.

II. Placement of a Codman Catheter

  A. Insert the Touhey needle (included in the Codman kit) into the scalp, 2 cm away from the incision, and tunnel it to the incision in the subgaleal space.

  B. Pass the Codman ICP monitor catheter through the Touhey needle. When the catheter is in the desired area, pull the needle out.

  C. Calibrate the ICP monitor according to the enclosed instructions.

  D. When the ICP monitor is calibrated, make a small hole through the dura using a sharp, 18-gauge needle.

  E. Test the monitor by lightly pressing on the tip of the catheter. A significant pulse pressure waveform should be evident.

  F. Insert the ICP monitor tip into the wound approximately 1.5–2.0 cm from the outer surface of the skull or until a good pressure waveform is seen on the monitor. The waveform should correlate with the pulse rate and should have respiratory variability.

  G. When a good pressure waveform is obtained, pull excess wire from the wound through the distal segment of the ICP monitor.

H. Close the dermis-epidermis layer with interrupted 3–0 nylon sutures.

I. Insert a 3–0 nylon U stitch where the distal portion of the ICP monitor exits the skin. Also, place several sutures throughout the length of the wire to secure it to the scalp.

J. Apply bacitracin ointment and a sterile dressing.

K. Start the patient on gram-positive prophylactic antibiotics (e.g., cefazolin) until the catheter is removed.

III. **Placement of a Ventricular Drainage Catheter**

A. Using a sharp, 18-gauge needle, make a small hole into the underlying dura. Extend this opening using a blunt needle. Clean any periosteum over the dura.

B. Make a small punch incision lateral to the ventricular incision. Tunnel a small mosquito clamp through the punch incision to the ventricular incision under the subgaleal layer. This will be used to tunnel the distal end of the catheter.

C. With the stylet inside the ventricular catheter, place the ventricular catheter into the wound.

D. Maintain a perpendicular alignment between the catheter and the skull. Pay attention to the 5- and 10-cm marks on the catheter.

   1. The direction of the catheter insertion should be perpendicular to the skull.
   2. An alternative is to **direct the catheter to the point where the external auditory meatus and the medial canthus intersect.** This point theoretically places the catheter close to the foramen of Monro.

E. Slowly insert the catheter through the brain parenchyma, noticing the soft, no-resistance texture of the brain as the catheter is inserted.

F. At approximately 4–5 cm, if there is no significant shift, there should be a change of resistance when the catheter reaches the ependymal surface of the ventricles.

   1. When entering the ventricle, if there is increased ICP, a column of cerebrospinal fluid (CSF) may be noticed within the catheter and stylet.
   2. If no CSF is evident, advance the catheter until the 7-cm mark is reached.

G. Remove the stylet, lower the catheter below the level of the incision, and assess CSF drainage. Pull the ventricular catheter back, leaving approximately 6 cm in length.

H. Tunnel the catheter out of the punch incision with the mosquito clamp.

I. Attach the catheter to the pressure transducer.

J. Close both incisions with interrupted 3–0 nylon sutures.

K. Apply sterile dressing.

L. Send CSF daily for culture to assess the sterility of the system. After 5 days of drainage, the rate of CSF infection increases, at which point changing the ventricular system through a new hole should be seriously considered.

36

Intubation

I. **Indications**
  A. Decreased PO_2
  B. Increased PCO_2
  C. Inability to protect the airway
  D. Altered mental status
  E. Depressed respiratory drive
  F. Anticipated cardiovascular or respiratory collapse
  G. Inability to stabilize the airway
II. **Contraindications**
  A. **Oral intubation**
    1. Tracheal fracture
    2. Tracheal disruption
  B. **Nasal intubation**
    1. Cerebrospinal fluid rhinorrhea
    2. Nasal fracture
    3. Deviated septum or nasal occlusion
    4. Coagulopathy
    5. Previous transphenoidal hypophysectomy
    6. Previous posterior pharyngeal flap for the repair of craniofacial defects
    7. Pregnancy
III. **Assessment for Ease of Intubation**
  A. Assessment of the following factors may help to **predict a difficult intubation.**
    1. Assess the visibility of the pharynx.
    2. Assess the mobility of the atlanto-occipital joint.
      a. Mobility is estimated by the angle traversed by the occlusal surface of the maxillary teeth when the head is extended from the neutral position.
      b. The normal joint extends 35°. If reduced by one third, then intubation may be difficult.
    3. Estimate the mentohyoid distance. In a normal adult, this distance is estimated as three finger breadths. If less than three finger breadths, intubation may be difficult.

    4. Assess the excursion of the temporomandibular joint. Adults with a normal mouth opening can fit three fingers vertically.

  B. Common reasons for **failure of intubation** include:

    1. Abnormal anatomy (e.g., anteriorly placed larynx, large tongue)

    2. Poor visualization (e.g., tumor obstructing the view, poor light source, excessive bleeding)

    3. Trismus (never give any paralytics without assessing this possibility)

    4. Not using a stylet in the endotracheal tube

    5. Patient is a laryngectomee (always make sure the patient has an airway)

IV. Anesthesia

  A. An induction agent and neuromuscular blocking agent are used to ease intubation. Sedatives are then given as appropriate to make the patient comfortable.

    1. Induction agents include:

      a. Thiopental 4–6 mg/kg

      b. Etomidate 0.3 mg/kg

      c. Ketamine 1–3 mg/kg

    2. Neuromuscular blocking agents (see p 753)

    3. Sedatives include:

      a. Diazepam

      b. Lorazepam

      c. Midazolam

  B. Resuscitation drugs should be available at the bedside and include:

    1. Atropine

    2. Phenylephrine

    3. Ephedrine

    4. Epinephrine

V. Procedure

  A. Determining the **method of intubation** (see Figure 19-2)

  B. Oral intubation

    1. Check the endotracheal tube cuff for leaks.

    2. Check the laryngoscope to make sure the light is working.

    3. Preoxygenate with 100% oxygen by bag-valve-mask ventilation.

    4. Have an assistant apply cricoid pressure.

    5. Grasp the laryngoscope in the left hand.

    6. Place the thumb and second finger of the right hand on the right upper and lower molars and open the mouth with a scissors-like motion.

    7. Place the laryngoscope blade in the right side of the mouth. Protect the teeth.

    8. Advance the blade toward the glottis. Keep the tongue on the left.

    9. With the left wrist in the unbroken position, lift the laryngoscope handle upward and caudally to expose the vocal cords. Avoid applying pressure on the upper teeth.

10. Place the styletted tube into the right side of the mouth and through the vocal cords.
11. Place the endotracheal tube just below the cords and inflate the balloon with 5–10 ml of air.
12. Hold the tube at the lips.
13. Give several breaths, watch for chest expansion, and listen for equal bilateral breath sounds and absence of sounds over the gastric area. An end-tidal carbon dioxide monitor also may be attached to assure the placement in the tracheal tree.
    a. If the esophagus is intubated, remove the tube and oxygenate the patient.
    b. Occasionally, the esophageal tube may be left in place as a guide for tracheal intubation and then removed.
14. Tape the tube securely to the face. Place an oral airway in an awake patient.
15. Obtain a chest x-ray to check the position of the endotracheal tube.

C. Nasal intubation

1. Check the endotracheal tube cuff for leaks.
2. Preoxygenate with 100% oxygen by bag-valve-mask ventilation.
3. Use nasal airways to dilate the nares, and use an endotracheal tube one size smaller than the largest dilator.
4. Coat the endotracheal tube with lidocaine jelly or water-soluble lubricant.
5. With the concave side facing the palate, pass the endotracheal tube into the nose and past the inferior turbinate. It may be necessary to increase the angle on the tube to get it into the pharynx.
6. Watch the tube for fogging as it approaches the vocal cords.
7. Ask the patient to take deep breaths, and on inspiration advance the endotracheal tube beyond the vocal cords.
8. Place the endotracheal tube just below the cords and inflate the balloon with 5–10 ml of air.
9. Hold the tube at the nose.
10. Check tube position and secure the tube.

Local Anesthetic Blocks

I. **Local Anesthetic Agents** (Table 37-1)

> **Epinephrine should never be used in areas
> of end arterial perfusion (e.g., fingers, toes,
> nose, ears, penis) or in areas of infection.**

II. **General Procedure**
   A. Prepare and drape the area in a sterile fashion.
   B. Stretch the skin and inject the anesthetic agent in the desired location.
      1. It is best to inject along an incision line or near the edges of a wound.
      2. Make sure to draw back before injecting to confirm that the needle is not intravascular.
   C. To minimize discomfort, inject slowly with a small-caliber needle (25 gauge) or add sodium bicarbonate to the anesthetic solution (e.g., 1 ml 10% sodium bicarbonate in 9 ml of 1% lidocaine).

III. **Specific Procedures**
   A. **Digital block**
      1. Advance a 3/4-inch, 25-gauge needle into the two web spaces surrounding the finger. The needle should be advanced in a horizontal plane, parallel to the hand and fingers.
      2. Inject each of the interdigital web spaces with 3 ml of 1% lidocaine.

> **The digital nerves of the thumb
> are in a more volar location.**

      3. Infiltrate an additional 3 ml at the dorsum of the metacarpophalangeal joint to block the radial digital nerve.
      4. Allow 5–20 minutes for the anesthetic to take effect. If still insufficient, inject another 2 ml in each web space.

Table 37-1. Local Anesthetic Agents

Local Anesthetic	Onset of Action	Maximum Dose (mg/kg)	Maximum Dose with Epinephrine (mg/kg)	Duration of Action (hr)	Duration of Action with Epinephrine (hr)
Lidocaine (1%–2%)*	Rapid	6	9	0.5–2.0	1–4
Bupivacaine (0.25%–0.50%)*	Slow	2.5	3.5	2–4	4–8
Procaine	Slow	6	9	0.25–0.50	0.5–1.0

*1% = 10 mg/ml.

B. Wrist block

1. It is possible to isolate the individual nerves for different situations.

2. Inject 4 ml of 2% lidocaine into the following four sites for a complete block or individually if desired.

   a. Median nerve

   (1) Locate the palmaris longus. Use the space created by the opposition of the thumb and fifth finger and wrist flexion.

   (2) Inject radial to the palmaris longus at the level of the wrist flexion crease.

   b. Ulnar nerve

   (1) Locate the flexor carpi ulnaris by fifth-finger abduction and wrist flexion.

   (2) Inject radial to the flexor carpi ulnaris at the level of the wrist flexion crease.

   c. Radial nerve

   (1) Locate the anatomic snuff box by thumb abduction.

   (2) Inject over the radial styloid at the base of the snuff box.

   d. Dorsal cutaneous branch of the ulnar nerve—inject over the ulnar styloid prominence.

38

Lumbar Puncture

I. **Functions**
    A. **Diagnostic** uses include sampling cerebrospinal fluid (CSF) and measuring intrathecal pressure.
    B. **Therapeutic** uses include draining CSF and administering intrathecal medications.

II. **Contraindications**
    A. Coagulopathy
    B. Intracranial mass (e.g., tumor, hematoma, noncommunicating hydrocephalus, abscess, papilledema)
    C. Tethered cord

III. **Patient Positioning**
    A. **Lateral decubitus** positioning is necessary for measuring intrathecal opening pressure.
        1. The patient should lie on his or her side and flex the back as much as possible.
        2. The patient's knees should be drawn to the chest and the neck should be flexed, bringing the chin to the chest.
        3. The patient's back should be hanging off of the bed slightly.
        4. The person performing the lumbar puncture should sit at the bedside at the patient's back.
        5. An assistant should stand opposite the person performing the lumbar puncture and should help the patient to flex the back.
    B. **Sitting** position may be preferable for obese patients or for large-volume taps.
        1. The patient should sit on the side of the bed with the legs hanging down.
        2. A bedside table should be placed in front of the patient at nipple level.
        3. The patient should lean forward onto the table, resting his or her head on crossed arms.
        4. The patient should flex the back as much as possible.

IV. **Puncture Site**

A. A puncture should be made at an **intervertebral space** (e.g., L3-L4, L4-L5, L5-S1).
B. The following steps should be used to locate an intervertebral space.
  1. Observe and palpate the spinous processes to identify midline.

> **When identifying midline, use caution in interpreting skin folds because these can stray from the midline with gravity.**

  2. Remember that the intercristal line, connecting the superior posterior iliac crests, usually crosses the midline at L4.
  3. Identify an accessible intervertebral space and mark it with a skin indentation or ink.

V. Procedure

> **In general, a computed tomography scan of the head to rule out a mass lesion should precede the lumbar puncture.**

A. Prepare the skin with iodine solution, allowing a generous margin around the site.
B. Drape the back with a fenestrated sterile drape, exposing the site, and secure it to the patient with tape.
C. Anesthetize the patient with 1% lidocaine.
  1. First make a skin wheal.
  2. Then infiltrate subcutaneous tissue and lumbodorsal fascia.
D. Insert an 18-, 20-, or 22-gauge spinal needle with a stylet at the site. Direct it superiorly, making an angle of 75° with the skin.
E. Palpate the spinous processes to ensure that the needle always remains in midline.
F. Advance the needle into the CSF.
  1. The ligamentum flavum should be felt as a momentary resistance.
  2. If bone is encountered, retract the needle into the subcutaneous tissue and make another attempt at a slightly different angle.
G. Remove the stylet periodically. If CSF remains bloody without clearing or fails to flow, replace the stylet, withdraw the needle, and make a new attempt.
H. Measure the opening pressure.
  1. Attach the manometer to the needle.
  2. Have the patient straighten his or her legs.
  3. Note the CSF height in the column.
I. Collect CSF in multiple tubes as required.
  1. Cell count is usually checked in tubes 1 and 4.
  2. The remaining tubes are used for protein level, glucose level, Gram stain, antigen studies, culture, and sensitivities.

J. Measure the closing pressure following the same procedure used to measure the opening pressure.

K. Replace the stylet and remove the needle.

L. Place a sterile, dry dressing.

M. Instruct the patient to lie flat for 4–12 hours to reduce the incidence of headache.

N. Perform serial neurologic examinations and check the vital signs to detect herniation or hemorrhage.

39

Mini Mental Status

Examination

I. **Procedure**
   A. **Orientation**
      1. Ask the patient for the year, season, date, day, and month (1 point for each correct answer; maximum of 5 points).
      2. Ask the patient for the state, country, town, hospital, and floor (1 point for each correct answer; maximum of 5 points).
   B. **Registration**
      1. Name three objects, taking 1 second to say each one. Then ask the patient to repeat all three objects (1 point for each correct response; maximum of 3 points).
      2. Have the patient repeat the objects until the patient has learned all three. Record the number of trials.
   C. **Attention and calculation**
      1. Serial 7s—ask the patient to count by 7 (7, 14, 21, 28, 35) [1 point for each correct response; stop after five answers].
      2. Alternatively, have the patient spell the word "world" backward.
   D. **Recall.** Ask the patient for the three objects identified previously (1 point for each correct response; maximum of 3 points).
   E. **Language**
      1. Show the patient a pencil and a watch and ask the patient to identify each (1 point for each correct response; maximum of 2 points).
      2. Have the patient repeat the following: "No ifs, ands, or buts" (1 point).
      3. Have the patient follow a three-stage verbal command (1 point for each correct response; maximum of 3 points):

          a. "Take a paper in your right hand."
          b. "Fold the paper in half."
          c. "Put the paper on the floor."
    4. Have the patient read and obey the following commands:
          a. Close your eyes (1 point).
          b. Write a sentence (1 point).
          c. Copy the design (1 point) [Figure 39-1].
  F. Level of consciousness (assess along a continuum)
    1. Alert
    2. Drowsy
    3. Stupor
    4. Coma
II. Scoring
  A. A perfect score is 30.
  B. Any score below 25 indicates the presence of significant cognitive dysfunction.

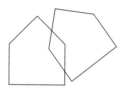

Figure 39-1. Design that the patient is asked to copy during testing.

40

Needle Biopsies

I. Fine-Needle Biopsy of Thyroid, Breast, Lymph Node, and Soft Tissue Lesions

   A. Position the patient.

   1. For a thyroid lesion, position the patient supine with a roll behind the shoulders to allow for neck extension.

   2. Patients with upper quadrant breast lesions should be seated upright.

   3. Patients with lower quadrant breast lesions should be in the supine position.

   4. Positioning for patients with lymph node or soft tissue lesions depends on the location of the lesion.

   B. Prepare the area with an alcohol pad.

   C. Palpate the lesion and immobilize it between two fingers on the nondominant hand.

   D. With the dominant hand, advance a 25-gauge needle with a 10-ml syringe attached.

   E. Upon entering the lesion, note the consistency (e.g., firm, soft, rubbery, doughy, gritty) and apply 10 ml of suction with a syringe.

   F. While maintaining suction, move the needle back and forth in different paths through the lesion.

   G. Before removing the needle from the lesion, release the plunger on the syringe.

   H. Remove the needle and apply pressure to the site.

   I. Detach the needle from the syringe, draw up 10 ml of air into the syringe, and then reconnect the needle to the syringe.

   J. Touch the needle to a glass slide at a 45°-90° angle and expel the contents of the needle onto the slide.

   K. Press a second glass slide down on the first and draw out material to the feathered edge.

   L. Air dry the smear or apply cytologic fixative.

   M. Repeated sequences may be necessary to increase yield.

   N. Send for cytology if a significant amount of fluid is aspirated.

II. Core Needle Biopsy

A. Position the patient so that the lesion can be fixed with one hand.

B. Prepare and drape the area in a sterile fashion.

C. Administer local anesthesia (i.e., lidocaine) to the overlying skin and subcutaneous tissues using 25- and 22-gauge needles, respectively.

D. Using a scalpel, make a 5-mm incision in the skin.

E. Fully retract the obturator so the specimen notch is covered.

F. Insert the needle into the lesion. The specimen notch must be within the borders of the lesion.

G. Hold the obturator in place and pull outward on the T-shaped cannula. This action opens the specimen notch.

H. Quickly advance the cannula over the obturator to sever the tissue that has prolapsed into the specimen notch.

I. Remove the needle with the cannula over the obturator.

J. Advance the obturator to reveal the specimen, which can be removed.

K. Apply dressing to the wound and hold pressure.

41

Paracentesis

I. **Indication.** Paracentesis is used to remove fluid from the abdominal cavity for diagnostic and therapeutic purposes.

II. **Location.** The best location for drainage may be determined by physical examination or with the help of ultrasound.

III. **Procedure**

   A. Have the patient void before the procedure or place a Foley catheter.

   B. Apply povidone-iodine solution to the area and then place sterile drapes.

   C. Anesthetize the skin with 1% lidocaine using a 25-gauge needle, and then switch to a 22-gauge needle to anesthetize the depth of the abdominal wall to the peritoneum.

   D. Using an IV catheter (needle with sheath), advance the needle through the abdominal wall, aspirating as it advances. It is best to have the needle at an oblique angle to reduce ascites leakage following paracentesis.

   E. Alternatively, a Z-path can be formed with the catheter by penetrating the skin, drawing the catheter to one side, and piercing the muscle wall in this new location.

   F. When there is a free flow of fluid, advance the catheter over the needle and remove the needle.

   G. Withdraw fluid.

      1. For diagnostic studies, attach a syringe to the catheter and slowly withdraw the fluid.

      2. For therapeutic purposes, a large volume of fluid may be removed by attaching IV tubing to the catheter and using gravity drainage or vacuum bottles. Alternatively, a large central venous catheter may be inserted into the abdomen using the Seldinger technique.

   H. If the drainage slows, reposition the patient so that the catheter is in a more dependent position.

Never reintroduce a dilator, needle, or guide wire.

42

Pericardiocentesis

I. **Monitoring.** The patient's vital signs, central venous pressure, and electrocardiogram (ECG) should be monitored before, during, and after the procedure.

II. **Procedure**

   A. Surgically prepare the xiphoid and subxiphoid areas.

   B. Locally anesthetize the puncture site.

   C. Attach a 35-ml empty syringe with a three-way stopcock to a 16- or 18-gauge, 6-inch or longer needle with a catheter.

   D. Assess the patient for any mediastinal shift by examination or x-ray.

   E. Puncture the skin 1–2 cm inferior to the left xiphocondral junction at a 45° angle with the skin.

   F. Carefully advance the needle cephalad and aim toward the tip of the left scapula.

   G. If the needle is advanced too far (i.e., into the ventricular muscle) an injury pattern with extreme ST-T wave changes or widened and enlarged QRS complex appears on the ECG (Figure 42-1). The pericardiocentesis needle should be withdrawn until the baseline ECG reading is restored.

   H. When the needle tip enters the blood-filled pericardial sac, aspirate as much nonclotted blood as possible.

   1. During aspiration, the epicardium approaches the inner pericardiac surface and the needle tip; thus, an ECG injury pattern may reappear.

   2. If an injury pattern appears, the needle should be removed slightly or withdrawn.

   I. At this time, a decision is made as to whether or not to leave the catheter in place for subsequent drainage until definitive treatment is rendered. If the catheter is going to be left in place, remove the needle and syringe, place a stopcock on the catheter, and secure the catheter in place.

   J. Should the cardiac tamponade recur, the stopcock may be reopened and the pericardial sac drained.

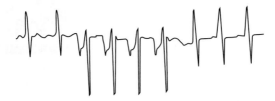

Figure 42-1. Negative deflection seen on electrocardiogram during pericardiocentesis.

43

Peritoneal Lavage,

Diagnostic

I. Indications

  A. Blunt abdominal trauma with hypotension at the scene (perform en route or in the emergency department)

  B. Computed tomography (CT) unavailable to assess abdominal compartment

> **Only patients who are hemodynamically stable should be considered for abdominal CT.**

  C. Abdominal stab wounds

  D. Unexplained hypotension

II. Contraindications

  A. An existing need for emergent celiotomy is an absolute contraindication.

  B. Relative contraindications include:

    1. Previous abdominal surgery (may try the open technique)

    2. Morbid obesity

    3. Advanced cirrhosis

    4. Pre-existing coagulopathy

    5. Pregnancy (perform open and above the umbilicus)

III. Procedure

  A. Decompress the urinary bladder by the insertion of a Foley catheter.

  B. Decompress the stomach by the insertion of a nasogastric (NG) tube. Keep the NG tube to suction.

  C. Prepare the abdomen using povidone-iodine solution and place sterile drapes.

  D. Inject a local anesthetic midline and one third the distance from the umbilicus to the symphysis pubis.

1. An incision should be made just above the umbilicus in a pregnant patient.
2. Use lidocaine with epinephrine to prevent blood contamination from the skin and subcutaneous tissues.

E. Place the catheter using the open or percutaneous technique.
   1. **Open technique**
      a. Vertically incise the skin and subcutaneous tissues below the umbilicus down to the fascia.
      b. Grasp the fascial edges with clamps, then elevate and incise the peritoneum.
      c. Insert the catheter into the peritoneum.
      d. Advance the catheter to the pelvis.
      e. After the catheter is removed, close the open technique with #0 or #1 suture and then use staples on the skin.
   2. **Percutaneous technique**
      a. Make a small, 1-cm vertical incision below or just above the umbilicus.
      b. Grasp the skin edges with towel clamps.
      c. Lift the skin with the clamps, place the needle through the incision, and enter the fascia until two "pops" are felt as the needle passes through the two fascial layers.
      d. Draw back on the needle with a syringe. Air should be aspirated with good placement.
      e. Place the wire through the needle and remove the needle.
      f. Place the dilator over the guidewire, dilate the fascial opening, and remove the dilator.
      g. Place the catheter over the wire and direct it toward the pelvis.

F. Connect the catheter to a syringe and aspirate.
   1. If gross blood (10 ml) is obtained, the procedure is complete. Plan for an immediate celiotomy.
   2. If gross blood is not obtained, continue with the following procedure.
      a. Instill 10 ml/kg of warmed Ringer's lactate or normal saline (up to 1 L) into the peritoneal cavity and allow it to sit for a few minutes. Gently agitate the abdomen.
      b. Drain the fluid by placing the infusion bag of fluid on the floor. At least half of the instilled fluid should be drained.

IV. Samples to be Sent to the Laboratory

A negative lavage does not rule out retroperitoneal, hollow viscus, or diaphragmatic injuries.

A. Positive erythrocyte count
   1. Greater than 100,000 red blood cells (RBCs)/mm^3 in patients with blunt abdominal trauma
   2. Greater than 150,000 RBCs/mm^3 in hemodynamically stable patients with pelvic fracture

3. Greater than 5000 RBCs/mm^3 for patients with pericostal stab wounds
4. Greater than 1000 RBCs/mm^3 for patients with abdominal stab wounds

B. Positive leukocyte count ($>$ 500 white blood cells/mm^3)

C. Presence of **stool, food particles, amylase, lipase, alkaline phosphatase, food fibers,** or **bacteria** (indicates a positive result and intra-abdominal injury)

44

Pulmonary Artery

Catheter Placement

I. **Preparation**
   A. Widely prepare the skin with povidone-iodine solution.
   B. Drape out the insertion site using sterile drapes or table sheets.
   C. Wear a mask, cap, and sterile gown at all times.

II. **Placement of the Cordis Sheath**
   A. The cordis sheath can be placed in the internal jugular or subclavian veins. The least torturous routes to the right heart are through the right internal jugular and left subclavian veins.
   B. Follow the procedure for subclavian or internal jugular central line placement (see Chapter 49).

III. **Placement of a Pulmonary Artery (PA) Catheter**
   A. Placement of a PA catheter should be supervised by a senior team member.
   B. Prepare and drape the area of the cordis sheath in a sterile fashion.
   C. The patient should be supine; the patient does not need to be in the Trendelenburg position.
   D. Remove the PA catheter and syringe from the package in sterile fashion.
   E. Attach the syringe with 1.0–1.5 ml of air and inflate the balloon. The balloon should obscure the tip of the catheter to prevent the possible puncture of a vessel or the heart by the catheter.
   F. Place the sterile sheath on the catheter and move it to the proximal position.
   G. Attach the catheter ports to the monitor setup and flush each port.
   H. With attention to the retained curve of the catheter and the anatomic curve through the right heart into the PA, insert the catheter into the cordis sheath to a length of 20 cm.
   I. Fully inflate the balloon and start advancing the catheter (Figure 44-1).

1. First, a right atrial wave appears.
2. Second, the large ventricular wave appears.
3. Third, the PA wave, which has a notch and double peaks, appears.
4. Fourth, the waveform flattens (wedge).

J. Stop and deflate the balloon, at which point the PA waveform should reappear.

K. Check the position by reinflating the balloon and making sure there is a flat waveform for the pulmonary capillary wedge pressure. There may be respiratory variation in the wave.

L. Attach the end of the sterile sheath to the cordis sheath so the entire catheter remains sterile.

M. Clearly note the length at which the catheter wedges. The catheter usually should not need to be advanced beyond 60 cm.

N. If there is difficulty positioning the PA catheter, do not hesitate to deflate the balloon, pull back to 20 cm, and start over. Removal of the PA catheter to reorient it may be necessary.

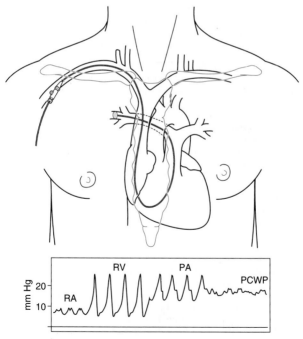

Figure 44-1. Diagram for pulmonary artery catheter placement.

> **A simple trick to aid in the floating of the catheter is to sequentially sit the patient up. This helps float the catheter by the flow of blood. If this fails, turn the patient so the right side is elevated compared to the left side.**

    O. If there is trouble obtaining a good wedge, the balloon might be in the left PA. It is best to have it in the right PA; however, this may be impossible. Obtain a chest x-ray to document the position of the catheter.

> **During PA catheter placement, arrhythmias may occur. Preparations for this possibility should be made before catheter placement. Arrhythmias may require balloon deflation, withdrawal of the catheter to 20 cm, and initiation of Advanced Cardiac Life Support. Recurrent ventricular tachycardia may be treated prophylactically with lidocaine before catheter placement.**

IV. Normal Readings (Table 44-1)

Table 44-1. Normal Pulmonary Artery Catheter Readings*	
Central venous pressure	2–8 mm Hg
Right ventricle systolic/diastolic	25/2 mm Hg
Pulmonary artery systolic/diastolic	15–30/5–12 mm Hg
Mean pulmonary artery pressure	5–12 mm Hg
Cardiac output	4–7 L/min
Systemic vascular resistance	800–1200 dyne/sec/cm^{-5}

*These values must be used in conjunction with the clinical setting.

45

Suprapubic Cystostomy

Tube Placement

I. Preparation
A. Position the patient flat in bed at a comfortable working height.
B. Fill the bladder to avoid injury to other organs.
   1. Using a Foley catheter with the tip in the urethra or bladder, gently fill the bladder with normal saline.
   2. If Foley catheterization is impossible, allow time to pass until the bladder fills with urine.
C. Localize the bladder, if possible.
   1. Use ultrasonography, if available, and mark the skin.
   2. Attempt to palpate the bladder and mark the skin.
   3. Localization of the bladder using a long spinal needle can aid in catheter placement, especially in obese patients or patients with previous abdominal surgery.
D. Shave the hair from the suprapubic region.
E. Prepare the skin of the suprapubic region with povidone-iodine solution.
F. Choose a location in the midline, 2–3 cm superior to the symphysis pubis.

II. Procedure
A. Anesthetize the skin and subcutaneous tissue using 1% lidocaine solution.
B. Make a stab incision through the skin with an 11-blade scalpel.
C. Pierce the fascia in the midline using a spinal needle with a syringe attached, aiming in the direction of the anus.
D. Carefully advance the spinal needle while pulling back on the syringe plunger until urine is aspirated.
E. The spinal needle may be left in place as a guide or it may be removed.

F. Using the tract identified by the spinal needle, introduce the cannula and trocar needle, aiming in the direction of the anus.

G. Carefully advance the cannula and trocar needle while pulling back on the syringe plunger until urine is aspirated.

H. Remove the trocar needle while maintaining the cannula position at all times.

I. Slide the suprapubic tube through the cannula into the bladder.

J. Remove the cannula while maintaining the suprapubic tube position at all times.

K. Secure the catheter to the skin using several nonabsorbable sutures.

L. Place a sterile dressing over the site and attach the catheter to a drainage bag.

46

Thoracentesis

I. Preparation

  A. A chest x-ray is a helpful guide and should be reviewed by the person performing the procedure. The effusion should be assessed for evidence of loculation, free flow, and quantity.

  B. Ultrasound may be helpful.

II. Procedure

  A. Position the patient.

    1. Sit the patient on the edge of the bed with feet hanging to the floor.

    2. Rest the patient's extended arms and head on a bedside table.

  B. Use a percussion technique or ultrasound to determine the bottom of the unaffected lung field or the meniscus of the affected lung zone.

  C. Prepare the patient's back with povidone-iodine solution and drape a sterile field.

  D. With a sterile pen or the tip of a needle, locate the posterior rib two interspaces below the top of the effusion. Be careful not to go below the eighth intercostal space.

  E. Administer 1% lidocaine locally to the area or just below the tip of the scapula. Then proceed with anesthetizing the subcutaneous tissue and muscle down to the periosteum of the rib.

  F. Slowly move the needle over the rib until it enters the pleural space and withdraw some fluid. Remove the needle and insert a large-bore needle (14- to 18-gauge) in a similar fashion.

  G. Insert the wire through the needle into the chest and remove the needle over the wire.

  H. Place the dilator over the wire to enlarge the tract and then remove the dilator over the wire.

  I. Place a catheter over the wire and, when in place, remove the wire.

> **Keep the end of the catheter covered
> to prevent air from entering the chest.**

J. Remove fluid.
   1. The catheter allows movement of the patient into different positions to optimize fluid recovery and may be used with a vacuum apparatus or with multiple syringes.
   2. Alternatively, the large-bore needle introduced earlier may be an angiocatheter. When the needle is removed, fluid may be removed through the remaining catheter.
K. After all the fluid is removed, the catheter may be removed while a simultaneous occlusive dressing is applied.
L. Obtain a chest x-ray to assess the remaining fluid and to rule out a pneumothorax.

47

Thoracotomy, Emergent

I. Indication: Traumatic Cardiac Arrest

A. Emergent thoracotomy is effective for a patient with penetrating chest trauma who has signs of life in the field or has a transport time less than 10 minutes and presents with electromechanical dissociation.

B. Emergent thoracotomy is ineffective for patients with hypovolemic cardiac arrest or electromechanical dissociation secondary to blunt trauma.

II. Technique (Figure 47-1)

> **Warm saline lavage of the heart may be lifesaving.**

A. Before the procedure, obtain an airway and IV access. It is also helpful to have a nasogastric tube in place.

B. Prepare the left side of the chest with povidone-iodine.

C. Rapidly incise the skin and subcutaneous tissues in the left fifth intercostal space (below the pectoralis in men and below the breast in women).

D. Incise the intercostal muscles and costal cartilages superiorly (2 cm lateral to the sternum to avoid the internal mammary artery).

E. Insert the Finochietto retractor (rib spreader) and spread the ribs.

F. Release the inferior pulmonary ligament and retract the left lung into the apex of the pleural space.

G. Incise the pericardium vertically, anterior to the phrenic nerve, and open it longitudinally in a sharp fashion. Internal cardiac compression may be performed by compressing the heart between both hands or between the right hand and the sternum.

H. Bluntly dissect the thoracic aorta circumferentially from the posterior mediastinum. Cross-clamp the thoracic aorta. It helps to have a nasogastric tube in the esophagus, which lies directly anterior to the aorta.

I. If blood pressure returns, transport the patient to the operating room.

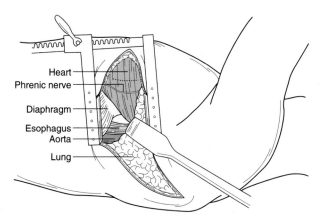

Heart
Phrenic nerve
Diaphragm
Esophagus
Aorta
Lung

Figure 47-1. Anatomy of the left thorax for emergent thoracotomy. (Adapted with permission from Chen H, Sola JE, Lillemoe KD: *Manual of Common Bedside Surgical Procedures*. Baltimore, Williams & Wilkins, 1995, p 127.)

48

Tracheostomy,

Percutaneous

I. **Indications**. Percutaneous tracheostomy is indicated when the patient has a need for prolonged ventilatory support. It may easily be performed in the ICU.

II. **Contraindications.** Percutaneous tracheostomy is contraindicated in the following patients:
   A. Patients who have had an emergency placement of a tracheostomy tube
   B. Patients with enlarged thyroids or nonpalpable cricoid cartilage
   C. Pediatric patients

III. **Patient Preparation**
   A. Place the patient in the tracheostomy position.
   B. Place a pillow or roll under the patient's shoulders to permit full extension of the head and neck.
   C. Elevate the head of the bed by 30°.
   D. Use sedation and ventilator changes to control respirations. Continuous oxygen saturation monitoring is required.
   E. Loosen the endotracheal tube fixation tape.
   F. Prep and drape the anterior neck region.

IV. **Procedure**
   A. Palpate the landmark structures (thyroid notch, cricoid cartilage). The tube will ultimately be placed between the cricoid cartilage and the first tracheal ring, or between the first and second tracheal rings.
   B. Mark the skin incision, which will extend from the lower edge of the cricoid cartilage approximately 1–1.5 cm in the midline.
   C. Infiltrate the proposed incision with 1% lidocaine with epinephrine.
   D. Deflate the cuff of the endotracheal tube and withdraw the tube approximately 1 cm or just below the vocal cords.

E. After making the skin incision, use a curved mosquito clamp to dissect vertically and horizontally down to the pretracheal space. With the tip of a finger, gently dissect the front of the trachea in the midline and identify the cricoid cartilage. Displace the isthmus of the thyroid downward if present. (NOTE: The skin incision may also be made after the J-wire is in place.)

NOTE: The following steps may be performed under direct vision with the use of a bronchoscope. It is helpful to identify the entrance of the needle, wire, and dilators and then to check the position of the tracheostomy tube relative to the carina.

F. Inject additional local anesthetic into this area.
  1. With the plunger on the syringe pulled back, insert the needle in a posterior caudad direction in the midline, seeking the tracheal air column. Once the trachea is entered, bubbles will appear in the syringe.
  2. With the needle tip in the trachea, inject 1 cc of lidocaine and remove the needle.
  3. Attach the syringe with lidocaine to the 17-gauge sheath introducer needle. Using the technique described above, locate the tracheal air column.
  4. Once the needle is in the trachea, have the respiratory therapist gently move the endotracheal tube to ensure that it was not impaled by the needle. If the needle is seen and felt to move, withdraw the needle and have the respiratory therapist pull the endotracheal tube back.
G. When free flow of air is obtained, remove the inner needle and advance the outer sheath a few millimeters. Aspirate from the sheath to ensure that there is air return.
H. Place the J wire through the sheath and into the trachea; remove the sheath introducer. There is a nub on the wire to identify how far to advance the wire (the nub is meant to stay at skin level).
I. Using a slight twisting motion, advance the 11 Fr introducing dilator over the wire to dilate the initial access site into the trachea. Remove the dilator while maintaining the wire in position.
J. Following the direction of the arrow on the guiding catheter, advance the 8 Fr guiding catheter over the J wire to the skin level mark. Advance the guiding catheter and J wire as a unit into the trachea until the safety ridge on the guiding catheter is at the skin level. Align the proximal end of the guiding catheter at the mark on the proximal portion of the J wire.
K. Begin to serially dilate the access site into the trachea.
  1. First, advance the 12 Fr dilator over the J wire/guiding catheter assembly.

2. To align the dilator on the assembly, position the proximal end of the dilator at the single positioning mark on the guiding catheter.
3. While maintaining these references between the assembly and dilator, advance them as a unit, using a twisting motion, to the skin level mark on the dilator.
4. Advance and pull back the dilator assembly a few times to perform effective dilation of the tracheotomy.
5. Remove the blue dilator, leaving the assembly in place.

L. Continue the dilation procedure by advancing in sizing sequence on the dilators, as done in Step K above.

M. Slightly overdilate the tracheotomy to a size that is appropriate for the desired tracheostomy tube (24 Fr for 6 mm inner diameter, 28 Fr for 7 mm, 32 Fr for 8 mm, and 36 Fr for 9 mm).

N. Choose the appropriate dilator for introduction of the tracheostomy tube (18 Fr for 6 mm, 21 Fr for 7 mm, 24 Fr for 8 mm, and 28 Fr for 9 mm).

O. Lubricate the appropriate dilator. Place the tracheostomy tube on the dilator so its tip is approximately 2 cm back from the distal tip of the dilator. Make sure the balloon is totally deflated. Lubricate the tracheostomy tube and dilator assembly.

P. Advance the preloaded tracheostomy dilator assembly over the guiding assembly to the safety ridge, and then advance them as a unit into the trachea. As soon as the deflated balloon enters the trachea, withdraw the blue dilator and guiding catheter assembly.

Q. Advance the tracheostomy tube to its flange.

R. Connect the tracheostomy tube to the ventilator and inflate the cuff. Test ventilation and then remove the endotracheal tube. Suction through the tracheostomy to check for bleeding. The bronchoscope may be used to check position and to aid in suctioning.

S. Place nylon sutures to hold the tracheostomy tube in place. Tie the straps in place.

49

Vascular Access

I. **Subclavian Venipuncture**
  A. Place the patient in the supine position with 15°–30° of Trendelenburg positioning (i.e., head down) to distend the neck veins and prevent an air embolus. A roll between the shoulder blades or gentle traction on the ipsilateral arm is often helpful to level out the clavicles.
  B. Turn the patient's head away from the site if the cervical spine has been cleared.
  C. Prepare the skin around the venipuncture site with povidone-iodine solution and drape the area in sterile fashion.
  D. Inject local anesthetic at the venipuncture site, two finger breadths inferior to the junction of the middle and medial thirds of the clavicle and along the clavicle.

> **Always draw back before injection of anesthesia to assure that the needle is not in a vessel.**

  E. Introduce a large-caliber needle attached to a 10-cc syringe into the skin. Hold the needle and syringe parallel to the frontal plane.
  F. Direct the needle medially, slightly cephalad and toward the sternal notch. Touch the needle to the clavicle and walk down the clavicle until the needle can pass just below the clavicle.
  G. Continue to aim toward the sternal notch or 1 cm above it and slowly advance the needle while gently applying back pressure to the syringe.
  H. When a free flow of blood appears in the syringe, remove the syringe and cap the end with your finger to prevent an air embolism.

> **If the blood is pulsatile, the artery was entered. Withdraw the needle and hold pressure for 10 minutes.**

I. Pass the wire through the needle with the J tip oriented to the desired direction. Advance the wire as tolerated and always hold on to the wire.
   1. If there are premature beats noted on the cardiac monitor, the wire is in the appropriate direction.
   2. If resistance is met, withdraw the guidewire and reattach the syringe to adjust the position or withdraw the needle and start over.
J. Remove the needle over the guidewire.
K. Using an 11-blade scalpel, make a small incision at the skin puncture site.
L. With the guidewire in place, pass the tunnel dilator over the wire.
M. Advance the catheter over the wire until the wire extends out of the open end of the catheter. Then slide the catheter through the skin incision and into place.
N. Aspirate blood from all ports to ensure good flow.
O. Suture the catheter in place with 2–0 or 3–0 silk and place sterile dressing.
P. Obtain a chest x-ray to check placement and to rule out pneumothorax. The tip of the catheter should sit at the junction of the superior vena cava and right atrium.

II. Internal Jugular Venipuncture

A. Middle approach

1. Place patient in the supine position with 15°–30° of Trendelenburg to distend the neck veins and prevent an air embolus.
2. Turn the patient's head away from the site if the cervical spine has been cleared.
3. Locate the triangle formed by the clavicle and the two heads of the sternocleidomastoid muscle (Figure 49-1).
4. Prepare the skin around the venipuncture site with povidone-iodine solution and drape the area in sterile fashion.
5. Inject local anesthetic at the venipuncture site.
6. Palpate the carotid pulse and apply gentle traction medially with the other hand.
7. Use a 20- or 22-gauge finder needle on a 10-cc syringe to locate the internal jugular vein by directing the needle caudally, parallel to the sagittal plane and at a 30° angle to the frontal plane, aiming toward the ipsilateral nipple. If no blood is encountered, some medial or lateral adjustment may be needed. Always know the location of the carotid artery.
8. Once the vein is located, introduce a large-caliber needle attached to a 10-cc syringe into the skin in the same direction (i.e., along the same path) as the finder needle.
9. Once the vein is entered with the large-caliber needle, remove the finder needle.
10. Proceed with steps I-P under subclavian venipuncture (see p 716).

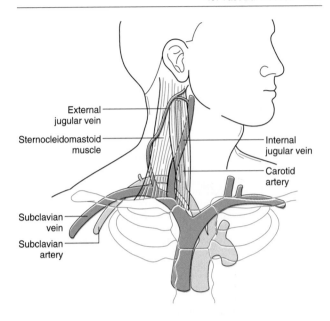

Figure 49-1. Anatomy of the internal jugular and subclavian veins for central venous access.

B. Anterior approach

1. Place patient in the supine position with 15°–30° of Trendelenburg to distend the neck veins and prevent an air embolus.
2. Turn the patient's head away from the site if the cervical spine has been cleared.
3. Locate the medial aspect of the sternocleidomastoid muscle and the carotid artery as it runs along the muscle (see Figure 49-1).
4. Prepare the skin around the venipuncture site (i.e., lateral to but at the level of the cricoid cartilage) with povidone-iodine solution and drape the area in sterile fashion.
5. Inject local anesthetic at the venipuncture site, which is approximately midway up the sternocleidomastoid muscle.
6. Use a 20- or 22-gauge finder needle on a 10-cc syringe to locate the internal jugular vein.
   a. Insert the needle at a 30° angle to the frontal plane and caudally along the middle of the medial edge of the sternocleidomastoid muscle.

   b. Pass the needle in the direction of the ipsilateral nipple, retracting the carotid artery medially with the other hand.

7. Once the vein is located, introduce a large-caliber needle attached to a 10-cc syringe into the skin in the same direction (i.e., along the same path) as the finder needle.

8. Once the vein is entered with the large-caliber needle, remove the finder needle.

9. Proceed with steps I-P under subclavian venipuncture (see p 716).

C. Posterior approach

1. Place patient in the supine position with 15°–30° of Trendelenburg to distend the neck veins and prevent an air embolism.

2. Turn the patient's head away from the site if the cervical spine has been cleared.

3. Identify the lateral border of the sternocleidomastoid muscle where the external jugular vein crosses it, which is approximately 4–5 cm above the clavicle (see Figure 49-1).

4. Anesthetize the region along the sternocleidomastoid muscle and 5 cm superior to the clavicle (i.e., 0.5 cm above the external jugular vein).

5. Introduce a large-caliber needle and direct it inferiorly and anteriorly toward the suprasternal notch.

6. Once venous blood is encountered, place the large-caliber needle in the same direction as the finder needle. Once the vein is entered, remove the finder needle. Then remove the syringe from the large needle.

   a. If the vein is not entered on the first pass, maintain negative pressure on the syringe while slowly withdrawing the needle. Medial and lateral adjustment of the needle direction may be required.

   b. If the carotid artery is entered, remove the needle and hold pressure for 10 minutes.

7. Proceed with steps I-P under subclavian venipuncture (see p 716).

III. Femoral Venipuncture (Figure 49-2)

A. Place patient in the supine position.

B. Prepare the skin around the puncture site with povidone-iodine solution and drape the area in sterile fashion.

C. Locate the femoral vein by palpating the femoral artery. The vein lies just medial to the artery.

D. Inject local anesthetic at the venipuncture site.

E. Introduce a large-caliber needle with a 10-cc syringe attached into the skin directly over the vein, aimed cranially and posteriorly.

F. Advance the needle while withdrawing the plunger of the syringe until there is free flow of blood into the syringe.

G. Advance the guidewire through the needle and remove the needle.

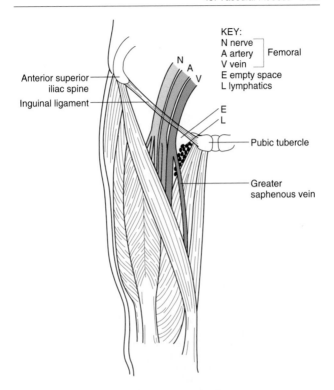

Figure 49-2. Orientation of the femoral vessels. (Adapted with permission from Chen H, Sola JE, Lillemoe KD: *Manual of Common Bedside Surgical Procedures.* Baltimore, Williams & Wilkins, 1995, p 70.)

    H. Advance the dilator only into the subcutaneous tissue (approximately 4–5 cm) and remove. Use a scalpel at the skin entry site to facilitate dilator placement.

    I. Insert the catheter over the wire into the vein and remove the guidewire.

    J. Draw back on each port and then flush each port.

    K. Suture the catheter in place with a 2–0 or 3–0 silk. The patient should be at bed rest while the catheter is in place. There is a risk of an arterial-venous fistula occurring due to erosion of the catheter into the artery.

IV. Intraosseous Puncture and Infusion (Figure 49-3)

    A. Place patient in the supine position. Select an uninjured lower extremity, place sufficient padding under the knee to effect a 30° angle, and allow the patient's heel to rest on the stretcher.

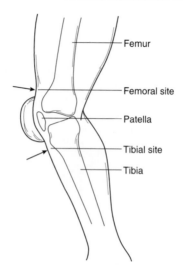

Figure 49-3. Site for intraosseous puncture.

B. Identify the anteromedial aspect of the proximal tibia, approximately one finger breadth below the tibial tuberosity. It may also be identified using the lower medial third of the femur with the same patient positioning.

C. Prepare the skin around the puncture site with povidone-iodine solution and drape the area in sterile fashion.

D. Inject local anesthetic if the patient is awake.

E. At a 90° angle, insert a short, large-caliber bone marrow aspiration needle or a short, 18-gauge spinal needle into the skin with the needle bevel facing the foot.

F. Using a gentle twisting motion, advance the needle through the bone cortex and into the bone marrow.

G. Remove the stylet and attach the needle to a 10-cc syringe with 6 cc of saline.

    1. Gently withdraw on the syringe. There should be aspiration of bone marrow.

    2. Inject the 6 cc of saline.

H. Connect the needle to large-caliber IV tubing.

V. Venous Cutdown

  A. Consider the anatomy.

    1. The primary site is the greater saphenous vein at the ankle, which is located at a point approximately 2 cm anterior and superior to the medial malleolus (Figure 49-4).

    2. The secondary site is the antecubital medial basilic vein, which is located 2.5 cm lateral to the medial epicondyle of the humerus at the flexion crease of the elbow.

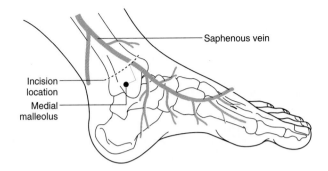

Figure 49-4. Course of the saphenous vein at the ankle.

    B. Prepare the skin of the puncture site with povidone-iodine solution and drape the area in sterile fashion.
    C. Make a full-thickness, transverse skin incision to a length of 2.5 cm.
    D. By blunt dissection, identify the vein and dissect it free from any accompanying structures.
    E. Elevate and dissect the vein for a distance of 2 cm.
    F. Ligate the distal, mobilized vein, leaving the suture in place for traction.
    G. Pass a tie around the vein cephalad.
    H. Make a small, transverse venotomy and gently dilate the vein with the closed tip of a hemostat.
    I. Introduce a plastic cannula through the venotomy and secure it in place with the tie around the vein and cannula.
    J. Attach IV tubing to the cannula.
    K. Close the incision with interrupted sutures and apply sterile dressing.

VI. Peripherally Inserted Central (PIC) Catheter
    A. Place a tourniquet on the arm.
    B. Identify the vein in the forearm that is continuous with the basilic or cephalic vein.
    C. Prepare the area with povidone-iodine solution and a sterile drape.
    D. Measure the catheter from the insertion site to the superior vena cava. The catheter may need to be cut before placement.
    E. Flush the catheter with saline or heparin flush.
    F. Anesthetize the insertion site with a small amount of lidocaine.
    G. Insert the introducer needle into the vein. At the first flash of blood, advance the plastic introducer over the needle, then remove the needle.
    H. Insert the Silastic catheter through the plastic introducer.

I. Once inside the vein, remove the tourniquet and advance the catheter to the desired length.

J. Once the catheter is in position, remove the guidewire and the introducer catheter.

K. Attach the catheter hub and suture in place.

L. Apply sterile dressing.

M. Obtain a chest x-ray to confirm placement.

VII. Radial Artery Catheterization

A. Perform Allen's test to assure adequate hand arterial supply from the ulnar artery.

1. Occlude both radial and ulnar arteries.

2. Release the ulnar artery and check for the hand to fill with blood.

3. If the hand color does not return within 5 seconds, choose another site.

B. Place the patient's arm on a table with the ventral surface exposed. Dorsiflex the wrist and place a towel or gauze roll under the dorsal surface of the wrist. It is often helpful to tape the patient's hand and arm to an arm board.

C. Prepare the area with povidone-iodine solution and drape in sterile fashion.

D. Palpate the radial pulse at the distal radius between your index and middle fingers.

E. Using an 18- to 22-gauge angiocatheter or a specialized arterial catheter with a wire, insert the needle between your fingers at a 45° angle and advance it toward the palpated pulse. Once blood is seen in the needle, advance the catheter or wire.

F. Remove the needle and compress the artery to prevent bleeding while attaching the arterial monitoring apparatus. If there is no bleeding, slowly remove the catheter and watch for blood return.

1. If blood return occurs, slowly advance the catheter.

2. It is helpful to attach the catheter to the monitoring apparatus and flush the catheter as it advances. This often floats the catheter into position.

G. Once the catheter is working well, suture it in place.

H. Place sterile dressing.

VIII. Femoral Artery Catheterization

A. Place patient in the supine position.

B. Locate the femoral artery pulse at the midpoint of the inguinal ligament and follow its course approximately 1–2 cm distally (see Figure 49-2).

C. Prepare the skin around the puncture site with povidone-iodine solution and drape the area in sterile fashion.

D. Inject local anesthetic at the arterial puncture site.

E. Introduce a large-caliber needle with a 10-cc syringe attached. Begin directly over the artery, pointing in the direction of the head and posteriorly.

F. Advance the needle while withdrawing the plunger of the syringe until there is a free flow of blood into the syringe.

G. Insert the guidewire into the needle and then remove the needle.

H. Use a scalpel at the skin entry site to facilitate dilator entry.

I. Advance the dilator only into the subcutaneous tissue (approximately 4–5 cm).

J. Insert the catheter over the wire into the artery and remove the guidewire.

K. Attach a pressure monitor to the catheter.

L. Suture the catheter in place with 2–0 or 3–0 silk. The patient should be at bed rest while the catheter is in place. There is a risk of an arterial-venous fistula occurring due to erosion of the catheter through the artery.

IX. Dorsalis Pedis Artery Catheterization

A. Prepare and drape the dorsal surface of the foot.

B. Locate the dorsal pedis pulse lateral to the extensor hallucis longus at the proximal first metatarsal (Figure 49-5).

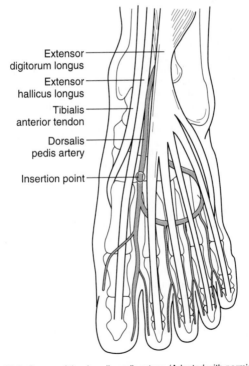

Figure 49-5. Course of the dorsalis pedis artery. (Adapted with permission from Chen H, Sola JE, Lillemoe KD: *Manual of Common Bedside Surgical Procedures.* Baltimore, Williams & Wilkins, 1995, p 67.)

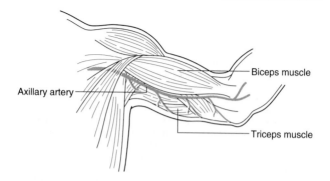

Figure 49-6. Course of the axillary artery. (Adapted with permission from Chen H, Sola JE, Lillemoe KD: *Manual of Common Bedside Surgical Procedures*. Baltimore, Williams & Wilkins, 1995, p 74.)

    C. Anesthetize the skin with lidocaine.
    D. With the bevel up on a 20-gauge angiocatheter, enter the skin at a 45° angle and advance proximally toward the pulse.
    E. Once blood return is evident, hold the needle in place and advance the catheter.
    F. Remove the needle and hold pressure on the artery.
    G. Connect the catheter to the monitoring apparatus.
    H. Suture the catheter in place with 3–0 silk.
X. Axillary Artery Cannulation (Figure 49-6)
    A. Instruct the patient to lie supine with the shoulder externally rotated and the arm fully abducted.
    B. Shave, prepare, and drape the axilla.
    C. Administer anesthetic along the course of the artery.
    D. Using an 18-gauge insertion needle with a 5-ml syringe attached, advance the needle while aspirating at a 45° angle to the skin. If no arterial blood is encountered, slowly withdraw the needle and watch for the flash of blood.
    E. Once the artery is punctured, advance the J wire through the needle, with the tip directed toward the heart.
    F. Once the wire is easily passed, remove the needle and maintain control of the wire.
    G. Using a scalpel, enlarge the puncture site.
    H. Advance the catheter over the wire.
    I. Attach the catheter to the monitoring system and assess arterial waveform.
    J. Using a 2–0 or 3–0 silk, suture the catheter to the skin.

Appendix **A**

Equations

CARDIOPULMONARY CRITICAL CARE

1. **Central venous pressure (CVP)** [normal = 0–8 mm Hg]
2. **Mean pulmonary arterial pressure (PA)** [normal = 10–20 mm Hg]
3. **Pulmonary capillary wedge pressure (PCWP)** [normal = 4–12 mm Hg]
4. **Mean arterial pressure (MAP)** [normal = 80–90 mm Hg]

$$MAP = DBP + \frac{SBP - DBP}{3}$$

5. **Stroke volume (SV)** [normal = 50–60 ml]

$$SV = \frac{CO}{HR}$$

6. **Stroke volume index (SVI)** [normal = 35–40]

$$SVI = \frac{CI}{HR}$$

7. **Cardiac output (CO)** [normal = 4–8 L/min]

$$CO = SV \times HR$$

8. **Cardiac index (CI)** [normal = 3.5–4.0 L/min/m^2]

$$CI = \frac{CO}{BSA}$$

9. **Right ventricular stroke work (RVSW)** [normal = 6–10 g/beat/m^2]

$$RVSW = SVI \times (PA - CVP) \times 0.0136$$

10. **Left ventricular stroke work (LVSW)** [normal = 43–56 g/beat/m^2]

$$LVSW = SVI \times (MAP - PCWP) \times 0.0136$$

11. **Systemic vascular resistance (SVR)** [normal = 800–1200 dynes/sec/cm^{-5}]

$$SVR = \frac{80 \times (MAP - CVP)}{CO}$$

12. **Pulmonary vascular resistance (PVR)** [normal = 100–200 dynes/sec/cm^{-5}]

$$PVR = \frac{80 \times (MAP - PCWP)}{CO}$$

13. **Myocardial oxygen consumption (MVO$_2$)**

$$MVO_2 = \frac{SBP \times HR}{100}$$

14. **Partial pressure of oxygen in the alveoli (PAO$_2$)**

$$PAO_2 = (760 - 47) \times \% FIO_2 - \frac{PaCO_2}{0.8}$$

15. **Capillary oxygen content (Cc'O$_2$)**

$$Cc'O_2 = (PaO_2 \times 0.0031) + Hgb \times 1.34 \times \% O_2 \text{ saturation}$$

16. **Arterial oxygen content (CaO$_2$)** [normal = 20 ml O$_2$/dl]

$$CaO_2 = (PaO_2 \times 0.0031) + [Hgb \times 1.34 \times SaO_2]$$

Note: CaO$_2$ = plasma O$_2$ content + Hgb-bound O$_2$

17. **Mixed venous oxygen saturation (S$\bar{v}$O$_2$)** [normal = > 65%]

18. **Mixed venous oxygen content (C$\bar{v}$O$_2$)** [normal = 13 ml/100 ml]

$$CvO_2 = (PvO_2 \times 0.0031) + [Hgb \times 1.39 \times SvO_2]$$

19. **Oxygen delivery (DO$_2$)** [normal = 600–1000 ml/min]

$$DO_2 = CaO_2 \times CO \times 10$$

20. **Arteriovenous oxygen saturation difference (AVDO$_2$)** [normal = 3.5–4.5 ml/100 ml]

$$AVDO_2 = CaO_2 - CvO_2$$

21. **Oxygen availability (O$_2$ AVI)** [normal = 500–600 ml/min/m^2]

$$O_2 AVI = CI \times CaO_2 \times 10$$

22. **Oxygen consumption ($\dot{V}$O$_2$)** [normal = 110–150 ml/min/m^2]

$$VO_2 = (CaO_2 - CvO_2) \times CO \times 10$$

23. **Oxygen extraction ratio (O$_2$ER)** [normal = 25%]

$$O_2ER = \frac{CaO_2 - C\bar{v}O_2}{CaO_2}$$

OXYGENATION

1. **Respiratory quotient (RQ)** [normal = 0.8]

$$RQ = \frac{CO_2\ produced}{O_2\ consumed}$$

2. **Barometric pressure (P_B)** [normal = 760 mm Hg at sea level]
3. **Partial pressure of water (P_{H_2O})** [normal = 47 mm Hg at 37°C]
4. **Partial pressure of inspired oxygen (PIO_2)** [normal = 150 mm Hg at sea level]

$$PIO_2 = FIO_2 \times (P_B - P_{H_2O})$$

5. **Partial pressure of alveolar oxygen (PAO_2)** [range: 100 mm Hg on room air, 673 mm Hg on 100% O_2]

$$PAO_2 = \frac{FIO_2 \times (P_B - P_{H_2O}) - PaCO_2}{RQ}$$

6. **Partial pressure of arterial oxygen (PaO_2)** [normal = 70–100 mm Hg]
7. **Alveolar-arterial oxygen gradient (A-a)** [normal = 2–22 on room air, 10–60 on 100% O_2]

$$A\text{-}a = [(P_B - P_{H_2O}) \times FIO_2 - PaCO_2\ (1.25)] - PaO_2$$

VENTILATION

1. **Partial pressure of arterial carbon dioxide ($PaCO_2$)** [normal = 46 mm Hg]
2. **Minute ventilation (V_E)** [normal = 6 L/min; estimate 90 ml/kg and increase 5% for each °F increase in temperature]

$$V_E = TV \times RR$$

3. **Pulmonary capillary blood oxygen content**

$$O_2\ content = 1.36 \times (Hgb) \times (SaO_2) \times (FIO_2) +$$
$$0.003 \times (P_B - PH_2O - PaCO_2) \times (FIO_2)$$

4. **Shunt fraction (intrapulmonary; Q_{sp}/Q_t)** [normal = < 0.10]

$$Q_{sp}/Q_t = \frac{Cc'O_2 - CaO_2}{Cc'O_2 - C\bar{V}O_2}$$

LUNG MECHANICS

1. **Static compliance (C_{stat})** [normal = 50–85 ml/cm H_2O]

$$C_{stat} = \frac{TV}{Plateau\ pressure - PEEP}$$

2. **Dynamic compliance (C_{dyn})**

$$C_{dyn} = \frac{TV}{PIP - PEEP}$$

LUNG CAPACITIES

1. **Total lung capacity** (volume in lungs at end of maximum inspiration; TLC) [normal = 4–6 L]

$$TLC = VC + RV$$

2. **Vital capacity** (maximum volume expelled by forced effort after maximum inspiration; VC) [normal: female = 50–60 ml/kg, male = 70 ml/kg; decreases 250 ml/yr after age 20]

$$VC = IRV + ERV + TV$$

3. **Inspiratory capacity** (maximum volume inspired from rest; IC) [normal = 1.0–2.4 L]

$$IC = IRV + TV$$

4. **Functional residual capacity** (volume in lungs at end tidal expiration; FRC) [normal = 1.8–3.4 L]

$$FRC = ERV + RV$$

5. **Tidal volume** (volume inspired and expired with each breath; TV) [normal = 6–7 ml/kg]

6. **End reserve volume** (maximum expired volume from end tidal expiration; ERV) [normal = 25% of vital capacity]

7. **Residual volume** (volume remaining in lungs after maximum expiration; RV) [normal = 1.0–2.4 L]

FLUID BALANCE

1. **Free-water deficit in hypernatremia**

$$Deficit = 0.6 \times weight\ (kg) \times \left[\frac{plasma\ Na}{140} - 1 \right]$$

2. **Free-water excess in hypernatremia**

$$Excess = 0.6 \times weight\ (kg) \times \left[1 - \frac{plasma\ Na}{140} \right]$$

3. **Fractional excretion of sodium (FE$_{Na}$)**

$$FE_{Na} = \frac{urine\ [Na^{+2}]}{plasma\ [Na^{+2}]} \times \frac{plasma\ [creatinine]}{urine\ [creatinine]} \times 100$$

4. **Creatinine clearance** (estimate of glomerular filtration rate; Cl$_{creat}$) [ml/min]

$$*Cl_{creat} = \frac{(140 - age) \times (weight\ in\ kg)}{72 \times (serum\ creatinine)}$$

$$Cl_{creat} = \frac{urine\ creatinine}{serum\ creatinine} \times \frac{urine\ volume}{time\ (min)}$$

*Multiply by 0.85 in females.

5. **Renal failure index (RFI)**

$$RFI = \frac{urine\ Na \times serum\ creatinine}{urine\ creatinine}$$

6. **Estimated serum osmolality** (normal = 290 mOsm/kg H_2O)

$$Estimated\ serum\ osmolality = 2\ (Na) + \frac{glucose}{18} + \frac{BUN}{2.8} + \frac{mannitol}{18} +$$

$$\frac{ethyl\ alcohol}{4.6} + \frac{ethylene\ glycol}{6.2} + \frac{methanol}{3.2}$$

7. **Corrected sodium for hyperglycemia**

$$Corrected\ Na = 0.016\ (measured\ glucose - 100) + measured\ Na$$

8. **Calculated sodium deficit**

$$Calculated\ Na\ deficit = 0.6 \times (weight\ in\ kg) \times (140 - Na) +$$
$$140 \times (volume\ deficit\ in\ L)$$

9. **Corrected calcium**

$$Corrected\ Ca = serum\ Ca + (4 - albumin) \times (0.8)$$

10. **Free-water clearance**

$$Free\text{-}water\ clearance = urine\ volume - \left[\frac{urine\ osmolality}{(plasma\ osmolality) \times (urine\ volume)} \right]$$

11. **Maintenance fluids:**

$$First\ 10\ kg\ body\ weight = 100\ ml/kg/24\ hr$$
$$Second\ 10\ kg\ body\ weight = 50\ ml/kg/24\ hr$$
$$Weight > 20\ kg\ body\ weight = 20\ ml/kg/24\ hr$$

12. **Calculated stool osmolality**

$$Calculated\ stool\ osmolality = 2 \times stool\ (Na + K)$$

NUTRITION

1. **Basal energy expenditure (BEE)** [BEE = Kcal/day, weight = kg, height = cm, age = years]

$$Male\ BEE = 66 + (13.7 \times weight) + (5 \times height) - (6.7 \times age)$$

$$Female\ BEE = 665 + (9.6 \times weight) + (1.8 \times height) - (4.7 \times age)$$

2. **Nitrogen balance**

$$Nitrogen\ balance = \frac{total\ protein\ intake}{6.25} - (urinary\ urea\ nitrogen + 4)$$

3. **Ideal body weight (IBW)**

$$Male\ IBW = 50\ kg\ for\ first\ 5\ feet + 2.3\ kg\ for\ each\ additional\ inch$$

$$Female\ IBW = 45.5\ kg\ for\ first\ 5\ feet + 2.3\ kg\ for\ each\ additional\ inch$$

4. **Oxygen consumption index** (normal = 90–120 ml/min/m²)

$$O_2\ consumption\ index = \frac{(Ca_{O_2} - C\bar{v}_{O_2}) \times CO \times 10}{BSA}$$

5. **Resting energy expenditure (REE)**

$$REE = (3.9 \times O_2\ consumption) + (1.1 \times CO_2\ production)$$

CEREBRAL PERFUSION PRESSURE

Cerebral perfusion pressure (CPP) [normal = 70–100 mm Hg]

$$CPP = MAP - ICP$$

ACID-BASE EQUATIONS

1. **Anion gap** (normal = 12–16)

$$Anion\ gap = (Na + K) - (Cl + HCO_3^-)$$

2. **Bicarbonate deficit**

$$Bicarbonate\ deficit = (0.4 \times weight\ in\ kg) \times (HCO_3^-\ desired - HCO_3^-\ measured)$$

3. **Metabolic acidosis**

$$Expected\ P_{CO_2} = 1.5 \times HCO_3^- + 8\ (\pm 2)$$

4. **Metabolic alkalosis**

$$Expected\ P_{CO_2} = 0.7 \times HCO_3^- + 20 (\pm 1.5)$$

5. **Respiratory acidosis**

$$Acute\ compensated = pH\ change\ of\ 0.008\ units$$
$$for\ each\ 1\ mm\ Hg\ change\ in\ P_{CO_2}$$

$$Chronic\ compensated = pH\ change\ of\ 0.003\ units$$
$$for\ each\ 1\ mm\ Hg\ change\ in\ P_{CO_2}$$

6. **Respiratory alkalosis**

$$Acute\ compensated = pH\ change\ of\ 0.008\ units$$
$$for\ each\ 1\ mm\ Hg\ change\ in\ P_{CO_2}$$

$$Chronic\ compensated = pH\ change\ of\ 0.017\ units$$
$$for\ each\ 1\ mm\ Hg\ change\ in\ P_{CO_2}$$

Appendix **B**

Notes and Orders

ADMISSION AND POSTOPERATIVE ORDERS

1. Admit to Dr. _____ (attending)
   Service:
   Ward/ICU:
   Resident's name and pager number:
2. Diagnosis (postoperative)
3. Condition (e.g., stable, fair, poor, critical)
4. Vitals (frequency)
   • Neurologic checks
   • Vascular and pulse checks
5. Allergies
6. Activity (e.g., bed rest, out of bed to chair, ambulatory with assistance, ad lib)
7. Call physician for:
   • Temperature > _____
   • Pulse > _____, < _____
   • Systolic blood pressure > _____, < _____
   • Respiratory rate > _____, < _____
   • Mental status changes
   • Urine output < _____ (normal is 1/2 cc/kg/hr)
   • Change in neurologic status
   • Change in vascular examination
8. Nursing
   • Strict ins and outs (record q _____ hr)
   • Daily weights
   • Venodyne boots while in bed
   • Foley catheter to gravity
   • Nasogastric tube to low continuous wall suction, to gravity, or clamped
   • Nasogastric tube flushed with 30 cc q 4 hr
   • Manipulation restrictions (e.g., nasogastric tube, Foley catheter, drains)
   • Wound care and dressing changes
   • Drain orders (e.g., culture, laboratory studies, dressings)

- Chest tube instructions (e.g., to 20 cc wall suction, to waterseal)
- Incentive spirometry q 1 hr

9. Diet
   - Instructions (e.g., NPO, clear fluids, full liquids, soft, regular)
   - Dietary restrictions (e.g., cardiac, renal, diabetic, low fat, low cholesterol, no concentrated sweets)
10. Intravenous fluid (type and rate)
11. Symptomatic and scheduled medications
    - Antibiotics
    - Stress ulcer prophylaxis
    - Deep venous thrombosis prophylaxis (i.e., heparin 5000 units SQ q 8–12 hr or sequential compression devices)
    - Pain medications
    - Sleep medications
    - Nausea medications
    - Fever medications
    - Itching medications
    - Constipation
    - Hypertension
    - Daily medications (as allowed)
    - Anticoagulation
    - Bowel preparation
    - Oxygen requirements
12. Vascular orders
    - Sheep skin to foot of bed
    - Bed cradle to foot of bed
    - Lanolin to feet, calves, and shins
    - Elevate or immobilize extremity
13. Electrocardiogram
14. Radiology
15. Laboratory tests (e.g., serum labs, urine analysis, arterial blood gas, pulmonary function tests, blood bank specimen)

PREOPERATIVE NOTE

1. Date of procedure
2. Preoperative diagnosis
3. Procedure planned
4. Surgeon (attending)
5. Checklist to be completed:
   - ☐ Pertinent test results (e.g., radiology, cardiac work-up)
   - ☐ Laboratory results (e.g., complete blood count, platelets, partial thromboplastin time, prothrombin time, electrolytes, blood urea nitrogen/creatinine, liver function tests, thyroid function tests)
   - ☐ Urine analysis
   - ☐ Blood bank specimen (reserve appropriate number of units of blood products)
   - ☐ Arterial blood gas (if appropriate)
   - ☐ Pulmonary function tests (if appropriate)

- ☐ Chest x-ray
- ☐ Electrocardiogram
- ☐ Consent on chart for appropriate procedure
- ☐ Anesthesia preoperative note on chart
- ☐ List of medications
- ☐ Allergies
- ☐ Preoperative orders on the chart
    - ☐ NPO after midnight
    - ☐ Antibiotics on call to operating room (adjust for allergies)
    - ☐ Bowel preparation (if necessary)
    - ☐ IV fluid after NPO
    - ☐ Patient to shower
    - ☐ Other (e.g., hold heparin, hold medications)

BRIEF OPERATIVE NOTE

1. Preoperative diagnosis
2. Postoperative diagnosis
3. Procedure
4. Surgeon (attending)
5. Assistants (residents, students)
6. Type of anesthesia (e.g., general, spinal, epidural, regional, local, sedation)
7. Anesthesiologist
8. Total fluids in (e.g., crystalloid, blood, fresh frozen plasma, platelets)
9. Total fluids out (e.g., urine, estimated blood loss)
10. Drains (e.g., Penrose, Jackson Pratt, Davol, Foley, nasogastric tube)
11. Specimens
    - Pathology and/or microbiology
    - Frozen sections and results
12. Surgical findings (diagram if necessary)
13. Intraoperative x-rays and interpretation of x-rays
14. Complications
15. Disposition
16. Dictation

OPERATIVE REPORT

1. Name of patient
2. Medical record number
3. Dictating physician
4. Date of dictation
5. Attending surgeon and service
6. Date of procedure
7. Preoperative diagnosis
8. Postoperative diagnosis
9. Procedure performed
10. Surgeon and assistants
11. Type of anesthesia
12. Estimated blood loss

13. Fluid and blood products administered during procedure
14. Specimens (e.g., pathology, microbiology, frozen sections)
15. Drains and tubes placed
16. Complications
17. Consultants intraoperatively
18. Indication for surgery
19. Surgical findings (list)
20. Description of operation
    - Patient position
    - Skin preparation and draping
    - Location and type of incision
    - Details of procedure (e.g., normal and abnormal findings, intraoperative studies, hemostatic and closure techniques, dressing applied)
    - Patient's condition and disposition
    - Needle and sponge counts
21. Send a copy of the report to the surgeons and referring physicians.

CRITICAL CARE PROGRESS NOTE

1. Resuscitation code status (date)
2. Date
3. Hospital course
   - ICU day
   - Postoperative day
   - Hospital day
4. History (e.g., reason for admission, ongoing issues)
5. Events in past 24 hours
6. Medications (e.g., drips, antibiotics, routine, preadmission)
7. Vital signs (e.g., temperature, heart rate, pulse, blood pressure, respiratory rate)
8. Fluid status
   - Total in (e.g., IV fluid, total parenteral nutrition, tube feeds, blood products)
   - Total out (e.g., urine, nasogastric tube, drains, blood, dialysis)
9. Neurologic status
   - Sedation, analgesia, paralysis
   - Intracranial pressure, cerebral perfusion pressure
   - Glasgow Coma Scale
   - Examination findings
10. Respiratory status
    - Vent settings (e.g., mode, rate, tidal volume, FIO_2, peep, pressure support)
    - Arterial blood gas (most recent and worst in past 24 hours)
    - Ventilation parameters (e.g., minute ventilation, compliance, peak airway pressures)
    - Wean mode
    - Examination findings
    - Chest x-ray findings
11. Cardiac status
    - Vasoactive medications and drips

- Cardiac parameters (e.g., central venous pressure, peak airway pressure, pulmonary capillary wedge pressure, cardiac output, cardiac index, SvO_2, MvO_2)
- Lactic acid (trend)
- Most recent electrocardiogram
- Creatine phosphokinase with MB fraction and troponin I level
- Examination findings

12. Renal status
    - Continuous veno-venous hemofiltration, dialysis
    - Net fluid

13. Gastrointestinal tract status
    - Incision and dressings
    - Drains
    - Examination findings

14. Nutrition
    - Status [e.g., NPO, PO, total parenteral nutrition, tube feed (include tube type)]
    - Nutrition parameters (e.g., total calories, protein, carbohydrates, amino acids, volume)
    - Swallow study
    - Stool caliber (e.g., diarrhea)
    - Insulin order

15. Extremities
    - Deep venous thrombosis prophylaxis (e.g., SQ heparin, Venodyne boots, inferior vena cava filter)
    - Examination findings (e.g., sensory, motor, reflexes)
    - Pulses
    - Drains and dressings

16. Infectious disease
    - Cultures and sensitivities
    - Sites and durations of arterial and venous lines
    - Wounds

17. Radiology
    - Computed tomography scans
    - Supine films
    - Abdominal x-rays
    - Ultrasounds

18. Hematology
    - Complete blood count (e.g., white blood cells, hemoglobin, hematocrit, platelet count)
    - Coagulation (prothrombin time, partial thromboplastin time, international normalized ratio)
    - Disseminated intravascular coagulopathy screen (e.g., fibrin split products, platelet count, fibrinogen)

19. Chemistries
    - Electrolytes (e.g., Na, K, CO_2, Cl, Mg^{+2}, PO_4, Ca^{+2})
    - Renal function (e.g., blood urea nitrogen, creatinine)
    - Urine electrolytes (e.g., Na, K, Cl, creatinine, osmolarity)
    - Hepatobiliary findings (e.g., aspartate aminotransferase, alanine aminotransferase, alkaline phosphatase, lactate dehydrogenase, amylase, lipase)

- Nutrition (e.g., glucose, albumin, prealbumin)
- Drug levels (e.g., phenytoin, phenobarbital, carbamazepine, digoxin)

20. Assessment
21. Plan (include neurology, respiratory, cardiac, fluid and electrolytes, renal, gastrointestinal, hematology, extremities, nutrition, infectious disease, radiology)

POSTOPERATIVE NOTE

1. Date and time (usually 5–6 hours after surgery)
2. _(Age)_ -year-old male/female status post _(procedure)_
3. Vital signs [e.g., temperature (maximum and present), heart rate, blood pressure, respiratory rate, oxygen saturation]
4. Total ins and outs (operating room + recovery room + ward = totals)
5. Physical examination findings
6. Comments
   - Surgical incision
   - Drains
   - Dressing
7. Postoperative laboratory results
8. Assessment
9. Plan

DISCHARGE SUMMARY

1. Patient name
2. Hospital ID number
3. Attending physician
4. Admission date
5. Discharge date
6. Diagnosis
7. Reason for admission
   - History of present illness
   - Past medical and surgical history
   - Medications
   - Allergies
   - Physical examination
   - Admission laboratory results, electrocardiogram, x-rays
8. Hospital course
   - Relevant test results
   - Procedures
   - Complications
9. Discharge plan
   - Follow-up plan
   - Home nursing visits or care
   - List of medications at discharge
   - Instructions
10. Physician dictating

Appendix C

APACHE II
Severity of Disease
Classification System

APACHE* II SEVERITY OF DISEASE CLASSIFICATION SYSTEM

Physiologic Variable	High Abnormal Range			+1	0	Low Abnormal Range			
	+4	+3	+2	+1	0	+1	+2	+3	+4
Temperature—rectal (°C)	≥41°	39°–40.9°		38.5°–38.9°	36°–38.4°	34°–35.9°	32°–33.9°	30°–31.9°	≤29.9°
Mean arterial pressure (mm Hg)	≥160	130–159	110–129		70–109		50–69		≤49
Heart rate (ventricular response)	≥180	140–179	110–139		70–109		55–69	40–54	≤39
Respiratory rate (nonventilated or ventilated)	≥50	35–49		25–34	12–24	10–11	6–9		≤5
Oxygenation: DO_2 or PaO_2 (mm Hg)									
a. FiO_2 ≥0.5; record DO_2	≥500	350–499	200–349		<200				
b. FiO_2 <0.5, record only PaO_2					PO_2 >70	PO_2 61–70		PO_2 55–60	PO_2 < 55
Arterial pH	≥7.7	7.6–7.69		7.5–7.59	7.33–7.49		7.25–7.32	7.15–7.24	<7.15
Serum sodium (mMol/L)	≥180	160–179	155–159	150–154	130–149		120–129	111–119	≤110
Serum potassium (mMol/L)	≥7	6–6.9		5.5–5.9	3.5–5.4	3–3.4	2.5–2.9		<2.5
Serum creatinine (mg/100 mL) (double point score for acute renal failure)	≥3.5	2–3.4	1.5–1.9		0.6–1.4		<0.6		
Hematocrit (%)	≥60		50–59.9	46–49.9	30–45.9		20–29.9		<20
White blood cell count (total/mm³) (in 1,000s)	≥40	20–39.9		15–19.9	3–14.9		1–2.9		<1
Glasgow coma score (GCS); Score=15 minus actual GCS									

(A) Total Acute Physiology Score (APS)

Sum of the 12 individual variable points

Serum HCO_3 (venous–mMol/L) (not preferred, use if no arterial blood gases)	≥52	41–51.9	32–40.9	22–31.9	18–21.9	15–17.9	<15

(B) Age Points

Assign points to age as follows:

Age (y)	Points
≤44	0
45–54	2
55–64	3
65–74	5
≥75	6

(C) Chronic Health Points

If the patient has a history of severe organ-system insufficiency or is immunocompromised, assign points as follows:

a. For nonoperative or emergency postoperative patients—5 points

b. For elective postoperative patients—2 points

APACHE II Score =

Sum of (A) + (B) + (C) = _____

DEFINITIONS

Organ insufficiency or immunocompromised state must have been evident prior to this hospital admission and conform to the following criteria:

LIVER: Biopsy-proven cirrhosis and documented portal hypertension; past episodes of upper GI bleeding attributed to portal hypertension; or prior episodes of hepatic failure/encephalopathy/coma; CARDIOVASCULAR: New York Heart Association Class IV; RESPIRATORY: Chronic restrictive, obstructive, or vascular disease resulting in severe exercise restriction, ie, unable to climb stairs or perform household duties; or documented chronic hypoxia, hypercapnia, secondary polycythemia, severe pulmonary hypertension (>40 mm Hg), or respirator dependency; RENAL: Receiving chronic dialysis; IMMUNOCOMPROMISED: The patient has received therapy that suppresses resistance to infection, eg, immunosuppression, chemotherapy, radiation, long-term or recent high-dose steroids, or has a disease that is sufficiently advanced to suppress resistance to infection, eg., leukemia, lymphoma, AIDS.

---

*APACHE = Acute Physiology and Chronic Health Evaluation.

(Adapted from Knaus WA, Draper EA, Wagner DP, Zimmerman JE: APACHE II: A severity of disease classification system. *Crit Care Med* 13:818–829, 1985.)

Appendix D

Pharmacy

ALPHA AND BETA AGONISTS (Tables D-1 and D-2)

Table D-1. Cardiovascular Effects of Sympathomimetic Drugs

Drug	Dose	HR	Inotrope	Constrictor	Dilator	Dopaminergic
Dopamine	1–5 μg/kg/min	2+	2+	0	2+	4+
	> 5 μg/kg/min	2+	2+	2–3+	0	2+
Dobutamine	1–10 μg/kg/min	1+	4+	1+	2+	0
Epinephrine	1–10 μg/min	4+	4+	4+	3+	0
Norepinephrine	2–8 μg/min	2+	2+	4+	0	0
Isoproterenol	1–4 μg/min	4+	4+	0	4+	0
Phenylephrine	20–200 μg/min	0	0	4+	0	0

All potencies are expressed on a scale of 0–4+.
HR = heart rate.

Table D-2. Potency of Sympathomimetic Drugs

Drug	Intravenous Drip Rates*				
	Alpha 1†	Alpha 2†	Beta 1‡	Beta 2‡	Dopa§
Dopamine (μg/kg/min)	>10	>10	3–10	3–10	1–2
Dobutamine (μg/kg/min)	—	—	5–10	>10	—
Epinephrine (μg/min)	>10	>10	4–10	1–2	—
Norepinephrine (μg/min)	4–10	4–10	4–10	—	—
Isoproterenol (μg/min)	—	—	2–10	2–10	—
Phenylephrine (μg/min)	0.15–0.75	0.15–0.75	—	—	—

*Values indicate intravenous drip rates in the units indicated for each drug.
†Alpha agonists vasoconstrict peripheral arterioles and veins.
‡Beta 1 agonists increase contractility and chronotropy and enhance atrioventricular conduction. Beta 2 agonists vasodilate the mesenteric and skeletal beds, bronchodilate, and increase chronotropy (reflex pathway).
§Dopamine vasodilates the renal and mesenteric beds.

ANESTHETICS, LOCAL

Table D-3. Local Anesthetic Agents

	Onset	Duration	Maximum Dose	Equivalent Concentration
Lidocaine	< 2 min	0.5–1 hr	5 mg/kg	1%
Lidocaine + epinephrine	< 2 min	2–6 hr	7 mg/kg	1%
Mepivacaine	3–5 min	0.75–1.5 hr	—	1%
Bupivacaine*	5 min	2–4 hr	2 mg/kg*	0.25%
Bupivacaine + epinephrine	> 5 min	3–7 hr	3 mg/kg*	0.25%
Etidocaine	3–5 min	5–10 hr	—	0.5%
Procaine	2–5 min	0.25–1 hr	7 mg/kg	2%
Chloroprocaine	6–12 min	0.5 hr	—	2%

*Bupivacaine should not be used in children < 12 years of age.

ANTIMICROBIAL AGENTS: COMPARISON OF SPECTRA (Tables D-4, D-5, and D-6)

Table D-4. Comparison of Antimicrobial Spectra: Penicillins, Imipenem, Aztreonam, Metronidazole, and Fluoroquinolones

Organisms	Pen G	Pen V	Methicillin	Nafcillin/Oxacillin	Cloxacillin	Dicloxacillin	Amp/Amox	Amox/Clav	Amp/Sulb	Ticarcillin	Ticar/Clav	Pip/Tazo	Mezlocillin	Piperacillin	Imipenem	Meropenem	Aztreonam	Metronidazole	Ciprofloxacin	Ofloxacin	Lomefloxacin	Pefloxacin	Levofloxacin	Sparfloxacin	Trovafloxacin	Grepafloxacin
Gram-Positive:																										
Strep, Group A,B,C,G	+	+	+	+	+	+	+	+	+	+	+	+	+	+	+	+	○	○	+|	+|	○	○	+	+	+	+
Strep. pneumoniae	+	+	+	+	+	+	+	+	+	+	+	+	+	+	+	+	○	○	+|	+|	○	○	+	+	+	+
Viridans strep, milleri	+	+	+	+	+	+	+	+	+	+	+	+	+	+	+	+	○	○	○	○			+	+	+	+
Enterococcus faecalis	+	+	○	○	○	○	+	+	+	+|	+|	+	+	+	+	+|	○	○	→	→		○	+	+	+	+
Enterococcus faecium	+|	+|	○	○	○	○	+	+	+	+|	+|	+|	+|	+|	+|	○	○	○	○	○		○	○	+|	+|	+|
Staph. aureus (MSSA)	○	○	+	+	+	+	○	+	+	○	+	+	○	○	+	+	○	○	+	+	+	+	+	+	+	+
Staph. aureus (MRSA)	○	○	○	○	○	○	○	○	○	○	○	○	○	○	○	○	○	○	○	○	○	○	+|	+|	+|	+|
Staph. epidermidis	○	○	+|	+|	+|	+|	+|	+	+	+|	○	○	○	○	+	+	○	○	+	+	○	+	+	+	+	+
C. jeikeium	○	○	○	○	○	○	○	○	○	○	○	○	○	○	○		○	○	○	○	+	+	+|	○	○	
L. monocytogenes	+	○	○	○	○	○	+	+	+	+	+	+	+	+	+	+	○	○	+		+	+	+	+|	+	+
Gram-Negative:																										
N. gonorrhoeae	○	○	○	○	○	○	○	+	+	+	+	+	+	+	+	+	+	○	+	+	+	+	+	+	+	+
N. meningitidis	+	○	○	○	○	○	+	+	+	+	+	+	+	+|	+	+	+	○	+	+	+	+	+	+	+	+
M. catarrhalis	○	○	○	○	○	○	○	+	+	○	+	+	○	+|	+	+	+	○	+	+	+	+	+	+	+	+
H. influenzae	○	○	○	○	○	○	+|	+	+	+|	+	+	+|	+|	+	+	+	○	+	+	+	+	+	+	+	+
E. coli	○	○	○	○	○	○	+|	+	+	+|	+	+	+	+	+	+	+	○	+	+	+	+	+	+	+	+
Klebsiella sp.	○	○	○	○	○	○	○	+	+	○	+	+	+	+	+	+	+	○	+	+	+	+	+	+	+	+
Enterobacter sp.	○	○	○	○	○	○	○	○	○	+|	+	+	+	+	+	+	+	○	+	+	+	+	+	+	+	+
Serratia sp.	○	○	○	○	○	○	○	○	○	○	+	+	+	+	+	+	+	○	+	+	+	+	+	+	+	+
Salmonella sp.	○	○	○	○	○	○	+|	+	+	+	+	+	+	○	+	+	+	○	+	+	+	+	+	+	+	+

Shigella sp.	0	0	0	0	±	+	+	+	+	+	+	+	+	+	+	+	+	+
Proteus mirabilis	0	0	0	0	+	+	+	+	+	+	+	+	+	+	+	+	+	+
Proteus vulgaris	0	0	0	0	+	+	+	+	+	+	+	+	+	+	+	+	+	+
Providencia sp.	0	0	0	0	+	+	+	+	+	+	+	+	+	+	+	+	+	+
Morganella sp.	0	0	0	0	±	+	+	+	+	+	+	+	+	+	+	+	+	+
Citrobacter sp.	0	0	0	0	0	+	+	+	+	+	+	+	+	+	+	+	+	+
Aeromonas sp.	0	0	0	0	0	+	+	+	+	+	+	+	+	+	+	+	+	+
Acinetobacter sp.	0	0	0	0	0	+	+	+	±	+	+	0	±	+	+	+	+	+
Ps. aeruginosa	0	0	0	0	0	+	+	+	+	+	+	+	+	0	+	+	+	+
B. (Ps.) cepacia*	0	0	0	0	0	±	0	0	0	0	0	0	0	0	±			
S. (X.) maltophilia*	0	0	0	0	±	0	0	0	+	±	0	0	0		+	+	+	
Y. enterocolitica	0	0	0	0	0	+	+	+	+	+	+	+	+	+	+	+	+	+
Legionella sp.	0	0	0	0	0	0	0	0	0	0	0		+	+				
P. multocida	+	+	+	+	+	+	+	+	+	+	+	0	+	+	+	+	+	+
H. ducreyi	+	0	0	+	0	0			+	+								
Miscellaneous																		
Chlamydia sp.	0	0	0	0	0	0	0	0	0	0				0		0		+
M. pneumoniae	0	0	0	0	0	0	0	0	0	+			+	+		+		+
Anaerobes:																		
Actinomyces	+	0	0	+	+	±	+	+	+	0	+		±	0		0		0
Bacteroides fragilis	0	0	0	0	0	+	+	+	+	+	0		0	0		0		0
P. melaninogenica*	+‡	0	0	+	+	+	+	+	+	+	0		0	0		+		0
Clostridium difficile	±‡	0	0	±‡	+‡	±‡	+‡	‡	+‡	+	0		±‡	+‡		+‡		±‡
Clostridium (not difficile)	+	0	0	+	+	+	+	+	+	+	0		±‡	+		+		±‡
Peptostreptococcus sp.	+	+	+	+	+	+	+	+	+	+	0		±‡	+		+		±‡

Adapted with permission from Gilbert DN, Muellering RC, Sande MA: *The Sanford Guide to Antimicrobial Therapy.* Virginia, Antimicrobial Therapy, Inc., 1998, p 52.

Amox/Clav = amoxicillin clavulanate; Amp/Sulb = ampicillin sulbactam; Pip/Tazo = piperacillin tazobactam; Ticar/Clav = ticarcillin clavulanate; + = usually effective clinically or >60% susceptible; ± = clinical trials lacking or 30%–60% susceptible; 0 = not effective clinically or <30% susceptible.

*B. melaninogenicus → Prevotella melaninogenica, Pseudomonas cepacia → Burkholderia cepacia, Xanthomonas → Stenotrophomonas.

†B. melaninogenicus → Prevotella melaninogenica, not in systemic infection.

‡Most strains ±, can be used in urinary tract infection, not in systemic infection.

†No clinical evidence that penicillins or fluoroquinolones are effective for C. difficile enterocolitis (but they may cover this organism in mixed intra-abdominal and pelvic infections).

Table D-5. Comparison of Antimicrobial Spectra: Cephalosporins

Generation	Agent	Strep Group A,B,C,G	Strep. pneumoniae‡	Viridans strep	Enterococcus faecalis	Staph. aureus (MSSA)	Staph. aureus (MRSA)	Staph. epidermidis	C. jeikeium	L. monocytogenes	N. gonorrhoeae	N. meningitidis	M. catarrhalis	H. influenzae	E. coli	Klebsiella sp.	Enterobacter sp.	Serratia sp.	Salmonella sp.	Shigella sp.	Proteus mirabilis	Proteus vulgaris	Providencia sp.
Oral Agents	Cefpodoxime-Prox.	+	+	+		+		+|			+		+	+	+		○	○			+	+|	
Oral Agents	Cefetamet-Piv.	+	+	+|	○	○	○				+|		+	+	+		○	○	+		+	+	+
Oral Agents	Ceftibuten	+	+|	○	○	○	○	○	○	○	+|	+|	+	+	+	+	+|	+|	+	+	+	+	+
Oral Agents	Cefixime	+	+	○	○	○	○	○	○	○	+	+|	+	+	+	+	○	+|	+	+	+	+	+
Oral Agents	Loracarbef†	+	+	○	+	○	+|	○	○		+|	+|	+	+	+	+					+		
Oral Agents	Cefurox. axetil	+	+	○	+	○	+|	○	○		+|	+|	+	+	+	+	○	○	+	+	+	○	+
Oral Agents	Cefprozil	+	+	○	○	+	○	+|	○	○	+|	+|	+	+	+	+	○	○	+	+	○	○	
Oral Agents	Cefaclor	+	+	○	+	○	+|	○	○		+|	+|	+	+	+	+	○	○			+	○	○
Oral Agents	Cephalexin	+	+	○	+	○	+|	○	○		○	○	○	○	+	○	○	○	○	○	+	○	○
Oral Agents	Cefadroxil	+	+	○	+	○	+|	○	○		○	○	+		+	○	○			+	○	○	
3rd Generation	Cefepime	+	+	○	+	○	+|		○		+	+|	+	+	+	+	+	+	+	+	+	+	+
3rd Generation	Ceftazidime	+	‡	‡	○	+	○	+|	○	○	+|	+|	+	+	+	+	+	+	+	+	+	+	+
3rd Generation	Cefoperazone	+	+	+	+	○	+|	○	○		+|	+|	+	+	+	+	+	+	+	+	+	+	+
3rd Generation	Ceftriaxone	+	+	○	+	○	+|	○	○		+	+	+	+	+	+	+	+	+	+	+	+	+
3rd Generation	Ceftizoxime	+	+	○	○	+|	○	○			+|	+|	+	+	+	+	+	+	+	+	+	+	+
3rd Generation	Cefotaxime	+	+	○	○	+|	○	○			+|	+	+	+	+	+	+	+	+	+	+	+	+
2nd Generation	Cefuroxime	+	+	○	+	○	+|	○	○		+|	+	+	+	+	+	+|	○	+	+	+	○	+
2nd Generation	Cefoxitin	+	+	○	+	○	+|	○	○		+|	+|	+	+	+	○	○	+	+	+	+	+	
2nd Generation	Cefotetan	+	+	○	+	○	+|	○	○		+|	+|	+	+	+	+|	+	+	+	+	+	+	
2nd Generation	Cefonicid	+	+	○	+	○	+|	○	○		+|	+|	+	+	+	+	○				+	+	+
2nd Generation	Cefmetazole	+	+	○	+	○	+|	○	○		+|	+|	+	+	+	○	○	+	+	+	+	+	
2nd Generation	Cefamandole	+	+	○	+	○	+|	○	○		+|	+|	+	+	+	○	○	+	○	+	+|	+	
1st Generation	Cephalothin	+	+	○	+	○	+|		○		+	○	+	+	+	○	○	+	+	○	○		
1st Generation	Cefazolin	+	+	○	○	+|	○	○			+	○	+	+	+	○	○	+	○	○			

Morganella sp.	0	0	+	+	+	+	+	±	+	+	+	+	+	+	0	0	0	0	±		0	0	0	0
C. freundii									0				0	+								0		
C. diversus									+				+	+								+		
Citrobacter sp.		0	±	±	+	±	±	±	+	+	+	+	+	+		0	±	0	±		+	+	±	+
Aeromonas sp.	0	0	±	+	+	+	±	+	+	+	+	+	+	+							+	+	+	
Acinetobacter sp.	0	0	0	0	0	0	0	0	+	+	+	0	+	±	0	0	0	0	0		0	0		
Ps. aeruginosa	0	0	0	0	0	0	0	0	±	±	±	+	+	+	0	0	0	0	0		0	0		0
B. (Ps.) cepacia*	0	0	0	0	0	0	0	0	+	+	+	+	+	±	0	0	0	0	0		0	+		
S. (X.) maltophilia*	0	0	0	0	0	0	0	0	0	0	0	±	±	0	0	0	0	0	0		0	0		
Y. enterocolitica	0	0				±	±	±	+	+	+	±	±	+							+	+	+	
Legionella sp.	0	0	0	0	0	0	0	0	0	0	0	0	0		0	0	0	0	0	0	0			
P. multocida			+							+	+	+				0					+			
H. ducreyi		+					+		+	+	+		+								+			
Anaerobes:																								
Actinomyces										+	+													
Bacteroides fragilis	0	0	0	+§	0	+§	+	0	0	±	0	0	0	0		0	0	0	0		0	0	0	
P. melaninogenica*			+	+		+	+	+	+	+	±	+	+	0			+	+	+		+		+	
Clostridium difficile						+	0		0	0		0		0										
Clostridium (not difficile)			+	+	+	+	+	+	+	+	+	+	+					+	+		0			
Peptostreptococcus sp.			+	+	+	+	+	+	+	+	+	+	+	+		+	+	+	+		+			

Adapted with permission from Gilbert DN, Muellering RC, Sande MA: *The Sanford Guide to Antimicrobial Therapy.* Virginia, Antimicrobial Therapy, Inc., 1998, p 53.

MRSA = methicillin-resistant *Staphylococcus aureus;* MSSA = methicillin-sensitive *S. aureus;* + = usually effective clinically or > 60% susceptible; ± = clinical trials lacking or 30%–60% susceptible; 0 = not effective clinically or < 30% susceptible; blank = data not available.

B. melaninogenicus → Prevotella melaninogenica, Psuedomonas cepacia →Burkholderia cepacia, Xanthomonas → Stentrophomonas

†A 1-carbacephem best classified as a cephalosporin.

‡Ceftaz 8–16x less active than cefotax/ceftriax, effective only versus Pen-sens. strains (*AAC* 39:2193, 1995). Oral cefuroxime, cefprozil, cefpodoxime most active in vitro versus resistant *S. pneumoniae* (*PIDJ* 14:1037, 1995).

§Cefotetan and cefmetazole are less active against *B. ovatus, B. distasonis,* and *B. thetaiotamicron.*

Table D-6. Comparison of Antimicrobial Spectra: Aminoglycosides, Macrolides, Glycopeptides, and Urinary Tract Agents

Class	Drug	Strep Group A,B,C,G	Strep. pneumoniae	Enterococcus faecalis	Enterococcus faecium	Staph. aureus (MSSA)	Staph. aureus (MRSA)	Staph. epidermidis	C. jeikeium	N. gonorrhoeae	M. catarrhalis‡	H. influenzae	Aeromonas	E. coli	Klebsiella sp.	Enterobacter sp.	Serratia marcescens	Proteus vulgaris
	Quinupristin/dalfopristin	+	+	o	+	+	+	+	+	+	+	+|			o	o	o	
Urinary Tract Agents	Metronidazole	o	o	o	o	o	o	o	o	o	o	o	o	o	o	o	o	o
	Rifampin	+	+	+|	o	+	o	+	+	+	+	+	o	o	o	o	o	o
	Enoxacin	o	+|	o	o	+	o	+	o	+		+		+	+	+		+
	Norfloxacin	o	o	o	o	+|	o	+|	o	+	+	+		+	+	+	+	+
	Nitrofurantoin	+	+	+|	o	+	o		o	+				+	+|	+|	o	o
	TMP/SMX	++	+	++	o	+	o	+|	o	+|	+	+|	+	+	+		+|	o
	Trimethoprim	+	+|	+	o	+|	o	+	o	o	+|		+	+	+|	o	o	
Glycopeptides	Fusidic Acid	+|	+|	+		+	+	+	+	+			o	o	o	o	o	
	Teicoplanin	+	+	+	+|	+	+	+|	+			o	o	o	o	o		
	Vancomycin	+	+	+	+|	+	+	+	+	o			o	o	o	o	o	
	Minocycline	+	+	o	o	+	o	o	o	+|	+	+		+|	o	o	o	o
	Doxycycline	+|	+	o	o	+|	o	o	o	+|	+	+	+	+|	o	o	o	o
Macrolides	Clarithromycin	+	+			+	o		o	+|	+	+		o	o	o	o	o
	Azithromycin	+	+	o		+	o	+|	o	+|	+	+		o	o	o	o	o
	Dirithromycin	+	+	o	o	+|	o	+|	o	+|	+	+|	o	o	o	o	o	o
	Erythromycin	+	+	o	o	+|	o	+|	o	+|	+	+|		o	o	o	o	o
	Clindamycin	+	+	o	o	+	o	o	o	o	o	o		o	o	o	o	o
	Chloramphenicol	+	+	+|	+|	+|	o	o	o	+	+	+	+	+	+|	o	o	+|
Amino-Glycosides	Netilmicin	o	o	S	o	+	o	+|	o	o	+	+		+	+	+	+	+
	Amikacin	o	o	S	o	+	o	+|	o	o	+	+		+	+	+	+	+
	Tobramycin	o	o	S	o	+	o	+|	o	o	+	+		+	+	+	+	+
	Gentamicin	o	o	S	S	+	o	+|	o	o	+	+	o	+	+	+	+	+

Acinetobacter sp.					0	+	0	0	0	0	0	0		0	0	±|	0	0	0	0	0
Ps. aeruginosa					+	+	+	+	0	0	0	+		0	0	0	0	0	0	+	+
B. (Ps.) cepacia‡	0	+	0	0		+	+	+	0	0	0	0		0	+	+	0	+	0	0	0
S. (X) maltophilia‡	+	0	0	0	+	+	+	+	0	0	0	0		+	0	0	0	0	0	+	+
Y. enterocolitica	+	+	0	0	+	+	+		0	0	0	0			+	+	±	0	0		±
F. tularensis	+								0	0	0	+					0				
Brucella sp.	+					+	+		+	+	+	+			+	+					
Legionella sp.						+	+	0	+	0	+	0							+		
H. ducreyi	0		0		0	+	+	+	0	+	+		+							+	
V. vulnificus		0		+	+				+	+	±	+			0	0				0	+
Miscellaneous:																					
Chlamydia trachomatis	0	0	0	0	±	0	+	+	+	+	+	+		0	0	0	0	0	0	0	0
M. pneumoniae	0	0	0	0		+	+	+	+	±	+	+		0	0	0	+	+	0	+	+
Rickettsia sp.	0	0	+					±	+	+	+	+		0	+	+	+	±	0	+	0
Mycobacterium avium												+								+	
Anaerobes:																					
Actinomyces	0	0	0	0	+	+	+	+	+	+	+	+		+	+	+	0	0	0	0	+
Bacteroides fragilis	0	0	0	0	+	+	+	0	±	±	±	±		0	0	0	+	+	±	+	+
P. melaninogenica‡	0	0	0	0	+	+	+	+	+	+	+	+		+	0	0	+	+	+	+	+
Clostridium difficile	0	0	0	0					±						0	0			+	+	
Clostridium (*not difficile*)§	0	0	+					+	+	+	+	+		+	0	0	+	+	+	+	

Adapted with permission from Gilbert DN, Muellering RC, Sande MA: *The Sanford Guide to Antimicrobial Therapy.* Virginia. Antimicrobial Therapy, Inc., 1998, p 54.

MRSA = methicillin-resistant *Staphylococcus aureus*; *MSSA* = methicillin-sensitive *S. aureus*; *S* = potential synergy in combination with penicillin, ampicillin, vancomycin, or teicoplanin; *TMP/SMX* = trimethoprim/sulfamethoxazole; + = usually effective clinically or > 60% susceptible; ± = clinical trials lacking or 30%–60% susceptible; 0 = not effective clinically or < 30% susceptible; blank = data not available.

*In vitro results discrepant, (i.e., + in one study, 0 in another) [*JAC 31* (Suppl. C):39, 1993]
†Although active in vitro, TMP/SMX is not clinically effective for Group A strep pharyngitis or for infections due to *E. faecalis*.
‡*B. melaninogenicus* → *Prevotella melaninogenica*, *Pseudomonas cepacia* → *Burkholderia cepacia*, *Xanthomonas* → *Stentrophomonas*
§Vancomycin, metronidazole given PO active versus *C. difficile*; IV vancomycin is not effective.

CARDIAC DRUGS (Table D-7)

Table D-7. Hemodynamic Trends of Common Cardiac Drugs

Drugs	BP	HR	CO	SV	SVR	PCWP
Dopamine < 6 µg/kg/min	0 to ↓	↑	↑↑	↑	0 to ↓	0
> 6 µg/kg/min	↑↑	↑	↑↓		↑	↓
Dobutamine	0 to ↑	0 to ↑	↑↑	↑↑	↓	↓
Amrinone	0	0	↑↑	↑	↓↓	↓↓
Epinephrine	↑	↑↑	↑	0 to ↑	↑↓	0 to ↓
Norepinephrine	↑↑	0 to ↓	0 to ↓	0 to ↓	↑	↑
Digoxin	0 to ↓	0 to ↓	↑	↑	0	↓
Isoproterenol	↓	↑↑	↑↑	0 to ↑	↓	↓
Diltiazem IV	↓	0 to ↓	0 to ↑	0 to ↑	↓	0
Nifedipine IV	↓↑	↑	↑↑	0	↓↓	0
ACE inhibitors	↓	0	0 to ↑	↑↑	↓	↓↓
Nitroglycerin IV	↓	↑	↑	↓	↓	↓
Tridil	↓	↑	↑	↓	↓	↓
Intra-aortic balloon pump	↓	0	↑		↓	↓

ACE = angiotensin-converting enzyme; BP = blood pressure; CO = cardiac output; HR = heart rate; PCWP = pulmonary capillary wedge pressure; SV = stroke volume; SVR = systemic vascular resistance; 0 = no effect; ↑ = increase; ↓ = decrease.

CORTICOSTEROIDS (Table D-8)

Table D-8. Relative Potencies of Corticosteroids

Drug	Equivalent Anti-inflammatory Dose (mg)	Relative Anti-inflammatory Potency	Relative Mineralo-corticoid Activity	Duration of Action (hr)
Hydrocortisone	20.0	1.0	1.0	8–12
Cortisone	25.0	0.8	0.8	8–12
Prednisone	5.0	4.0	0.8	12–36
Prednisolone	5.0	4.0	0.8	12–36
Methylprednisolone	4.0	5.0	0.5	12–36
Triamcinoline	4.0	5.0	0	12–24
Dexamethasone	0.75	25.0	0	36–72
Betamethasone	0.60	25.0	0	36–72
9-Alphafluorocortisol	—	10	125	18–36

INSULIN PREPARATIONS (Table D-9)

Table D-9. Insulin Preparations			
Mixture	**Onset**	**Peak**	**Duration**
Regular, Humulin R	0.5–1 hr	2–4 hr	5–7 hr
Semilente	1–3 hr	2–8 hr	12–16 hr
NPH, Humulin N	3–4 hr	6–12 hr	24–48 hr
Lente, Humulin L	1–3 hr	8–12 hr	24–48 hr
Ultralente, Humulin U	4–6 hr	18–24 hr	36 hr
Humalog (insulin lispro)	< 0.25 hr	0.5–1.5 hr	5–7 hr

70/30 insulin preparation is 70% regular insulin and 30% NPH.

NEUROMUSCULAR BLOCKING AGENTS (Table D-10)

Table D-10. Neuromuscular Blocking Agents

Drug	Bolus	Infusion	Onset	Duration	Cautions
Succinylcholine*	1 mg/kg	—	1 min	5–10 min	Hyperkalemia, renal failure, sepsis, burns, Mildly vagolytic
Pancuronium	0.06–0.15 mg/kg	0.01–0.15 mg/kg/hr (guide by clinical exam)	1–2 min	45–90 min	
Atracurium	0.4–0.5 mg/kg	0.3–0.6 mg/kg/hr (guide by clinical exam)	1–2 min	30 min	May cause histamine release
Vecuronium	0.08–0.15 mg/kg	0.01–0.10 mg/kg/hr	1–2 min	30 min	Minimal hemodynamic effect; caution in hepatic failure
Mivacurium	0.15 mg/kg	5–15 µg/kg/min	1 min	15–20 min	Dose-related decrease in blood pressure

*Succinylcholine is the only depolarizing agent. It is used for rapid-sequence induction.

PAIN MANAGEMENT (Tables D-11, D-12, and D-13)

Table D-11. Nonopioid Analgesics

Nonopioids	Route	Time to Peak (hr)	Onset (hr)	Duration (hr)	Max. Dose/ 24 hr (mg)
Aspirin	PO	0.5–2.0	0.5–1.0	2–4	3600
Diflunisal	PO	2–3	1–2	8–12	2000
Fenoprofen	PO	1–2	1	4–6	3200
Ibuprofen	PO	1–2	0.5	4–6	3200
Naproxen	PO	2–4	1	4–7	1500
Indomethacin	PO	1–2	0.5	4–6	200
Sulindac	PO	2–4	2	12	400
Ketorolac	IM	1	0.5–1.0	4–6	120
Acetaminophen	PO	0.5–1.0	0.5	2–4	1200

Table D-12. Common Opioid Analgesics

Opioids	Route	Dose (mg)	Time to Peak (hr)	Onset (hr)	Duration (hr)
Morphine	IV	2.5	0.125	0.5–1.0	2–4
Codeine	IM	15–60	0.25–0.50	1–5	4–6
Hydromorphone	IV/IM	1–4	0.30–0.51	2–3	4–5
Oxycodone	PO	5	0.5	1–2	3–6
Methadone	PO	2.5–10.0	0.5–1.0	1.5–2.0	4–8
Propoxyphene	PO	32–65	0.25–1.00	1–2	3–6
Meperidine	IM	0.3–0.6	0.12	1	6–8

Table D-13. Patient–Controlled Analgesia (PCA)

Agonists	Bolus Dose (mg)	Lockout (min)	Continuous Infusion (mg/hr)
Fentanyl	0.015–0.050	3–10	0.02–0.10
Hydromorphone	0.10–0.50	5–15	0.2–0.5
Meperidine	5–15	5–15	5–40
Methadone	0.5–3.0	5–20	—
Morphine	0.5–3.0	5–20	1–10
Sufentanil	0.003–0.200	3–10	0.004–0.030

VASOPRESSORS (Table D-14)

Table D-14. Sympathomimetic Drugs

Drug	Dose	Receptor	Action	Side Effects	Miscellaneous
Epinephrine	Begin with 2 µg/min, double q 5–15 min until desired effect	Balanced α and β agonists	Chronotropic; inotropic; vasoconstrictor; ↑ MAP, CO, and SVR	Hypertensive effect in patients on β blockers	↑ myocardial oxygen delivery over consumption
Norepinephrine	Begin with 2 µg/min, double q 5–15 min until desired effect	α Agonist with mild β1	Vasoconstrictor β1 (chronotropic effect at doses < 10 µg/min)	High doses ↑ risk of tissue ischemia and hypertension	Often used with low-dose dopamine, CO remains stable until high doses
Isoproterenol	Begin with 2 µg/min, titrate to desired heart rate	β1 and β2	Chronotropic inotropic vasodilation/bronchodilation	↑ heart rate leads to ↑ CO	↑ heart rate and CO in the setting of bradycardia or torsades de pointes to ↓ QT interval
Neo-Synephrine	Begin with 2 µg/min, double q 5–15 min until desired effect	Pure α agonist	Vasoconstrictor	↑ in afterload may ↓ CO	↑ BP in setting of SVT; use with IV nitroglycerin to ↓ preload and coronary vasodilation while maintaining BP in patient with acute cardiac ischemia

continued

Table D-14. Sympathomimetic Drugs

Dopamine				
Low dose	2–5 µg/kg/min	β1	Stimulates renal dopaminergic c receptors, enhances GFR, promotes sodium excretion	↑ potential for arrhythmias
High dose	>10 µg/kg/min	α	Intense vasoconstriction (similar to norepinephrine)	↑ potential for arrhythmias
				If > 10–20 µg/kg/min needed, add epinephrine or norepinephrine and wean dopamine
Dobutamine	Begin with 2–5 µg/kg/min; titrate to effect	β1	Inotropic systemic vasodilator	↑ CO by ↑ SV
				May cause hypotension in a hypovolemic patient due to secondary peripheral vasodilation

BP = blood pressure; CO = cardiac output; GFR = glomerular filtration rate; MAP = mean arterial pressure; SV = stroke volume; SVR = systemic venous resistance.

Appendix **E**

Drug Index

acetaminophen
- Antipyretic, analgesic
- Dose
  - Adult: 325–1000 mg PO q 4–6 hr (max of 4 g/day)
  - Pediatric: 10 mg/kg/dose q 6–8 hr
- Use with caution in hepatic impairment.

acetazolamide (Diamox)
- A carbonic anhydrase inhibitor with mild diuretic properties.
- Causes loss of bicarbonate, resulting in alkalinization of urine.
- Contraindications: hepatic failure, end-stage renal disease, and adrenocortical insufficiency
- Dose
  - Adult (disease dependent)
    - Diuretic: 250–375 mg PO/IV qd-qod
    - Metabolic alkalosis: 500 mg PO/IV q 8 hr
    - Renal insufficiency (increase dosing interval):
      - If creatinine clearance is 10–50, dose q 12 hr.
      - If creatinine clearance < 10 ml/min, avoid use if possible.
  - Pediatric
    - Diuretic: 5 mg/kg/dose PO/IV qd-qod
    - Urine alkalinization: 5 mg/kg/dose bid-tid
- Elimination: excreted unchanged in urine.
- Peak effect occurs 15 minutes after IV dose.

acetylcysteine (Mucomyst)
- A mucolytic and antidote for acetaminophen overdose.
- Dose
  - Adult
    - Mucolytic: 3–5 ml of 10%–20% solution in nebulizer tid-qid/prn (10% use undiluted; 20% dilute with normal saline)
    - Acetaminophen overdose: 140 mg/kg loading dose PO or per NG tube; maintenance requires 17 doses of 70 mg/kg PO or per NG tube q 4 hr
  - Pediatric
    - Acetaminophen overdose: same as adult dose
    - Meconium ileus: 5–30 ml of 10% solution PO/PR 3–6 x/day

• Mucolytic: 3–5 ml of 20% solution in nebulizer tid-qid/prn

adenosine

- An antiarrhythmic that slows cardiac conduction at AV node and is a potent vasodilator of peripheral coronary arteries.
- Indications: diagnosis and treatment of types of supraventricular tachycardia (e.g., atrioventricular nodal re-entrant tachycardia, Wolff-Parkinson-White syndrome). [Note: patients on theophylline may not respond.]
- Contraindications: second- or third-degree atrioventricular block, sick sinus syndrome, atrial fibrillation/flutter, ventricular tachycardia
- Dose
  - Adult
    - Initial: 6-mg IV rapid push (start with 3 mg if given via central vein)
    - No response in 1–2 min: 12 mg IV; may repeat × 1
    - Half-life < 10 sec
  - Pediatric
    - 0.1 mg/kg IV push
    - May increase by 0.05 mg/kg q 2 min [max of 0.25 mg/kg (or 12 mg)]
- Complications: patient may become severely bradycardic or asystolic.

albuterol (Ventolin, Proventil)

- β_2-selective stimulant; bronchodilator
- Indication: treatment of reactive airway disease
- Dose
  - Adult
    - Nebulizer: 0.25–0.50 ml of 0.5% solution in 3 ml normal saline q 4–6 hr. [Some patients may require higher doses and/or more frequent intervals (i.e., q 1–2 hr).]
    - Metered-dose inhaler: two inhalations q 4–6 hr prn

aminocaproic acid (Amicar)

- Indications: excessive bleeding resulting from systemic hyperfibrinolysis and urinary fibrinolysis, provided that DIC is not the cause
- Mechanism of action: Inhibits fibrinolysis by inhibition of plasminogen activator substances and, to a lesser extent, through antiplasmin activity
- Dose: Bolus 5 g PO/IV, then 1–1.25 g PO/IV q 1 hr as needed (not to exceed 30 g/24 hr). To control bleeding following TURP or intractable bladder hemorrhage, administer 0.5% solution by continuous bladder irrigation at 30 ml/hr.
- Adverse Reactions: Thrombosis

aminophylline

- Respiratory agent with bronchodilating and diaphragmatic stimulating actions.
- Physiology: increases cAMP levels in tissues leading to increased levels of catecholamines.
- Dose [Note: aminophylline = 80% theophylline; or 500 mg aminophylline = 400 mg theophylline]
  - Adult

- Load: 5–6 mg/kg IV over 30 min
- Maintenance
  - Adult smoker: 0.9 mg/kg/hr
  - Adult nonsmoker: 0.6 mg/kg/hr
  - CHF, cirrhosis, ascites: 0.3 mg/kg/hr
- IV dose (mg/hr): daily PO dose of theophylline divided by 20
- Pediatric
  - Load: 5–6 mg/kg IV over 20 min
  - Maintenance:
    - ≤ 24 days: 0.10 mg/kg/hr IV
    - > 24 days: 0.14 mg/kg/hr IV
    - 6 weeks–6 months: 0.5 mg/kg/hr IV
    - 6 months–1 year: 0.6–0.7 mg/kg/hr IV
    - 1–9 years: 1.0–1.2 mg/kg/hr IV or 20 mg/kg/day PO divided q 6 hr
    - 9–12 years and smokers: 0.9 mg/kg/hr or 16 mg/kg/day PO divided q 6 hr
    - > 12 years and healthy nonsmokers: 0.7 mg/kg/hr IV
- Therapeutic blood level range: 10–20 μg/ml for asthma
- Elimination: metabolized by the liver; change dose in liver dysfunction
- Adverse reactions: GI upset, diarrhea, nausea, vomiting, nervousness, headache, tremor, tachycardia, muscle cramps
- Drug interactions: use with caution in patients on drugs that inhibit cytochrome P_{450} (i.e., ciprofloxin, cimetidine, erythromycin, fluconazole).

amiodarone
- Physiology
  - Inhibits adrenergic stimulation
  - Prolongs action of the potential and refractory periods
  - Decreases AV node conduction and sinus node function
- Indication: type III antiarrhythmic used in the management of recurrent ventricular fibrillation or hemodynamically unstable ventricular tachycardia.
- Dose
  - Adult
    - Ventricular arrhythmias: 800–1600 mg PO daily for 1–3 weeks, then 600–800 mg daily for 1–3 weeks, then 200–400 mg daily
    - Atrial fibrillation: 600 mg PO daily for 1 week, then 400 mg daily for 2 weeks; after 3 weeks attempt cardioversion and then maintain if converted on 200 mg PO daily
  - Pediatric
    - < 1 year: 600–800 mg/1.73 m^2/24 hr divided q 12–24 hr, then reduce to 200–400 mg/1.73 m^2/24 hr
    - > 1 year: 10–15 mg/kg/day divided q 12–24 hr × 7–14 days until adequate control, then reduce to 5 mg/kg/day divided q 12–24 hr
- Therapeutic level: 0.5–2.5 mg/L
- Elimination: metabolized by liver with active metabolites
- Drug interactions: significantly interacts with warfarin, causing an

increased anticoagulant effect, and with digoxin, causing decreased clearance.
- Monitoring parameters: ECG; thyroid, liver, and pulmonary function tests

amoxicillin
- Spectrum: *Streptococcus* sp, *Escherichia coli*, *Proteus* sp, *Helicobacter pylori*
- Indications: otitis media, sinusitis, respiratory and urinary tract infections
- Dose
  - Adult: 250–500 mg PO q 8 hr
  - Pediatric: 20–50 mg/kg/day PO divided q 8 hr
  - Renal failure: 250 mg PO q 24 hr

amoxicillin/clavulanate (Augmentin)
- Spectrum: *Staphylococcus* sp, *Streptococcus* sp, gram-negative cocci, anaerobes and β-lactamase-producing *Moraxella catarrhalis*, *Haemophilus influenza*, *Neisseria gonorrhea*
- Indications: otitis media; sinusitis; respiratory tract, urinary tract, or skin and soft tissue infections
- Dose (based on amoxicillin dose)
  - Adult: 250–500 mg PO tid or 875 mg bid
  - Pediatric < 40 kg: 20–40 mg/kg/day divided q 8 hr

amphotericin B
- Indication: treatment of severe systemic infections and meningitis caused by *Candida albicans*, *Histoplasma capsulatum*, *Cryptococcus neoformans*, *Aspergillus* sp, *Blastomyces dermatitidis*, *Torulopsis glabrate*, and *Coccidioides immitis*; fungal peritonitis, or bladder irrigation.
- Dose (for most infections)
  - Adult
    - Systemic illness (most infections require cumulative dose of 1 g)
      - 1 mg IV test dose over 30 min; observe for signs and symptoms of allergic reaction
      - Loading dose: 0.5–0.6 mg/kg over 4–6 hr; may premedicate
      - Use 1.0–1.5 mg/kg/day for aspergillus or CNS infection.
    - Amphotericin B lipid complex
      - Indicated for aspergillus, candidiasis, and cryptococcal meningitis.
      - May have less nephrotoxicity than conventional amphotericin therapy.
      - Dose: 5 mg/kg/day over 2–4 hr
      - Note: different formulations exist and they are not interchangeable.
    - Bladder irrigation
      - 50 mg in 1 L of sterile water run as continuous irrigation at 42 cc/hr
      - Length of treatment: 3–5 days
  - Pediatric
    - IV: mix in D_5W to 0.1 mg/ml (peripheral IV) or 0.2 mg/ml (central line)
    - Test dose: 0.1 mg/kg up to a 1 mg max

- Initial dose: 0.25 mg/kg/day
- May increase by 0.25–0.50 mg/kg/day to approximately 1 mg/kg/day qd or 1.5 mg/kg/day qod (max of 1.5 mg/kg/day)

ampicillin

- Spectrum: *Streptococcus* sp, *Listeria* sp, *Escherichia coli*, *Proteus* sp, *Salmonella* sp, *Shigella* sp
- Prehydration may decrease nephrotoxicity.
- Dose
  - Adult: 250–3000 mg IV q 6 hr (max 12 g/day)
  - Pediatric ($\geq$ 7 days)
    - < 1.2 kg: 50–100 mg/kg/day IV/IM divided q 12 hr
    - 1.2–2.0 kg: 75–150 mg/kg/day IV/IM divided q 8 hr
    - > 2 kg: 100–200 mg/kg/day IV/IM divided q 6 hr
  - Pediatric (child): 100–400 mg/kg IV/IM q 6–8 hr
  - Renal failure: change dosing to q 12–24 hr

ampicillin/sulbactam (Unasyn)

- Spectrum: *Staphylococcus* sp, *Streptococcus* sp, Enterobacteriaceae, *Klebsiella* sp, anaerobes, *Haemophilus influenzae*
- Indications: skin and soft tissue (e.g., bite wounds), gynecologic, intra-abdominal, and upper respiratory tract infections
- Dose
  - Adult: 1.5–3.0 g IV q 6 hr
  - Pediatric: 100–200 mg/kg IV/IM q 6 hr
  - Renal failure: change dosing to q 12–24 hr

amrinone (Inocor)

- Positive inotrope with vasodilator effects; inotropic effects additive with digoxin
- Indication: treatment of CHF, low output states, or adjunctive therapy for pulmonary hypertension
- Dose
  - Adult
    - Initial: 0.75 mg/kg bolus over 2–3 min; may be repeated 30 min later
    - Maintenance: 5–10 µg/kg/min
    - Refractory CHF: doses up to 40 µg/kg/min
  - Pediatric
    - Initial: 0.75 mg/kg bolus over 2–3 min; may be repeated 30 min later.
    - Maintenance: child, 5–10 µg/kg/min; neonate, 3–5 µg/kg/min
- Adverse effects: thrombocytopenia, hepatotoxicity, hypotension

atenolol (Tenormin)

- Indication: β_1-selective adrenergic blocker used in the treatment of angina, hypertension, and postmyocardial infarction.
- Dose
  - Adult
    - IV (in acute myocardial infarction): 2.5–5.0 mg over 5 min; may repeat in 10 min
    - PO: 25–100 mg qd
  - Pediatric: 1.0–1.2 mg/kg/dose PO qd (max of 2 mg/kg)

atropine
- Indications: anticholinergic agent used to inhibit secretions, sinus bradycardia, and exercise-induced bronchospasm.
- Dose
  - Adult
    - Preanesthesia: 0.5 mg/dose
    - CPR: 0.5–1.0 mg/dose IV q 5 min (max of 2 mg/dose)
    - Bronchospasm: 0.05 mg/kg/dose in 2.5 ml normal saline (max of 1 mg/dose)
  - Pediatric
    - Preanesthesia: 0.01 mg/kg IV/SQ q 4–6 hr (max of 0.4 mg/dose)
    - CPR: 0.02 mg/dose IV q 5 min (max of 0.5 mg/dose)
    - Bronchospasm: 0.05 mg/kg/dose in 2.5 ml normal saline q 8 hr via nebulizer (max of 1 mg/dose)

aztreonam
- Spectrum: aerobic, gram-negative bacilli bacteria
- Dose
  - Adult: 1–2 g IV q 6–8 hr
  - Pediatric
    - Neonate: 30 mg/kg/dose q 12 hr if < 2 kg or q 8 hr if > 2 kg
    - Children: 90–120 mg/kg/day IV divided q 6–8 hr
  - Renal failure (increase dosing intervals and administer after dialysis)
    - If creatinine clearance is 30–50 ml/min, dose q 12 hr.
    - If creatinine clearance is 10–30 ml/min, dose q 24 hr.
    - If creatinine clearance < 10 ml/min, dose q 48 hr.

bretylium
- Physiology (type III antiarrhythmic)
  - Increases fibrillation threshold, action potential duration, and effective refractory period
  - Positive inotrope
- Indication: second-line agent for treatment of ventricular tachyarrhythmias resistant to lidocaine
- Dose
  - Adult
    - Initial: 5 mg/kg IV; may increase to 10 mg/kg IV over 8 min
    - Maintenance: 1–2 mg/min IV; 25%–50% of dose for creatinine clearance 10–50 ml/min and 25% of dose for creatinine clearance < 10 ml/min
    - Maximum: 30 mg/kg
  - Pediatric
    - Initial: 5–10 mg/kg/dose IV; may repeat q 10–20 min for a total dose of 30 mg
    - Maintenance: 5 mg/kg/dose IV q 6–8 hr

bumetanide (Bumex)
- A potent loop diuretic that inhibits sodium and chloride resorption in the loop of Henle and proximal tubule.
- Indication: management of edema secondary to CHF or hepatic or renal disease

- Contraindication: patients on aminoglycosides
- Dose (Note: 1 mg bumetanide = 40 mg furosemide)
  - Adult
    - PO: 0.5–2.0 mg qd
    - IV: 0.5–1.0 mg over 1–2 min; may repeat q 2–3 hr (max of 10 mg/day)
  - Pediatric: 0.015–0.100 mg/kg/dose qd-qod if ≥ 6 months

carbamazepine (Tegretol)

- Indication: an anticonvulsant used in prophylaxis of generalized tonic-clonic, partial and mixed-partial, or generalized seizures.
- Dose
  - Adult
    - Initial: 200 mg PO bid
    - May increase to 400 mg PO tid-qid based on serum levels.
  - Pediatric
    - < 6 years
      - 5–10 mg/kg/day PO divided bid-qid
      - Increase q 5–7 days up to 20 mg/kg/day
    - 6–12 years
      - 10 mg/kg/day PO divided bid (max of 100 mg bid)
      - Increase q 7 days by 100 mg/day divided tid-qid until desired effect or level
      - Maintenance of 20–30 mg/kg/day PO divided bid-qid (max of 1 g/day)
    - > 12 years
      - Initially 200 mg PO bid
      - Increase q 7 days by 200 mg/day divided tid-qid until desired effect
      - Maintenance of 600–1200 mg/day PO divided bid-qid
- Interaction with other drugs:
  - Decreases serum levels of theophylline, warfarin, cyclosporine, phenytoin, and haloperidol.
  - Erythromycin, cimetidine, isoniazid, and calcium channel blockers increase its serum level.

cefazolin (Kefzol, Ancef)

- First-generation cephalosporin
- Spectrum: *Staphylococcus* sp, *Streptococcus* sp, *Klebsiella* sp, *Escherichia coli*
- Dose
  - Adult: 1–2 g IV q 8 hr (max of 6 g/day)
  - Pediatric
    - Neonate ≤ 7 days: 20 mg/kg IV q 12 hr
    - Neonate > 7 days: ≤ 2 kg, 20 mg/kg IV q 12 hr; > 2 kg, 30 mg/kg IV q 8 hr
    - > 1 month: 50–100 mg IV divided q 8 hr
  - Renal failure (increase dosing intervals)
    - If creatinine clearance is 10–30 ml/min, dose q 12 hr.
    - If creatinine clearance is < 10 ml/min, dose q 24 hr.

cefoperazone (Cefobid)

- Third-generation cephalosporin

- Spectrum: gram-negative bacilli including Enterobacteriaceae, *Acinetobacter* sp, *Pseudomonas* sp
- Indications: nosocomial pneumonia, sepsis, skin and soft tissue infection
- Dose
  - Adult: 1–2 g IV q 12 hr
  - Pediatric: 150 mg/kg/day IV divided q 8 hr
  - Can increase prothrombin time. Give vitamin K weekly.

cefotaxime (Claforan)
- Third-generation cephalosporin
- Spectrum: *Staphylococcus* sp, *Streptococcus* sp, Enterobacteriaceae, *Acinetobacter* sp, *Escherichia coli, Klebsiella* sp
- Has good penetration into body fluids and tissues, including aqueous humor, ascites, bone, and CSF.
- Dose
  - Adult: 1–2 g IV q 6–8 hr (up to 12 g/day)
  - Pediatric: 50–200 mg/kg/day IV/IM divided q 6–8 hr
  - Renal failure (increase dosing intervals)
    - If creatinine clearance is 10–50 ml/min, dose q 8–12 hr.
    - If creatinine clearance is < 10 ml/min, dose q 24 hr.

cefotetan (Cefotan)
- A second-generation cephalosporin with excellent penetration of body fluids, especially intra-abdominal, gynecologic, and skin infections.
- Spectrum: *Staphylococcus* sp, *Streptococcus* sp, gram-negative cocci, Enterobacteriaceae, anaerobes
- Indication: excellent choice for surgical prophylaxis.
- Dose
  - Adult: 1–3 g IV q 12 hr
  - Pediatric: 20–40 mg/kg IV q 12 hr
  - Renal failure: normal dose, but give qd

cefoxitin (Mefoxin)
- Second-generation cephalosporin
- Spectrum: gram-negative cocci, Enterobacteriaceae, *Salmonella* sp, anaerobes
- Dose
  - Adult: 1–2 g IV q 6–8 hr
  - Pediatric: 80–160 mg/kg/day IV divided q 6 hr (max dose of 12 g/day)
  - Renal failure: change dosing to q 24–48 hr

ceftazidime (Fortaz)
- A third-generation cephalosporin with excellent penetration into respiratory, abdominal, and CSF spaces.
- Spectrum: gram-negative pathogens including *Escherichia coli, Klebsiella* sp, Enterobacteriaceae, *Acinetobacter* sp, *Pseudomonas* sp
- Dose
  - Adult: 1–2 g IV q 8–12 hr
  - Pediatric
    - Neonate
      - ≤ 7 days: 50 mg/kg IV q 12 hr
      - > 7 days and < 1.2 kg: 50 mg/kg IV q 12 hr

- > 7 days and > 1.2 kg: 50 mg/kg IV q 8 hr
- Infant/child: 90–150 mg/kg/day divided q 8 hr (max dose of 6 g/day)
- Meningitis: 75 mg/kg IV q 8 hr
- Renal failure (increase dosing intervals)
  - If creatinine clearance is 30–50 ml/min, dose q 12 hr.
  - If creatinine clearance is 10–30 ml/min, dose q 24 hr.
  - If creatinine clearance is < 10 ml/min, dose q 48 hr.

ceftizoxime (Cefizox)
- Third-generation cephalosporin
- Spectrum: *Staphylococcus* sp, *Streptococcus* sp, Enterobacteriaceae, *Acinetobacter* sp, *Pseudomonas* sp
- Dose
  - Adult: 1–4 g IV q 8–12 hr (max 12 g/day)
  - Pediatric: 150–200 mg/kg/day divided q 6–8 hr
  - Renal failure: change dosing to q 24 hr

ceftriaxone (Rocephin)
- A third-generation cephalosporin with a broad spectrum, except *Pseudomonas* sp, and excellent CSF penetration.
- Spectrum: *Streptococcus* sp, *Klebsiella* sp, Enterobacteriaceae, gram-negative cocci, *Acinetobacter* sp, *Escherichia coli*
- Dose
  - Adult: 1.0–2.0 g IV/IM q 12–24 hr (for suspected gonorrhea, use 250 mg IM × 1 dose)
  - Pediatric
    - 50–75 mg/kg/day IV divided q 12–24 hr
    - Meningitis: 100 mg/kg/day IV divided q 12–24 hr

cefuroxime (Zinacef)
- Second-generation cephalosporin
- Spectrum: *Staphylococcus* sp, *Streptococcus* sp, gram-negative cocci, Enterobacteriaceae, *Haemophilus* sp, *Escherichia coli, Klebsiella* sp
- Dose
  - Adult
    - IV: 0.75–1.50 g q 8 hr
    - PO: 250–500 mg bid
  - Pediatric
    - Neonate: 20–50 mg/kg/day divided q 12 hr
    - Infant/child: 75–150 mg/kg/day IV divided q 8 hr
      - Otitis: 15 mg/kg PO bid
      - Pharyngitis: 10 mg/kg PO bid
  - Renal failure (increase dosing intervals)
    - If creatinine clearance is 10–20 ml/min, dose q 12 hr.
    - If creatinine clearance is < 10 ml/min, dose qd.

cephalexin (Keflex)
- First-generation cephalosporin
- Spectrum: *Staphylococcus* sp, *Streptococcus* sp, *Escherichia coli, Klebsiella* sp
- Dose
  - Adult: 250–500 mg PO q 6 hr
  - Pediatric: 25–100 mg/kg/day PO divided q 6–12 hr

chlorpromazine (Thorazine)
- Indication: treatment of intractable hiccups, nausea and vomiting, and psychosis
- Dose
  - Adult
    - Hiccups: 25–50 mg PO tid-qid
    - Nausea and vomiting: 10–25 mg PO q 4–6 hr, 25–50 mg IM/IV q 4–6 hr, or 25–50 mg PR q 6–8 hr
  - Pediatric
    - > 6 months: 2.5–6.0 mg/kg/day IM/IV divided q 6–8 hr or PO q 4–6 hr
    - < 5 years: max of 40 mg/day
    - 5–12 years: max of 75 mg/day

cimetidine (Tagamet)
- H_2-receptor antagonist
- Indications: treatment of peptic ulcer disease, pathologic hypersecretory states, gastroesophageal reflux disease, and for stress ulcer prophylaxis
- Dose
  - Adult
    - Acute
      - 800 mg PO qhs or 400 mg PO bid
      - 300 mg PO ac and qhs
    - Maintenance: 400 mg PO qhs
    - IV
      - Intermittent: 300 mg IV q 6–8 hr
      - Continuous: 150 mg IV load, then 37.5 mg/hr
  - Pediatric
    - Neonate/infants: 10–20 mg/kg/day IM/IV/PO divided q 6 hr
    - Children: 20–40 mg/kg/day PO/IV/IM divided q 6 hr
- Drug interactions: multiple interactions involving the P_{450} enzyme system, especially with warfarin, cyclosporin, phenytoin, and triazolam.

ciprofloxacin
- Fluoroquinolone
- Spectrum: gram-positive bacteria including *Staphylococcus aureus, Staph. epidermidis,* and *Listeria monocytogenes;* gram-negative bacteria including *Pseudomonas* sp, *Escherichia coli, Klebsiella* sp, Enterobacteriaceae, *Salmonella* sp, *Shigella* sp, *Campylobacter* sp, and *Neisseria gonorrhoeae*
- Dose
  - Adult: 250–750 mg PO bid; 200–400 mg IV q 12 hr
  - Pediatric (Note: not recommended in children less than 18 years due to risk of transient arthropathy.)
    - 10–20 mg/kg/day IV divided q 12 hr
    - 20–30 mg/kg/day PO divided q 12 hr (max of 1.5 g/day)
  - Renal failure: 50% of dose

cisatracurium
- Nondepolarizing neuromuscular blocker that is an isomer of atracurium, which minimally stimulates histamine release

- Indication: used in hepatic and renal insufficiency or failure
- Pharmacokinetics
  - Onset of action: 2–3 min
  - Duration of action from single bolus: 20–40 min
- Dose
  - Initial bolus: 0.1–0.2 mg/kg/hr IV
  - Continuous infusion: 0.12–0.2 mg/kg IV
- Drug interactions: Aminoglycosides, diuretics, and magnesium prolong the duration of action of cisatracurium.
- Independent of any organ for metabolism or elimination

clindamycin (Cleocin)

- Spectrum: *Staphylococcus* sp, *Streptococcus* sp, all anaerobes, excellent coverage for oral flora
- Dose
  - Adult: 150–450 mg PO q 6 hr; 150–900 IV q 8 hr
  - Pediatric
    - Neonates ≤ 7 days
      - ≤ 2 kg: 5 mg/kg/dose q 12 hr
      - > 2 kg: 5 mg/kg/dose q 8 hr
    - Neonates > 7 days
      - ≤ 2 kg: 5 mg/kg/dose q 12 hr
      - 1.2–2.0 kg: 5 mg/kg/dose q 8 hr
      - > 2 kg: 5 mg/kg/dose q 6 hr
    - Children
      - 20–30 mg/kg/day PO divided q 6 hr
      - 25–40 mg/kg/day IV divided q 6–8 hr
  - Renal failure: no change

codeine

- Narcotic, analgesic, antitussive
- Dose
  - Adult
    - Analgesic: 15–60 mg/dose IM/SQ/PO q 4–6 hr prn
    - Antitussive: 10–20 mg/dose q 4–6 hr prn (max 120 mg/day)
  - Pediatric
    - Analgesic: 0.5–1.0 mg/kg/dose IM/PO/SQ q 4–6 hr
    - Antitussive
      - Child 2–6 years: 2.5–5.0 mg/dose q 4–6 hr to a max of 30 mg/day
      - Child 6–12 years: 5–10 mg/dose q 4–6 hr to a max of 60 mg/day

dantrolene

- Indication: treatment of malignant hyperthermia and spasticity
- Dose
  - Adult
    - Acute: 1–2 mg/kg IV bolus; repeat q 15 min to a max of 10 mg/kg
    - Maintenance: 1–2 mg/kg PO qid for 3 days
  - Pediatric: same as adult
  - Prophylaxis before surgery: 4–8 mg/kg/day divided q 6–8 hr × 2 days

Darvocet
- Analgesic
- Preparations
  - N-50: 50 mg propoxyphene napsylate and 325 mg acetaminophen
  - N-100: 100 mg propoxyphene napsylate and 650 mg acetaminophen
- Dose: 50–100 mg propoxyphene PO q 4 hr prn for pain

desmopressin (DDAVP)
- Indication: treatment of central diabetes insipidus and bleeding disorders (e.g., uremia, von Willebrand's disease)
- Dose
  - Adult
    - Bleeding: 0.3 µg/kg diluted in 50 ml normal saline, injected slowly IV over 15–30 min
    - Central diabetes insipidus
      - Intranasal 10–40 µg/day divided bid/tid
      - IV/SQ 2–4 µg/day divided bid
  - Pediatric
    - Bleeding: same as adult
    - Central diabetes insipidus (3 months–12 years): 5–30 µg/day intranasal divided qd-bid

dexamethasone (Decadron)
- Corticosteroid with potent anti-inflammatory actions (see Table D-7)
- Dose
  - Adult
    - Cerebral edema: 10 mg IM/IV initially, then 6 mg IM/IV q 6 hr
    - Dexamethasone suppression test (see Chapter 14)
  - Pediatric
    - Cerebral edema: load with 1–2 mg/kg/dose PO/IV/IM × 1 then maintenance of 1.0–1.5 mg/kg/day divided q 4–6 hr
    - Airway edema: 0.5–2.0 mg/kg/day PO/IV/IM divided q 6 hr (begin 24 hours before extubation and continue for 4–6 doses after extubation)

dextran
- A colloidal plasma volume expander that causes a decrease in platelet function and has a mild anticoagulant effect.
- Dose: 20–25 ml/hr
  - The dose is empiric and is not based on weight.
  - There is no way to monitor effect.
- Use with caution in patients with CHF and renal failure.

diazepam (Valium)
- Benzodiazepine, anxiolytic, anticonvulsant
- Dose
  - Adult
    - Status epilepticus: 5–10 mg IV q 10–15 min to a max of 30 mg
    - Sedative/muscle relaxant: 2–10 mg IM/IV q 3–4 hr or PO q 6–12 hr
  - Pediatric

- Status epilepticus
  - Neonate: 0.30–0.75 mg/kg IV q 15–30 min × 2–3
  - > 1 month: 0.2–0.5 mg/kg IV q 15–30 min
  - Maximum dose: < 5 years, 5 mg; ≥ 5 years, 10 mg
- Sedative/muscle relaxant: 0.04–0.20 mg/kg q 2–4 hr to a max of 0.6 mg/kg q 8 hr
- Complications: possible hypotension and respiratory depression
- Long half-life

digoxin (Lanoxin)
- Cardiac glycoside
- Physiology
  - Inhibits Na/K ATPase with increased intracellular calcium leading to increased contractility.
  - Blocks AV conduction with an increase in the refractory period and a decrease in conduction velocity.
- Indication: management of atrial fibrillation and CHF
- Dose
  - Adult
    - Inpatient dosing: 0.25–0.50 mg IV initially, then 0.25 mg IV q 6–8 hr until rate is controlled or total dose of 0.75–1.00 mg is given in 24 hr
    - Begin maintenance dose of 0.125–0.250 mg PO/IV daily based on patient size and digoxin levels.
  - Pediatric
    - Premature
      - Initial: 10 µg/kg PO or 7.5 µg/kg IV/IM, then 5 µg/kg PO or 3.75 µg/kg IV/IM q 8–18 hr × 2 doses
      - Maintenance: 2.5 µg/kg PO bid or 1.5–2.0 µg/kg IV/IM bid
    - Full term
      - Initial: 15 µg/kg PO or 10 µg/kg IV/IM, then 7.5 µg/kg PO or 5 µg/kg IV/IM q 8–18 hr × 2 doses
      - Maintenance: 4–5 µg/kg PO bid or 3–4 µg/kg IV/IM bid
    - < 2 years
      - Initial: 20–25 µg/kg PO or 15–20 µg/kg IV/IM, then 10.0–12.5 µg/kg PO or 7.5–10.0 µg/kg IV/IM q 8–18 hr × 2 doses
      - Maintenance: 5–6 µg/kg PO bid or 3.75–4.50 µg/kg IV/IM bid
    - 2–10 years
      - Initial: 15–20 µg/kg PO or 10–15 µg/kg IV/IM, then 7.5–10.0 µg/kg PO or 5.0–7.5 µg/kg IV/IM q 8–18 hr × 2 doses
      - Maintenance: 4–5 µg/kg PO bid or 3–4 µg/kg IV/IM bid
    - > 10 years: same as adults
- Therapeutic level: 0.8–2.0 ng/ml

diltiazem (Cardizem)
- Calcium channel blocker
- Indication: used to convert paroxysmal supraventricular tachycardia to sinus rhythm and to control ventricular rate during atrial fibrillation/flutter.
- Dose (IV)

- Initial: 0.15–0.25 mg/kg over 2 min; if no response, wait 15 min and increase bolus to a max of 0.35 mg/kg over 2 min.
- Maintenance: constant infusion 5–20 mg/hr
- Note: each time the infusion needs to be adjusted, the patient usually requires a new bolus.
- Results in atrial fibrillation or flutter, which usually occurs in 2–7 min.
- Note: patient should have continuous ECG monitoring and BP checks during drug administration.

diphenhydramine (Benadryl)
- Antihistamine with anticholinergic and sedative properties
- Dose
  - Adult: 10–50 mg PO/IM/IV q 6–8 hr to a max of 400 mg/day
  - Pediatric: 5 mg/kg/day PO/IV/IM divided q 6 hr to a max of 300 mg/day
- Use with caution in elderly patients and patients with bronchial asthma, hyperthyroidism, hypertension, and cardiovascular disease due to atropine-like effect. May be a sedative in the elderly.

divalproex (Depakote)
- Indication: an anticonvulsant used in the management of simple and complex absence seizures, mixed types, myoclonic and generalized tonic-clonic seizures.
- Dose
  - 15 mg/kg/day PO
  - Increase at weekly intervals by 5–10 mg/kg/day to a max of 60 mg/kg/day.
  - If dose exceeds 250 mg/day, give in divided doses.

dobutamine (Dobutrex)
- β_1 agonist
- Physiology
  - Increases inotropy, and to lesser extent heart rate
  - Decreases SVR (reflexly)
  - BP remains stable
  - Produces dose-related increase in cardiac output up to a dose of 40 μg/kg/min
- Indication: cardiogenic shock, severe CHF, s/p myocardial infarction with low cardiac output/index
- Contraindication: hypertrophic cardiomyopathy, atrial fibrillation or flutter
- Dose
  - Adult
    - Mixture: 250 mg in 250 ml (15 gtts = 1 mg)
    - Initial: 1–2 μg/kg/min IV, then 2.5–15.0 μg/kg/min IV
    - Can be increased to 40 μg/kg/min if necessary
  - Pediatric: same as adult
- Note: tolerance develops in 72 hours.
- May increase insulin requirements.

dopamine
- Stimulates both dopaminergic and adrenergic receptors.
- Indication: shock, poor perfusion of vital organs, decreased splanchnic perfusion, low cardiac output

- Dose-dependent actions
  - Adult
    - Mixture: 200 mg in 250 ml D_5W (15 gtts = 200 μg)
    - 1–3 μg/kg/min [ra] dopaminergic-mediated increase in renal blood flow
    - 5–10 μg/kg/min [ra] a β-adrenergic receptor mediated increase in cardiac inotropy
    - 10–15 μg/kg/min [ra] an α-adrenergic mediated increase in SVR with some β-adrenergic effect
    - > 15 μg/kg/min of pure α agonist [ra] ↑ SVR, afterload, and peripheral vasoconstriction
  - Pediatric: same as adult

droperidol
- Antiemetic, sedative
- Dose: 0.03–0.07 mg/kg/dose IV q 4–6 hr prn nausea; may increase to 0.10–0.15 mg/kg/dose

edrophonium (Tensilon)
- Indication: an anticholinesterase useful in the reversal of neuromuscular blockade or the diagnosis of myasthenia gravis.
- Dose
  - Adult
    - 2 mg IV test dose
    - 8 mg after 45 sec (if no reaction); may repeat 10 mg q 5–10 min to a max of 40 mg
  - Pediatric
    - Neonates: 0.1 mg single dose
    - Infants/children
      - Initial: 0.04 mg/kg/dose × 1 (max of 1 mg if < 34 kg or 2 mg if ≥ 34 kg)
      - No response after 1 minute: 0.16 mg/kg/dose for total of 2 mg/kg
      - Total maximum dose: 5 mg if < 34 kg; 10 mg if ≥ 34 kg
- Complications: may induce cholinergic crisis, arrhythmias, or bronchospasm. Hypersensitivity (i.e., fasciculations and intestinal cramping) is an indication to stop treatment.

enoxaparin (Lovenox)
- Low molecular weight heparin
- Does not alter PTT and is not reversed by protamine
- Dose
  - DVT prophylaxis 40 mg SQ qd (30 mg SQ q 12 hr) for hip/knee surgery
  - Treatment of DVT or PE: 1 mg/kg SQ q 12 hr
  - Treatment of acute coronary syndromes (unstable angina, NQW MI): 1 mg/kg SQ q 12 hr or 1.5 mg/kg SQ qd

epinephrine (Adrenaline)
- A sympathomimetic that directly stimulates α and β receptors.
- Physiology
  - Increases BP, SVR, HR, coronary and cerebral blood flow.
  - Positive inotrope that increases oxygen demand and ectopy.
  - Can produce profound peripheral vasoconstriction, especially in splanchnic and renal buds.

- Metabolic effects include lactic acidosis, hyperglycemia, and ketoacid accumulation.
- Dose
  - Adult
    - Mixture: 2 mg in 250 ml (15 gtts = 2 μg)
    - IV drip: 2–20 μg/min (0.025–0.300 μg/kg/min)
    - Status asthmaticus (in patients < 30 years) and anaphylaxis: 0.3–0.5 mg IV of 1:10,000 solution; may repeat q 5–10 min
    - Cardiopulmonary arrest: 0.5–1.0 mg of 1:10,000 solution IV; may be repeated q 3–5 min (may be given down endotracheal tube)
  - Pediatric
    - Neonate
      - Asystole/bradycardia: 0.01–0.03 mg/kg of 1:10,000 solution (0.1–0.3 ml/kg) IV or via endotracheal tube q 3–5 min
    - Infant/child
      - Bradycardia/asystole: start with 0.01 mg/kg (0.1 ml/kg) of 1:10,000 solution IV or 1:1000 via endotracheal tube, then 0.1 mg/kg (0.1 ml/kg) of 1:1000 solution via IV or endotracheal tube q 3–5 min
      - Bronchospasm: 0.01 mg/kg/dose SQ of 1:1000 solution (max of 0.3 ml) q 15 min × 3–4 doses or q 4 hr prn
    - IV drip: 2–20 μg/min (0.025–0.300 μg/kg/min)
    - Croup: 0.05 ml/kg/dose diluted with 2.5 ml normal saline given via nebulizer over 15 min (may give q 1–2 hr)

erythromycin
- Spectrum: *Staphylococcus* sp, *Streptococcus* sp, gram-positive bacilli, gram-negative cocci, *Legionella* sp
- Dose
  - Adult: 250–500 mg PO q 6–12 hr; 15–20 mg/kg IV by continuous infusion or over 30–60 min q 6 hr as promotility agent, 250 mg PO tid before meals
  - Pediatric: 30–50 mg/kg/day PO divided q 6–8 hr

esmolol (Brevibloc)
- Ultra short acting (9 min half-life) β_1-selective β-blocker
- Indication: acute treatment of angina and arrhythmias
- Dose
  - Adult
    - Load 100–500 μg/kg over 1 min, then 25–100 μg/kg/min for 4 min.
    - May repeat loading dose and increase maintenance dose by 25–50 μg/kg/min q 5 min.
    - Most patients respond to an infusion rate of 150–500 μg/kg/min. Adjust infusion as tolerated clinically.
    - As clinical effect is approached, discontinue bolus and increase infusion.
  - Pediatric: same as adult
- Note: levels are increased by morphine.

famotidine (Pepcid)
- H_2-receptor antagonist

- Indication: peptic ulcer disease, pathologic hypersecretory states, gastroesophageal reflux disease
- Dose
  - Adult
    - Acute: 40 mg PO/IV qhs or 20 mg PO/IV bid
    - Maintenance: 20 mg PO qhs
    - Hypersecretory conditions: 20 mg PO q 6 hr
  - Pediatric
    - IV: 0.6–0.8 mg/kg/day divided q 8–12 hr to a max of 40 mg/day
    - PO: 1.0–1.2 mg/kg/day divided q 8–12 hr to a max of 40 mg/day

fluconazole (Diflucan)
- Indication: an azote antifungal agent useful in treating candidiasis and cryptococcal infections.
- Dose
  - Adult
    - Oropharyngeal or esophageal candidiasis
      - Load: 200 mg PO/IV
      - Maintenance: 100 mg PO/IV qd for 2–3 weeks
    - Systemic disease or acute cryptococcal meningitis
      - Load: 400–800 mg PO/IV (double the maintenance dose)
      - Maintenance: 200–400 mg PO/IV qd for 10–12 weeks
      - Unstable patient with suspected fungemia: increase dose to 800 mg
  - Pediatric (3–13 years)
    - Load: 10 mg/kg
    - Maintenance: 3–6 mg/kg PO/IV qd (start 24 hr after loading dose)
  - Must follow liver function and enzymes

flumazenil (Romazicon)
- Benzodiazepine antagonist
- Physiology: inhibits P_{450} enzymes.
- Dose
  - Adult
    - Reversal of conscious sedation or general anesthesia
      - Initial: 0.2 mg IV over 15 sec
      - May repeat at 1-min intervals to a max of 1 mg
      - Management of suspected benzodiazepine overdose
      - Initial: 0.2 mg IV over 30 sec
      - May repeat with 0.3–0.5 mg at 1-min intervals to a max of 3 mg
  - Pediatric
    - Initial: 0.1 mg
    - No response in 30–60 sec: repeat with 0.1–0.2 mg
    - May repeat dose to total of 1–3 mg in 1 hr
- Use with caution in patients on warfarin, cyclosporin, and phenytoin because these drugs will increase the level.
- Note: patients should have a secure airway and IV access.

folic acid
- Dose
  - Adult: 1–3 mg/dose PO/IM/IV/SQ divided qd-tid, then 0.5 mg/day
  - Pediatric
    - Infant: 15 µg/kg PO/IM/IV/SQ (max of 50 µg/day), then 30–45 µg/day
    - Child: 1 mg PO/IM/IV/SQ, then 0.1–0.4 mg/day

furosemide (Lasix)
- A diuretic that acts at the loop of Henle.
- Indication: fluid diuresis and hypertension
- Dose
  - Adult
    - Initial: 10–20 mg PO/IV (max of 600 mg daily) [Note: patients who have not had furosemide will need a smaller dose than patients who are on it chronically.]
    - Continuous infusion: start at 0.05 mg/kg/hr and titrate to effect. An initial bolus is helpful before continuous infusion.
  - Pediatric (infants and children)
    - PO: 2 mg/kg q 6–8 hr prn; may increase by 1–2 mg/kg/dose
    - IV/IM: 1 mg/kg q 6–12 hr prn; may increase by 1 mg/kg/dose
    - Maximum dose: 6 mg/kg/dose PO/IV/IM
- IV peak diuretic effect is 30 min with a 2-hr duration of effect.

gentamicin
- Spectrum: Enterobacteriaceae, *Pseudomonas* sp, *Klebsiella, E. coli, Proteus* sp.
- Dose (Note: adjust doses per peak and trough levels.)
  - Adult
    - Load: 1.5–2.0 mg/kg
    - Maintenance: 1.7 mg/kg q 8 hr for CrCl > 70
      1.7 mg/kg q 12 hr for CrCl 50–70
      1.7 mg/kg q 24 hr for CrCl 30–49
      1.4 mg/kg q 24 hr for CrCl 20–29
      1.4 mg/kg q 48 hr for CrCl 10–19
      1.4 mg/kg P hemodialysis session
    - Single daily dose: 5.1 mg/kg. Monitor random level 18 hr after dose; level should be < 1.0.
  - Pediatric (children): 7.5 mg/kg/day divided q 8 hr
  - Renal failure: dosed q 24–48 hr based on random levels. Approximately 30% eliminated by hemodialysis.

glucagon
- Physiology: exerts effects by stimulating adenylcyclase to produce increased cAMP, thereby promoting hepatic glycogenolysis and gluconeogenesis.
- Indications: management of hypoglycemia and severe β-adrenergic blocking agent overdose
- Dose
  - Hypoglycemia
    - Adults: 0.5–1.0 mg IV/PO/SQ; repeat in 20 min prn
    - Neonates: 0.3 mg/kg/dose to a max of 1 mg/dose
    - Children: 0.025–0.1000 mg/kg/day; repeat in 20 min prn (not to exceed 1 mg/dose)

- β-Blocker overdose
  - Bolus: 3–10 mg IV; repeat in 10 min if necessary
  - May follow bolus with an infusion of 1–5 mg/hr or 0.02 mg/kg/hr.
- Use with caution in patients with insulinoma or pheochromocytoma.

haloperidol (Haldol)
- Antipsychotic and sedative
- Dose (adjust in liver disease)
  - Adult
    - Regimen for levels of agitation
      - Mild: 0.5–2.0 mg IV
      - Moderate: 2–5 mg IV
      - Severe: 5–10 mg IV (may dose up to 80 mg/24 hr)
      - PO: twice the IV dose
      - Allow 20–30 min between doses and use reduced doses in elderly patients.
      - Once patient is controlled, add total dose in 24 hr and divide q 6–8 hr.
    - Sundowning: ≥ 0.5 mg PO/IM q 4–6 hr prn
    - Continuous drip for control: 10 mg/hr IV, then increase by 1 mg q 20 min until control is achieved
  - Pediatric (3–12 years)
    - Agitation: 0.01–0.03 mg/kg PO qd
    - Psychosis: 0.05–0.15 mg/kg/day PO divided bid/tid
    - Tourette's syndrome: 0.050–0.075 mg/kg/day PO divided bid/tid; may increase dose by 0.5 mg/day

heparin
- The goal is to achieve therapeutic levels quickly and safely (Tables E-1 and E-2).

hydrocortisone (Solu-Cortef)
- A corticosteroid with increased mineralocorticoid effects.
- Adult dose (see p 163)
- Pediatric dose
  - Status asthmaticus: 4–8 mg/kg (max of 250 mg) loading dose, then 8 mg/kg/day IV divided q 6 hr
  - Anti-inflammatory: 0.8–4.0 mg/kg/day divided q 6 hr

Table E-1. Heparin Therapy: Empiric Dosing Schedule*

PTT	Bolus (IU)	Hold (min)	Rate Change (IU/hr)
<50	5000	0	↑ by 120
50–59	0	0	↑ by 120
60–85	0	0	No change
86–95	0	0	↓ by 80
96–120	0	30	↓ by 80
>120	0	60	↓ by 160

* Give 5000 IU IV bolus, 1280 IU/hr infusion, check PTT q 6 hr until stable, and adjust according to the values in this table.

Table E-2. Heparin Therapy: Weight-Based Regimen*

PTT	× Control	Bolus (IU/kg)	Hold (min)	Rate change (IU/kg/hr)
<35	<1.2	80	0	↑ by 4
35–45	>1.2–1.5	40	0	↑ by 2
46–70	>1.5–2.3	0	0	No change
71–90	>2.3–3.0	0	0	↓ by 2
>90	>3.0	0	60	↓ by 3

* Give 80 IU/kg IV bolus, 18 IU/kg/hr IV infusion, check PTT q 6 hr until stable, and adjust according to the values in this table.

- Physiologic replacement:
  - 12.5 mg/M^2 PO qd 3
  - 7.5 mg/M^2 PO q 3 d
  - 25 mg/M^2/day divided tid
  - Stress dose: 25–50 mg/M^2/day as continuous IV infusion

hydromorphone (Dilaudid)
- Narcotic, analgesic
- Dose
  - Adult: 1–4 mg/dose PO/IV/SQ/IM q 4–6 hr
  - Pediatric
    - IV: 0.015 mg/kg/dose q 4–6 hr
    - PO: 0.03–0.08 mg/kg/dose q 4–6 hr

hydroxyzine (Atarax, Vistaril)
- Antihistamine, anxiolytic
- Dose
  - Adult: 25–100 mg/dose IM q 4–6 hr or PO tid-qid
  - Pediatric: 0.5–1.0 mg/kg IM q 4–6 hr or 0.5 mg/kg PO q 6 hr

imipenem-cilastatin (Primaxin)
- Antibiotic spectrum: gram-positive cocci, gram-negative cocci and bacilli, anaerobes
- Dose
  - Adult: 250–1000 mg IV q 6–8 hr (max 4 g/day or 50 mg/kg/day)
  - Pediatric: 50–100 mg/kg/day IV divided q 6–8 hr (max 4 g/day)
  - Renal failure: 125–250 mg IV q 12 hr. (Note: use with caution in renal failure due to increased likelihood of seizures.)

insulin
- Preparations (Table E-3)
- Route of administration: SQ route is used on the wards while IV can be used in the ICU.
- Dose
  - Adult
    - Insulin-dependent diabetics: total requirements are roughly 1 unit/kg/day. This is usually divided by regular and NPH mixtures. Dosages should vary according to "fingerstick blood glucose."
    - Continuous drip: 1 mg/hr IV and titrate as needed

Table E-3. Insulin Preparations

Mixture*	Onset (hr)	Peak (hr)	Duration (hr)
Humulin R (regular)	0.5–1.0	2–4	5–7
Semilente	1–3	2–8	12–16
Humulin N (NPH)	3–4	6–12	24–48
Humulin L (lente)	1–3	8–12	24–48
Humulin U (ultralente)	4–6	18–24	36
Humalog (insulin lispro)	<0.25	0.5–1.5	5–7

NPH = neutral protamine Hagedorn.
*A 70/30 mixture is 70% NPH insulin and 30% regular insulin.

- Intermittent dosing: SQ route with dose varying with patient insulin tolerance. Interval varies with type of insulin preparation.
- Pediatric (regular insulin)
  - Ketoacidosis: 0.1 U/kg IV bolus, then 0.1 U/kg/hr as continuous IV infusion
  - Usual diabetic maintenance (NPH insulin)
    - Children: 0.5–1.0 U/kg/day
    - Adolescents: 0.8–1.2 U/kg/day (give 2/3 before breakfast and 1/3 before dinner)
- Sliding scale insulin (Table E-4)
  - Order according to fingerstick values q 4–12 hr depending on clinical situation.
  - Use regular insulin for replacement IV or SQ depending on clinical situation.

isoproterenol (Isuprel)
- A β-adrenergic agonist with chronotropic and inotropic properties.
- Indications
  - Inotropic support when myocardial oxygen is normal
  - Bradycardia and shock (increasing HR increases cardiac output)
  - Shock with severe aortic insufficiency
  - Heart block (temporarily accelerates HR)
- Contraindication: myocardial ischemia
- Dose
  - Adult
    - Mixture: 1 mg in 250 ml (15 gtts = 1 µg)
    - 0.5–20 µg/min IV to a max of 30 µg/min (2–5 µg/kg/min)
  - Pediatric
    - Initial: 0.1–2.0 µg/kg/min
    - Maintenance: increase dose by 0.1 µg/kg/min q 5–10 min to a max of 2 µg/kg/min and desired effect
- Complication: causes muscle bed vasodilation, which can unmask relative hypovolemia and result in hypotension. Be prepared for volume replacement.

Table E-4. Adult Sliding Scale for Regular Insulin

Glucose Level (mg/dl)	Units of Insulin		
	Conservative	Moderate	Aggressive
<200	0	1	1
200–250	2	3	4
251–300	4	5	6
301–350	6	7	10
351–400	9	11	13
>400	11 and call M.D.	13 and call M.D.	15 and call M.D.

isosorbide dinitrate (Isordil)
- An oral nitrate that is a vasodilator of veins and coronary vessels.
- Dose
  - Short-acting: 10–40 mg PO qid
  - Long-acting: 40–80 mg PO bid-tid

ketorolac (Toradol)
- Nonopioid analgesic, nonsteroidal anti-inflammatory
- Dose (Note: use should be limited to 5 days.)
  - Adult
    - Maintenance: 30 mg IM q 6 hr for patients < 65 years and 15 mg IM q 6 hr for patients ≥ 65 years
    - PO: 10 mg q 6 hr
  - Pediatric: 0.5 mg/kg IV/IM q 6 hr (max of 120 mg/day or 30 mg q 6 hr)

labetalol (Normodyne, Trandate)
- A nonselective β-blocker that also selectively blocks α_1 receptors.
- Indication: treatment of hypertension (does not increase HR)
- Contraindications: CHF, reactive airway disease, severe bradycardia, and second- to third-degree heart block
- Dose
  - Adult
    - Continuous infusion: start at 2 mg/min
    - Intermittent: 20 mg IV over 2 min and additional doses of 40–80 mg given at 10-min intervals (max of 300 mg)
    - PO: 100 mg bid; may be increased q 2–3 days in increments of 100 mg bid
    - Discontinue: must taper dose
  - Pediatric
    - Initial: 0.2–1.0 mg/kg bolus, then 0.4–1.0 mg/kg/hr IV infusion to a max of 3 mg/kg/hr
    - Intermittent: 0.3–1.0 mg/kg q 10 min to a max of 20 mg/dose

lactulose
- Laxative
- Indication: severe constipation or hepatic encephalopathy
- Dose
  - Adult
    - Constipation: 15–30 ml PO qd-bid

- Hepatic encephalopathy
  - Acute episode: 30–45 ml PO q 1–2 hr until 2–3 soft stools per day
  - Maintenance: 15–60 ml PO/PR bid-qid
  - Rectal: 300 ml diluted in 700 ml water in 30–60 min retention enema
- Pediatric
  - Constipation: 7.5 ml PO qd
  - Hepatic encephalopathy
    - Infant: 2.5–10.0 ml/day PO divided tid-qid
    - Children: 40–90 ml/day PO divided tid-qid

lepirudin (Refludan)
- Recombinant hirudin derived from yeast
- Indicated as anticoagulant in patients with heparin-induced thrombocytopenia (HIT) and thromboembolic disease to prevent further thromboembolic complications
- Mechanism of action: Binds thrombin and neutralizes its effects, and irreversibly halts its effects in clotting. It essentially affects all thrombin dependent coagulation assays.
- Pharmacokinetics: Half-life of 1.2 hr (72 min)
- Dose
  - Adult: Bolus 0.4 mg/kg IV, then initiate continuous infusions at 0.15 mg/kg/hr
  - Dose adjustments are made by checking aPTT every 4 hr. The target aPTT is 1.5–2.5 times normal. If aPTT is too low, increase infusion rate by 20%. If aPTT is too high, hold infusion for 2 hr and restart infusion at 50% of original rate.
  - Pediatrics: Safety and efficacy not established.
- Adverse Reactions: Bleeding. There is no known antidote. Blood transfusions may be necessary for acute life-threatening bleeding episodes.

levothyroxine (Synthroid)
- Thyroxine replacement
- Indication: hypothyroid or myxedema coma
- Dose
  - Adult
    - PO: 12.5–50.0 μg qd with increases of 25–50 μg q 2–4 weeks until euthyroid or symptoms resolve
    - IM/IV: 50% of PO dose qd
    - Usual dose: 100–200 μg qd
    - Myxedema coma or hypothyroid with angina: 200–500 μg PO × 1 dose, then 100–300 μg next day if needed
  - Pediatric
    - 0–6 months: 8–10 μg/kg/day qd
    - 6–12 months: 6–8 μg/kg/day qd
    - 1–5 years: 5–6 μg/kg/day qd
    - 6–12 years: 4–5 μg/kg/day qd
    - > 12 years: 2–3 μg/kg/day qd
    - IM/IV: 50%–75% of PO dose

lidocaine (Xylocaine)
- Type Ib antiarrhythmic

- Physiology
  - Decreases automaticity and conduction in ischemic and infarcted tissue.
  - Increases fibrillation threshold.
- Indication: treatment of ventricular arrhythmias and prophylaxis in anterior wall myocardial infarctions
- Dose
  - Adult
    - Acute therapy
      - Bolus: 1 mg/kg IV bolus, then additional boluses of 0.5 mg/kg q 5–8 min to total of 3 mg/kg
      - Infusion: begin at 1–4 mg/kg/min
    - Prophylaxis
      - Load: 1 mg/kg
      - Infusion: begin at 1–4 mg/kg/min
    - Anesthetic: max of 7 mg/kg/dose (with epinephrine) or 4.5 mg/kg/dose (without epinephrine) q 2 hr (max total dose of 500 mg)
  - Pediatric
    - Antiarrhythmic
      - Bolus: 1 mg/kg slow IV bolus, may repeat q 5–10 min prn to a max of 3.0–4.5 mg/kg/hr
      - Infusion: 20–50 µg/kg/min IV
    - Anesthetic: same as adult
  - Endotracheal tube: 2.5 × IV dose
  - Reduce dosage in the following cases:
    - Liver disease (to max of 2 mg/min)
    - Age > 70 years
    - After 3–4 days of treatment due to decreased clearance

lorazepam (Ativan)
- A short-acting benzodiazepine with sedative and amnestic properties.
- Indication: sedation and prevention of alcohol withdrawal
- Dose (must individualize dosing interval)
  - Adult
    - Status epilepticus: 4 mg/dose; may repeat in 5–15 min
    - Premedication: 0.05 mg/kg IM 2 hr before procedure (max 4 mg/dose)
    - Sedation: 2–4 mg/kg q 2–12 hr
  - Pediatric
    - Status epilepticus: 0.05–0.10 mg/kg IV (max of 4 mg/dose); may repeat 0.05 mg/kg in 15–20 min × 1 dose
    - Premedication: same as adult
    - Anxiolytic/sedation: 0.05 mg/kg PO/IV q 4–8 hr
- Note: has a 16-hour half-life and the onset is within 15–20 minutes.

mannitol
- An osmotic agent that increases effective intravascular volume and diuresis.
- May be used to reduce reperfusion injury and to prevent dye-induced ATN.
- Dose

- Adult: 25–75 g or 1–2 g/kg of 20% solution IV over 30–60 min; may repeat q 6 hr prn
- Pediatric
  - Anuria/oliguria: 0.2 g/kg IV over 3–5 min; discontinue if no diuresis within 2 hr
  - Cerebral edema: 0.25 g/kg IV push, repeated q 5 min prn; may increase to 1 g/kg/dose
  - Neurosurgery preoperative: 1.5–2.0 g/kg IV over 0.5–1 hr
- Complications: watch for signs of CHF, pulmonary edema, or circulatory collapse.

meperidine (Demerol)
- Opioid analgesic
- Indication: pain management (better agent for biliary pain)
- Dose
  - Adult
    - IV: 50–100 mg q 3–6 hr prn pain
    - PO: 100–250 mg q 3–6 hr prn pain
  - Pediatric: 1.0–1.5 mg/kg/dose q 3–4 hr prn pain
- Avoid in elderly patients and patients with renal failure.

methylprednisolone (Solu-Medrol)
- Dose
  - Adult (see p 162)
  - Pediatric
    - Status asthmaticus: 1–2 mg/kg IV loading dose, then 2 mg/kg/day IV divided q 6 hr
    - Anti-inflammatory: 0.16–0.80 mg/kg/day IV divided q 6–12 hr

metoclopramide (Reglan)
- GI stimulant and antiemetic
- Indication: decreased gastric emptying or small bowel transit
- Dose
  - Gastroparesis (severe): 10 mg IV over 1–2 min bid-qid
  - Gastroparesis (mild): 10 mg PO 30 min before meals and hs
  - Gastroesophageal reflux: 10–15 mg PO 30 min before meals and hs

metolazone (Zaroxolyn)
- A diuretic that affects electrolyte absorption in the proximal and distal renal tubules. It often works synergistically with furosemide.
- Dose
  - Adult
    - Edema: 5–20 mg PO qd
    - Hypertension: 2.5–5.0 mg PO qd
  - Pediatric (children): 0.2–0.4 mg/kg/day PO divided qd-bid

metoprolol (Lopressor)
- β_1-selective β-blocker
- Indication: treatment of angina, hypertension, and atrial fibrillation
- Dose
  - Acute: 5 mg IV q 5 min to total of 15 mg
  - Maintenance: 50–100 mg PO bid or 5–10 mg IV q 6 hr

metronidazole (Flagyl)
- Spectrum: anaerobes (including *Clostridium difficile*)

- Dose
  - Adult: 500 mg IV/PO q 6–8 hr; 250–500 mg PO q 6 hr
  - Pediatric: 35–50 mg/kg/day PO divided q 8 hr; 30 mg/kg/day IV q 6–12 hr
  - Renal failure: 50% of dose
  - *Clostridium difficile:* oral dosing preferred

mezlocillin

- Spectrum: *Staphylococcus* sp, *Streptococcus* sp, *Neisseria* sp, *Enterobacter* sp, *Klebsiella* sp, *Escherichia coli, Morganella* sp, *Proteus* sp, *Serratia* sp, *Acinetobacter* sp, *Enterococcus* sp, *Pseudomonas* sp
- Dose
  - Adult: 1.5–4.0 g IV q 4–6 hr (max of 24 g/day)
  - Pediatric
    - Neonate IV/IM
      - < 1.2 kg: 150 mg/kg/day divided q 12 hr
      - ≥ 1.2 kg and ≤ 7 days: 150 mg/kg/day divided q 12 hr
      - ≥ 1.2 kg and > 7 days: 225 mg/kg/day divided q 8 hr
  - Renal failure: change dosing to q 8–12 hr

midazolam (Versed)

- A short-acting benzodiazepine used as a short-term sedative for procedures, anesthesia, or when there is a need to obtain frequent neurologic examinations.
- Dose
  - Adult: 0.5–2.0 mg/dose IV over 2 min; repeat for clinical effect (higher doses may be needed)
  - Pediatric
    - Preoperative sedation: 0.08 mg/kg IM or 0.3 mg/kg PR
    - Sedation for procedures
      - 0.05–0.10 g/kg IV over 2 min; repeat prn (max of 0.2 mg/kg)
      - 0.05–0.07 mg/kg of IV form given PO
    - Intermittent mechanical ventilation
      - Intermittent dose (infant/children): 0.05–0.15 mg/kg q 1–2 hr prn
- Complications: respiratory depression and apnea
- Titrate slowly and have oxygen and resuscitative equipment nearby.
- Drug effect may be reversed by flumazenil.

morphine

- Opioid analgesic
- Dose (This dosing schedule is a guide; each patient is different.)
  - Adult
    - PO: 10–30 mg q 4 hr prn (immediate release) or 15–30 mg q 8–12 hr (controlled release)
    - IM/IV/SQ: 2–15 mg q 2–6 hr prn
    - Infusion: 0.8–10.0 mg/hr
  - Pediatric (infants and children)
    - PO: 0.2–0.5 mg/kg q 4–6 hr prn (immediate release) or 0.3–0.6 mg/kg q 12 hr (controlled release)
    - IM/IV/SQ: 0.1–0.2 mg/kg q 2–6 hr prn
    - Infusion: 0.025 mg/kg/hr; increase based on patient response

naloxone (Narcan)
- A narcotic antagonist that reverses opioid effects including respiratory depression, sedation, and hypotension.
- Dose (Must continuously reevaluate the patient's clinical condition and redose when necessary.)
  - Adult: 0.4–2.0 mg q 2–3 min × 1–3 (max of 2 mg/dose)
  - Pediatric
    - < 20 kg: 0.1 mg/kg IM/IV/SQ/endotracheal tube; repeat q 2–3 min prn
    - ≥ 20 kg or > 5 years: 2 mg/dose; may repeat q 2–3 min prn
- Duration of action is 1–3 hours, but many narcotics have longer duration.

nifedipine (Procardia)
- Calcium channel blocker
- Indication: treatment of angina and hypertension
- Dose
  - Adult: 10 mg PO for urgent treatment of hypertension (PO gives a more even absorption and effect)
  - Pediatric
    - Hypertension: 0.25–0.50 mg/kg PO/SL q 6–8 hr prn
    - Hypertrophic cardiomyopathy: 0.6–0.9 mg/kg/day PO/SL divided q 6–8 hr (max of 180 mg/day)

nitroglycerin (IV)
- Physiology
  - Relaxes vascular smooth muscle (venous > arterial) and dilates coronary arteries.
  - Decreases preload > afterload, myocardial oxygen demand, ventricular filling pressures, and pulmonary vascular resistance.
  - Increases cardiac output and coronary blood flow.
- Indication: myocardial ischemia/infarct and pulmonary hypertension
- Dose
  - Adult
    - Mix 50 mg in 250 ml D_5W (200 μg/ml)
    - Bolus: 50 μg
    - Initial: 5–20 μg/min; may increase in increments of 5–20 μg/min
    - Maximum dose: approximately 400 μg/min
  - Pediatric: 0.25–0.50 μg/kg/min IV infusion; may increase by 1 μg/kg q 3–5 min to effect (max of 5 μg/kg/min)
- Note: tolerance can develop.

nitroglycerin (paste; Nitropaste)
- Indication: treatment of angina and hypertension
- Dose: apply 1–2 inches topically to the chest wall q 4–6 hr
- A sliding scale can be written based on the number of inches (0.5–2.0 inches topical) for different BP levels.

nitroglycerin (SL tablets; Nitrostat)
- Indication: treatment of acute onset of angina
- Preparations: 1/100, 1/150, 1/400
  - For most patients, prescribe 1/150 grain.
  - If patient is very sensitive to the drug, prescribe 1/400.

- Dose
  - Angina: 1 tablet SL q 5 min; up to 3 tablets if necessary

nitroprusside (Nipride)
- Relaxes vascular smooth muscle (arterial > venous), leading to vasodilation and pulmonary artery vasodilation.
- Indication:
  - Treatment of severe hypertension (i.e., extremely elevated SVR)
  - Afterload reducing agent in acute myocardial infarction, hypertensive emergencies, or acute left ventricular failure without hypotension
- Dose
  - Adult
    - Mixture: 50 mg in 250 ml D_5W (200 μg/ml)
    - Initial dose: 0.3–0.5 μg/kg/min; max of 2–3 μg/kg/min for 72 hours (titrate to specific SBP)
  - Pediatric dose: same as adult
- Complications
  - Nitroprusside is decomposed to cyanide, which is converted in the liver and kidneys to thiocyanate; therefore, it is necessary to monitor thiocyanate levels, especially in patients with liver or renal disease.
  - Thiocyanate levels > 20 mg/dl are toxic while levels < 10 mg/dl are tolerated.

norepinephrine (Levophed)
- Physiology
  - Strong α-adrenergic stimulator
  - Increases SVR, BP, and peripheral vascular resistance in all vascular beds, including the renal arteries
  - Decreases cardiac output and perfusion of skin, viscera, kidney, skeletal muscle, and brain
- Indication: treatment of shock and sepsis
- Dose
  - Adult
    - Mixture: 4 mg in 250 ml (15 gtts = 4 μg or 16 μg/ml)
    - Shock: initial infusion of 8–12 μg/min
    - Milder forms of hypotension: 2–4 μg/min; required maintenance dose of 2–4 μg/min
  - Pediatric: 0.05–0.10 μg/kg/min; titrate to effect or max of 2 μg/kg/min
- May use with dopamine to restore flow to kidneys.
- Note: Administer through a large vein. If it extravasates, give phentolamine.

nystatin
- Antifungal agent; oral solution used for thrush
- Dose
  - Adult: 5–15 ml (500,000–1,500,000 U) swish and swallow qid
  - Pediatric
    - Preterm infant: 0.5 ml (50,000 U) to each side of mouth qid

- Term infant: 1 ml (100,000 U) to each side of mouth qid

omeprazole (Prilosec)
- Gastric proton pump inhibitor
- Indication: peptic ulcer disease, gastroesophageal reflux, gastric hypersecretory states
- Dose
  - Adult
    - Acute duodenal ulcer, severe esophagitis, or severe gastroesophageal reflux: 20 mg PO qd × 4–8 weeks
    - Pathologic hypersecretory conditions
      - Initial: 60 mg PO qd
      - Increase as needed to shut down gastric acid secretion.
      - Doses > 80 mg should be divided.
  - Pediatric: 0.7–3.3 mg/kg PO qd

ondansetron (Zofran)
- Antiemetic
- Indication: severe nausea and vomiting, especially associated with chemotherapy or anesthesia
- Dose
  - Adult: 0.15 mg/kg IV by slow infusion; may repeat q 4–6 hr
  - Pediatric
    - < 4 years: 2 mg PO q 4 hr prn
    - 4–11 years: 4 mg PO q 4 hr prn or 0.15 mg/kg/dose IV q 4 hr
    - > 12 years: 8 mg PO q 4 hr prn or 0.15 mg/kg/dose IV q 4 hr

oxacillin (Bactocill)
- Spectrum: *Staphylococcus* sp, *Streptococcus* sp
- Dose
  - Adult: 1–2 g IV q 4 hr or 500–1000 mg PO q 4–6 hr
  - Pediatric: 100–200 mg/kg/day IV divided q 6 hr
  - Renal failure: no change

pancuronium (Pavulon)
- A neuromuscular blocking agent that relaxes skeletal muscle.
- Dose
  - Adult
    - Mixture: 20 mg in 100 ml normal saline
    - Initial: 0.04–0.10 mg/kg IV push
    - Maintenance: 0.01–0.02 mg/kg IV push given q 20–60 min prn
  - Pediatric
    - Neonate
      - Initial: 0.02 mg/kg IV; may repeat q 5–10 min × 2 doses prn
      - Then 0.03–0.09 mg/kg IV q 0.5–4 hr prn
    - > 1 month
      - Initial: 0.04–0.10 mg/kg IV
      - Then 0.02–0.10 mg/kg IV q 0.5–1 hr prn
    - Defasciculating dose: 0.005–0.010 mg/kg IV
- Contraindications: renal failure, tachycardia
- When using a paralyzing agent, it is necessary to keep a twitch

monitor on the patient and titrate dosing to maintain 1–2 twitches.

penicillin
- Spectrum: *Streptococcus* sp, Spirochetes, gram-positive anaerobes (except *Clostridium difficile*)
- Dose
  - Adult: 0.5–4.0 million units IV/IM q 4 hr
  - Pediatric: 25,000–250,000 units/kg/day IV/IM divided q 4–8 hr
  - Renal failure: 20%–50% of normal dose

pentobarbital (Nembutal)
- Barbiturate
- Indication: induce coma to minimize uncontrollable seizures
- Dose
  - Load: 10–15 mg/kg over 1–2 hr
  - Maintenance: begin at 1 mg/kg/hr; increase as needed to 3 mg/kg/hr
- Use an electroencephalogram to estimate effect on seizure activity.

Percocet
- Opioid analgesic
- Dose
  - 1 tablet = 5 mg oxycodone and 325 mg acetaminophen
  - Adult and pediatric: 1–2 tablets PO q 3–6 hr prn pain

Percodan
- Opioid analgesic
- Dose
  - 1 tablet = 5 mg oxycodone and 325 mg aspirin
  - Adult and pediatric: 1–2 tablets PO q 4–6 hr prn pain

phentolamine (Regitine)
- Potent antagonist of α receptor
- Physiology
  - Decreases BP, SVR, and myocardial oxygen demand
  - Increases cardiac output and renal blood flow
- Indication: treatment of pheochromocytoma or α-adrenergic (Levophed) skin infiltration
- Dose
  - Adult
    - Infusion: 0.3–2.0 mg/min IV infusion
    - Diagnosis of pheochromocytoma
      - Inject 5 mg into supine, resting patient.
      - If SBP > 35 mm Hg and DBP > 24 mm Hg, it is a positive test for pheochromocytoma.
  - Pediatric
    - Treatment of extravasation
      - Neonate: solution of 0.25–0.50 mg/ml with normal saline; inject SQ 0.2 ml × 5 around site
      - Infant/child: solution of 0.5–1.0 mg/ml with normal saline; inject SQ 0.2–1.0 ml × 5 around site
    - Diagnosis of pheochromocytoma
      - Inject 0.1 mg/kg (max 5 mg) into supine, resting patient.
      - If SBP > 35 mm Hg and DBP > 24 mm Hg, it is a positive test.

phenylephrine (Neo-Synephrine)
- Stimulates α receptors; powerful peripheral vasoconstriction
- Physiology
  - Increases SVR and BP
  - Decreases renal perfusion
- Dose
  - Adult
    - Mixture: 30 mg in 250 ml (15 gtts = 30 μg)
    - 10–50 μg/min (1–4 g/kg) IV (max of 180 μg/min)
    - 2–5 mg IM/SQ q 1–2 hr prn
    - 0.1–0.5 mg IV q 10–15 min prn
    - 1–4 μg/kg/min continuous IV infusion; titrate to effect
  - Pediatric
    - 0.1 mg/kg IM/SQ q 1–2 hr prn (max of 5 mg)
    - 5–20 μg/kg IV q 10–15 min prn
    - 0.1–0.5 μg/kg/min continuous IV infusion; titrate to effect
- Contraindications: severe vasoconstriction, hypovolemia, ventricular tachycardia, severe hypertension, pheochromocytoma
- Complications: may cause tremor, insomnia, or palpitations. Use with caution with hypertension, arrhythmias, hyperthyroidism, and hyperglycemia.

phenytoin (Dilantin)
- An anticonvulsant used for seizure treatment and prophylaxis, including post head injury.
- Dose
  - Adult
    - IV load: 15–20 mg/kg at max rate of 50 mg/min
    - Maintenance: 100 mg PO/IV tid-qid
    - PO and IV doses are the same.
  - Pediatric
    - Status epilepticus: 15–20 mg/kg IV (max 1 g/day)
    - Antiseizure maintenance: 5–10 mg/kg/day IV/PO divided qd-tid
      - Neonate: 5–8 mg/kg/day
      - 6 months–3 years: 8–10 mg/kg/day
      - 4–6 years: 7.5–9.0 mg/kg/day
      - 7–9 years: 7–8 mg/kg/day
      - Bolus to adjust up serum level = 0.7 mg/kg × (target level − measured level)
      - 10–16 years: 6–7 mg/kg/day
- Therapeutic level: 10–20 μg/ml: level adjustment based on albumin
  - *Adjusted level = measured level ÷ [(02 × albumin) + 0.2]*
  - For renal failure:
  - *Adjusted level = measured level ÷ [(0.2 × albumin) + 0.1]*
- Drug interactions: steroids, warfarin, quinidine, digoxin

piperacillin/tazobactam (Zosyn)
- Spectrum: *Staphylococcus* sp, *Streptococcus* sp, gram-negative cocci, *Pseudomonas* sp, Enterobacteriaceae, and anaerobes
- Dose
  - Adult: 3.375 g IV q 6 hr

- Pediatric
  - < 6 months: 150–300 mg/kg/day IV divided q 6–8 hr
  - > 6 months: 300–400 mg/kg/day IV divided q 6 hr
- Renal failure: 2.25 g IV q 8 hr

prednisone
- Dose
  - Adult: (see p 163)
  - Pediatric dose
    - Anti-inflammatory: 0.5–2.0 mg/kg/day PO or 25–60 mg/M^2/day PO divided q 6–12 hr
    - Physiologic replacement: 4–5 mg/M^2/day PO divided bid

procainamide (Pronestyl)
- Type Ia antiarrhythmic agent
- Indication: treatment of ventricular and supraventricular arrhythmias
- Dose
  - Adult
    - Load: 100 mg q 3–5 min to max of 1.5 g or IV infusion at max rate of 20 mg/min
    - Maintenance: 2–4 mg/min (Watch for increased QRS complex duration and hypotension.)
  - Pediatric
    - Continuous IV infusion: 2–6 mg/kg IV over 5 min loading dose, then 20–80 μg/kg/min (max of 100 mg/dose or 2 g/day)
    - IM: 20–30 mg/kg/day divided q 4–6 hr (max of 4 g/day)
    - PO: 15–50 mg/kg/day divided q 3–6 hr (max of 4 g/day)
- Active metabolite: N-acetyl procainamide
- Monitoring: follow QRS complex and correcte°–d QT intervals as well as procainamide and N-acetyl procainamide levels to avoid cardiotoxicity.

prochlorperazine (Compazine)
- Antiemetic
- Dose
  - Adult
    - PO: 5–10 mg tid-qid
    - PR: 25 mg bid
    - IM: 5–10 mg q 4–6 hr
    - IV: 5–10 mg q 3–4 hr
  - Pediatric (> 10 kg or > 2 years)
    - PO/PR: 0.4 mg/kg/day divided tid-qid
    - IM: 0.10–0.15 mg/kg tid-qid

propofol (Diprivan)
- An IV sedative-hypnotic with immediate onset. Awakening may occur within 8 minutes if drug is discontinued.
- Dose: 2.0–2.5 mg/kg; titrate 40 mg q 10 sec IV push or 0.1–0.2 mg/kg/min constant IV infusion
- Contraindication: egg allergy
- Complications: apnea and hypotension (Patient should be normovolemic before dosing.)

propranolol (Inderal)
- Indication: class II antiarrhythmic that has β-adrenergic blocking characteristics.
- Dose
  - Adult
    - Arrhythmia: 1 mg IV q 5 min to a max of 5 mg; or 10–30 mg PO tid-qid, increasing prn to daily range of 40–320 mg
    - Hypertension: 40 mg PO bid; increase by 10–20 mg/dose q 3–5 days to a daily max of 640 mg
    - Thyrotoxicosis: 1–3 mg IV over 10 min (may repeat in 4–6 hr); or 10–40 mg PO q 6 hr
  - Pediatric
    - Arrhythmia: 0.01–0.10 mg/kg/dose IV over 10 min; repeat in 6–8 hr
    - Hypertension: 0.5–1.0 mg/kg/day divided q 6–12 hr; may increase to a max of 8 mg/kg/day
    - Thyrotoxicosis
      - Neonates: 2 mg/kg/day divided q 6–12 hr
      - Children: 1–3 mg IV over 10 min (may repeat in 4–6 hr); or 10–40 mg PO q 6 hr

protamine
- Heparin antidote
- Dose
  - General guideline: 1 mg neutralizes 115 U porcine intestinal heparin or 90 U beef lung heparin.
  - Time of heparin and antidote administration
    - If protamine is given immediately, give 100%–150% of dose.
    - If protamine is given within 0.5–1.0 hr, give 50% of dose.
    - If protamine is given at ≥ 2 hours, give 25% of dose.
    - The maximum dose is 50 mg IV at 5 mg/min.

quinidine sulfate (Quinidex), quinidine gluconate (Quinaglute)
- Type Ia antiarrhythmic agent
- Dose
  - Adult
    - Quinidine sulfate: 200–400 mg q 6 hr
    - Quinidine gluconate: 324–648 mg q 8–12 hr
  - Pediatric
    - Test dose: 2 mg/kg PO (max of 200 mg)
    - Quinidine sulfate: 15–60 mg/kg/day PO divided q 6 hr
    - Quinidine gluconate (not recommended for children): 2–10 mg/kg IV q 3–6 hr prn
- ECG monitoring
  - Follow corrected QT intervals and QRS complex for toxicity.
  - Quinidine prolongs PT interval in patients on warfarin and increases digoxin levels.

ranitidine (Zantac)
- H_2-receptor antagonist
- Indication: ulcer prophylaxis
- Dose
  - Adult

- PO: 150 mg bid or 300 mg qd
- IV: 50 mg q 8 hr
- Pediatric
  - Neonates
    - PO: 2–4 mg/kg/day divided q 8–12 hr
    - IV: 2 mg/kg/day divided q 6–8 hr
  - Infants/children
    - PO: 4–5 mg/kg/day divided q 8–12 hr
    - IV: 2–4 mg/kg/day divided q 6–8 hr

spironolactone (Aldactone)
- A potassium-sparing diuretic that competitively inhibits aldosterone.
- Dose
  - Adult
    - Maintenance: 25–100 mg/day PO divided bid-qid to a max of 200 mg/day
    - Diagnosis of primary aldosteronism: 400 mg PO qd × 4 days or 3–4 weeks
  - Pediatric
    - Children: 1.0–3.3 mg/kg/day PO divided bid-qid
    - Diagnosis of primary aldosteronism: 125–375 mg/m^2/day PO in divided doses
- Complication: increased risk of digoxin toxicity

succinylcholine
- A short-acting, depolarizing neuromuscular blocker.
- Dose
  - Adult: 1 mg/kg IV
  - Pediatric: 1–2 mg/kg IV (3–4 mg/kg IM) initial dose, then 0.3–0.6 mg/kg IV q 5–10 min prn

sucralfate (Carafate)
- A glucose polymer that binds to ulcer base (i.e., antiulcer agent).
- Indications: ulcer prophylaxis and stress gastritis
- Dose
  - Adult
    - Acute therapy: 1 g PO qid on an empty stomach
    - Maintenance: 1 g PO bid
  - Pediatric: 40–80 mg/kg/day PO divided q 6 hr

thiamine
- Vitamin (B$_1$)
- Dose
  - Adult
    - Deficiency: 5–30 mg IM/IV tid × 2 weeks, followed by 5–30 mg/day divided qd-tid × 1 month
    - Wernicke's encephalopathy: 50 mg IV and 50 mg IM × 1 dose, then 50 mg IM qd until patient is on normal diet
  - Pediatric
    - Deficiency: 10–25 mg IM/IV qd or 10–50 mg PO qd × 2 weeks, followed by 5–10 mg qd × 1 month
    - Wernicke's encephalopathy: 50 mg IV and 50 mg IM × 1 dose, then 50 mg IM qd until patient is on normal diet

ticarcillin/clavulanate (Timentin)
- Spectrum: *Staphylococcus* sp, *Streptococcus* sp, gram-negative cocci, Enterobacteriaceae, anaerobes, *Pseudomonas* sp
- Dose
  - Adult: 3 g IV q 4–6 hr
  - Pediatric (infant/child): 200–300 mg/kg/day IV divided q 4–6 hr
  - Renal failure: 2 g IV q 12 hr

tobramycin
- Spectrum: some *Staphylococcus* sp, Enterobacteriaceae, *Pseudomonas* sp, *Xanthomonas* sp
- Dose
  - Adult
    - Loading: 1.5–2.0 mg/kg IV, then 1.2–1.7 mg/kg q 8 hr
    - Single daily dose: 5.1 mg/kg daily
  - Pediatric: 4–5 mg/kg/day divided q 8 hr
  - Renal failure: dose q 24–48 hr and based on random levels

trimethoprim/sulfamethoxazole (Bactrim, Septra)
- Spectrum: *Staphylococcus* sp, *Enterococcus* sp, Enterobacteriaceae, *Pneumocystis carinii, Shigella* sp
- Dose
  - Adult: 1 double-strength tablet PO bid; 8–10 mg/kg/day of trimethoprim IV divided q 6–12 hr
  - Pediatric: 8 mg/40 mg/kg/day PO divided q 12 hr

Tylenol with Codeine
- Analgesic
- Preparations
  - Tylenol #1: 7.5 mg codeine + 300 mg acetaminophen
  - Tylenol #2: 15 mg codeine + 300 mg acetaminophen
  - Tylenol #3: 30 mg codeine + 300 mg acetaminophen
  - Tylenol #4: 60 mg codeine + 300 mg acetaminophen
- Dose
  - Tylenol #1: 1–4 tablets PO q 4–6 hr prn pain
  - Tylenol #2: 1–3 tablets PO q 4–6 hr prn pain
  - Tylenol #3: 1–2 tablets PO q 4–6 hr prn pain
  - Tylenol #4: 1 tablet PO q 4–6 hr prn pain

vancomycin
- Spectrum: *Staphylococcus* sp, *Streptococcus* sp, *Enterococcus* sp, *Clostridium difficile*
- Dose
  - Adult: 15 mg/kg IV q 12 hr
  - Pediatric: 40–60 mg/kg/day IV divided q 6 hr
  - Renal failure: 1 g q 4–7 days based on level

vasopressin (Pitressin)
- Physiology
  - Low dose has antidiuretic effect.
  - High dose stimulates smooth muscle contractions and decreased blood flow to splanchnic and coronary vessels as well as the skin.
- Indication: treatment of bleeding esophageal varices and neurogenic diabetes insipidus

- Consider giving with nitrates to decrease peripheral and coronary vasoconstriction.
- Dose
  - Adult
    - GI hemorrhage
      - Initial: 0.2–0.4 units/min
      - Maintenance: 0.2–0.6 units/min
    - Diabetes insipidus
      - SQ/IM: 5–10 U divided q 6–12 hr
      - Continuous infusion: start at 0.5 mU/kg/hr; double dose q 30 min to a max of 10 mU/kg/hr
  - Pediatric
    - Aqueous: 2.5–10.0 U SQ/IM bid-qid
    - Tannate (not to be given IV or SQ): 1.25–2.50 U IM q 2–3 days
    - Diabetes insipidus
      - SQ/IM: 2.5–10.0 U
      - Continuous infusion: start at 0.5 mU/kg/hr; double dose q 30 min to a max of 10 mU/kg/hr
    - GI hemorrhage (aqueous)
      - Uncontrolled bleeding: 0.2–0.4 U/min continuous IV infusion; titrate to effect (max of 0.9 U/min)
      - Controlled bleeding: taper infusion by 0.1 unit q 6–12 hr

vecuronium (Norcuron)
- A nondepolarizing neuromuscular blocking agent that competes for cholinergic receptors at motor end plates.
- Dose
  - Adult
    - Bolus: 0.08–0.10 mg/kg IV
    - Maintenance: 0.010–0.015 mg/kg q 30–60 min depending on effect
  - Pediatric
    - Neonate: initial 0.1 mg/kg IV, then 0.03–0.15 mg/kg IV q 1 hr prn
    - 7 weeks–1 year: initial 0.08–0.10 mg/kg IV, then 0.05–0.10 mg/kg IV q 1 hr prn
    - > 1 year: initial 0.08–0.10 mg/kg IV, then 0.05–0.10 mg/kg IV q 1 hr prn; may administer continuous infusion at 0.1 mg/kg/hr IV
- Vecuronium is one third more potent than pancuronium.
- Drug interactions
  - Succinylcholine increases the effects of vecuronium and prolongs its actions.
  - Aminoglycosides may prolong duration of action.
  - Action is reversed by neostigmine, edrophonium, and pyridostigmine.

verapamil (Calan, Isoptin)
- Calcium channel blocker
- Indication: treatment of supraventricular arrhythmias, diastolic dysfunction, and angina
- Contraindications
  - CHF

- Hypotension
- Shock
- Secondary or tertiary AV block and right to left shunting
- Patients with ejection fraction < 30%
- Patients on β blockers
- Sick sinus syndrome
- Ventricular tachycardias
- Dose
  - Adult
    - IV
      - Bolus: 2.5–10.0 mg IV over 2–3 min; may repeat if indicated
      - Initial infusion: 0.375 mg/min × 30 min
      - Maintenance infusion: 0.125 mg/min
    - PO: 40–160 mg tid
  - Pediatric
    - 0–1 year: 0.1–0.2 mg/kg IV over 2–3 min; may repeat after 30 min × 1 dose
    - 1–15 years
      - IV: 0.1–0.3 mg/kg over 2–3 min; may repeat after 30 min × 1 dose (max of 5 mg)
      - PO: 4–10 mg/kg/day divided tid
- Cautions
  - Use with extreme caution in infants.
  - Verapamil can cause apnea, bradycardia, AV block, or hypotension.
  - Have calcium and isoproterenol on hand to treat hypotension and bradycardia.
  - Do not use within a few hours before or after administration of β blockers.
- Reversal
  - Calcium chloride: 5–10 ml of 10% solution
  - Calcium gluconate: 10–20 ml of 10% solution

Vicodin
- Analgesic
- Preparations
  - Vicodin: 5 mg hydrocodone + 500 mg acetaminophen
  - Vicodin ES: 7.5 mg hydrocodone + 750 mg acetaminophen
- Dose
  - Vicodin: 1–2 tablets PO q 4–6 hr prn pain
  - Vicodin ES: 1 tablet PO q 4–6 hr prn pain

Vitamin K (Phytonadione)
- Indication: replacement therapy for lack of production or permanent or temporary reversal of warfarin.
- Dose
  - Normalize prothrombin time without acute need for warfarin therapy: 10 mg SQ qd × 3 days
  - Temporarily normalize prothrombin time with thought of warfarin anticoagulation in near future: 1 mg SQ/IV

warfarin (Coumadin)
- An anticoagulant that inhibits production of vitamin K.
- Dose: variable among patients (i.e., dependent on a stable protime and international normalized ratio)

Drug Ledger

	Drug	Indication	Adult Dose	Pediatric Dose
1.				
2.				
3.				
4.				
5.				
6.				
7.				
8.				
9.				
10.				
11.				
12.				
13.				
14.				
15.				
16.				
17.				
18.				
19.				
20.				

21. _____

22. _____

23. _____

24. _____

25. _____

26. _____

27. _____

28. _____

29. _____

30. _____

31. _____

32. _____

33. _____

34. _____

35. _____

36. _____

37. _____

38. _____

39. _____

40. _____

41. _____

42. _____

43. _____

44. _____

45. _____

46. _____

47. _____

48. _____

49. _____

50. _____

51. _____

52. _____

53. _____

54. _____

55. _____

56. _____

57. _____

58. _____

59. _____

60. _____

61. _____

62. _____

63. _____

64. _____

65. _____

66. _____

67. _____

68. _____

69. _____

70. _____

Hospital Directory

	Hospital #1	Hospital #2
Admitting office		
Cafeteria		
Cardiac cath lab		
Departments		
• Anesthesiology		
• Cardiology		
• Dermatology		
• Gastroenterology		
• Genetics		
• Hematology		
• Infectious diseases		
• Nephrology		
• Nutrition		
• Obstetrics and gynecology		
• Occupational therapy		
• Oncology		
• Ophthalmology		
• Pain management		
• Pathology		

	Hospital #1	Hospital #2
• Cytology		
• Frozen section		
• Surgical pathology		
• Pediatrics		
• Perinatology		
• Personnel health		
• Physical therapy		
• Psychiatry		
• Pulmonary medicine		
• Radiation therapy		
• Rehabilitation		
• Respiratory therapy		
• Social work		
• Speech and swallowing service		
• Vascular laboratory		
Diagnostic imaging		
• CT scan		
• Emergency room		
• File room		
• Fluoroscopy suite		
• Interventional radiology		
• MRI		
• Nuclear medicine		
• Pediatric radiology		

	Hospital #1	Hospital #2
• Portable		
• Reading rooms		
• Ultrasonography		
Dialysis		
EEG laboratory		
Emergency department		
• Main desk		
• Radiology		
• Trauma room		
• Triage		
EMG laboratory		
Endoscopy suite		
Hospital information		
Intensive care units		
• Cardiac		
• Labor and delivery		
• Medical		
• Newborn		
• Neurologic		
• Pediatric		
• Respiratory		
• Surgical		
• Step-down unit		
Laboratories		

	Hospital #1	Hospital #2
• Blood bank		
• Chemistry		
• Hematology		
• Immunology		
• Microbiology		
• Virology		
Medical records		
Nursing office		
Operating room		
• Adult		
• Labor and delivery		
• Pediatric		
• Outpatient		
• Scheduling		
Outpatient clinics		
• Emergency department		
• General surgery		
• Medicine		
• Neurology		
• Obstetrics and gynecology		
• Orthopaedic		
• Plastic		
• Primary care		
• Trauma		

	Hospital #1	Hospital #2
• Vascular surgery		
Page operator		
Parking		
Pharmacy		
• Nutrition		
• Outpatient		
• Medical		
• Surgical		
• Pediatric		
Postanesthesia care units		
• Adult		
• Pediatric		
• Outpatient		
Preoperative testing unit		
Pulmonary function laboratory		
Resident education office		
Security		
Surgery service chiefs		
• Cardiac		
• Chairman		
• Emergency medicine		
• Gastrointestinal		
• General		
• Neurosurgery		

	Hospital #1	Hospital #2
• Oncology		
• Orthopaedics		
• Otolaryngology		
• Pediatric		
• Plastic		
• Residency director		
• Thoracic		
• Transplant		
• Trauma		
• Urology		
• Vascular		
Wards		
• Gynecology		
• Medical		
• Neurology		
• Nursery		
• Obstetrics		
• Pediatric		
• Rehabilitation		
• Surgical		

PHONE BOOK

Name	Office	Home	Beeper	E-Mail	Other
1.					
2.					
3.					
4.					
5.					
6.					
7.					
8.					
9.					
10.					

PHONE BOOK

Name	Office	Home	Beeper	E-Mail	Other
11.					
12.					
13.					
14.					
15.					
16.					
17.					
18.					
19.					
20.					

PHONE BOOK

Name	Office	Home	Beeper	E-Mail	Other
21.					
22.					
23.					
24.					
25.					
26.					
27.					
28.					
29.					
30.					

PHONE BOOK

Name	Office	Home	Beeper	E-Mail	Other
31.					
32.					
33.					
34.					
35.					
36.					
37.					
38.					
39.					
40.					

PHONE BOOK

Name	Office	Home	Beeper	E-Mail	Other
41.					
42.					
43.					
44.					
45.					
46.					
47.					
48.					
49.					
50.					

PHONE BOOK

Name	Office	Home	Beeper	E-Mail	Other
51.					
52.					
53.					
54.					
55.					
56.					
57.					
58.					
59.					
60.					

NOTES

NOTES

NOTES

Index

References in *italics* indicate figures; those followed by "t" denote tables